Clinical Diagnosis and Assessment of HIV/AIDS

Clinical Diagnosis and Assessment of HIV/AIDS

Editor: Roger Mostafa

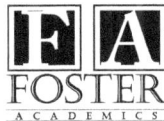

FA FOSTER
ACADEMICS

www.fosteracademics.com

www.fosteracademics.com

FA FOSTER
ACADEMICS

Cataloging-in-Publication Data

Clinical diagnosis and assessment of HIV/AIDS / edited by Roger Mostafa.
    p. cm.
Includes bibliographical references and index.
ISBN 978-1-63242-532-4
1. AIDS (Disease). 2. HIV (Viruses). 3. AIDS (Disease)--Diagnosis.
4. HIV infections--Diagnosis. I. Mostafa, Roger.
RA643.8 .C55 2018
614.599 392--dc23

Foster Academics,
118-35 Queens Blvd., Suite 400,
Forest Hills, NY 11375, USA

ISBN 978-1-63242-532-4 (Hardback)

Contents

Preface

HIV/AIDS is transmitted from one person to another by sexual contact, blood transfer or breast milk. It causes the failure of the immune system. It has a number of symptoms such as fever, rash, enlarged glands and headache. From theories to research, case studies related to all contemporary topics of relevance to this field have been included in this book. It is a vital tool for all those who are researching or studying HIV/AIDS, as it gives incredible insights into emerging trends in diagnostic and assessment techniques.

The researches compiled throughout the book are authentic and of high quality, combining several disciplines and from very diverse regions from around the world. Drawing on the contributions of many researchers from diverse countries, the book's objective is to provide the readers with the latest achievements in the area of research. This book will surely be a source of knowledge to all interested and researching the field.

In the end, I would like to express my deep sense of gratitude to all the authors for meeting the set deadlines in completing and submitting their research chapters. I would also like to thank the publisher for the support offered to us throughout the course of the book. Finally, I extend my sincere thanks to my family for being a constant source of inspiration and encouragement.

Editor

Clinical Reactivations of Herpes Simplex Virus Type 2 Infection and Human Immunodeficiency Virus Disease Progression Markers

Bulbulgul Aumakhan[1]*, Charlotte A. Gaydos[2], Thomas C. Quinn[2,3], Chris Beyrer[1], Lorie Benning[1], Howard Minkoff[4], Daniel J. Merenstein[5], Mardge Cohen[6], Ruth Greenblatt[7], Marek Nowicki[8], Kathryn Anastos[9], Stephen J. Gange[1]

1 Johns Hopkins Bloomberg School of Public Health, Baltimore, Maryland, United States of America, 2 Johns Hopkins University School of Medicine, Baltimore, Maryland, United States of America, 3 Laboratory of Immunoregulation, Division of Intramural Research, National Institute of Allergy and Infectious Diseases, National Institutes of Health, Bethesda, Maryland, United States of America, 4 Maimon des Medical Center and SUNY Downstate, Brooklyn, New York, United States of America, 5 Georgetown University Medical Center, Washington, D. C., United States of America, 6 Cook County Medical Center, Chicago, Illinois, United States of America, 7 Schools of Pharmacy and Medicine, University of California San Francisco, San Francisco, California, United States of America, 8 University of Southern California, Los Angeles, California, United States of America, 9 Albert Einstein College of Medicine, Bronx, New York, United States of America

Abstract

Background: The natural history of HSV-2 infection and role of HSV-2 reactivations in HIV disease progression are unclear.

Methods: Clinical symptoms of active HSV-2 infection were used to classify 1,938 HIV/HSV-2 co-infected participants of the Women's Interagency HIV Study (WIHS) into groups of varying degree of HSV-2 clinical activity. Differences in plasma HIV RNA and CD4+ T cell counts between groups were explored longitudinally across three study visits and cross-sectionally at the last study visit.

Results: A dose dependent association between markers of HIV disease progression and degree of HSV-2 clinical activity was observed. In multivariate analyses after adjusting for baseline CD4+ T cell levels, active HSV-2 infection with frequent symptomatic reactivations was associated with 21% to 32% increase in the probability of detectable plasma HIV RNA (trend p = 0.004), an average of 0.27 to 0.29 log10 copies/ml higher plasma HIV RNA on a continuous scale (trend p<0.001) and 51 to 101 reduced CD4+ T cells/mm^3 over time compared to asymptomatic HSV-2 infection (trend p<0.001).

Conclusions: HIV induced CD4+ T cell loss was associated with frequent symptomatic HSV-2 reactivations. However, effect of HSV-2 reactivations on HIV disease progression markers in this population was modest and appears to be dependent on the frequency and severity of reactivations. Further studies will be necessary to determine whether HSV-2 reactivations contribute to acceleration of HIV disease progression.

Editor: Landon Myer, University of Cape Town, South Africa

Funding: Data in this manuscript was collected by the Women's Interagency HIV Study (WIHS) Collaborative Study Group with centers (Principal Investigators) at New York City/Bronx Consortium (Kathryn Anastos); Brooklyn, NY (Howard Minkoff); Washington, DC Metropolitan Consortium (Mary Young); The Connie Wofsy Study Consortium of Northern California (Ruth Greenblatt); Los Angeles County/Southern California Consortium (Alexandra Levine); Chicago Consortium (Mardge Cohen); Data Coordinating Center (Stephen Gange). The WIHS is funded by the National Institute of Allergy and Infectious Diseases (UO1-AI-35004, UO1-AI-31834, UO1-AI-34994, UO1-AI-34989, UO1-AI-34993, and UO1-AI-42590) and by the Eunice Kennedy Shriver National Institute of Child Health and Human Development (UO1-HD-32632). The study is co-funded by the National Cancer Institute, the National Institute on Drug Abuse, and the National Institute on Deafness and Other Communication Disorders. Funding is also provided by the National Center for Research Resources (UCSF-CTSI Grant Number UL1 RR024131). The contents of this publication are solely the responsibility of the authors and do not necessarily represent the official views of the National Institutes of Health. The funders had no role in study design, data collection and analysis, decision to publish, or preparation of the manuscript.

Competing Interests: The authors have declared that no competing interests exist.

* E-mail: baumakhan@hivresearch.org

Introduction

Individuals with human immunodeficiency virus (HIV) infection are often found to be co-infected with herpes simplex virus type 2 (HSV-2) – the causative agent of genital herpes (GH).

Genital herpes has a widely variable clinical course. Some individuals manifest severe forms of disease with the frequent development of painful and typical mucocutaneous lesions while others experience mild or atypical forms with manifestations that

can easily go unnoticed [1]. In rare situations, the herpes virus can disseminate systemically and cause devastating complications in many internal organs [2–4]. The effect of this clinical heterogeneity on the course of HIV is not clear.

The nature and precise mechanisms of interaction between these two sexually transmitted pathogens are still incompletely understood with studies often producing conflicting results leading to ongoing debate on whether HSV-2 is indeed a significant risk factor for HIV acquisition, transmission or disease progression.

Some experts argue that there is sufficient evidence of viral synergy between these two sexually transmitted pathogens to call for immediate actions to control HSV-2 [5]. Others argue that recent trials demonstrating no effect of HSV suppressive therapy on HIV acquisition and transmission [6–8] suggest that HSV-2 based interventions will have little to no effect on HIV epidemic [9].

We attempted to investigate this interaction within Women's Interagency HIV Study (WIHS), the nation's largest cohort study of HIV natural history by evaluating the association of the type (symptomatic vs. asymptomatic) and severity (frequency of symptomatic recurrences) of HSV-2 infection with HIV disease progression markers (plasma HIV RNA and CD4+ T cell count) among highly active antiretroviral therapy (HAART) naïve HIV/HSV-2 co-infected participants of WIHS.

Methods

Ethics Statement

This study was conducted under IRB approval of WIHS Data Management and Analysis Center (Principal Investigator – Stephen Gange). IRB number: H.34.97.05.19.A2. Written informed consent was obtained from all participants.

Study population

The study population consisted of 2,056 HIV infected participants recruited into WIHS between 1994 and 1995. WIHS is an ongoing multicenter cohort study of HIV natural history in women across six sites in the U.S. (Los Angeles, CA; Washington, DC; the San Francisco Bay area, CA; New York City/Bronx, NY; Brooklyn, NY; and Chicago, IL). Complete physical and gynecological examination with collection of biologic specimens was done on women semiannually since 1994. Gynecological examination included assessment for genital tract infections, including ulcers and intraepithelial dysplasia as previously described [10]. Detailed review of the WIHS study population and methods have been previously published [11].

Study follow up

Study follow up was restricted to the first three WIHS visits (1.5 years of follow up). Less than 3% of participants were treated with HAART during that time period. To avoid possible selection and survival biases participants with only one (n = 221) or two (n = 237) study visits as well as those on HAART (n = 40) were excluded.

Exposure assessment

1) Laboratory assessment of HSV serostatus. Serologic reactivity to HSV-1 and HSV-2 was determined by a commercially available type-specific glycoprotein G-based enzyme immunoassay (gG-EIA, Gull Laboratories, Salt Lake City, Utah, USA) at enrollment as previously described [12,13]. Negative and equivocal results were confirmed by Western Blot as previously described [13–15]. The sensitivity of the gG-EIA for HSV-1 is 95% and the specificity is 96%. For HSV-2, the sensitivity is 98% and the specificity is 97% [12,13].

2) Clinical assessment of HSV-2 infection and classification of study groups. Clinicians' assessment of genital herpes was based on visualization of ulcers and/or vesicles in the genital area during pelvic exam. Clinicians were either women's health nurse practitioners or physician gynecologists. All have been trained to complete the WIHS protocol. An interval history of genital sores was collected by self-report at each study visit. Participants were classified into groups based on the type of HSV-2 infection (symptomatic or asymptomatic) and frequency of visits with genital lesions observed over the duration of the initial

three visits. This classification was based on the assumption that the likelihood of having active and more severe HSV-2 infection will be highest in clinically symptomatic women presenting with herpetic lesions at least once during the specified study period as opposed to women who remain clinically asymptomatic during the same time period. This assumption also stems from the results of preliminary work in which the presence and quantity of HSV-2 DNA in lower genital tract was highest in symptomatic women presenting with typical herpetic lesions (~30%) compared to women clinically asymptomatic over extended periods of time or women with other lesions (<10%) when cervicovaginal lavage samples from a subset of WIHS women (n~400) were tested by polymerase chain reaction (Aumakhan, unpublished thesis). Based on this assumption and data, a participant who was HSV-2 seropositive but negative for potential indicators of active HSV-2 infection, such as presence of any genital lesions and negative for a history of genital sores over the duration of this study was considered as having asymptomatic HSV-2 infection and considered as having symptomatic HSV-2 infection if she had at least one visit (out of three) at which she presented with genital lesions identified by clinicians as herpetic and/or had a positive history of GH sores in between the visits. The degree of HSV-2 clinical activity among symptomatic women was then graded from: a) mild symptomatic (only self report positive but no lesions at any study visit), b) mild to moderate (lesions at only one of the study visits), c) moderate (lesions at two visits), and d) severe symptomatic (lesions at all three study visits). Women with lesions not identified as herpetic and negative for a history of genital sores were considered as having symptoms not highly suggestive of active HSV-2 infection and thus, excluded.

Outcome assessment

HIV RNA plasma load was quantified by an isothermal nucleic acid sequence-based amplification assay (NASBA/Nuclisens, Merieux, Durham, North Carolina, USA), which had a lower limit of quantification (LOQ) of 4,000 copies/ml. CD4+ T cells were quantified using standard flow cytometry methods.

Statistical analysis

Plasma HIV RNA load was stratified into two categories with the cutpoint at the LOQ: ≤4,000 and >4,000. HIV RNA values below the LOQ were summarized using proportions, and values above the LOQ were log_{10} transformed for comparison purposes. Univariate analyses were carried out comparing selected characteristics between defined study groups. Proportions were compared using the chi square test. Continuous variables were summarized with medians and compared using the Wilcoxon rank-sum (Mann-Whitney) test. The Generalized Estimating Equations (GEE) method with robust variance estimation was used to explore the mean differences in plasma HIV RNA and CD4+ T cell counts between the study groups. To explore the cumulative association of repeated HSV-2 episodes on HIV markers, linear regression for continuous and Poisson extensions of log binomial models [16] for dichotomous outcomes were implemented at the third or last follow up visit. Multivariate models adjusted for selected demographic and risk variables known to be associated with HIV risk and disease progression as well as variables that were statistically different in crude comparisons and included age, race, injection and noninjection drug use, number of lifetime sexual partners, use of herpes medications and antiretroviral therapy, as well as baseline CD4+ T cell count. The asymptomatic group was the reference group in all models. Analyses were carried out with STATA, version 10 (Stata Corporation, College Station, Texas, USA). Statistical significance was defined as a p-value of <0.05.

Results

a) Study groups

Ninety four percent of the source cohort (n = 1,938) had known baseline HSV-2 serostatus and of those 78% (n = 1,510) were HSV-2 seropositive (Figure 1). After excluding women with incomplete follow up as well as those on HAART there were 1,012 women eligible for the study. Of 1,012 women, 262 (n = 26%) were classified as asymptomatic for HSV-2 infection and 388 (n = 38%) as symptomatic according to the definitions described earlier. Women with lesions not identified by clinicians as herpetic as well as negative for an interval history of genital sores (n = 362, 36%) were excluded. By degree of HSV-2 clinical activity, of 388 symptomatic women 101 (26%) had positive history of GH but no lesions identified at any of the three study visits, 125 (32%) presented with genital lesions once (1 lesion-visit or 1 L-V); 92 (24%) - twice (2 lesion-visits or 2 L-V); and 70 (18%) had lesions observed at all three visits (3 lesion-visits or 3 L-V).

b) Comparison of demographic, risk and clinical characteristics by study groups

Table 1 displays distribution of selected baseline characteristics by main study groups: symptomatic vs. asymptomatic. Overall, symp-

tomatic women were younger than asymptomatic women (median age 36 years vs. 38 years, p = 0.001). White women tended to be symptomatic as opposed to their African American counterparts (71% vs. 57%, p = 0.026). In addition, symptomatic women were more likely to be on combination antiretroviral therapy (35% vs. 26%, p = 0.013). However, the biggest difference was observed in the use of herpes treatment: 19% of symptomatic women vs. 3% of asymptomatic women reported use of herpes medications at baseline visit (p<0.0001). There were no statistically significant differences observed in HIV risk exposure, number of sexual partners, or proportion of HSV-1 seropositivity between the groups. Demographic, risk and clinical characteristics were not significantly different when explored by subgroups of HSV-2 clinical activity or the frequency of lesion-visits within the symptomatic cohort.

c) Comparison of HIV disease progression markers by study groups

Table 2 presents values of HIV markers by the main study groups as well as by subgroups of HSV-2 clinical activity. A gradient trend was observed such that the values of HIV markers became progressively worse as the level of HSV-2 clinical activity progressively increased from mild symptomatic to severe symptomatic with frequent reactivations. Specifically, symptomatic

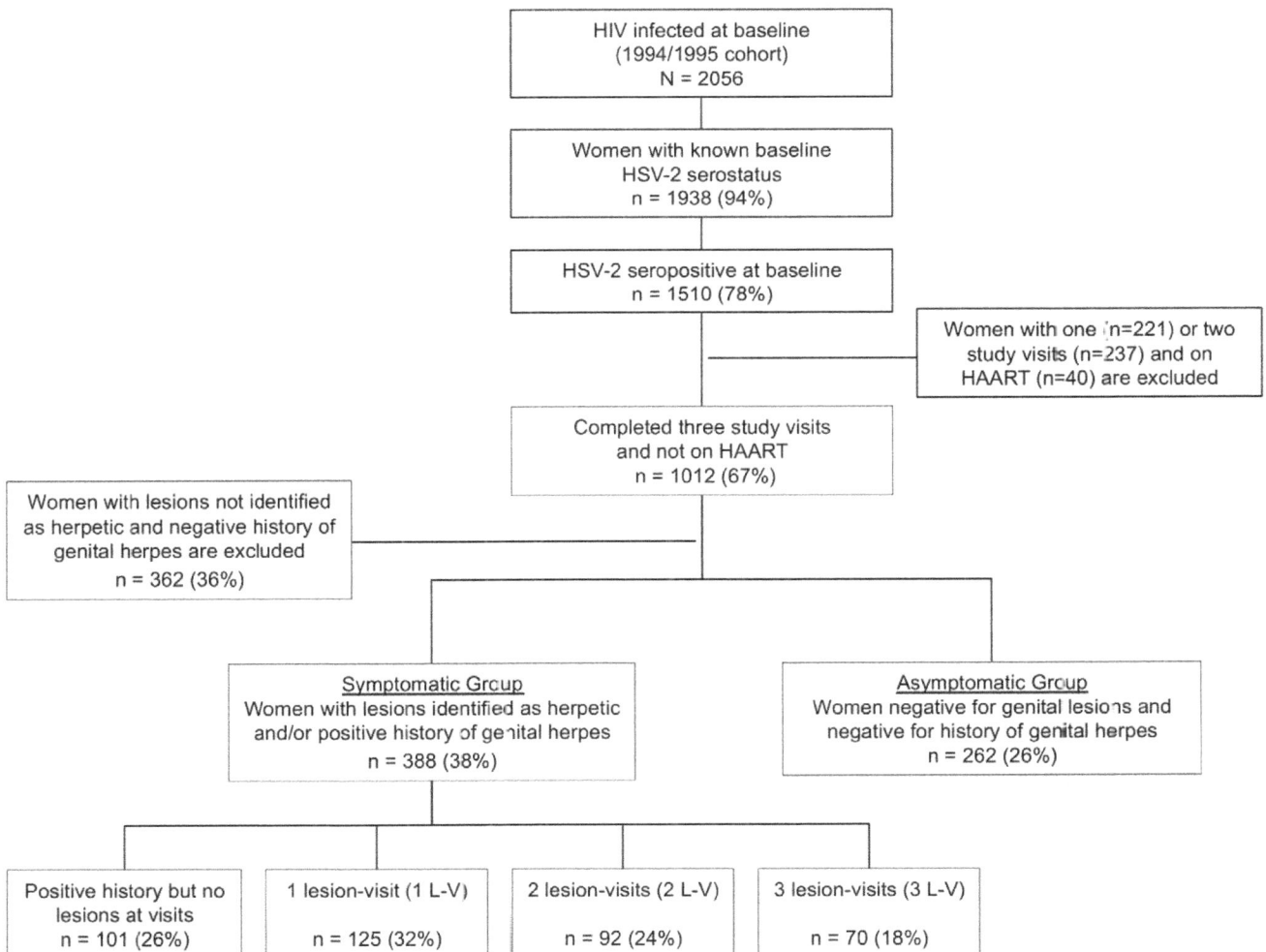

Figure 1. Flowchart of study participants and description of exposure groups.

Table 1. Comparison of demographic, risk and clinical characteristics by study groups.

Characteristic/Study Group		Asymptomatic (n = 262)	Symptomatic (n = 388)	P
Median age at baseline (IQR), years		38 (33–43)	36 (31–40)	0.001
Median age at 1ˢᵗ sex (IQR), years		15 (13–17)	15 (13–17)	0.459
Race/Ethnicity, n (%)	African-American	175 (67%)	228 (59%)	0.026
	Latina/Hispanic	53 (20%)	91 (23%)	
	White	24 (9%)	61 (16%)	
	Other	10 (4%)	8 (2%)	
HIV risk exposure category, n (%)	Intravenous drug use	98 (38%)	116 (30%)	0.183
	Heterosexual risk	96 (37%)	166 (43%)	
	Transfusion risk	8 (3%)	17 (4%)	
	Not known	60 (23%)	89 (23%)	
Number of lifetime sexual partners, n (%)	0–1	8 (3%)	11 (3%)	0.428
	2–4	44 (17%)	47 (12%)	
	5–9	42 (16%)	69 (18%)	
	10–49	85 (33%)	121 (31%)	
	≥50	81 (31%)	138 (36%)	
	Not known	2 (<1%)	2 (<1%)	
HSV-1 seropositive, n (%)		204 (78%)	277 (71%)	0.065
Use of herpes treatment at baseline, n (%)		8 (3%)	74 (19%)	<0.001
Use of antiretroviral therapy at baseline, n (%)	None	113 (43%)	128 (33%)	0.013
	Mono	82 (31%)	125 (32%)	
	Combination	67 (26%)	135 (35%)	

Note: IQR, interquartile range; P, p-value.

women with outbreaks of genital lesions at all three visits had more than 3-fold unfavorable differences in outcome HIV markers compared to asymptomatic women who had none (p<0.001). Interestingly, among these symptomatic women only 5 had lesions identified as herpetic at all three visits but they had the highest viral load values with median plasma HIV RNA of 490,000 copies/ml (interquartile range [IQR]: 205,000–3,865,000) and lowest CD4 T cell counts with median CD4+ T cell number of only 14 (IQR: 4–94).

d) Association between frequency of lesion-visits and the probability of detectable plasma HIV RNA

Crude GEE analyses demonstrated a 21%, 25% and 50% increased probability of detectable plasma HIV RNA in women

with lesions at one, two and three visits respectively (Table 3). Corresponding adjusted estimates were 11%, 13% and 21% (Table 4, trend p-value = 0.005). Similarly, an 8% to a 32% increase was observed when Poisson extension of log binomial regression was carried out to estimate the cumulative effect of repeated lesion-visits on the probability of detectable plasma HIV RNA at the last or 3ʳᵈ study visit (Table 5, trend p-value = 0.004).

e) Association between frequency of lesion-visits and mean differences in the levels of detectable plasma HIV RNA and CD4+ T cell levels

In the crude GEE models women with lesions at all three visits were observed to have up to 0.42 (Table 3) and in adjusted

Table 2. Comparison of baseline HIV disease markers by study groups.

Characteristic/Study Group	Asymptomatic (N = 262)	Symptomatic (N = 388)				P*
		SR GH† (N = 101)	1 L-V‡ (N = 125)	2 L-V (N = 92)	3 L-V (N = 70)	
Number/Total (%) with HIV pVL ≤4,000 copies/ml	107/258 (41%)	36/99 (36%)	34/125 (27%)	22/88 (25%)	9/69 (13%)	<0.001
Median HIV pVL (IQR), copies/ml**	25,000 (12,000–100,000)	42,000 (13,000–1000,000)	46,000 (19,000–140,000)	76,500 (23,000–180,000)	92,000 (20,500–245,000)	<0.001
Median CD4+ T cell count (IQR), cells/mm³	418 (285–593)	391 (270–567)	347 (179–542)	282 (147–430)	138 (19–365)	<0.001

Note: IQR, interquartile range; SR GH, self reported genital herpes; L-V, lesion-visit; †positive self report of genital herpes only; ‡number of visits with lesions.
* P - p-value for overall comparison of symptomatic group vs. asymptomatic group.
** among women with HIV pVL >4,000 copies/ml.

Table 3. Crude prevalence risk ratios (PRs) of detectable plasma HIV RNA and mean differences in plasma HIV RNA and CD4+ T cell counts (from the GEE analysis with robust variance estimation) by degree of HSV-2 clinical activity.

Grade	N	Detectable plasma HIV RNA (>4,000 copies/ml)		Mean difference (Δ) in log10 plasma HIV RNA		Mean difference (Δ) in CD4+ T cell counts	
		Crude PR (95% CI)	P	Crude mean Δ (95% CI)	P	Crude mean Δ (95% CI)	P
Asymptomatic	262	1.0 (reference)		0.00 (reference)		0.00 (reference)	
SR GH †	101	1.07 (0.92, 1.25)	0.388	+0.10 (−0.05, 0.25)	0.201	−46 (−108, 17)	0.150
1 L-V‡	125	1.21 (1.06, 1.38)	0.005	+0.19 (0.05, 0.32)	0.006	−95 (−152, 37)	0.001
2 L-V	92	1.25 (1.09, 1.44)	0.002	+0.28 (0.12, 0.44)	0.001	−176 (−235, −116)	<0.001
3 L-V	70	1.50 (1.34, 1.68)	<0.001	+0.42 (0.25, 0.58)	<0.001	−273 (−336, −212)	<0.001

Note: GEE, Generalized Estimating Equations; CI, confidence interval; PR, prevalence ratio; P, p-value; SR GH, self reported genital herpes; L-V, lesion-visit; †positive self report of genital herpes only; ‡number of visits with lesions.

models up to 0.29 $\log_{10}$ copies/ml higher mean plasma HIV RNA levels compared to women in the asymptomatic group who had no lesion-visits (Table 4, trend p-value <0.001). The average difference in CD4+ T cell counts was up to 273 cells less among women with lesions at all three visits in the crude models compared to women in asymptomatic group (Table 3) but only up to 51 cells less in the multivariate models adjusted for baseline CD4+ T cell count (Table 4, trend p-value <0.001). This difference was up to 101 cells less when linear regression was carried out at the 3rd visit (Table 5, trend p-value <0.001).

Discussion

Our findings indicate that the levels of HIV replication and immunocompromise are associated with the presence of active HSV-2 infection. Specifically, two sides of the observed association deserve further evaluation: 1) HIV induced CD4+ T cell loss directly correlated with the degree of HSV-2 activity or frequent symptomatic HSV-2 reactivations; and 2) active HSV-2 infection with frequent HSV-2 reactivations was, in turn, associated with modestly elevated plasma HIV RNA levels and reduced CD4+ T cell count over time, compared to women remaining clinically asymptomatic after adjusting for baseline CD4+ T cell levels.

Immunological determinants of HSV-2 infection severity are not completely understood and there are few data on the associations between innate/acquired immune responses and frequencies of HSV-2 reactivation. Moreover, data regarding the relative importance of CD8+ T cells vs. CD4+ T cells as pure effector cells in controlling HSV-2 infection remains controversial [17–21]. The correlation of CD4+ T cell depletion with frequency/severity of symptomatic recurrences observed in this study suggests that CD4+ T cells are perhaps one of the important immunologic correlates of protection against HSV-2 reactivations.

While it appears that T cell mediated immunity is of key importance in keeping HSV-2 in check, infiltration and persistence of the same T cells as well as other inflammatory cells at the site of inflammation may in fact provide a perfect milieu for HIV to infect additional CD4+ T cells and thus, enhance HIV replication. Recent in situ study of the cellular infiltrates of HSV-2 lesions demonstrated that CD4+ T cells accumulated at the site of lesions had enriched CCR5 expression and were in close proximity to dendritic cells (DCs) expressing DC-SIGN or CD123 of DCs, the receptor known for the ability to transfer HIV to CD4+ T cells [22]. This may present a risk for enhanced local HIV replication and the potential for its systemic dissemination, which perhaps depends on the extent and duration of local inflammation elicited by host immune responses. Indeed, a modest but consistent trend towards elevated plasma HIV RNA levels in symptomatic women compared to asymptomatic women was observed even after adjusting for baseline CD4+ T cell levels.

Table 4. Adjusted* prevalence risk ratios (PRs) of detectable plasma HIV RNA and mean differences in plasma HIV RNA and CD4+ T cell counts (from the GEE analysis with robust variance estimation) by degree of HSV-2 clinical activity.

Grade	N	Detectable plasma HIV RNA (>4,000 copies/ml)		Mean difference (Δ) in log10 plasma HIV RNA		Mean difference (Δ) in CD4+ T cell counts	
		Adjusted PR (95% CI)	P	Adjusted mean Δ (95% CI)	P	Adjusted mean Δ (95% CI)	P
Asymptomatic	262	1.0 (reference)		0.00 (reference)		0.00 (reference)	
SR GH†	101	1.05 (0.90, 1.22)	0.509	+0.11 (−0.03, 0.25)	0.130	−5 (−23, 13)	0.595
1 L-V‡	125	1.11 (0.98, 1.27)	0.105	+0.15 (0.02, 0.27)	0.026	−19 (−39, −30)	0.047
2 L-V	92	1.13 (0.98, 1.30)	0.083	+0.16 (0.01, 0.31)	0.034	−32 (−51, −13)	0.001
3 L-V	70	1.21 (1.06, 1.39)	0.005	+0.29 (0.13, 0.44)	<0.001	−51 (−81, −21)	0.001
		Trend P=0.005		Trend P<0.001		Trend P<0.001	

Note: GEE, Generalized Estimating Equations; CI, confidence interval; PR, prevalence ratio; P, p-value; SR GH, self reported genital herpes; L-V, lesion-visit; *adjusted for baseline CD4+ T cell count, herpes medications and type of antiretroviral therapy used at the visit, age, race, lifetime number of sexual partners, injection and noninjection drug use; †positive self report of genital herpes only; ‡number of visits with lesions.

Table 5. Adjusted* prevalence risk ratios (PRs) of detectable plasma HIV RNA and mean differences in plasma HIV RNA and CD4+ T cell counts (from the cross-sectional log binomial and linear regression models at the 3rd visit) by degree of HSV-2 clinical activity.

Grade	N	Detectable plasma HIV RNA (>4,000 copies/ml) Adjusted PR (95% CI)	P	Mean difference (Δ) in log10 plasma HIV RNA Adjusted mean Δ (95% CI)	P	Mean difference (Δ) in CD4+ T cell counts Adjusted mean Δ (95% CI)	P
Asymptomatic	262	1.0 (reference)		0.00 (reference)		0.00 (reference)	
SR GH[†]	101	1.08 (0.89, 1.30)	0.449	+0.18 (−0.006, 0.37)	0.057	−13 (−50, 23)	0.471
1 L-V[‡]	125	1.11 (0.94, 1.32)	0.212	+0.19 (0.02, 0.37)	0.028	−42 (−76, −8)	0.015
2 L-V	92	1.14 (0.96, 1.37)	0.139	+0.21 (0.02, 0.41)	0.029	−64 (−103, −26)	0.001
3 L-V	70	1.32 (1.12, 1.56)	0.001	+0.27 (0.07, 0.46)	0.007	−101 (−144, −59)	<0.001
		Trend P=0.004		Trend P=0.004		Trend P=<0.001	

Note: CI, confidence interval; PR, prevalence ratio; P, p-value; SR GH, self reported genital herpes; L-V, lesion-visit; *adjusted for baseline CD4+ T cell count, herpes medications and type of antiretroviral therapy used at the visit, age, race, lifetime number of sexual partners, injection and noninjection drug use; [†]positive self report of genital herpes only; [‡]number of visits with lesions.

However, it is possible that these changes may have been due to incomplete adjustment of immunosuppression by CD4+ T cells. Despite that, the observed difference of 0.29 log10 copies/ml in plasma HIV RNA load in women with frequent lesion-visits compared to women who had none is very similar to the 0.25 log10 reduction in mean plasma HIV RNA observed in the recent acyclovir suppressive therapy trial [23] which translated into a 16% reduction in HIV disease progression [24]. The fact that the acyclovir experimental trial and our observational study in which most participants did not use acyclovir or other herpes medications found similar magnitude changes in HIV viral load, leads us to speculate whether the frequency and severity of HSV-2 reactivations were responsible for the magnitude of the observed effect in the trial. It is unlikely that the small to modest changes in HIV disease markers associated with HSV-2 reactivations observed in this population will negatively affect the development of AIDS or overall mortality, particularly in the HAART era. On the other hand, these seemingly small viral load changes and reductions in disease progression may not be innocuous. A recent systematic review and meta- analysis of small viral load changes in treatment naïve HIV positive adults showed that even small increases in plasma HIV RNA levels can eventually lead to faster disease progression and a higher risk of ongoing HIV transmission [25]. Although it is possible that the reductions in HIV RNA load observed in clinical trials may have been mediated through the recently discovered inhibitory effect of acyclovir on HIV reverse transcriptase, this effect was noted to be dependent on the ability of HSV-2 and other herpesviruses to provide sufficient amounts of activated acyclovir [26]. This would likely only be achieved if there is sufficient replication of HSV-2 and of other herpesviruses present in the host at the time. Multiple other trials observed similar or greater magnitude reductions in plasma HIV RNA levels with suppressive herpes therapy [27–30].

The magnitude of CD4+ T cells lost due to frequent symptomatic HSV-2 reactivations after adjustment for baseline CD4+ T cell levels was not high and may seem to be negligible. However, it is possible that the CD4+ T cell values at the lesion-visits may in fact represent the "elevated" values due to increased activation of CD4+ and other immune cells in response to HSV-2 reactivation which may exacerbate CD4+ T cell loss. In support of this possibility is the observation of higher CD4+ T cell counts among treatment naïve HIV-1/HSV-2 co-infected adults in early

HIV infection [31] which may reflect vigorous immune response to HSV-2 reactivations in a not yet deeply immunosuppressed host. Indeed, the trend of CD4+ T cell loss was slight but persisted across the visits and by the time of the last visit those with lesions at all three visits had the lowest mean CD4+ T cell counts compared to those who had none.

A main limitation of the study is the possible misclassification bias due to use of self reported lesions as one of the indicators for the presence of active HSV-2 infection. The WIHS women have not been specifically educated for HSV-2 which can considerably increase the recognition of mild or atypical symptoms [32,33]. This would be particularly relevant to the asymptomatic group as subsequent follow up data revealed that nearly 75% (n = 196) of 262 asymptomatic women experienced symptoms suggestive of HSV-2 reactivation during extended follow up. Thus, the results of this study are likely to be underestimated as the study did not use HSV-2 uninfected women as controls in whom the possibility of clinical and subclinical reactivations should be minimal if not absent. Another limitation is the absence of laboratory confirmation of genital HSV-2 reactivations in these women. However, laboratory confirmation of HSV-2 reactivations alone is not optimal as HSV-2 detection is influenced by multiple factors such as the intermittent nature of HSV-2 shedding, shedding from multiple anatomic locations as well as the laboratory methodology used. Other limitations include the use of semiannual data that precluded direct assessment of recurrences between the visits and possibly limited generalizability to those with incident HIV and HSV-2 infections where viral and host immune response dynamics are different from those with established infections.

In summary, HIV induced CD4+ T cell loss was associated with symptomatic and frequent HSV-2 reactivations. Symptomatic HSV-2 infection with frequent reactivations, in turn, was associated with modestly elevated HIV replication and reduced CD4+ T cell count over time. Long term studies will be necessary to clarify the exact role the frequency and severity of HSV-2 reactivations play in the natural history of HIV infection, particularly in developing countries where there is no universal access to HAART therapy. In addition, since HSV-2 is most active immediately after HSV-2 acquisition it may be worth to investigate whether early herpes suppressive therapy will delay the need for initiation of HAART in both developing and developed country settings among individuals with frequent HSV-2 reactivations.

Acknowledgments

The authors would like to greatly acknowledge Drs. Larry Moulton and Anna Wald for constructive criticism and suggestions as well as Warren Sateren, MPH for editorial support and helpful comment.

Author Contributions

Conceived and designed the experiments: BA CAG TCQ CB SG. Performed the experiments: BA. Analyzed the data: BA LB SG. Contributed reagents/materials/analysis tools: LB HM DJM MC RG MN KA SG. Wrote the paper: BA CAG TCQ CB KA SG.

References

1. Ashley RL, Wald A (1999) Genital herpes: Review of the epidemic and potential use of type-specific serology. Clin Microbiol Rev 12(1): 1–8.
2. Chretien F, Belec L, Wingerstmann L, de Truchis P, Baudrimont M, et al. (1997) Central nervous system infection due to herpes simplex virus in AIDS. Arch Anat Cytol Pathol 45(2-3): 153–158.
3. Haanpaa M, Paavonen J (2004) Transient urinary retention and chronic neuropathic pain associated with genital herpes simplex virus infection. Acta Obstet Gynecol Scand 83(10): 946–949.
4. Tran TH, Stanescu D, Caspers-Velu L, Rozenberg F, Liesnard C, et al. (2004) Clinical characteristics of acute HSV-2 retinal necrosis. Am J Ophthalmol 137(5): 872–879.
5. Van de Perre P, Segondy M, Foulongne V, Ouedraogo A, Konate I, et al. (2008) Herpes simplex virus and HIV-1: Deciphering viral synergy. Lancet Infect Dis 8(8): 490–497.
6. Watson-Jones D, Weiss HA, Rusizoka M, Changalucha J, Baisley K, et al. (2008) Effect of herpes simplex suppression on incidence of HIV among women in tanzania. N Engl J Med 358(15): 1560–1571.
7. Celum C, Wald A, Hughes J, Sanchez J, Reid S et al. (2008) Effect of aciclovir on HIV-1 acquisition in herpes simplex virus 2 seropositive women and men who have sex with men: A randomised, double-blind, placebo-controlled trial. Lancet 371(9630): 2109–2119.
8. Cowan FM, Pascoe SJ, Barlow KL, Langhaug LF, Jaffar S, et al. (2008) A randomised placebo-controlled trial to explore the effect of suppressive therapy with acyclovir on genital shedding of HIV-1 and herpes simplex virus type 2 among zimbabwean sex workers. Sex Transm Infect 84(7): 548–553.
9. Cheng RG, Nixon DF (2009) Herpes simplex virus and HIV-1: Deciphering viral synergy. Lancet Infect Dis 9(2): 74; author reply74–5.
10. Greenblatt RM, Bacchetti P, Barkan S, Augenbraun M, Silver S, et al. (1999) Lower genital tract infections among HIV-infected and high-risk uninfected women: Findings of the women's interagency HIV study (WIHS). Sex Transm Dis 26(3): 143–151.
11. Barkan SE, Melnick SL, Preston-Martin S, Weber K, Kalish LA, et al. (1998) The women's interagency HIV study. WIHS collaborative study group. Epidemiology 9(2): 117–125.
12. Ashley RL, Wu L, Pickering JW, Tu MC, Schnorenberg L (1998) Premarket evaluation of a commercial glycoprotein G-based enzyme immunoassay for herpes simplex virus type-specific antibodies. J Clin Microbiol 36(1): 294–295.
13. Ameli N, Bacchetti P, Morrow RA, Hessol NA, Wilkin T, et al. (2006) Herpes simplex virus infection in women in the WIHS: Epidemiology and effect of antiretroviral therapy on clinical manifestations. AIDS 20(7): 1051–1058.
14. Ashley R, Cent A, Maggs V, Nahmias A, Corey L (1991) Inability of enzyme immunoassays to discriminate between infections with herpes simplex virus types 1 and 2. Ann Intern Med 115(7): 520–526.
15. Ashley RL, Militoni J, Lee F, Nahmias A, Corey L (1988) Comparison of western blot (immunoblot) and glycoprotein G-specific immunodot enzyme assay for detecting antibodies to herpes simplex virus types 1 and 2 in human sera. J Clin Microbiol 26(4): 662–667.
16. Spiegelman D, Hertzmark E (2005) Easy SAS calculations for risk or prevalence ratios and differences. Am J Epidemiol 162(3): 199–200.
17. Koelle DM, Corey L (2008) Herpes simplex: Insights on pathogenesis and possible vaccines. Annu Rev Med 59: 381–395.
18. Koelle DM, Posavad CM, Barnum GR, Johnson ML, Frank JM, et al. (1998) Clearance of HSV-2 from recurrent genital lesions correlates with infiltration of HSV-specific cytotoxic T lymphocytes. J Clin Invest 101(7): 1500–1508.
19. Posavad CM, Koelle DM, Shaughnessy MF, Corey L (1997) Severe genital herpes infections in HIV-infected individuals with impaired herpes simplex virus-specific CD8+ cytotoxic T lymphocyte responses. Proc Natl Acad Sci U S A 94(19): 10289–10294.
20. Harandi AM, Svennerholm B, Holmgren J, Eriksson K (2001) Differential roles of B cells and IFN-gamma-secreting CD4(+) T cells in innate and adaptive immune control of genital herpes simplex virus type 2 infection in mice. J Gen Virol 82(Pt 4): 845–853.
21. Milligan GN, Bernstein DI, Bourne N (1998) T lymphocytes are required for protection of the vaginal mucosae and sensory ganglia of immune mice against reinfection with herpes simplex virus type 2. J Immunol 160(12): 6093–6100.
22. Zhu J, Hladik F, Woodward A, Klock A, Peng T, et al. (2009) Persistence of HIV-1 receptor-positive cells after HSV-2 reactivation is a potential mechanism for increased HIV-1 acquisition. Nat Med 15(8): 886–892.
23. Celum C, Wald A, Lingappa JR, Magaret AS, Wang RS, et al. (2010) Acyclovir and transmission of HIV-1 from persons infected with HIV-1 and HSV-2. N Engl J Med 362(5): 427–439.
24. Lingappa JR, Baeten JM, Wald A, Hughes JP, Thomas KK, et al. (2010) Daily aciclovir for HIV-1 disease progression in people dually infected with HIV-1 and herpes simplex virus type 2: A randomised placebo-controlled trial. Lancet.
25. Modjarrad K, Chamot E, Vermund SH (2008) Impact of small reductions in plasma HIV RNA levels on the risk of heterosexual transmission and disease progression. AIDS 22(16): 2179–2185.
26. Lisco A, Vanpouille C, Margolis L (2009) A missed point in deciphering the viral synergy between herpes simplex virus and HIV. Lancet Infect Dis 9(9): 522–523.
27. Baeten JM, Strick LB, Lucchetti A, Whittington WL, Sanchez J, et al. (2008) Herpes simplex virus (HSV)-suppressive therapy decreases plasma and genital HIV-1 levels in HSV-2/HIV-1 coinfected women: A randomized, placebo-controlled, cross-over trial. J Infect Dis 198(12): 1804–1808.
28. Nagot N, Ouedraogo A, Foulongne V, Konate I, Weiss HA, et al. (2007) Reduction of HIV-1 RNA levels with therapy to suppress herpes simplex virus. N Engl J Med 356(8): 790–799.
29. Delany-Moretlwe S, Lingappa JR, Celum C (2009) New insights on interactions between HIV-1 and HSV-2. Curr Infect Dis Rep 11(2): 135–142.
30. Dunne EF, Whitehead S, Sternberg M, Thepamnuay S, Leelawiwat W, et al. (2008) Suppressive acyclovir therapy reduces HIV cervicovaginal shedding in HIV- and HSV-2-infected women, chiang rai, thailand. J Acquir Immune Defic Syndr.
31. Barbour JD, Sauer MM, Sharp ER, Garrison KE, Long BR, et al. (2007) HIV-1/HSV-2 co-infected adults in early HIV-1 infection have elevated CD4+ T cell counts. PLoS ONE 2(10): e1080.
32. Koelle DM, Wald A (2000) Herpes simplex virus: The importance of asymptomatic shedding. J Antimicrob Chemother 45 Suppl T3: 1–8.
33. Wald A, Zeh J, Selke S, Warren T, Ryncarz AJ, et al. (2000) Reactivation of genital herpes simplex virus type 2 infection in asymptomatic seropositive persons. N Engl J Med 342(12): 844–850.

2

Multidimensional Patient-Reported Problems within Two Weeks of HIV Diagnosis in East Africa: A Multicentre Observational Study

Victoria Simms[1,2]*, Nancy Gikaara[3], Grace Munene[3], Mackuline Atieno[3], Jeniffer Kataike[3], Clare Nsubuga[3], Geoffrey Banga[3], Eve Namisango[3], Suzanne Penfold[1], Peter Fayers[4], Richard A. Powell[3], Irene J. Higginson[2], Richard Harding[2]

1 London School of Hygiene and Tropical Medicine, London, United Kingdom, 2 Cicely Saunders Institute, King's College London, London, United Kingdom, 3 African Palliative Care Association, Kampala, Uganda, 4 Department of Population Health, University of Aberdeen, Aberdeen, United Kingdom

Abstract

Objectives: We aimed to determine for the first time the prevalence and severity of multidimensional problems in a population newly diagnosed with HIV at outpatient clinics in Africa.

Methods: Recently diagnosed patients (within previous 14 days) were consecutively recruited at 11 HIV clinics in Kenya and Uganda. Participants completed a validated questionnaire, the African Palliative Outcome Scale (POS), with three underpinning factors. Ordinal logistic regression was used to evaluate risk factors for prevalence and severity of physical, psychological, interpersonal and existential problems.

Results: There were 438 participants (62% female, 30% with restricted physical function). The most prevalent problems were lack of help and advice (47% reported none in the previous 3 days) and difficulty sharing feelings. Patients with limited physical function reported more physical/psychological (OR = 3.22) and existential problems (OR = 1.54) but fewer interpersonal problems (OR = 0.50). All outcomes were independent of CD4 count or ART eligibility.

Conclusions: Patients at all disease stages report widespread and burdensome multidimensional problems at HIV diagnosis. Newly diagnosed patients should receive assessment and care for these problems. Effective management of problems at diagnosis may help to remove barriers to retention in care.

Editor: Kara K. Wools-Kaloustian, Indiana University, United States of America

Funding: The project was funded by USAID (www.usaid.gov) through Cooperative Agreement GPO-A-00-03-00003-00, under the authority provided to the University of North Carolina. The funders had no role in study design, data collection and analysis, decision to publish, or preparation of the manuscript.

Competing Interests: The authors have declared that no competing interests exist.

* E-mail: Victoria.simms@lshtm.ac.uk

Introduction

A very high proportion of people newly diagnosed with HIV lose contact with health care services and do not initiate antiretroviral therapy (ART) at the most appropriate time, leading to increased mortality and morbidity[1]. Improved linkage of services and retention in care is a priority in order to optimise treatment outcomes[2]. Correct management of patients at diagnosis is the gateway to other health services including ART. Unaddressed social, emotional and informational needs at the time of HIV diagnosis are thought to be a cause of avoidant coping strategies such as denial[3]. Depressive symptoms are very common for HIV positive people presenting for a test, and impact upon CD4 test uptake[4]. Common physical and psychological symptoms (pain, vomiting, fatigue, confusion and hopelessness) are reported as impediments to ART adherence[5,6]. A multidimensional approach to patient assessment at diagnosis which incorporates physical, psychological, emotional, social and informational elements would enable early management of these

problems, which could help to remove some of the barriers that prevent patients from remaining in care[4].

From an early stage[7], HIV has a multidimensional impact on patient wellbeing, with negative physical[8,9], psychological[10,11], social[12,13] and spiritual[14] repercussions, but very little is known about patient-reported experience at the specific time of HIV diagnosis[15]. Retrospective research is the most common method, but is unsuitable due to severe bias in the recall of emotionally significant events[16]. An alternative option is to measure outcomes just prior to diagnosis in patients later identified as HIV positive[4], but this approach, while suitable for research, is not realistic in terms of clinical practice.

A systematic review of multidimensional problems reported by newly diagnosed HIV patients[15] found only two prospective studies that recruited an outpatient sample within two weeks after diagnosis in a resource-poor setting (typifying the majority of new HIV diagnoses[17]), and both had methodological flaws. One was a comparative study of military personnel in Nigeria which identified lowered physical, mental, role and social functions associated with HIV diagnosis using the MOS-HIV questionnaire, but did not represent the wider population[18]. The other, a cross-sectional survey in India, found high prevalence of pain, physical symptoms, and emotional, spiritual and work-related problems, but used convenience sampling and an unvalidated questionnaire[19].

This study aimed to measure prevalence, severity and risk factors for multidimensional problems in the first two weeks after HIV diagnosis in a sample of outpatients in sub-Saharan Africa.

Methods

Ethics statement

Ethical approval was obtained from Ugandan National Council for Science and Technology (UNCST, Ref. SS 1964, the Kenyan Medical Research Institute (Ref. KEMRI/RES/7/3/1) and the College Research Ethics Committee at King's College London (Ref. CREC/06/07-140). All participants gave informed written consent prior to data collection.

Study design

The data were collected as part of a previously described mixed-methods evaluation of care and support[20]. Patients presenting with a new HIV diagnosis at eleven HIV comprehensive care clinics attached to urban district or national hospitals in Kenya and Uganda were recruited consecutively in 2008. The clinics are described in detail in two evaluation reports[21,22]. In Kenya two clinics were in the west, three in central Kenya and one in Mombasa. In Uganda, three clinics were in Kampala and two in southern towns. The total length of recruitment time at all clinics was 819 working days. All eligible patients were approached for consent. Eligibility criteria were: self-report that their first positive HIV diagnosis had occurred within the previous 14 days, aged 18 or over, not requiring hospital admission. Participants were interviewed four times at monthly intervals. Cross-sectional data from the day of recruitment are presented here.

Problems were recorded using the African Palliative Care Association (APCA) African Palliative Outcome Scale(POS), a multidimensional instrument designed[23] and validated in Africa[24]. A demographic questionnaire was also completed. The date and results of CD4 count and World Health Organization HIV stage were abstracted from patient records.

Recruitment and data collection was conducted by clinic health care workers, who received training and regular two-weekly support visits from research assistants. The questionnaires were translated and back-translated by experts into Swahili, Luo, Luganda and Runyakitara. The African POS had previously been validated in English and Luganda, among other languages[24]. The Swahili, Luo and Runyakitara translations were new. All translations were piloted with patients before use. Data were double-entered into a predesigned EpiData 3.1 database with validation checks, and exported to Stata 10.0 for analysis.

The POS consists of ten items addressing physical and psychological symptoms, spiritual, practical and emotional concerns, and psychosocial needs[24]. Seven items are completed by the patient and three by a family carer, but in this study it was anticipated that few patients would have a carer present and so only the patient-report items were analysed. POS scores were reversed where necessary so that 0 always represented the best response (no problem) and 5 the worst. Independent variables were gender; age group (18–28, 29–35, 36–59); country; physical function (measured with the ECOG scale[25], converted to 0 = best, 1 = middle, 2–4 = worst); education (no formal education, primary, secondary, diploma/degree); wealth quintile (calculated

using the Demographic Health Surveys Wealth Index method[26]); CD4 count (0–100, 101–200, 201–350 and 351+); and time since HIV diagnosis (0 days, 1–2 days, 3–7 and 8–14 days). Patients were defined as ART eligible if they had a CD4 of 350 or below, or a WHO score 3 or 4, following the 2010 WHO guidelines for ART initiation[27], although when the data were collected in 2008 Kenya and Uganda had not yet adopted the eligibility threshold of 350.

Analysis plan

The study outcomes are the three factors which have been identified underpinning the seven patient-completed items of the POS: physical/psychological wellbeing (questions 1, 2 and 3), interpersonal wellbeing (questions 4 and 7), and existential wellbeing(questions 5 and 6)[28]. These factors were generated by summing the scores for the appropriate questions. The ranges of the interpersonal and existential outcomes were 0–10, and of the physical/psychological outcome was 0–15, but preliminary analysis showed that no participants scored above 12.

For multivariate analysis each outcome was divided into three categories, coded 'mild problems' (0–4), 'medium problems' (5–7) and 'severe problems' (8–10 or 8–12). All independent variables were analysed as either ordinal (wealth quintile, education, physical function, age group, CD4 count, time since diagnosis) or dichotomous (gender, country, ART eligibility). The independent variables were compared with each outcome using chi square tests and non-parametric tests for trend, before being combined in a multivariate model using ordinal logistic regression.

Results

Response rate was over 99%. Participants were 270 women (61.6%) and 168 men, aged 18–59 (mean 32.9); a little over half (56.4%, n = 247) were recruited in Kenya (Table 1). Age distribution was 20.3% aged 18–25, 63.0% aged 26–40 and 16.7% aged 41–59. The majority (69.9%, n = 306) were physically fully active (ECOG score 0), with 23.3% (n = 102) scoring 1 and 6.8%(n = 30) scoring more than 1. In terms of education, 19(4.3%) had none, 229(52.3%) primary education, 147(33.6%) secondary and 43(9.8%) a diploma or higher qualification. Six facilities recorded WHO stage for their 196 patients, with 26% Stage I, 36% Stage II, 31% Stage III and 7% Stage IV. A CD4 count was recorded for 303 participants (69.2%).

For all seven items, the majority of participants reported problems (Table 2). The items with the highest scores were those measuring need for help and advice, and difficulty sharing feelings. Almost half of participants (47.3%) reported receiving no help or advice in the previous three days and almost a third (32.0%) had not been able to tell anyone how they were feeling. Further, 19.2% reported a peace score of 4 or 5, indicating a severe problem, 10.7% reported severe worry, 10.0% had a severe problem finding life worthwhile, 6.2% had severe pain and 3.2% severe physical symptoms other than pain.

Reflecting the distributions of the individual items, physical/psychological problems were skewed to the left (45% mild problems, 43% moderate, 11% severe), as were existential problems (58% mild, 35% moderate, 7% severe). Interpersonal problems were skewed to the right (11% mild problems, 42% moderate, 46% severe).

In bivariate analysis, physical/psychological problems were associated with lower CD4 count, impaired physical function, poverty and less education at p<0.1. The presence or absence of a CD4 count was not associated with any of the three outcomes. Interpersonal problems were more common for those with better

Table 1. Demographic characteristics of the newly-diagnosed participants by country.

Category	Subcategory	Kenya	Uganda
N		247	191
Gender, number female (%)		157 (63.6)	113 (59.2)
Age (mean, SD)		32.8 (8.7)	33.0 (8.3)
Age groups (%)	18–28	49 (19.8)	40 (20.9)
	29–35	159 (64.4)	117 (61.3)
	36–59	39 (15.8)	34 (17.8)
Education (%)	None formal	7 (2.8)	12 (6.3)
	Primary	141 (57.1)	88 (46.4)
	Secondary	78 (31.6)	69 (35.5)
	Diploma/higher	21 (8.5)	22 (11.5)
Physical function (%)	Best	180 (72.9)	126 (66.0)
	Middle	55 (22.3)	47 (24.6)
	Worst	12 (4.9)	18 (9.4)
Days since diagnosis (%)	0	29 (11.7)	79 (41.4)
	1–2	53 (21.5)	45 (23.6)
	3–7	102 (41.3)	35 (18.3)
	8–14	63 (25.5)	32 (16.8)
Wealth quintiles (%)	Poorest	63 (25.5)	25 (13.1)
	Second	51 (20.7)	37 (19.4)
	Middle	40 (16.2)	47 (24.6)
	Fourth	43 (17.4)	46 (24.1)
	Wealthiest	50 (20.2)	36 (18.9)
Has a recorded CD4 count (%)		222 (89.9)	81 (42.4)
Baseline CD4 count (median, IQR)		249 (95–407)	326 (193–483)
Has record of WHO stage (%)		124 (50.2)	(74 (38.7)
WHO stage (%)	I	32 (25.8)	20 (27.0)
	II	34 (27.4)	37 (50.0)
	III	47 (37.9)	15 (20.3)
	IV	11 (8.9)	2 (2.7)
Has ART eligibility score (%)		227 (91.9)	92 (48.2)
ART eligible (%)		162 (71.4)	56 (60.9)

physical function, women, and individuals living in Uganda. Interpersonal problems were also associated with wealth quintile but in no clear direction. Existential problems were associated with residence in Uganda, impaired physical function, and younger age. ART eligibility was not associated with any outcome. A missing value for ART eligibility was associated with interpersonal problems, with country and with wealth quintile, so this variable was not included in the multivariate models.

Table 3 shows the results of multivariate models of each outcome. Physical/psychological problems were associated with impaired physical function (OR = 3.22, 95% CI 2.32–4.48) and to a lesser extent with poverty (OR = 0.85, 95% CI 0.74–0.98). Interpersonal problems were more common for women (OR = 1.51, 95% CI 1.03–2.24), and less common for people with more education (OR = 0.71, 95% CI 0.54–0.93) or impaired physical function (OR = 0.50, 95% CI 0.37–0.68). A longer time since diagnosis was also associated with fewer interpersonal problems (OR = 0.78, 95% CI 0.65–0.94). Existential problems were more common in Uganda than Kenya (OR = 2.40, 95% CI 1.58–3.63) and were also associated with impaired physical function (OR = 1.54, 95% CI 1.14–2.08), poverty (OR = 0.82, 05% CI 0.70–0.95) and weakly with younger age (OR = 0.80, 95% CI 0.63–1.02).

Discussion

Physical, psychological, existential and interpersonal problems are highly prevalent and severe in the first two weeks after HIV diagnosis. These problems are reported by patients to be barriers to retention in care[5,6]. The sample consists of young adults, mainly women, as is typical of HIV clinic patients. None of the outcomes was associated with CD4 count, showing that problems can occur at any CD4 level.

The area of existential wellbeing is difficult to define and measure[29], but it is important to patients. Existential and spiritual concerns following HIV diagnosis are evident in qualitative studies[30], and for patients with advanced HIV in South Africa and Uganda, meaning in life is a higher priority than physical comfort or activity[14]. The question 'are you/have you felt at peace?' used in this study is an independently validated measure[24,31]. Existential problems as measured by the POS are more severe among Ugandan than Kenyan participants. Possible causes of this effect include difference in care provision, questionnaire translation, cultural and health care context, or time passed since diagnosis (median four days in Kenya and one in Uganda). In Uganda almost two thirds of participants (63.9%) did

Table 2. Prevalence and severity of multidimensional problems within 14 days of HIV diagnosis.

POS item	% of individuals scoring (n = 438)					
Over the past three days	0 (no problem)	1	2	3	4	5 (worst possible)
1. Please rate your pain	33.1	22.6	24.9	13.2	5.3	0.9
2. Have any other symptoms been affecting how you feel?	34.3	28.5	22.8	11.2	2.1	1.1
3. Have you been feeling worried about your illness?	31.5	22.4	26.0	9.4	5.7	5.0
4. Have you been able to share how you are feeling with your family or friends?	11.6	7.1	12.8	15.5	21.0	32.0
5. Have you felt that life was worthwhile?	42.7	21.2	14.8	11.2	5.0	5.0
6. Have you felt at peace?	24.4	21.7	23.1	11.6	8.0	11.2
7. Have you had enough help and advice for your family to plan for the future?	8.7	6.9	7.8	12.1	17.4	47.3

Table 3. Results of ordinal logistic regression models.

Risk factor (reference group)	Physical/psychological problems		Interpersonal problems		Existential problems	
	OR (95% CI)	p	OR (95% CI)	p	OR (95% CI)	p
Gender (male)	1.29 (0.87–1.92)	0.203	1.51 (1.03–2.24)	0.037	1.19 (0.79–1.79)	0.404
Age (18–28)	1.20 (0.95–1.52)	0.120	0.90 (0.72–1.14)	0.396	0.80 (0.63–1.02)	0.075
Education (none formal)	0.86 (0.65–1.13)	0.271	0.71 (0.54–0.93)	0.014	1.14 (0.86–1.52)	0.353
Wealth quintile (poorest)	0.85 (0.74–0.98)	0.027	0.92 (0.80–1.06)	0.242	0.82 (0.70–0.95)	0.009
Physical function (best)	3.22 (2.32–4.48)	<0.001	0.50 (0.37–0.68)	<0.001	1.54 (1.14–2.08)	0.005
Country (Kenya)	1.13 (0.76–1.68)	0.530	1.10 (0.75–1.63)	0.619	2.40 (1.58–3.63)	<0.001
Time since diagnosis (0 days)	1.03 (0.86–1.24)	0.709	0.78 (0.65–0.94)	0.008	1.03 (0.85–1.24)	0.773

not have a CD4 count on record a month after diagnosis, compared to only 13.8% in Kenya. This suggests that Uganda has either a lack of service availability or weaker care linkages. It is also possible that more CD4 tests were carried out and the problem was with study data collection.

Interpersonal problems – inability to access help and advice for the family or to share feelings – were reported most frequently. Those with more education have fewer interpersonal problems, which comprise lack of help/advice and inability to share feelings. In many cases these problems should be managed with counselling, which is a required element of care for all newly diagnosed patients[32]. The results suggest that lack of education limits the benefits of counselling for the patient. This could be caused by communication difficulties (low literacy, perhaps limited English), uncertainty what questions to ask, or reluctance to challenge health workers perceived to have authority. Interpersonal problems are more common for women, which is consistent with a multi-centre HIV study in 13 European countries which found that women received less emotional support than men and were also less likely to benefit from it[33].

Physical/psychological and existential problems are exacerbated by physical restriction and poverty, but those with impaired physical function actually report fewer interpersonal problems. The association may be affected by status disclosure. Physically active people with more resources may be more capable of concealing their HIV status, and non-disclosure could limit their ability to share their feelings and impede their access to help. There is evidence that people with more advanced disease are more likely to disclose their status and that disclosure is motivated by the need for material support[34,35].

Strengths and limitations

The study benefits from a sample recruited very soon after diagnosis and assessed using a validated, patient-reported instrument. This study includes a more representative sample than previous research in this area[15,19] but its application to other contexts is limited. The clinics were purposively selected and are all in urban areas. Many patients were first tested for HIV at VCT services and referred to the clinic for care, which explains why only 25% of patients were seen on the day of diagnosis. Consecutive sampling can lead to selection bias if couples or friends with similar characteristics attend the clinic together. On the positive side, refusal was very low (<1%) and recall bias was minimised by data collection very soon after HIV diagnosis and limiting recall to a three-day period.

Risk factors are limited to one clinical and six demographic characteristics. This is reasonable because very little reliable information is available for this important patient group. CD4 count and WHO stage were both missing for large numbers of patients, especially in Uganda.

The African POS validation was conducted in palliative care facilities, not HIV clinics, and compared to the present study the patients had poorer physical function (only 11% scored 0 on the ECOG scale) and probably more advanced HIV, although CD4 count and viral load were not reported. However, the POS was designed for use at any stage of HIV infection, not only the end of life, and two of the validation facilities accepted referrals from the point of diagnosis. Only two of the five translations used in this study had been validated. The three new versions (Swahili, Luo and Runyakitara) were translated and back-translated according to best practice. The differences in existential well-being between Kenya and Uganda may be attributable to difficulties in translating this culturally variable concept.

The study has no HIV negative control group and so it does not identify the proportion of patient burden attributable to the physiological effects of HIV infection, to the psychological effects of HIV diagnosis, to indirect effects such as reduced income from illness, or to unrelated causes. From a public health perspective, the key finding is that multidimensional problems are a severe burden to newly diagnosed patients, and therefore they require effective care to improve wellbeing and aid retention whether the problems are related to HIV status directly, indirectly or not at all. Equally, the risk factors of poverty, physical restriction and limited education may be associated with multidimensional problems in the HIV negative population as well, but this would not affect the findings or conclusions of the study.

The odds ratios report the effect on the outcome of increasing the independent variable by one. For binary variables such as country, this represents the entirety of measured variation, whereas for ordinal variables such as education and wealth quintile it represents only a fraction, which limits the strength of associations for ordinal variables. Further details of problems such as duration, frequency and effect on daily living were not collected. Marital status, number of children, and HIV disclosure status were also not collected, and these demographic variables may have affected the outcomes.

Conclusions

Clinical recommendations following from these findings are that newly diagnosed outpatients should receive assessment, screening and care for physical symptoms and psychological, spiritual and social problems within days of HIV diagnosis. Effective interventions must be developed and evaluated. A randomised controlled trial of the effectiveness of nurse training on multidimensional patient outcomes is in progress in Kenya and South Africa. The findings from this trial may be useful in the development of diagnosis-specific care support.

Clinical staff must be aware of the possibility of communication difficulties, and ensure patients have the opportunity to get the help and advice they seek. Patients need to be equipped with the means to overcome barriers to continued care, whether financial, structural, emotional or psychological. Those who see no benefit from care initially may be unlikely to return[36]. Future research should investigate whether outcomes improve over time from diagnosis after engagement with HIV services and ART initiation.

Acknowledgments

Keira Lowther read and commented on the manuscript. The authors are grateful for the guidance provided by the United States Government (USG) Palliative Care Technical Working Group and to the Kenyan and Ugandan USG Country Teams. Finally we are grateful to the staff and patients at the participating facilities.

Author Contributions

Conceived and designed the experiments: VS IJH RH. Performed the experiments: NG GM MA JK CN GB EN RAP. Analyzed the data: VS PF SP. Wrote the paper: VS.

References

1. Rosen S, Fox MP (2011) Retention in HIV care between testing and treatment in sub-Saharan Africa: a systematic review. PLoS Med 8(7): e1001056. Available http://www.plosmedicine.org/article/info%3Adoi%2F10.1371%2Fjournal.pmed.1001056.Accessed 24 January 2013.
2. Tayler-Smith K, Zachariah R, Massaquoi M, Manzi M, Pasulani O, et al. (2010) Unacceptable attrition among WHO stages 1 and 2 patients in a hospital-based setting in rural Malawi: can we retain such patients within the general health system? Trans R S Trop Med Hyg 104(5): 313–319.
3. Meursing K, Sibindi F (2000) HIV counselling - a luxury or necessity? Health Policy Plan 15(1): 17–23.
4. Ramirez-Avila L, Regan S, Giddy J, Chetty S, Ross D, et al. (2012) Depressive symptoms and their impact on health-seeking behaviors in newly-diagnosed HIV-infected patients in Durban, South Africa. AIDS Behav 16(8): 2226–35.
5. Roura M, Busza J, Wringe A, Mbata D, Urassa M, et al. (2009) Barriers to sustaining antiretroviral treatment in Kisesa, Tanzania: a follow-up study to understand attrition from the antiretroviral program. AIDS Patient Care STDs 23(3): 203–210.
6. Harding R, Lampe FC, Norwood S, Date HL, Clucas C, et al. (2010) Symptoms are highly prevalent among HIV outpatients and associated with poor adherence and unprotected sexual intercourse. Sex Transm Infect 86(7): 520–524.
7. Willard S, Holzemer WL, Wantland DJ, Cuca YP, Kirksey KM, et al. (2009) Does "asymptomatic" mean without symptoms for those living with HIV infection? AIDS Care 21(3): 322–328.
8. Makoae LN, Seboni NM, Molosiwa K, Moleko M, Human S, et al. (2005) The symptom experience of people living with HIV/AIDS in Southern Africa. J Assoc Nurses AIDS Care 16(3): 22–32.
9. Collins K, Harding R (2007) Improving HIV management in sub-Saharan Africa: how much palliative care is needed? AIDS Care 19(10): 1304–6.
10. Marwick KFM, Kaaya SF (2010) Prevalence of depression and anxiety disorders in HIV-positive outpatients in rural Tanzania. AIDS Care 22(3): 415–419.
11. Kaharuza FM, Bunnell R, Moss S, Purcell DW, Bikaako-Kajura W, et al. (2006) Depression and CD4 cell count among persons with HIV infection in Uganda. AIDS Behav 10:(4 Suppl) S105–S11.
12. Collins DL, Leibbrandt M (2007) The financial impact of HIV/AIDS on poor households in South Africa. AIDS (Suppl 7): S75–S81.
13. Thomas F (2006) Stigma, fatigue and social breakdown: exploring the impacts of HIV/AIDS on patient and carer well-being in the Caprivi Region, Namibia. Soc Sci Med 63: 3174–3187.
14. Selman L, Higginson IJ, Agupio G, Dinat N, Downing J, et al. (2011) Quality of life among patients receiving palliative care in South Africa and Uganda: a multi-centred study. Health Qual Life Outcomes 9 (21). Available http://www.ncbi.nlm.nih.gov/pmc/articles/PMC3094195/.Accessed 24 January 2013.
15. Simms V, Higginson IJ, Harding R (2011) What palliative care-related problems do patients experience at HIV diagnosis? A systematic review of the literature. J Pain Sympt Managem 42(5): 734–753.
16. Levine LJ, Pizarro DA (2004) Emotion and memory research: a grumpy overview. Soc Cognit 22(5): 530–554.
17. UNAIDS (2010) Report on the global AIDS epidemic 2010. Geneva: UNAIDS.
18. Olley BO, Bolajoko AJ (2008) Psychosocial determinants of HIV-related quality of life among HIV-positive military in Nigeria. Int J STD AIDS 19(2): 94–98.
19. Wig N, Sakhuja A, Agarwal SK, Khakha DC, Mehta S, et al. (2008) Multidimensional health status of HIV-infected outpatients at a tertiary care center in north India. Indian J Med Sci 62(3): 87–97.

20. Harding R, Simms V, Penfold S, McCrone P, Moreland S, et al. (2010) Multicentre mixed-methods PEPFAR HIV Care & Support Public Health Evaluation: study protocol. BMC Pub Health 10: 584. Available http://www.biomedcentral.com/1471-2458/10/584.Accessed 24 January 2013.
21. Simms V, Harding R, Penfold S, Namisango, Downing J, et al. (2009) PEPFAR Public Health Evaluation - Care and Support: Phase 2 Uganda. University of North Carolina. Measure Evaluation website. Available http://www.cpc.unc.edu/measure/publications. Accessed 24 January 2013.
22. Harding R, Simms V, Penfold S, Namisango E, Downing J, et al. (2009) PEPFAR Public Health Evaluation - Care and Support: Phase 2 Kenya. University of North Carolina. Measure Evaluation website. Available http://www.cpc.unc.edu/measure/publications. Accessed 24 January 2013.
23. Powell RA, Downing J, Harding R, Mwangi-Powell F, Connor S (2007) Development of the APCA African Palliative Outcome Scale. J Pain Sympt Managem 33(2): 229–232.
24. Harding R, Selman L, Agupio G, Dinat N, Downing J, et al. (2010) Validation of a core outcome measure for palliative care in Africa: the APCA African Palliative Outcome Scale. Health Qual Life Outcomes 8(10). Available http://www.hqlo.com/content/8/1/10. Accessed 24 January 2013.
25. Oken MM, Creech RH, Tormey DC, Hpoton J, Davis TE, et al. (1982) Toxicity and response criteria of the Eastern Cooperative Oncology Group. Am J Clin Oncol 5:649–655.
26. Rutstein S, Johnson K (2004) The DHS Wealth Index. DHS Comparative Reports, Calverton, MD, , USA: ORC Macro, No. 6.
27. World Health Organization (2010) Antiretroviral therapy for HIV infection in adults and adolescents: recommendations for a public health approach. Geneva: World Health Organization.
28. Harding R, Selman L, Simms V, Penfold S, Agupio G, et al. (2012) How to analyse palliative care outcome data for patients in sub-Saharan Africa: an international multicentred factor analytic examination of the APCA African POS. J Pain Sympt Managem epublished ahead of print. Available http://www.sciencedirect.com/science/article/pii/S0885392412003557.Accessed 24 January 2013..
29. Selman L, Harding R, Gysels M, Speck P, Higginson IJ (2011)The measurement of spirituality in palliative care and the content of tools validated cross-culturally: a systematic review. J Pain Sympt Managem 41(4): 728–753.
30. Maman S, Cathcart R, Burkhardt G, Omba S, Behets F (2009) The role of religion in HIV-positive women's disclosure experiences and coping strategies in Kinshasa, Democratic Republic of Congo. Soc Sci Med 68(5): 965–970.
31. Steinhauser KE, Voils CI, Clipp EC, Bosworth HB, Christakis NA, et al. (2006) 'Are you at peace?' One item to probe spiritual concerns at the end of life. Arch Intern Med 166(1): 101–105.
32. World Health Organization (2010) A handbook for improving HIV testing and counselling services - field-test version. Geneva: World Health Organization.
33. Gordillo V, Fekete EM, Platteau T, Antoni MH, Schneiderman N, et al. (2009) Emotional support and gender in people living with HIV: effects on psychological well-being. J Behav Med 32: 523–531.
34. Holt R, Court P, Vedhara K, Nott KH, Holmes J, et al. (1998) The role of disclosure in coping with HIV infection. AIDS Care 10(1): 49–60.
35. Miller AN, Rubin DL (2007) Motivations and methods for self-disclosure of HIV seropositivity in Nairobi, Kenya. AIDS Behav 11(5): 687–697.
36. Merten S, Kenter E, Musheke M, Ntalasha H, Martin-Hilber A (2010) Patient-reported barriers and drivers of adherence to antiretrovirals in sub-Saharan Africa: a meta-ethnography. Trop Med Int Health (Suppl 1): 16–33.

3

HIV Prevalence and Incidence among Sexually Active Females in Two Districts of South Africa to Determine Microbicide Trial Feasibility

Annaléne Nel[1], Cheryl Louw[2], Elizabeth Hellstrom[3], Sarah L. Braunstein[4], Ina Treadwell[3], Melanie Marais[3], Martie de Villiers[2], Jannie Hugo[2], Inge Paschke[3], Chrisna Andersen[3], Janneke van de Wijgert[5]*

1 International Partnership for Microbicides, Silver Spring, Maryland, United States of America, 2 Madibeng Centre for Research, Brits, South Africa, 3 Be Part Yoluntu Centre, Mbekweni and Paarl, South Africa, 4 New York City Department of Health and Mental Hygiene, New York City, New York, United States of America, 5 Academic Medical Center of the University of Amsterdam and Amsterdam Institute for Global Health and Development, Amsterdam, The Netherlands

Abstract

Background: The suitability of populations of sexually active women in Madibeng (North-West Province) and Mbekweni (Western Cape), South Africa, for a Phase III vaginal microbicide trial was evaluated.

Methods: Sexually active women 18–35 years not known to be HIV-positive or pregnant were tested cross-sectionally to determine HIV and pregnancy prevalence (798 in Madibeng and 800 in Mbekweni). Out of these, 299 non-pregnant, HIV-negative women were subsequently enrolled at each clinical research center in a 12-month cohort study with quarterly study visits.

Results: HIV prevalence was 24% in Madibeng and 22% in Mbekweni. HIV incidence rates based on seroconversions over 12 months were 6.0/100 person-years (PY) (95% CI 3.0, 9.0) in Madibeng and 4.5/100 PY (95% CI 1.8, 7.1) in Mbekweni and those estimated by cross-sectional BED testing were 7.1/100 PY (95% CI 2.8, 11.3) in Madibeng and 5.8/100 PY (95% CI 2.0, 9.6) in Mbekweni. The 12-month pregnancy incidence rates were 4.8/100 PY (95% CI 2.2, 7.5) in Madibeng and 7.0/100 PY (95% CI 3.7, 10.3) in Mbekweni; rates decreased over time in both districts. Genital symptoms were reported very frequently, with an incidence of 46.8/100 PY (95% CI 38.5, 55.2) in Madibeng and 21.5/100 PY (95% CI 15.8, 27.3) in Mbekweni. Almost all (>99%) participants said that they would be willing to participate in a microbicide trial.

Conclusion: These populations might be suitable for Phase III microbicide trials provided that HIV incidence rates over time remain sufficiently high to support endpoint-driven trials.

Editor: Matthew P. Fox, Boston University, United States of America

Funding: This study was funded by the International Partnership for Microbicides (a not-for-profit public-private partnership). The funders were involved in study design, data collection and preparation of the manuscript.

Competing Interests: AN is employed by The International Partnership for Microbicides (IPM), a not-for-profit public-private partnership aiming to develop a safe and effective vaginal microbicide for HIV prevention. All other authors are employed by not-for-profit organizations receiving funding from IPM to assist IPM with achieving this goal. The study reported in this manuscript did not involve the use of any candidate vaginal microbicides governed by intellectual property right; it was an observational cohort study to determine HIV incidence rates in preparation for future clinical trials of vaginal microbicides.

* E-mail: j.vandewijgert@amc-cpcd.org

Introduction

At the end of 2009, about 7,000 new HIV infections occurred each day [1]. New HIV prevention tools, especially those that women can use, are therefore desperately needed. Microbicides are being developed for topical application inside the vagina or rectum to prevent infection with HIV and possibly other sexually transmitted infections (STIs) [2]. Microbicide research has been ongoing for about 20 years. Proof-of-concept for vaginal microbicides was obtained in 2010, when the CAPRISA 004 trial showed a 39% reduction in HIV incidence after 30 months of tenofovir gel use compared to placebo gel use [3]. Phase III clinical trials of candidate microbicides are often conducted in sub-Saharan Africa because this is where 70% of the new HIV

infections occur [1]. In preparation for such trials, estimates of HIV incidence in target populations are needed to determine adequate sample size and statistical power for demonstrating safety and efficacy [4].

South Africa has hosted, and is hosting, several microbicide and other HIV prevention intervention trials. While HIV prevalence data are available for many districts of South Africa, they are not available for all potential microbicide trial populations. HIV incidence data are hard to find [5]. Madibeng and Mbekweni are two districts of South Africa that had not yet participated in HIV prevention intervention trials when the studies described in this paper were conducted, and HIV prevalence and incidence where not yet known. Madibeng is a rural district municipality in North-West Province supported by mining (chrome, granite, and platinum), manufacturing (automotive, metal, and fuel), and agriculture. Mbekweni is a small urban township close to Paarl in the Western Cape; many of its residents are employed in the deciduous farming and wine-making industry. In both districts, the community is somewhat migratory because of unstable employment.

Methods

Study design and populations

HIV prevalence and incidence in two districts of South Africa, Madibeng and Mbekweni, were estimated in cross-sectional studies (targeting 800 women) followed by prospective cohort studies (targeting 300 women) to determine the suitability of the populations for participation in Phase III microbicide trials. Women were recruited from local family planning clinics in Madibeng and from family planning clinics, community events, and door-to-door visits in Mbekweni. The clinical research centers (CRCs) used recruitment strategies that they also plan to use in

future Phase III microbicide trials and these were CRC-specific. However, the same study procedures were followed at each CRC from the moment women visited the CRC to be screened for study participation. Women were eligible for the cross-sectional studies if they were 18–35 years, not HIV-positive or pregnant by self-report, not breastfeeding, and sexually active (defined as at least one penetrative vaginal coital act per month for the previous three months). At cross-sectional study visits, eligible women were tested for HIV antibodies using a rapid testing algorithm (Figure 1) and for pregnancy. Women who tested positive for HIV antibodies were also tested by BED capture enzyme immunoassay (BED) to determine the proportion of recent infections [6].

Women who tested HIV- and pregnancy-negative in the cross-sectional cohort studies, still met the entry criteria described above, and met additional entry criteria for the cohort studies were subsequently offered enrollment into the cohort studies. These additional entry criteria included using a reliable WHO-approved contraceptive method [7], not injecting non-therapeutic drugs, not participating in other studies, not suffering from specified chronic

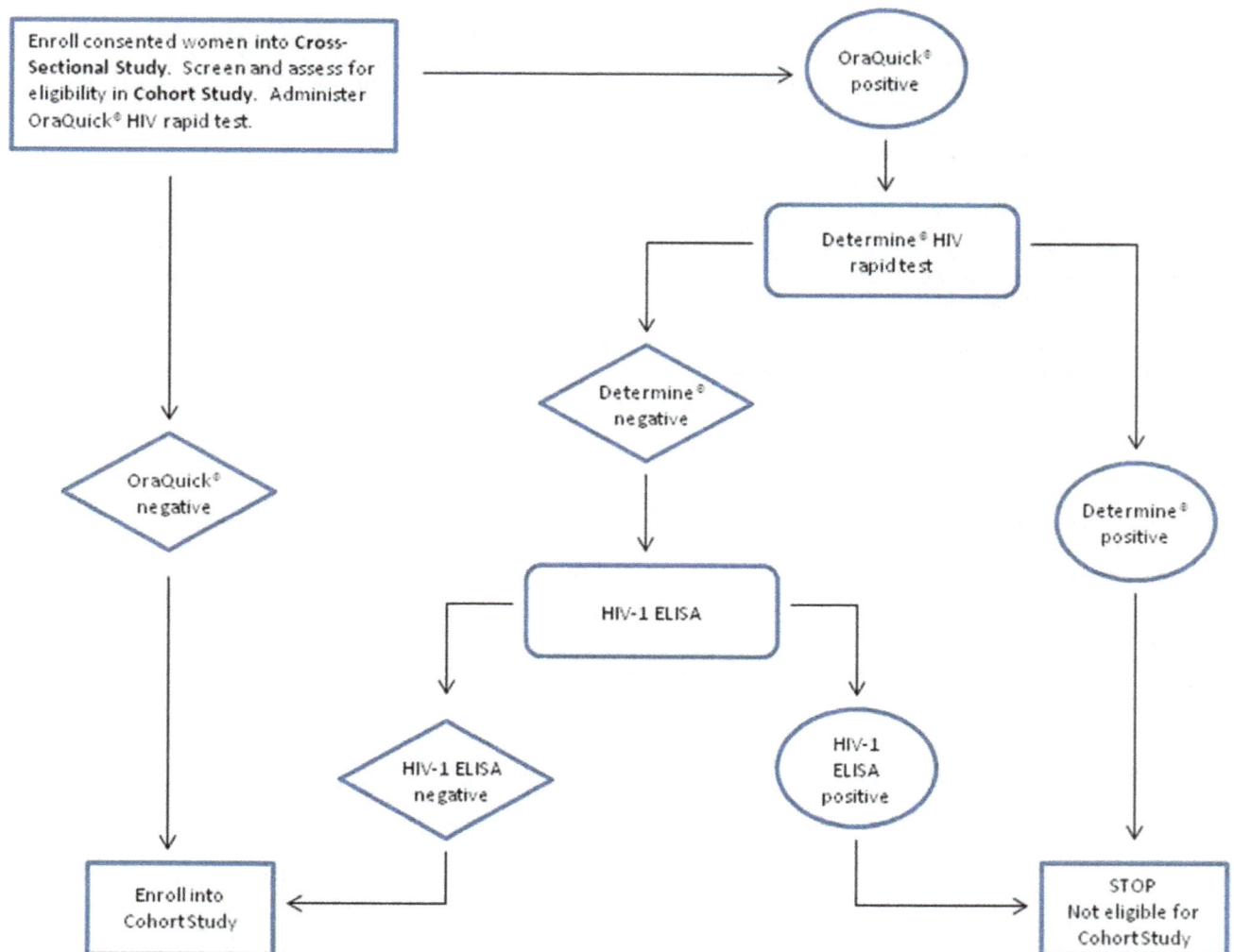

Figure 1. HIV testing algorithm. Approximately 800 women at each CRC were tested for HIV infection at screening as indicated. Those confirmed as seronegative and who met the entry criteria (299 at each CRC) were enrolled into the prospective cohort study and retested at 3, 6, 9, and 12 months after enrollment using the same algorithm. Participants who became HIV-positive while on study were referred to available sources of psychosocial and medical care and support. HIV-positive participants could continue on study for scheduled examinations per protocol with the exception of any further HIV testing and genital assessment, unless clinically indicated.

diseases or allergies, refraining from anal sex and planning to stay in the study area for the duration of the study. Follow-up visits occurred after 3, 6, 9 and 12 months. Screening continued until 800 women were enrolled in the cross-sectional studies and 300 HIV-negative women were enrolled in the cohort studies at each CRC.

All women in the cross-sectional and cohort studies (at all study visits) were interviewed regarding demographics, sexual behavior, and medical history; and received HIV risk reduction and contraceptive counseling, condoms, and syndromic management of sexually transmitted infections (STI) free of charge [8]. Confirmed HIV-positive women were referred for HIV care, and pregnant women were referred for antenatal care, but HIV-positive and pregnant women were retained in the study. The study was approved by Pharma-Ethics in South Africa. Written informed consent was obtained from all study participants.

Laboratory testing

Oral swabs from each participant were tested using OraQuick ADVANCE Rapid HIV-1/2 Antibody Test (OraSure Technologies, Inc., Bethlehem, PA, USA). Blood samples from women with positive OraQuick results were tested by Determine HIV-1/2 rapid test (Inverness Medical Professional Diagnostics, Princeton, NJ, USA), and by enzyme-linked immunosorbant assay (ELISA) if a tiebreaker was needed. Blood samples from women who were confirmed HIV-positive were also tested by BED assay (Calypte Biomedical Coorporation, Portland, OR, USA) according to the manufacturer's instructions. A specimen with a final normalized optical density value of less than or equal to 0.8 was considered to be from a patient who was infected less than 155 days ago [6].

Data Analysis and Statistics

Sample size calculations. In the cross-sectional studies, a sample size of 800 women would allow for a precision level of the HIV incidence estimate of 4.0/100 PY±3.5, 5.0/100 PY±3.7, and 6.0/100 PY±3.9 assuming an HIV prevalence of 25% and using the McWalter and Welte formula described below [9,10]. In the cohort studies, accumulation of 270 personyears (PY) of follow up (300 women for one year minus 10% PY lost to follow-up) would generate the following 95% confidence intervals around the observed HIV incidence rates: 11 seroconversions, 4.1 (95% CI 1.7, 6.5); 14 seroconversions, 5.2 (95% CI 2.5, 7.9); 17 seroconversions, 6.3 (95% CI 3.3, 9.3).

Statistical analysis. Data were double entered and analyzed using SAS version 9.2 (SAS Institute, Cary, NC). Descriptive statistics were used to summarize baseline demographic, behavioral and clinical characteristics. Categorical variables are expressed as percentages, and continuous data as medians with inter-quartile ranges.

HIV, pregnancy, and STI symptom incidence rates in the cohort studies were calculated based on a Poisson distribution with PY at risk in the denominator. A person's time at risk began at the enrollment visit and ended at the last study visit attended (usually the Month 12 visit) or when HIV infection or pregnancy occurred. HIV infection and pregnancy were assumed to have occurred at the mid-point between the last available negative test and first positive test. A woman who reached an HIV endpoint was no longer considered at risk for HIV but was still considered at risk for pregnancy, and vice versa. Incident genital symptom cases were defined as participants ever reporting a symptom during follow-up.

HIV incidence rates and 95% confidence intervals based on BED results in the cross-sectional studies were calculated using the formula, and accompanying spreadsheet, provided by McWalter and Welte [9,10]. Inputs in the formula include the total number of HIV-positive and HIV-negative individuals in the sample, the number of HIV-positive individuals who also tested positive on the BED assay, the BED window period (155 days), and an estimated BED false-recent rate of 5.2% [11]. Incidence estimates are expressed as an incidence rate (number of new HIV infections per 100 PY).

Age-adjusted logistic regression models were used to assess predictors of prevalent HIV infection and pregnancy, with p-values from the Wilcoxon-Mann-Whitney test for continuous variables and the Chi-square and Fisher's exact tests for categorical variables. Age-adjusted Cox proportional hazards regression models were used to assess predictors of HIV seroconversion and incident pregnancy.

Results

Disposition

Between April 2007 and March 2008, 798 women were enrolled in the cross-sectional study in Madibeng and 800 in Mbekweni; 299 women at each CRC were subsequently enrolled in the cohort studies. In the cohort studies, total PY of follow-up were 258.4 and 250.8 in Madibeng and Mbekweni, respectively. In Madibeng, 254 of 299 (85%) participants completed all scheduled visits; 17 women withdrew early from the cohort study, 15 were lost to follow-up, 13 missed a scheduled visit, and none died. In Mbekweni, 229 of 299 (77%) participants completed all scheduled visits; 23 women withdrew early from the cohort study, 22 were lost to follow-up, 25 missed a scheduled visit, and none died.

Demographic Characteristics

In the cross-sectional studies, the median age of study participants at each CRC was 24 years (Table 1). Most participants were black African, single, and had at least some high school education. Over 85% of participants at each CRC had one male sexual partner in the previous 3 months, and less than half (44–45%) used a condom during their last sex act. Twice as many participants in Mbekweni (32%) as Madibeng (16%) had a current sexual partner that they knew was HIV-positive. Anal sex was rarely reported at each CRC (<2%), but oral sex was more common (9–13%). The percentage of women cleansing the vagina before or after sex was higher in Madibeng than Mbekweni (6.5% vs 1.4% and 13.0% vs 0.9%, respectively). At each CRC, demographic and sexual behavior characteristics of cohort study participants at enrollment were similar to cross-sectional participants with one exception: in Madibeng, fewer women in the cohort than in cross-sectional study felt that they were at high risk for HIV (21% vs. 41%).

HIV prevalence

HIV prevalence was similar in the two districts: 24.1% (95% CI 12.1, 27.1) in Madibeng and 21.8% (95% CI 18.9, 24.7) in Mbekweni. Factors positively associated with prevalent HIV infection at both CRCs were: primary education as highest educational level achieved, inconsistent condom use in the last 7 days, self-assessment of HIV risk as high, suspected positive or unknown HIV serostatus of a current sexual partner, and presence of STI symptoms at baseline (Table 2). Being married or living together was negatively associated with HIV infection. Other risk factors were significantly associated with prevalent HIV infection at one CRC only (Table 2).

HIV incidence

HIV incidence rates based on seroconversions in the cohort studies are shown in Figure 2. Overall incidence rates for the 12-

Table 1. Baseline Characteristics of Study Participants.

Characteristic n (%)	Cross-Sectional Studies		Cohort Studies	
	Madibeng	Mbekweni	Madibeng	Mbekweni
	N = 798[1]	N = 800	N = 299[2]	N = 299[3]
Age in years (median)	24	24	23	23
Age in years				
18–20	202 (25.3)	172 (21.5)	95 (31.8)	90 (30.1)
21–25	316 (39.6)	283 (35.4)	120 (40.1)	110 (36.8)
26–30	159 (19.9)	195 (24.4)	53 (17.7)	57 (19.1)
31–35	121 (15.2)	150 (18.8)	31 (10.4)	42 (14.1)
Race				
Black African	744 (93.2)	711 (88.9)	270 (90.3)	292 (97.7)
Other	54 (6.8)	89 (11.1)	29 (9.7)	7 (2.3)
Marital status				
Married/living together	210 (26.3)	274 (34.3)	61 (20.4)	76 (25.4)
Separated/divorced	3 (0.4)	4 (0.5)	0	2 (0.7)
Widowed	0	1 (0.1)	0	0
Single	590 (73.9)	521 (65.1)	238 (79.6)	221 (73.9)
Education				
No school	2 (0.3)	1 (0.1)	1 (0.3)	0
Some/completed primary school	52 (6.5)	58 (7.3)	9 (3.0)	13 (4.3)
Some/completed high school	728 (91.2)	708 (88.5)	281 (94.0)	272 (91.0)
Some/completed tertiary school	16 (2.0)	33 (4.1)	8 (2.7)	14 (4.7)
Male sex partners in last 3 months				
1	685 (85.8)	759 (94.9)	256 (85.6)	287 (96.0)
2	85 (10.7)	38 (4.8)	32 (10.7)	11 (3.7)
3 or more	27 (3.4)	3 (0.4)	11 (3.7)	1 (0.3)
Male sex partners in last 7 days				
0	43 (5.4)	29 (3.6)	25 (8.4)	12 (4.0)
1	725 (91.4)	761 (95.1)	266 (89.6)	287 (96.0)
2 or more	25 (3.2)	10 (1.3)	6 (2.0)	0
Condom used during last sex act	355 (44.5)	348 (43.5)	138 (46.3)	153 (51.2)
Any chance that any current sex partner is HIV+				
Yes	123 (15.9)	246 (32.2)	34 (11.9)	104 (37.3)
No	413 (53.3)	216 (28.3)	175 (61.0)	45 (16.1)
Don't know	239 (30.8)	301 (39.5)	78 (27.2)	130 (46.6)
Willing to participate in microbicide trial	784 (98.6)	798 (99.9)	294 (98.3)	297 (99.7)
Ever had anal sex	15 (1.9)	12 (1.5)	6 (2.0)	4 (1.3)
Ever had oral sex	103 (12.9)	69 (8.6)	40 (13.4)	42 (14.0)
Ever vaginal cleansing before sex[4]	52 (6.5)	11 (1.4)	19 (6.4)	6 (2.0)
Ever vaginal cleansing after sex[4]	103 (13.0)	7 (0.9)	43 (14.4)	5 (1.7)
Self assessment of HIV risk				
No risk	49 (6.2)	3 (0.4)	28 (9.4)	0
Low risk	259 (32.6)	252 (31.7)	139 (46.5)	88 (29.4)
Moderate risk	87 (11.0)	26 (3.3)	37 (12.4)	3 (1.0)
High risk	327 (41.2)	484 (60.9)	64 (21.4)	204 (68.2)
Don't know	72 (9.1)	30 (3.8)	31 (10.4)	4 (1.4)

[1]Two women were not eligible and excluded.
[2]One woman was found to be less than 18 years of age after enrollment and was subsequently excluded.
[3]One woman enrolled twice using a different name; data from her second enrollment were excluded.
[4]Included disinfectants/soaps, cotton wool/wad of cloth, and traditional herbs (Mbekweni only).

Table 2. Determinants of Prevalent HIV Infection in the Cross-Sectional Studies[1].

Determinant	Madibeng (N = 192)		Mbekweni (N = 174)	
	% HIV+	Age-adjusted OR (95% CI)	% HIV+	Age-adjusted OR (95% CI)
Race				
Black African	24.7	2.1 (1.0, 4.7)	24.3	32.5 (4.5, 235.7)[2,3]
Other (reference)	14.8		1.1	
Marital status:				
Married/living together	24.3	0.6 (0.4, 0.9)[2]	21.5	0.6 (0.4, 0.9)[2]
Single, separated or divorced (reference)	24.0		21.9	
Highest level of education achieved[4]:				
Some/completed primary education	50.0	8.8 (1.1, 73.5)[2]	34.5	11.9 (1.5, 94.7)[2]
Some/completed high school	22.7	3.0 (0.4, 23.0)	21.5	8.0 (1.1, 59.1)[2]
Some/completed tertiary education (reference)	6.3		3.0	
Source of income:				
Woman herself (reference)	27.6		22.9	
Husband/partner	27.1	1.0 (0.6, 1.7)	20.4	0.8 (0.5, 1.2)
Family	18.1	1.1 (0.6, 2.0)	17.6	1.0 (0.7, 1.6)
Other	29.4	1.4 (0.8, 2.4)	40.3	2.9 (1.6, 5.3)[2]
Average monthly income[5]				
0-R500 (reference)	24.2		37.7	
R501-R1000	19.8	0.6 (0.4, 1.1)	29.2	0.7 (0.4, 1.2)
R1001-R2000	32.0	1.2 (0.8, 2.0)	22.1	0.5 (0.3, 0.9)[2]
>R2000	18.3	0.6 (0.3, 1.1)	12.7	0.2 (0.1, 0.5)[2]
Condom use in last 7 days				
Always (reference)	17.2		14.6	
Inconsistent	28.7	1.7 (1.0, 2.8)[2]	26.7	1.9 (1.1, 3.3)[2]
Never	25.0	1.1 (0.6, 1.8)	15.3	0.7 (0.4, 1.4)
Ever had anal sex				
Yes	46.7	3.3 (1.1, 9.9)[2]	16.7	0.6 (0.1, 3.0)
No (reference)	23.6		21.9	
Ever had oral sex				
Yes	21.4	0.9 (0.5, 1.4)	7.3	0.3 (0.1, 0.7)[2]
No (reference)	24.5		23.1	
Self assessment of HIV risk				
No/low risk (reference)	9.4		11.0	
Moderate risk	27.6	3.2 (1.7, 5.9)[2]	19.2	1.8 (0.6, 5.2)
High risk	35.8	5.1 (3.3, 8.1)[2]	26.5	2.7 (1.7, 4.2)[2]
Any chance that any current sex partner is HIV+				
Yes	50.4	5.5 (3.5, 8.8)[2]	26.0	2.2 (1.3, 3.5)[2]
No (reference)	13.2		13.9	
Don't know	28.5	2.3 (1.5, 3.4)[2]	22.9	1.9 (1.2, 3.1)[2]
Reported STI symptom at baseline				
Yes	31.0	1.6 (1.2, 2.3)[2]	41.8	3.1 (1.9, 5.1)[2]
No (reference)	20.7		19.6	

[1]Each row represents one bivariable model including age and the predictor of interest.
[2]Age-adjusted odds ratio significantly different for predictor vs. reference value (p<0.05);
[3]Only 7 women had a race other than black African (they were Cape coloured).
[4]Only 8 women in Madibeng and 14 women in Mbekweni had some/completed tertiary education.
[5]R = rand; 1 US dollar = 7.4 South African rands.

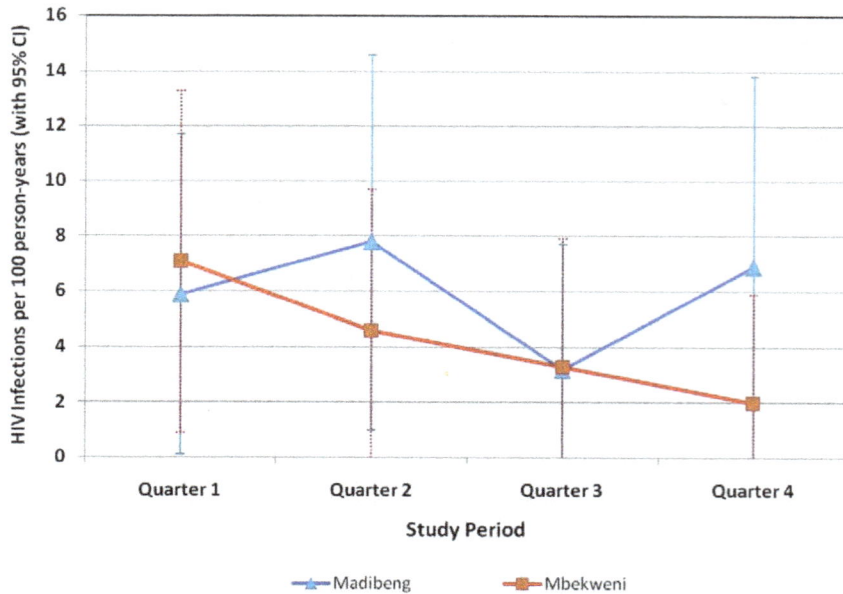

Figure 2. HIV incidence in the prospective cohort studies. Women enrolled in the 12-month cohort studies visited the CRC at 3, 6, 9, and 12 months after enrollment for HIV testing according to the algorithm presented in Figure 1. HIV incidence rates were calculated based on a Poisson distribution with PY at risk in the denominator. They are expressed as number of cases per 100 PY, with 95% confidence intervals (CI). HIV infection was assumed to have occurred at the mid-point between the last available negative test and first positive test.

month period were 6.0/100 PY (95% CI 3.0, 9.0) in Madibeng and 4.5/100 PY (95% CI 1.8, 7.1) in Mbekweni. Rates in Madibeng varied by study quarter, while rates in Mbekweni declined steadily, but number of events per quarter were small and confidence intervals wide (Figure 2). Positive predictors of seroconversion in Madibeng were ever having had anal sex (HR 8.5, 95% CI 1.9, 37.9); self-assessment of HIV risk as moderate/high versus none/low (HR 3.2, 95% CI 1.1, 9.1); and having two or more male sexual partners versus one in the 3-month period prior to screening (HR 7.4, 95% CI 2.7, 20.6). In Mbekweni, having a current sexual partner who is HIV-positive (HR 3.8, 95% CI 1.1, 13.0) was positively associated with HIV seroconversion.

HIV incidence rates estimated by cross-sectional BED testing were 7.1/100 PY (95% CI 2.8, 11.3) in Madibeng and 5.8/100 PY (95% CI 2.0, 9.6) in Mbekweni.

Pregnancy rates

In the cross-sectional studies, pregnancy prevalence was 2.5% (95% CI 1.4, 3.6) in Madibeng and 2.3% (95% CI 1.2, 3.3) in Mbekweni. In the cohort studies, overall pregnancy rates for the 12-month period were higher in Mbekweni (7.0/100 PY [95% CI 3.7, 10.3]) than Madibeng (4.8/100 PY [95% CI 2.2, 7.5]). In both districts, pregnancy rates decreased during the observation period (Figure 3). In Madibeng, decreased likelihood of condom use at last sex from baseline to follow-up was associated with incident pregnancy (6.0 [95% CI 1.6, 22.7], p<0.01). In Mbekweni, ever having cleansed the vagina before sex (reported at baseline) (7.7 [95% CI 1.7, 34.6], p<0.01); ever having cleansed the vagina after sex (reported at baseline) (12.6 [95% CI 2.7, 58.7], p<0.01); and not having used a condom in the last 7 days (reported during follow-up) (6.2 [95% CI 1.3, 29.6], p = 0.02) were predictors of incident pregnancy.

Genital symptom rates

In the cross-sectional studies, the prevalence of self-reported genital symptoms (including genital discharge, lower abdominal pain, vaginal pruritus, dysuria, genital odor, genital sores/ulcers, swelling in groin area, and others) was 32.7% (95% CI 29.5, 36.0) in Madibeng and 9.9% (95% CI 7.8, 12.0) in Mbekweni. In the cohort studies, the incidence of self-reported genital symptoms during the 12-month period was 46.8/100 PY (95% CI 38.5, 55.2) in Madibeng and 21.5/100 PY (95% CI 15.8, 27.3) in Mbekweni. Over half of participants who reported genital symptoms during follow-up, 87 of 121 (72%) in Madibeng and 30 of 54 (56%) in Mbekweni, also reported symptoms at enrollment. In both districts, the percentage of participants reporting genital symptoms at each visit decreased throughout the 12-month observation period to 6% at Madibeng and 3.7% at Mbekweni.

Willingness to participate in a microbicide trial

Almost all participants in each district (99–100%) reported that they are willing to participate in a microbicide trial.

Discussion

The HIV prevalence in our studies among sexually active adult women 18–35 years of age was estimated to be 22–24% in Madibeng and Mbekweni, which is higher than the 2009 UNAIDS estimates of 13.6% for 15–24 year-old and 17.8% for 15–49 year-old South African women [1]. We may have measured a higher HIV prevalence because our study populations were (semi-)urban or because women who suspected that they were at risk for HIV were more interested in participating in our studies to access counseling, testing, and prevention services. On the other hand, women who already knew that they were HIV-positive were not eligible for study participation, which would suggest an underestimation of the true HIV prevalence in our studies.

In the cohort studies, HIV incidence based on seroconversions over the 12-month follow-up period was 6.0/100 PY in Madibeng and 4.5/100 PY in Mbekweni. BED-based HIV incidence estimates from the cross-sectional studies were slightly higher: 7.1 and 5.8/100 PY in Madibeng and Mbekweni, respectively. It

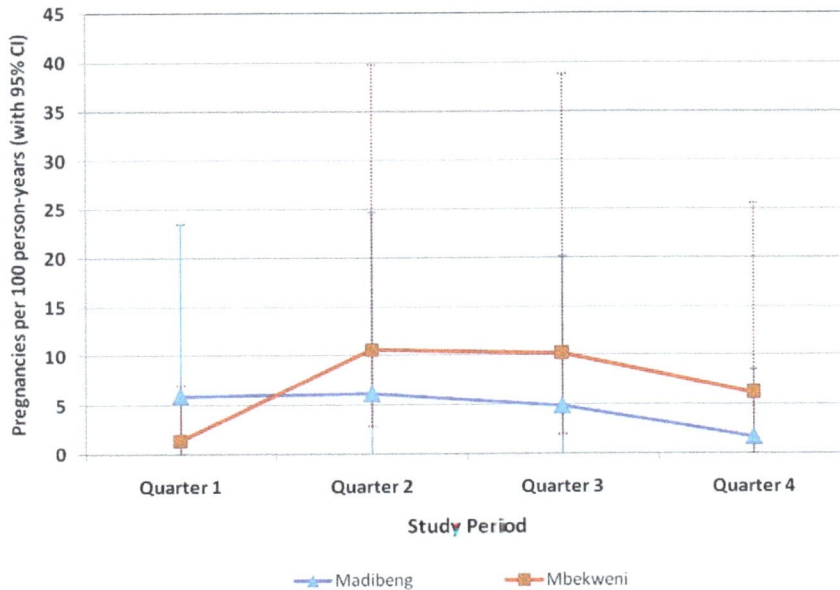

Figure 3. Pregnancy rates in the prospective cohort studies. Urine pregnancy tests were done at each study visit (screening, enrollment, and 3, 6, 9, and 12 months after enrollment in the cohort study). If test result was positive, the participant was to continue on study for follow-up per protocol. Estimated date of conception and estimated due date were to be recorded. If possible, follow-up was to continue for pregnancy outcome. Contraceptive counseling was provided and condoms were dispensed at each study visit.

should be noted, however, that the BED-based estimates were almost identical to the seroconversion rates in the first 6 months of the cohort studies (6.8 and 5.9/100 PY, respectively; data not shown). Data from the first 6 months of the cohort studies may be the most relevant for comparison with cross-sectional estimates because study participants may change their behavior in response to prevention messages and services received at the quarterly follow-up visits [12]. HIV seroconversion rates in Mbekweni indeed declined steadily during the 12 month follow-up period.

HIV incidence in both districts was high despite the fact that more than 85% of the women reported to only have had one sex partner in the past 3 months. This is most likely due to the high HIV prevalence in the communities: 12% of women in Madibeng and 37% of women in Mbekweni suspected that they had current sex partners that were HIV-positive. This proportion was most likely higher in Mbekweni than in Madibeng due to recent interventions in Mbekweni that promoted HIV testing. Furthermore, in both districts, condoms were not used consistently. In statistical models, determinants of both prevalent HIV infection at baseline and HIV seroconversion during the 12-month cohort studies were moderate or high perceived HIV risk, suspected positive or unknown serostatus of a current sexual partner, and ever having had anal sex. At entry into the cohort studies, women were asked to refrain from anal sex, and very few women reported anal sex throughout the studies (≤2% in both districts). However, anal sex is likely underreported in research studies due to social desirability bias [13]. Therefore, Phase III vaginal microbicide trial participants should be counselled on the increased HIV risk associated with anal sex, and the fact that vaginal microbicides are designed to protect women from vaginal acquisition of HIV only.

A few limitations of our data should be noted. The eligibility criteria for entry into our study limit generalizability of our results. The HIV prevalence rates in our paper apply to young, sexually active women who were not known to be HIV-infected or pregnant, and who agreed to be tested regularly for HIV. The

total number of seroconversions in each prospective cohort study (15 and 11 in Madibeng and Mbekweni, respectively) were low and the 95% confidence intervals were therefore wide. Models of determinants of HIV prevalence and HIV seroconversion were adjusted for age only to maximize statistical power, and residual confounding may therefore have been present. The 95% confidence intervals of the cross-sectional BED-based HIV incidence estimates were also wide. Furthermore, we did not measure local false-recent rates or window periods and could therefore not adjust our BED estimates as recommended by WHO [14].

The use of a reliable contraceptive method was a study requirement because this would also be a requirement for enrollment into a vaginal microbicide trial of a microbicide containing a new chemical entity. Despite this, pregnancy incidence rates were high in both districts (4.3 and 7.0/100 PY in Madibeng and Mbekweni, respectively). The number of pregnancies decreased throughout the studies, perhaps due to contraceptive counseling and provision of condoms at each study visit. However, contraceptive services at the CRCs should be strengthened further to keep pregnancy rates as low as possible during future microbicide trials [15].

The prevalence and incidence of self-reported genital symptoms were high in Madibeng (33%, 46.8/100 PY) and Mbekweni (10%, 21.5/100 PY), but since laboratory testing for STIs and vaginal infections was not done in these studies, conclusions cannot be drawn about the prevalence and incidence of STIs or vaginal infections in these communities. Almost all participants (over 99%) in both Madibeng and Mbekweni expressed strong interest in future microbicide trials.

In conclusion, the Madibeng and Mbekweni populations might be suitable for Phase III microbicide trials provided that HIV incidence rates over time remain sufficiently high to support endpoint-driven trials. However, contraceptive services should be strengthened to keep pregnancy rates as low as possible.

Acknowledgments

The authors gratefully acknowledge the study teams at the CRCs in Madibeng and Mbekweni, and the study team at the International Partnership for Microbicides, in particular Dr. Mercy Kamupira (Clinical Safety Physician), Neliëtte van Niekerk (Medical Writer), Dr. Paulina Kaptur (Scientific Writer) and Karen Bester (Project Manager).

Author Contributions

Conceived and designed the experiments: AN JvdW. Performed the experiments: CL EH IT MM MdV JH IP CA. Analyzed the data: SB JvdW. Wrote the paper: JvdW. Critically reviewed the manuscript: all authors.

References

1. UNAIDS (2010) UNAIDS Report on the Global AIDS Epidemic 2010. Geneva: UNAIDS. Available: http://www.unaids.org/globalreport/global_report.htm. Accessed 2011 July 23.
2. Elias C, Coggins C (1996) Female-controlled methods to prevent sexual transmission of HIV. AIDS 10(Suppl 3): S43–S51.
3. Abdool Karim Q, Abdool Karim SS, Frohlich JA, Grobler AC, Baxter C, et al. (2010) Effectiveness and safety of tenofovir gel, an antiretroviral microbicide, for the prevention of HIV infection in women. Science 329: 1168–1174.
4. van de Wijgert J, Jones H (2006) Commentary: Challenges in microbicide trial design and implementation. Stud Fam Plann 37: 123–129.
5. Braunstein S, van de Wijgert J, Nash D (2009) HIV incidence in sub-Saharan Africa: a review of available data with implications for surveillance and prevention planning. AIDS Reviews 11: 140–156.
6. Parekh BS, Kennedy MS, Dobbs T, Pau CP, Byers R, et al. (2002) Quantitative detection of increasing HIV type 1 antibodies after seroconversion: a simple assay for detecting recent HIV infection and estimating incidence. AIDS Res Hum Retroviruses 18: 295–307.
7. WHO Department of Reproductive Health (2010) Medical Eligibility Criteria for Contraceptive Use, 4th edition. Geneva: WHO. Available: http://www.who.int/reproductivehealth/publications/family_planning/9789241563888/en/Accessed 2011 July 23.
8. National Department of Health, South Africa (2008) First line comprehensive management and control of sexually transmitted infections (STIs): protocol for the management of a person with a sexually transmitted infection according to the Essential Drug List. Pretoria: National Department of Health.
9. McWalter TA, Welte A (2009) Relating recent infection prevalence to incidence with a sub-population of assay non-progressors. J Math Biol 60: 687–710.
10. Formula spreadsheet available at: http://www.sacema.com/page/assay-based-incidence-estimation. Accessed 2011 July 23.
11. Hargrove JW, Humphrey JH, Mutasa K, Parekh BS, McDougal JS, et al. (2008) Improved HIV-1 incidence estimates using the BED capture enzyme immunoassay. AIDS 22: 511–518.
12. Braunstein S, Nash D, Kim A, Ford K, Mwamarangwe L, et al. (2011) Dual testing algorithm of BED-CEIA and AxSYM Avidity Index assays performs best in identifying recent HIV infection in a sample of Rwandan sex workers. PloS ONE 6: e18402.
13. Baldwin JI, Baldwin JD (2000) Heterosexual anal intercourse: an understudied, high-risk sexual behavior. Arch Sex Behav 29: 357–373.
14. UNAIDS/WHO (2011) When and how to use assays for recent infection to estimate HIV incidence at a population level. Geneva: UNAIDS/WHO. Available: http://www.who.int/diagnostics_laboratory/hiv_incidence_may13_final.pdf. Accessed 2011 July 23.
15. Raymond EG, Taylor D, Cates W, Tolley EE, Borasky D, et al. (2007) Pregnancy in effectiveness trials of HIV prevention agents. Sex Transm Dis 34: 1035–1039.

4

Prevalence and Predictors of Major Depression in HIV-Infected Patients on Antiretroviral Therapy in Bamenda, a Semi-Urban Center in Cameroon

Bradley N. Gaynes[1]*, Brian W. Pence[2], Julius Atashili[3], Julie O'Donnell[4], Dmitry Kats[4], Peter M. Ndumbe[5]

1 Department of Psychiatry, University of North Carolina School of Medicine, Chapel Hill, North Carolina, United States of America, 2 Department of Community and Family Medicine, Duke Global Health Institute, and Center for Health Policy and Inequalities Research, Duke University, Durham, North Carolina, United States of America, 3 Department of Public Health and Hygiene, University of Buea, Buea, Cameroon, 4 Department of Epidemiology, Gillings School of Global Public Health, University of North Carolina, Chapel Hill, North Carolina, United States of America, 5 Department of Biomedical Sciences, University of Buea, and Department of Microbiology and Immunology, University of Yaounde I, Buea, Cameroon

Abstract

Recent blue-ribbon panel reports have concluded that HIV treatment programs in less wealthy countries must integrate mental health identification and treatment into normal HIV clinical care and that research on mental health and HIV in these settings should be a high priority. We assessed the epidemiology of depression in HIV patients on antiretroviral therapy in a small urban setting in Cameroon by administering a structured interview for depression to 400 patients consecutively attending the Bamenda Regional Hospital AIDS Treatment Center. One in five participants met lifetime criteria for MDD, and 7% had MDD within the prior year. Only 33% had ever spoken with a health professional about depression, and 12% reported ever having received depression treatment that was helpful or effective. Over 2/3 with past-year MDD had severe or very severe episodes. The number of prior depressive episodes and the number of HIV symptoms were the strongest predictors of past-year MDD. The prevalence of MDD in Cameroon is as high as that of other HIV-associated conditions, such as tuberculosis and Hepatitis B virus, whose care is incorporated into World Health Organization guidelines. The management of depression needs to be incorporated in HIV-care guidelines in Cameroon and other similar settings.

Editor: Geneviève Chêne, Institut National de la Santé et de la Recherche Médicale, France

Funding: This study was supported by grant R34 MH084673 of the National Institute of Mental Health, National Institutes of Health (NIH), Bethesda, MD, USA. BNG receives funding from the NC TRACS Institute, which is supported by grants UL1RR025747, KL2RR025746, and TLRR025745 from the NIH National Center for Research Resources and the National Center for Advancing Translational Sciences, NIH. BWP is an investigator with the Implementation Research Institute (IRI), at the George Warren Brown School of Social Work, Washington University in St. Louis, MO, through an award from the National Institute of Mental Health (R25 MH080916-01A2) and the Department of Veterans Affairs, Health Services Research & Development Service, Quality Enhancement Research Initiative (QUERI). This publication was made possible with help from the Duke University Center for AIDS Research (CFAR), an NIH-funded program (2P30 AI064518). The content is solely the responsibility of the authors and does not necessarily represent the official views of the NIMH or the NIH. The funders had no role in study design, data collection and analysis, decision to publish, or preparation of the manuscript.

* E-mail: bradley_gaynes@med.unc.edu

Introduction

More than 25 million people have died from HIV/AIDS, most of them in sub-Saharan Africa (SSA) where HIV/AIDS is the leading cause of mortality. [1] In 2010, SSA accounted for approximately two-thirds of global cases. [1] Despite recent global initiatives to improve the availability of and access to antiretroviral therapy (ART) in SSA, the continued high adult mortality due to HIV/AIDS in this region results in significant social and economic consequences.

Cameroon, located in central Africa, has an estimated 550,000 persons living with HIV and an HIV prevalence rate of 5.5%. [2] In a number of ways, Cameroon's experience with HIV is representative of many SSA countries. The HIV prevalence in Cameroon approximates the mean HIV prevalence in SSA (6.8%). [2] Further, as with the majority of low- and middle-income countries, and the majority of SSA nations, 20–39% percent of those eligible for ART receives the medications. [1]

Cameroon is also one of 22 priority countries identified in the World Health Organization's "Global Plan" as a key target because of the high estimated numbers of pregnant women living with HIV. [3]

Mental disorders, especially depression, are common in HIV-infected persons globally. The HIV/AIDS Costs and Services Utilization Study (HCSUS) study, a U.S. national study of HIV-infected individuals, found that nearly half (48%) of participants had a probable mental disorder. [4] The major mood and anxiety disorders are five to ten times more prevalent in HIV-positive individuals than in the general U.S. population, [5] with a similar increased risk found in SSA settings. [6] The most common psychiatric diagnoses among HIV-positive individuals are mood and anxiety disorders, particularly MDD and other depressive disorders. [5,6,7,8,9,10] Similar data are limited for persons with HIV in SSA generally and, to the best of our knowledge, are lacking for Cameroon.

Depression is associated with worse HIV-related outcomes. In individuals with HIV/AIDS, mental illness (MI) in general and depression in particular, have been consistently associated with negative HIV-related behaviors, particularly poor ART adherence, a critical consideration in HIV care where ART plays a central role in suppressing virus and protecting the immune system. [11,12,13,14,15,16,17] A recent meta-analysis of 95 studies encompassing 35,029 participants confirmed the consistent association of depression with poor ART adherence low-resource and high-resource settings. [18] Additionally, depression predicts a higher likelihood of engaging in unsafe needle-sharing and sexual behaviors that risk secondary transmission of HIV infection. [19,20] Depression has also been associated with poorer physical health, [21] decreased quality of life, [22] and AIDS-related mortality. [23] Thus, identifying those at risk of a depressive illness can highlight patients especially in need of active follow-up.

Recent prominent blue-ribbon panel reports have concluded that HIV treatment programs in less wealthy countries must integrate mental health identification and treatment into normal HIV clinical care and that research on mental health and HIV should be a high priority, especially in less wealthy countries. [24] Cameroon is one such country, and no prior studies of depression prevalence in HIV patients in Cameroon exist.

Accordingly, we sought:

- To determine the prevalence of clinically relevant depressive illness in HIV patients in a small urban setting in Cameroon, and

- To describe the severity of MDD in the patient population and to identify sociodemographic and clinical variables associated with a greater risk of depressive illness.

Methods

Ethical Approvals

This research was approved by the Institutional Review Boards of the University of North Carolina, Duke University, and the Cameroon National Ethics Committee.

Study Design/Population

Bamenda, a city in northwestern Cameroon and capital of the North West Province, has a population of 269,530, [25] making it the country's third most populated center. We conducted a cross-sectional study of HIV-infected patients on antiretroviral therapy (ART) attending the Bamenda Regional Hospital AIDS Treatment Center (BRHATC). This health facility is dedicated to the care of HIV-infected patients, the vast majority of whom are on ART. The center provides care to over 1,000 patients annually. Between May 2010 and October 2010, attendees of the BRHATC were informed of the study through thrice-weekly health education sessions. Patients were eligible if they were HIV-infected, on ART, were attending the BRHATC for any service (including counseling, clinical follow-up or drug refill), spoke English, and were willing to provide informed consent. Although more than 30 local languages exist, English is the language used for regular clinical care in the BRHATC and throughout the Northwest Region of Cameroon; more than 95% of clinic attendees can communicate effectively in English. Each participant could be eligible only once during the study period.

Our sampling goal was to recruit a study sample representative of HIV-infected patients receiving antiretroviral therapy at BRHATC. In the absence of a daily patient register to provide a sampling frame, study staff approached each patient consecu-

tively as the patients passed through a central point in the registration process (weight measurement) until a patient indicated willingness to participate in the study. The recruiting staff member then obtained written informed consent from the interested patient and completed the first part of data collection. The patient would then complete the second part of data collection with a second staff member while the recruiting staff member resumed approaching patients consecutively at registration.

Instruments

Lifetime and recent Major Depressive Disorder (MDD) were assessed using the World Health Organization's Composite International Diagnostic Instrument (CIDI), a lay-administered diagnostic instrument whose performance has been validated widely in multiple international settings, [26,27] including HIV settings. [6] The CIDI is a comprehensive, fully structured interview designed to be used by trained lay interviewers for the assessment of mental disorders in epidemiological and cross-cultural studies as well as for clinical and research purposes. We used the World Mental Health Survey Initiative Version of the CIDI (WMH-CIDI), which allows the assessment of mental disorders according to the definitions and criteria of ICD-10 and DSM-IV. [28,29] The diagnostic section of the interview expands upon earlier versions of the CIDI by adding detailed questions about disorder severity, impairment, service use, and treatment, and has improved generalizability with increased involvement of less wealthy countries. [29,30] This version has been successfully used in Sub-Saharan Africa (Nigeria). [29,30] We administered the Screening and Depression modules of the WMH-CIDI. Interviews were conducted in person by a health care professional who received formal CIDI training from a WHO-certified trainer.

Measures

Following standard CIDI scoring methodology, participants were assigned a diagnosis of a *lifetime episode of* MDD if they described ever experiencing a period meeting the following criteria: a period lasting at least two weeks characterized by at least 5 out of 9 core depressive symptoms, with at least one symptom being either depressed mood or anhedonia, and representing a change from previous functioning; the symptoms caused clinically significant distress or impairment in social, occupational, or other important areas of functioning; the symptoms were not better explained by substance use or a general medical condition; and the symptoms were not better explained by bereavement, or if secondary to bereavement, the episode either lasted more than two months or was characterized by at least one of the following: marked functional impairment, morbid preoccupation with worthlessness, suicidal ideation, psychotic symptoms, or psychomotor retardation.

On the CIDI, participants reporting any lifetime episode of MDD were asked if they had experienced any similar episodes in the past year, past 6 months, and past month. Participants reporting an episode in the past year or more recently completed a standard depressive severity rating scale called the Quick Inventory of Depressive Symptoms (QIDS) [31] that is embedded within the CIDI. The QIDS total score can range from 0–27 and has standard categories that correspond to very severe (21–27), severe (16–20), moderate (11–15), mild (6–10), and no (0–5) depressive symptoms. Participants were classified as having a diagnosis of a MDD in the past year, past 6 months, and past month if they endorsed a depressive episode in those time frames and received a score of 11 or above on the QIDS.

Participants additionally provided information on socio-demographics and on whether in the past 6 months they had experienced each of 13 symptoms commonly associated with HIV infection: [4] new or persistent headaches, fevers, oral pain, white patches in the mouth, rashes, nausea, trouble with eyes, sinus infection, numbness in the hands or feet, persistent cough, diarrhea, weight loss, or (for women only) abnormal vaginal discharge.

Statistical Analysis

Participant characteristics, prevalence of depression, and characteristics of depressive episodes are described with proportions or medians and interquartile ranges (IQR). We describe continuous variables with medians and interquartile ranges due to the skewed distributions of some of these variables. Logistic regression was used to examine potential predictors of a diagnosis of depression in the past 6 months and in the past year. Odds ratios (OR) from bivariable analyses are used to describe the association of each predictor variable with depression. Age (divided by 10) and number of reported HIV symptoms were each modeled as simple linear terms after confirmation of the appropriateness of this assumption. Thus the OR for age represents the predicted increase in the odds of depression associated with a 10-year increase in age, and the OR for HIV symptoms represents the predicted increase in the odds of depression associated with each additional HIV symptom reported. For multivariable logistic regression analyses, the number of variables to be included in each of the models was decided *a priori* based on prevalence of the outcome; variables were selected for inclusion based on prior knowledge of relationship to the outcome and on relevance to the study question. All statistical analyses were carried out using Stata statistical software (version 11.1; STATA Corp, College Station, Texas).

Results

General Characteristics of Study Population

Of the 400 HIV-infected participants enrolled in the study, nearly ¾ were female and most were between 34 and 47 years of age (median 41 years) (Table 1). Most had previously been married (44%) or were currently married or cohabitating (34%). The majority (61%) had no more than a primary level of education (≤6 years). Participants reported a median of 5 (IQR: 3–6) physical symptoms commonly associated with HIV infection.

Prevalence of MDD and Clinical Features

One in five participants met lifetime criteria for major depressive disorder (Table 2). The prevalence of MDD was 7% in the prior year, 5% in the prior 6 months, and 3% in the prior month.

For those who had experienced MDD in their lifetime, the median age at first onset of MDD was 34 years, and the median number of lifetime episodes was 2. The median length of the 1st episode was 122 days (approximately 4 months). Only 1/3 had ever spoken with a physician or other health professional about depression, and 1/8 (12%) reported ever having received treatment that was helpful or effective for their depression.

Characterizing the Most Recent Depressive Episode

Among those with MDD in the past year, the severity of the current episode (among those currently experiencing a major depressive episode) or the worst episode in the past year was pronounced, as reflected by a mean score of 16 on the QIDS instrument. As measured by the QIDS, 2/3 of patients depressed within the past year had either a severe (59%) or very severe (7%) episode (Figure 1).

Table 1. Characteristics of the overall study population (N [%] or median [IQR]).

	Study population, n = 400	
	N/median	%/IQR
Sex		
Male	103	26
Female	297	74
Age	41	34–47
Religion		
Christian	394	99
Other	5	1
Marital Status		
Married/cohabitating	137	34
Previously married	178	44
Never married	85	21
Education*		
Primary	245	61
Greater than primary	155	39
Daily expenditures**	1	1–3
Village of residence		
Urban	244	61
Rural	156	39
Competency in English***		
Excellent	158	40
Fair	242	60
HIV symptom score (possible range: 0–13)	5	3–6

*Primary = 6 years or fewer; greater than primary = more than 6 years.
**In US dollars, approximation based on reported weekly expenditures in FCFC.
***By interviewer assessment.

Table 2. Prevalence of depression diagnoses (N, % or median, IQR).

	Study population, n = 400	
	N/median	%/IQR
Depression Diagnosis		
Past Month	11	3
Past 6 Months	20	5
Past Year	29	7
Lifetime	84	21
Number of lifetime episodes	2	1–3
Lifetime Diagnosis, n = 84		
Age at 1st onset, years	34	25–40
Length of 1st episode, days	122	30–1095
Ever talk to MD/other professional	28	33
Ever receive effective depression treatment	10	12
Past-year Diagnosis, n = 29		
QIDS score	16	14–18

QIDS CATEGORY for Participants with Past-Year Depression

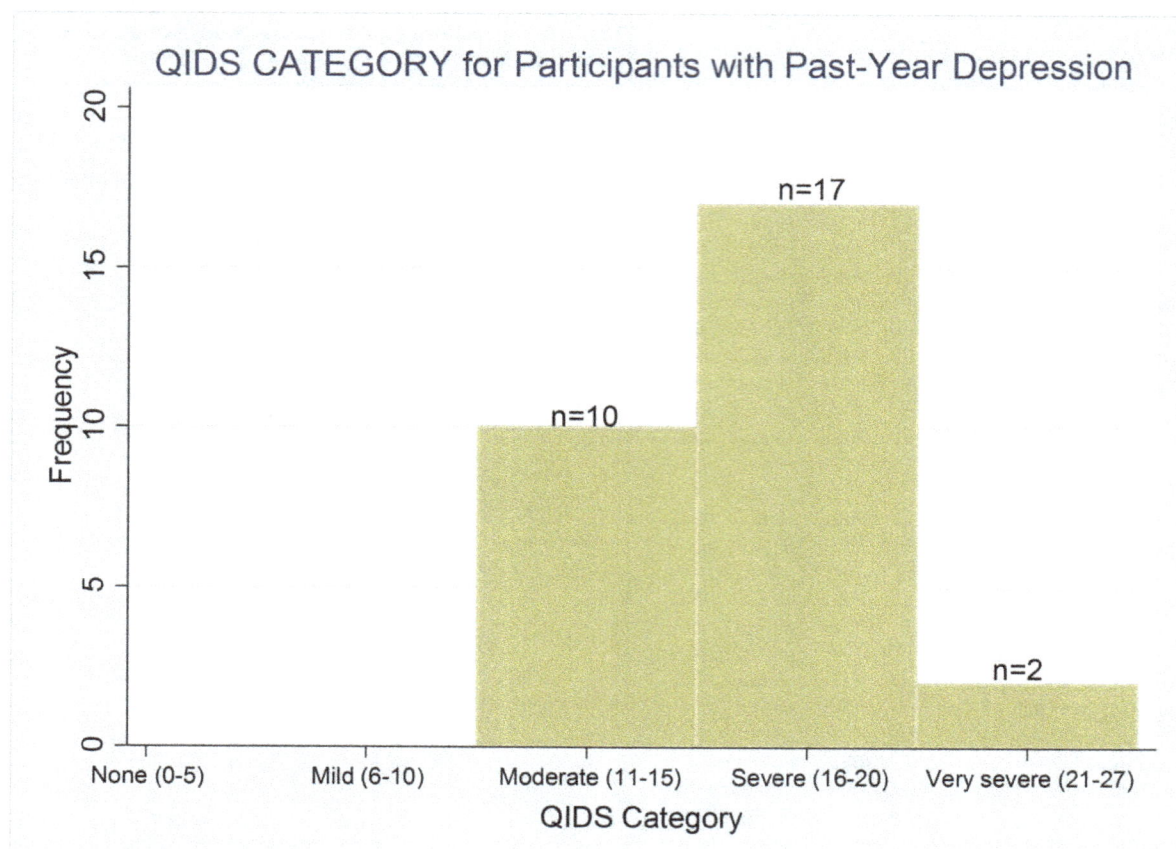

Figure 1. Categorized distribution of scores on the Quick Inventory of Depressive Symptomatology (QIDS) tool among participants with past-year depression.

We further delineated the specific depressive symptoms endorsed by depressed HIV-infected patients on the QIDS, as indicated by endorsing a symptom as present (Table 3). Among those with an episode in the past year, depressed mood and anhedonia were extremely common and nearly always presented together (97% of the sample reported each alone, and 100% had at least one of the two.) All depressed patients endorsed some type of insomnia (most commonly middle insomnia) and decreased attention/concentration. Nearly all endorsed feeling worthless or guilty and having a decreased level of energy (97% for each). Psychomotor retardation, weight change (nearly always weight loss), and appetite change (nearly always decreased appetite) were similarly frequently reported (93%, 93%, and 90% respectively). Restlessness and too much sleep were less frequently reported (73% and 59%, respectively). Thoughts of death or suicide were frequently endorsed by depressed HIV patients (86%).

For those patients who endorsed suicidal ideation, most reported having passive thoughts without active thoughts of harming themselves (Table 4). The great majority of those endorsing suicidal ideation reported thoughts that life was not worth living but had no thoughts of suicide, consistent with passive suicidal ideation (80%); 16% reported thoughts of suicide or death several times per week; and 4% endorsed plans or having recently made an attempt.

Correlates of Depression Diagnosis–bivariable Analysis

With bivariable analysis, we assessed whether common predictors were correlated with depressive diagnoses within the past year in this sample (Table 5). Females tended to be less likely than males to have depression, although this finding was not statistically significant. Older patients tended to be less likely to have MDD than younger ones. Those with education beyond the primary level tended to be twice as likely to have MDD as those with only primary education.

Two variables stood out as significant predictors of MDD within the past year. First, the number of HIV symptoms was positively associated with the odds of having MDD within the past year. Each additional HIV symptom was associated with approximately a 20% increased odds of MDD. Second, prior history of MDD was the strongest risk factor for MDD within the past year. For those with a history of one episode of MDD more than a year ago, the likelihood of MDD within the past year increased nearly seven-fold compared to those without such a history, while a prior history of two or more episodes of MDD increased the likelihood of MDD within the past year by more than twelve-fold.

Correlates of Depression Diagnosis–multivariable Analysis

Considering all these variables together in a multivariable analysis, findings remained consistent, with the number of prior depressive episodes and the number of HIV symptoms having significant associations with past-year MDD similar in magnitude

Table 3. Depressive symptoms endorsed.

	Current episode/worst episode in last year (n = 29)	
	N	%
Feeling sad	28	97
Anhedonia	28	97
Any insomnia	29	100
Initial insomnia	26	90
Middle insomnia	29	100
Terminal insomnia	24	83
Decreased attention/concentration	29	100
Feeling worthless/guilty	28	97
Decreased level of energy	28	97
Psychomotor retardation	27	93
Weight changes	27	93
Weight gain	2	7
Weight loss	25	86
Appetite changes	27	90
Decreased appetite	26	90
Increased appetite	0	0
Thoughts of death/suicide	25	86
Restlessness	21	72
Too much sleep	17	59

to those found in bivariable analyses (Table 6). Female patients and patients living in rural areas tended to be less likely to have MDD within the preceding year.

Discussion

In this sample of HIV-infected patients receiving antiretroviral therapy and attending a regional AIDS treatment center in Cameroon, 3% met criteria for a major depressive episode within the past month, 5% had an episode within the past 6 months, 7% had an episode in the past year, and 21% met criteria for major depressive disorder at some point in their life. These prevalence values are consistent with prior reports on the frequency of MDD in African HIV-infected populations receiving antiretroviral therapy as determined by structured diagnostic interviews in which functional impairment is part of the diagnosis, such as the CIDI. Maj et al. reported that past month prevalence of MDD in Nairobi, Kenya was 3.0% and 5.5% in asymptomatic and symptomatic HIV-infected patients, respectively; rates in Kinshasa, Democratic Republic of the Congo, were 0 and 4.4%,

respectively. [6] Current MDD was present in 2.7% of HIV-infected patients in a rural setting in Muleza, Tanzania. [32]

A small number of more recent studies have used as the diagnostic standard either the PRIME-MD mood module [33] or Mini International Neuropsychiatric Interview, [34,35,36,37,38] tools which do not consider functional impairment in diagnosing MDD. Accordingly, these studies may employ a more sensitive but less specific instrument to detect depression. These studies have reported a greater range of prevalence and higher rates of MDD, ranging from 8–34% in samples of HIV-infected individuals from Botswana, Nigeria, South Africa, and Uganda. [33,34,35,36,37,38] In any case, our findings, coupled with those already reported in the literature, identify depression as an illness in Cameroon with a prevalence as high as that of other HIV-associated conditions, such as tuberculosis (0.041%) [39] and Hepatitis B virus (8.3%), [40] which have care recommendations incorporated into World Health Organization guidelines. [41]

Further, the lifetime MDD prevalence of 21% in this sample was 2–3 times higher than what has been reported in urban sub-

Table 4. Description of Suicidal Ideation.

	Depression Diagnosis in Past Year with Suicidal Ideation (n = 25)	
	N	%
Life empty/not worth living	20	80
Thoughts of suicide/death several times/week	4	16
Thoughts of suicide/death several times/day w/plans or attempt	1	4

Table 5. Correlates of depression diagnosis – bivariable analysis.

	Depression Diagnosis in Past Year	
	OR	95% CI
Gender		
Male	REF	
Female	0.63	0.28, 1.41
Age*	0.82	0.50, 1.23
Marital Status		
Married/cohabiting	REF	
Previously married	1.12	0.46, 2.70
Never married	1.27	0.45, 3.54
Education		
Primary	REF	
Greater than primary	2.04	0.95, 4.36
Number of prior lifetime depressive episodes		
0	REF	
1	6.63	2.13, 20.59
2+	12.14	4.51, 32.67
HIV Symptoms**	1.19	1.05, 1.36
Village of residence		
Urban	REF	
Rural	0.81	0.37, 1.80

*Estimates for a 10-year increase in age.
**For each additional symptom.

Table 6. Correlates of depression diagnosis – multivariable analysis.

	Depression Diagnosis in Past Year	
	OR	95% CI
Gender		
Male	REF	
Female	0.61	0.23, 1.64
Age*	1.03	0.61, 1.73
Marital Status		
Married/cohabiting	REF	
Previously married	1.57	0.53, 4.62
Never married	1.24	0.36, 4.32
Education		
Primary	REF	
Greater than primary	1.03	0.38, 2.81
Number of prior lifetime depressive episodes		
0	REF	
1	5.42	1.65, 17.75
2+	11.38	4.04, 32.04
HIV Symptoms**	1.22	1.05, 1.42
Village of residence		
Urban	REF	
Rural	0.72	0.29, 1.81

*Estimates for a 10-year increase in age.
**For each additional symptom.

Saharan African settings, suggesting that the burden of depression in HIV patients may be greater than expected based on studies in major African cities. Indeed, in Nairobi, Kenya, 6.1% of asymptomatic patients and 9.7% of symptomatic patients had a lifetime history of MDD, and in Kinshasa (Democratic Republic of Congo), 3.8% and 7.3%, respectively, had a lifetime history of MDD. [6]

Identification and successful management of MDD by a health care professional, a key objective of blue-ribbon panel reports and the World Health Organization, [24] was uncommon. Discussion of depression with clinicians was low, with only 1/3 reporting having spoken with a health professional about the depression, and only 1/8 reported every receiving helpful or effective depression treatment.

Key variables discriminating between HIV-infected patients with and without depression were the number of prior lifetime episodes and the number of physical symptoms potentially related to HIV. In adjusted analyses, having one prior episode of MDD increased the risk of having a recent MDD episode by over five-fold, while having two or more prior episodes increased the risk of recent MDD by over eleven-fold. We found no other reports on how prior history of MDD in HIV patients affected the risk of a recent MDD. For clinicians, then, a key clinical piece of information in evaluating current depression is whether a patient has a history of depressive episodes.

Similarly, having a greater number of HIV symptoms increased the odds of having MDD within the past year. This finding is consistent with reports of prior studies suggesting an association between depression and severity of HIV illness. [42,43]

Depressive symptomatology in this population mirrored presentations of depression in other settings, and was notable for infrequent reports of weight gain or increased appetite. Middle insomnia, experienced by all depressed HIV patients in this sample, is a symptom that HIV clinicians might be able to address quickly and effectively with amitriptyline, the most commonly used and widely available antidepressant in Cameroon.

Suicidal ideation was common in depressed HIV patients (86%), but it was primarily passive, described as thoughts that life was not worth living rather than having active thoughts of self-harm. This high frequency of suicidal ideation in general with a low frequency of specifically active suicidal ideation is consistent with prior studies of depression in medical settings. [44]

Finally, the majority of individuals with MDD experienced severe rather than moderate depressive symptoms and were substantially impaired. Indeed, 2/3 met criteria for being severely or very severely depressed, which is a greater proportion than was reported in a rural sample in Tanzania (2/3 moderately depressed, 1/3 severely depressed). [32]

Our findings are limited by a number of issues. First, while consistent with prior reports, our prevalence of current depression was still smaller than we expected, limiting our ability to comprehensively assess variables predictive of major depressive disorder. We used a well validated and culturally translated instrument, and depression diagnoses were carefully reviewed by a psychiatrist, so the measurement of depression is likely to have high construct validity. The large majority of cases of depression were severe or very severe, so the predictors identified are likely to be good predictors of severe, clinically relevant depressive disorders with substantial impairment. Second, following our diagnostic reference standard, the CIDI, we collected a full report on depressive symptoms only on patients with MDD, so we could not identify depressive symptoms that distinguish between clinically depressed HIV patients and HIV patients with mild depressive symptoms who are not clinically depressed. Such information would be helpful to HIV clinicians to focus on key depressive symptoms that might differentiate those at higher risk of clinical depression. Third, these data are from a single site in a small urban center in Cameroon, which may limit their generalizability. However, findings here were generally consistent with what has been reported in other sub-Saharan Africa sites. Fourth, in the assessment of predictors of MDD, there may be some uncontrolled confounding because of the small number of variables that could be included in the multivariate analysis. Finally, most of the variables and measurements were self-reported, so their accuracy is dependent on the veracity of the participants.

Conclusions

This study of HIV-positive outpatients attending a hospital in a small urban center in Bamenda, Cameroon, found that 7% had depression at some point within the past year, most of which was severe or very severe. Identification and successful management of MDD by a health care professional was infrequent. Suicidal ideation was common, although usually passive. Important predictors of a major depressive episode in the past year were prior history of depression and a greater number of HIV symptoms. Future research can look at interventions to help HIV clinicians better identify and manage this common and complicating comorbidity. The management of depression (including screening and appropriate care) needs to be incorporated in HIV-care guidelines in Cameroon and other similar settings, as its prevalence is as high as those of other HIV-associated conditions such as tuberculosis and hepatitis B infection whose management is included in such guidelines.

Acknowledgments

We acknowledge with great appreciation the participation of our HIV clinicians, Dr. Gladys Tayong, Dr. Charles Kefie, and Dr. Awasum Charles; our psychiatric nurse, Mr. Fru Johnson; our Project Coordinators, Seema Parkash and Andrew Goodall; and our research assistants, Mrs. Shantal Asangi, Mr. Joseph Nyingcho, and Mrs. Irene Numfor.

Author Contributions

Conceived and designed the experiments: BNG BWP JA PN. Performed the experiments: BNG BWP JA. Analyzed the data: BNG BWP JA JKO DK. Wrote the paper: BNG BWP JA JKO DK PN.

References

1. UN AIDS (2011) UNAIDS World AIDS Day Report, 2011. Joint United Nations Programme on HIV/AIDS (UNAIDS). Available: http://www.unaids.org/en/media/unaids/contentassets/documents/unaidspublication/2011/JC2216_WorldAIDSday_report_2011_en.pdf. Accessed 2012 Mar 21.
2. UN AIDS (2009) AIDS epidemic update Joint United Nations Programme on HIV/AIDS (UNAIDS) and World Health Organization (WHO). Available: http://www.unaids.org/en/media/unaids/contentassets/dataimport/pub/report/2009/jc1700_epi_update_2009_en.pdf. Accessed 2012 Mar 21.
3. UN AIDS (2011) Global Plan towards The Elimination Of New HIV Infections among Children by 2015 and Keeping Their Mothers Alive 2011–2015. Joint United Nations Programme on HIV/AIDS (UNAIDS). Available: http://www.unaids.org/en/media/unaids/contentassets/documents/unaidspublication/2011/20110609_JC2137_Global-Plan-Elimination-HIV-Children_en.pdf. Accessed 2012 Mar 21.
4. Bing EG, Burnam MA, Longshore D, Fleishman JA, Sherbourne CD, et al. (2001) Psychiatric disorders and drug use among human immunodeficiency virus-infected adults in the United States. Arch Gen Psychiatry 58: 721–728.
5. Kessler R, McGonagle K, Zhao S, Nelson C, Hughes M, et al. (1994) Lifetime and 12-month prevalence of DSM-III-R psychiatric disorders in the United States: results from the National Comorbidity Survey. Arch Gen Psychiatry 51: 8–19.
6. Maj M, Janssen R, Starace F, Zaudig M, Satz P, et al. (1994) WHO Neuropsychiatric AIDS study, cross-sectional phase I. Study design and psychiatric findings. Arch Gen Psychiatry 51: 39–49. doi: 10.1001/archpsyc.51.1.39.
7. Kelly B, Raphael B, Judd F, Perdices M, Kernutt G, et al. (1998) Psychiatric disorder in HIV infection. Aust N Z J Psychiatry 32: 441–453.
8. Kilbourne AM, Justice AC, Rabeneck L, Rodriguez-Barradas M, Weissman S (2001) General medical and psychiatric comorbidity among HIV-infected veterans in the post-HAART era. Journal of Clinical Epidemiology 54: S22–S28.
9. Lyketsos CG, Hanson A, Fishman M, McHugh PR, Treisman GJ (1994) Screening for psychiatric morbidity in a medical outpatient clinic for HIV infection: the need for a psychiatric presence. Int J Psychiatry Med 24: 103–113.
10. Pence BW, Miller WC, Whetten K, Eron JJ, Gaynes BN (2006) Prevalence of DSM-IV-defined mood, anxiety, and substance use disorders in an HIV clinic in the Southeastern United States. J Acquir Immune Defic Syndr 42: 298–306.
11. Arnsten JH, Demas PA, Grant RW, Gourevitch MN, Farzadegan H, et al. (2002) Impact of active drug use on antiretroviral therapy adherence and viral suppression in HIV-infected drug users. J Gen Intern Med 17: 377–381.
12. Bartlett JA (2002) Addressing the challenges of adherence. J Acquir Immune Defic Syndr 29 Suppl 1: S2–10.
13. Ferrando SJ, Wapenyi K (2002) Psychopharmacological Treatment of Patients with HIV and AIDS. Psychiatric Quarterly 73: 33–49.
14. Gordillo V, del Amo J, Soriano V, Gonzalez-Lahoz J (1999) Sociodemographic and psychological variables influencing adherence to antiretroviral therapy. Aids 13: 1763–1769.
15. Laurence J, editor (2004) Medication adherence in HIV/AIDS. Larchmont, NY: Mary Ann Liebert, Inc.
16. Singh N, Squier C, Sivek C, Wagener M, Nguyen MH, et al. (1996) Determinants of compliance with antiretroviral therapy in patients with human immunodeficiency virus: prospective assessment with implications for enhancing compliance. AIDS Care 8: 261–269.
17. Spire B, Duran S, Souville M, Leport C, Raffi F, et al. (2002) Adherence to highly active antiretroviral therapies (HAART) in HIV-infected patients: from a predictive to a dynamic approach. Soc Sci Med 54: 1481–1496.
18. Gonzalez JS, Batchelder AW, Psaros C, Safren SA (2011) Depression and HIV/AIDS treatment nonadherence: a review and meta-analysis. J Acquir Immune Defic Syndr 58: 181–187.
19. Amirkhanian YA, Kelly JA, McAuliffe TL (2003) Psychosocial needs, mental health, and HIV transmission risk behavior among people living with HIV/AIDS in St Petersburg, Russia. Aids 17: 2367–2374.
20. Kelly JA, Murphy DA, Bahr GR, Koob JJ, Morgan MG, et al. (1993) Factors associated with severity of depression and high-risk sexual behavior among persons diagnosed with human immunodeficiency virus (HIV) infection. Health Psychol 12: 215–219.
21. Sikkema KJ, Watt MH, Meade CS, Ranby KW, Kalichman SC, et al. (2011) Mental health and HIV sexual risk behavior among patrons of alcohol serving venues in Cape Town, South Africa. J Acquir Immune Defic Syndr 57: 230–237.
22. Sherbourne CD, Hays RD, Fleishman JA, Vitiello B, Magruder KM, et al. (2000) Impact of Psychiatric Conditions on Health-Related Quality of Life in Persons With HIV Infection. Am J Psychiatry 157: 248–254.
23. Ickovics JR, Hamburger ME, Vlahov D, Schoenbaum EE, Schuman P, et al. (2001) Mortality, CD4 Cell Count Decline, and Depressive Symptoms Among HIV-Seropositive Women: Longitudinal Analysis From the HIV Epidemiology Research Study. JAMA 285: 1466–1474.
24. Freeman M, Patel V, Collins PY, Bertolote J (2005) Integrating mental health in global initiatives for HIV/AIDS. Br J Psychiatry 187: 1–3.
25. National Institute of Statistics of Cameroon (2010) 2005 Census. Yaounde: National Institute of Statistics of Cameroon. Available: http://www.statistics-cameroon.org/. Accessed 2012 Mar 30.
26. Kaaya SF, Fawzi MC, Mbwambo JK, Lee B, Msamanga GI, et al. (2002) Validity of the Hopkins Symptom Checklist-25 amongst HIV-positive pregnant women in Tanzania. Acta Psychiatr Scand 106: 9–19.
27. Robins LN, Wing J, Wittchen HU, Helzer JE, Babor TF, et al. (1988) The Composite International Diagnostic Interview. An epidemiologic Instrument suitable for use in conjunction with different diagnostic systems and in different cultures. Archives of General Psychiatry 45: 1069–1077.
28. Kessler RC, Abelson J, Demler O, Escobar JI, Gibbon M, et al. (2004) Clinical calibration of DSM-IV diagnoses in the World Mental Health (WMH) version of the World Health Organization (WHO) Composite International Diagnostic Interview (WMH-CIDI). International Journal of Methods in Psychiatric Research 13: 122–139.
29. Kessler RC, Ustun TB (2004) The World Mental Health (WMH) Survey Initiative Version of the World Health Organization (WHO) Composite International Diagnostic Interview (CIDI). International Journal of Methods in Psychiatric Research 13: 93–121.

30. Demyttenaere K, Bruffaerts R, Posada-Villa J, Gasquet I, Kovess V, et al. (2004) Prevalence, Severity, and Unmet Need for Treatment of Mental Disorders in the World Health Organization World Mental Health Surveys. JAMA 291: 2581–2590.

31. Rush AJ, Trivedi MH, Ibrahim HM, Carmody TJ, Arnow B, et al. (2003) The 16-Item quick inventory of depressive symptomatology (QIDS), clinician rating (QIDS-C), and self-report (QIDS-SR): a psychometric evaluation in patients with chronic major depression. Biol Psychiatry 54: 573–583.

32. Marwick KF, Kaaya SF (2010) Prevalence of depression and anxiety disorders in HIV-positive outpatients in rural Tanzania. AIDS Care 22: 415–419.

33. Lawler K, Mosepele M, Seloilwe E, Ratcliffe S, Steele K, et al. (2010) Depression among HIV-positive individuals in Botswana: a behavioral surveillance. AIDS Behav 15: 204–208.

34. Adewuya AO, Afolabi MO, Ola BA, et al (2008) Relationship between depression and quality of life in persons with HIV infection in Nigeria. Int J Psychiatry Med 38: 43–51.

35. Kinyanda E, Hoskins S, Nakku J, Nawaz S, Patel V (2011) Prevalence and risk factors of major depressive disorder in HIV/AIDS as seen in semi-urban Entebbe district, Uganda. BMC Psychiatry 11: 205.

36. Myer L, Smit J, Roux LL, Parker S, Stein DJ, et al. (2008) Common mental disorders among HIV-infected individuals in South Africa: prevalence, predictors, and validation of brief psychiatric rating scales. AIDS patient care and STDs 22: 147–158.

37. Olley BO, Gxamza F, Seedat S, Theron H, Taljaard J, et al. (2003) Psychopathology and coping in recently diagnosed HIV/AIDS patients–the role of gender. S Afr Med J 93: 928–931.

38. Spies G, Kader K, Kidd M, et al (2009) Validity of the K-10 in detecting DSM-IV-defined depression and anxiety disorders among HIV-infected individuals. AIDS Care 21: 1163–1168.

39. Kaiser Family Foundation (2010) U.S. Global Health Policy: an online gateway for the latest data and information on the U.S. role in global health. The Henry J. Kaiser Family Foundation (kff.org).Available: http://www.globalhealthfacts.org/data/country/profile.aspx?loc = 52&cat = 2&sn = 1. Accessed 2012 Mar 21.

40. Laurent C, Bourgeois A, Mpoudi-Ngole E, Kouanfack C, Ciaffi L, et al. (2009) High rates of active hepatitis B and C co-infections in HIV-1 infected Cameroonian adults initiating antiretroviral therapy. HIV Med 11: 85–89.

41. World Health Organization 2010 (2010) Antiretroviral therapy for HIV infection in adults and adolescents: recommendations for a public health approach, 2010 revision: World Health Organization. Available: http://www.who.int/hiv/pub/arv/adult2010/en/index.html. Accessed 2012 Mar 21.

42. Adewuya AO, Afolabi MO, Ola BA, Ogundele OA, Ajibare AO, et al. (2007) Psychiatric disorders among the HIV-positive population in Nigeria: a control study. J Psychosom Res 63: 203–206.

43. Freeman M, Nkomo, Kafaar Z, Kelly K (2007) Factors associated with prevalence of mental disorder in people living with HIV/AIDS in South Africa. AIDS Care: Psychological and Socio-medical Aspects of AIDS/HIV 19: 1201–1209.

44. Gaynes BN, Rush AJ, Trivedi M, Wisniewski SR, Balasubramani GK, et al. (2005) A direct comparison of presenting characteristics of depressed outpatients from primary vs. specialty care settings: preliminary findings from the STAR*D clinical trial. Gen Hosp Psychiatry 27: 87–96.

5

Cost Effectiveness of Screening Strategies for Early Identification of HIV and HCV Infection in Injection Drug Users

Lauren E. Cipriano[1]*, **Gregory S. Zaric**[2], **Mark Holodniy**[3,4,5], **Eran Bendavid**[4,5,6,7], **Douglas K. Owens**[3,4,7], **Margaret L. Brandeau**[1]

1 Department of Management Science and Engineering, Stanford University, Stanford, California, United States of America, 2 Richard Ivey School of Business, University of Western Ontario, London, Ontario, Canada, 3 Veterans Affairs Palo Alto Health Care System, Palo Alto, California, United States of America, 4 Department of Medicine, Stanford University, Stanford, California, United States of America, 5 Division of Infectious Diseases & Geographic Medicine, Stanford University, Stanford, California, United States of America, 6 Division of General Medicine Disciplines, Stanford University, Stanford, California, United States of America, 7 Center for Health Policy and Center for Primary Care and Outcomes Research, Department of Medicine, Stanford University, Stanford, California, United States of America

Abstract

Objective: To estimate the cost, effectiveness, and cost effectiveness of HIV and HCV screening of injection drug users (IDUs) in opioid replacement therapy (ORT).

Design: Dynamic compartmental model of HIV and HCV in a population of IDUs and non-IDUs for a representative U.S. urban center with 2.5 million adults (age 15–59).

Methods: We considered strategies of screening individuals in ORT for HIV, HCV, or both infections by antibody or antibody and viral RNA testing. We evaluated one-time and repeat screening at intervals from annually to once every 3 months. We calculated the number of HIV and HCV infections, quality-adjusted life years (QALYs), costs, and incremental cost-effectiveness ratios (ICERs).

Results: Adding HIV and HCV viral RNA testing to antibody testing averts 14.8–30.3 HIV and 3.7–7.7 HCV infections in a screened population of 26,100 IDUs entering ORT over 20 years, depending on screening frequency. Screening for HIV antibodies every 6 months costs $30,700/QALY gained. Screening for HIV antibodies and viral RNA every 6 months has an ICER of $65,900/QALY gained. Strategies including HCV testing have ICERs exceeding $100,000/QALY gained unless awareness of HCV-infection status results in a substantial reduction in needle-sharing behavior.

Discussion: Although annual screening for antibodies to HIV and HCV is modestly cost effective compared to no screening, more frequent screening for HIV provides additional benefit at less cost. Screening individuals in ORT every 3–6 months for HIV infection using both antibody and viral RNA technologies and initiating ART for acute HIV infection appears cost effective.

Editor: Jason Blackard, University of Cincinnati College of Medicine, United States of America

Funding: This work was supported by grant R01-DA15612 from the National Institute on Drug Abuse. LEC is supported by a doctoral fellowship from the Social Science and Humanities Research Council of Canada (http://www.sshrc-crsh.gc.ca) and the Seth Bonder Scholarship for Applied Operations Research in Health Services (http://www.informs.org). DKO and MH are supported by the Department of Veterans Affairs. The funders had no role in study design, data collection and analysis, decision to publish, or preparation of the manuscript.

Competing Interests: The authors have declared that no competing interests exist.

* E-mail: Lauren.Cipriano@gmail.com

Introduction

Approximately 16% of new HIV diagnoses and two-thirds of new hepatitis C virus (HCV) diagnoses in the U.S. are in injection drug users (IDUs) [1,2]. Co-infection among IDUs is common, affecting progression rates and treatment effectiveness for both diseases [3,4,5,6,7,8]. During the acute infection phase, standard antibody testing either cannot or has low sensitivity to detect these diseases; however, they can be detected with viral RNA tests [9,10]. Identification of individuals during this phase of infection may be important in averting infections and improving patient outcomes.

The acute phase of HIV infection, lasting approximately 3 months, is characterized by high viral load and high infectivity [11]. The proportion of new infections attributable to individuals with acute HIV infection is unknown, with estimates ranging from 11–50% of new sexually transmitted HIV infections [12,13]. Identification of individuals during the period of acute infection may reduce HIV transmission through behavior change and initiation of combination antiretroviral therapy (ART) which can reduce infectivity [14]. Additionally, initiating ART during acute infection may slow disease progression [14,15,16,17].

Treatment of chronic HCV with pegylated-interferon and ribavirin (PEG-IFN+RBV) is potentially curative but has high rates of undesirable side effects and is ineffective in 40–60% of patients [8,18,19,20]. Recent clinical trials demonstrated that combination therapy with a HCV protease inhibitor (PEG-IFN+RBV+PI) has higher efficacy in mono-infected genotype 1 patients who are not active IDUs [21,22,23]. In a non-IDU population, treatment with PEG-IFN+RBV+PI is cost effective in patients with moderate fibrosis [24]. During the acute phase of HCV infection, estimated to last up to 6 months, PEG-IFN+RBV treatment has substantially higher rates of sustained viral response than when treatment is initiated later in the course of the disease [25,26,27,28,29,30,31,32,33] and therefore it is possible that treatment during this phase of the disease may result in important benefits to patients and society.

Previous studies have found that HIV prevention and treatment programs targeted to IDUs, including opioid replacement therapy (ORT) and expanded access to ART, are cost effective and reduce transmission [34,35,36,37,38,39,40]. Although individuals in ORT reduce their risky behaviors, they continue to be at high risk for HIV and HCV [41]. Individuals in ORT are a readily accessible population for frequent screening and treatment initiation because of frequent interactions with health services. Screening for the short acute phase of HIV and HCV infection may identify enough individuals, resulting in improved health outcomes and reduced transmission, to be good value for the additional costs of viral RNA testing. We used a mathematical model to evaluate the potential population-level impacts–costs, effectiveness, and cost effectiveness–of various protocols and frequencies of screening IDUs in ORT for acute and chronic HIV and HCV infection. We considered two HIV and HCV screening technologies, conventional antibody testing and combined antibody and viral RNA testing, and several screening frequencies: once upon entry to ORT only; or upon entry to ORT and routinely thereafter, every 3, 6, or 12 months.

Methods

Model Overview

We developed a deterministic dynamic compartmental model to simulate the population of a representative large U.S. city with 2.5 million persons aged 15 to 59. We estimated values for all model parameters based on published literature, expert opinion, and model calibration (Table 1, Table S1). We validated the model's estimates of HIV and HCV incidence rates and the proportion of sexually transmitted HIV infections attributable to transmission from an individual in the acute phase of HIV infection to literature estimates (details in Appendix S1). We considered a 20-year time horizon, with calculations in monthly increments. We calculated expected survival, quality-adjusted survival, and expected lifetime health care costs by tracking the time spent in each health state and compared multiple scenarios. We took a societal perspective, considered costs and benefits over a lifetime horizon, and discounted outcomes at 3% annually [42]. We calculated incremental cost-effectiveness ratios (cost per life year (LY) and quality-adjusted life year (QALY) gained) by comparing each strategy to the next best non-dominated strategy. We conducted extensive sensitivity analysis to assess the robustness of model results.

Population Groups

We subdivided the population into three risk groups based on IDU status: current IDU, IDU in ORT, and non-IDU (Figure 1). Based on current estimates from large U.S. cities, we assumed that

approximately 1.2% of the modeled population are IDUs, with 6.5% HIV prevalence [43] and 35% HCV prevalence [44] among IDUs. We estimated HIV and HCV prevalence among non-IDUs using the U.S. adult population prevalence of 0.47% [45] and 1.7% [46], respectively. We calibrated the model to match estimates of HIV and HCV prevalence and incidence in IDUs and the general population (details in Appendix S1, Figure S1, Figure S2, and Figure S3).

We divided HIV infection status into uninfected, acute HIV infection, asymptomatic HIV, and symptomatic HIV/AIDS. We divided HCV infection status into uninfected, acute infection, asymptomatic chronic, symptomatic chronic, and end-stage liver disease. We grouped the four most common HCV genotypes into two groups based on similarity of treatment protocol and treatment response: genotypes 1 and 4 and genotypes 2 and 3. Further, we considered whether an individual is aware of his/her HIV or HCV infection status or is on HIV and/or HCV treatment. The model includes a compartment for every combination of IDU, HIV, and HCV status, and treatment and awareness, for a total of 756 compartments. Individuals transitioned between compartments according to rates defined by the dynamics of disease transmission and progression.

Data Sources and Assumptions

Population Dynamics. All individuals enter the model at age 15 as non-injection drug users (non-IDUs) without HIV or HCV infection. Individuals exit the population due to maturation (at age 60) or death. Annual baseline death rates vary by risk group to account for variation in drug-use-related mortality [47]. We estimated the mortality rate among non-IDUs using the average mortality rate for the 15–59 year old United States (U.S.) population [48,49]. We estimated the mortality rate among IDUs not in ORT to be 31.1 per 1000 person-years and estimated that IDUs in ORT have a 60% lower mortality rate than IDUs not in ORT [47,50,51].

Disease Progression and Mortality. We estimated HIV and HCV progression and mortality rates, and the impacts of co-infection on progression and treatment effectiveness from previous models of their natural history and progression as well as clinical and observational trials (Table 1, Table S1). We assumed that individuals with a CD4 count <500 cells/mm^3 were eligible to receive combination ART and that treatment with ART slowed the progression of HIV and reduced HIV infectivity. The duration of HCV therapy and treatment effectiveness differed by HCV genotype category and treatment type [2,22,23]. The effectiveness of a PEG-IFN+RBV+PI regimen to cure chronic genotype 1 HCV infection in mono-infected individuals was estimated from recent trials [22,23]. Treatment effectiveness of PEG-IFN+RBV for treatment of chronic HCV infection for genotypes other than type 1 and during the acute phase of HCV in mono- and HIV co-infected individuals was estimated based on recent trials [25,26,27,28,29,30,31,32].

Risk Behaviors. We estimated IDU risk behaviors using published reports from the Collaborative Injection Drug Users Study (CIDUS) [52,53,54]. We assumed that the injection-drug-using population would remain a stable proportion of the total population over the 20-year intervention horizon and that the proportion of the IDU population in ORT would be constant at 7% [55]. Without incremental interventions, we assumed that HIV-negative IDUs have a 4.0% annual probability and HIV-positive IDUs have a 6.7% annual probability of stopping injection behaviors [56]. We estimated that the annual rate of leaving ORT and stopping injection drug use was 1.8% and that each year 44.1% of individuals in ORT would quit ORT and return to drug

Table 1. Key input parameters.

Variable	Base value	Range		Source
Total population size, age 15–59	2,500,000			
Fraction of population that is IDU	1.2%	0.7%	1.8%	*[43]
Fraction of IDUs in ORT	7%	5%	15%	[55,136]
HIV Prevalence				
Overall (age 15–59)	0.47%			[45]
IDU	6.5%	2%	15%	* [137]
Non-IDU	0.40%	0.30%	0.45%	Calculated
Hepatitis C (HCV) Prevalence				
Overall (age 15–59)	1.7%	1.4%	2.0%	[46]
IDU	35%	14%	51%	[44]
Non-IDU	1.3%	1.2%	1.4%	Calculated
HCV Treatment Response				
Genotype 1 or 4:				
Acute HCV	62%	50%	70%	[25,26,27,28,29]
Acute HCV, HIV+	70%	50%	80%	[30,31,32,33]
Chronic HCV	PEG-IFN+RBV: 40%	30%	60%	[8,18,19,20]
	PEG-IFN+RBV+PI: 65%	40%	80%	[21,22,23]
Chronic HCV, HIV+	PEG-IFN+RBV: 30%	20%	50%	[8]
	PEG-IFN+RBV+PI: 65%	40%	80%	Assumed
Genotype 2 or 3:				
Acute HCV	62%	50%	70%	[25,26,27,28,29]
Acute HCV, HIV+	70%	50%	80%	[30,31,32,33]
Chronic HCV	82%	60%	88%	[19,20]
Chronic HCV, HIV+	66%	50%	80%	[8]
SEXUAL BEHAVIOR PARAMETERS				
Average number of sexual partners per year				
NON-IDU	2	1.1	3	[58]
IDU	4.3	2	8	[58,59]
HIV transmission (rate per partner-year)				
Acute HIV	0.20	0.10	0.70	Calculated
Asymptomatic HIV (CD4>500 cells/mm^3)	0.025	0.02	0.03	[79]
Symptomatic HIV (CD4<500 cells/mm^3)	0.05	0.04	0.075	[79]
Effect of ART on infection risk	0.1	0.01	0.5	[79,80,81,82,83,84,85,86]
HCV transmission (rate per partner-year)				
Acute and chronic HCV	0.0003	0	0.002	[138,139,140,141,142]
Effect of PEG-IFN+RBV or PEG-INF+RBV+PI on infection risk	0.1	0.01	0.5	Estimated, [143,144]
INJECTING BEHAVIOR PARAMETERS				
Average number of injections per year	700	500	1500	[65,145,146,147,148,149,150]
Fraction of injections that are shared	13%	10%	60%	[52,62,149,150,151,152,153,154,155]
Relative risk of shared-injecting behavior, in ORT	30%	50%	100%	[61,62]
HIV transmission (per injection with an HIV+ IDU)				
Acute HIV	1.0%	0.8%	1.2%	Assumed the same relative risk of transmission as for sexual contact
Asymptomatic HIV (CD4>500 cells/mm^3)	0.12%	0.09%	0.15%	[156,157]
Symptomatic HIV (CD4<500 cells/mm^3)	0.3%	0.25%	0.04%	[156,157]
Effect of ART on infection risk	0.50	0.1	1.0	[79]
HCV transmission (per injection with an HCV+ IDU)				
Acute and chronic HCV	0.4%	0.1%	4.0%	[158,159]
Effect of PEG-IFN+RBV or PEG-IFN+RBV+PI on infection risk	0.5	0.1	1.0	Estimated, [143,144]
COSTS				

Table 1. Cont.

Variable	Base value	Range	Source
Screening costs			
Counseling			
Pre-test counseling	12.76		[73]
Post-test, negative result	7.14		[73]
Post-test, positive result	13.84		[73]
HIV diagnostics (testing protocol details are described in Table S2)			
Antibody (negative)	12.96		CMS [94], CPT4 86701
Antibody (positive)	67.14		CMS [94], CPT4 86701 (3 times) +86689
RNA amplification (negative)	124.24		CMS [94], CPT4 87535
RNA amplification (positive)	276.74		CMS [94], CPT4 87535 (2 times) +86689
HCV diagnostics			
Antibody (negative)	20.84		CMS [94], CPT4 86803
Antibody (positive)	85.13		CMS [94], CPT4 86803 (3 times) +86804
RNA amplification (negative)	62.54		CMS [94], CPT4 87521
RNA amplification (positive)	147.69		CMS [94], CPT4 87521 (2 times) +86804

ART – antiretroviral therapy; HIV – human immunodeficiency virus; HCV – hepatitis C virus; ORT – opioid replacement therapy; CMS – Center for Medicare and Medicaid Services; CPT4 - Current Procedural Terminology, 4th Edition.
*The proportion of the population that is IDU and the HIV prevalence among IDUs was estimated as the unweighted average of the 21 Metropolitan Statistical Areas (MSAs) with populations between 1.5 and 5 million. Across these cities there is very wide variation in both parameters, so we performed extensive sensitivity analysis on these inputs. The cities included were (Population; % of population that are IDU; Prevalence of HIV in IDU): Boston–Brockton–Nashua, MA–NH (4.2 million, 1.6%, 4.5%), Washington, DC–MD–VA–WV (3.6 million, 0.8%, 9.0%), Philadelphia, PA–NJ (3.4 million, 1.7%, 8.8%), Atlanta, GA (3.0 million, 0.5%, 14.9%), Houston, TX (3.0 million, 1.1%, 6.4%), Detroit, MI (3.0 million, 0.9%, 6.4%), Dallas, TX (2.6 million, 1.3%, 3.4%), Phoenix–Mesa, AZ (2.3 million, 1.2%, 3.6%), Riverside–San Bernardino, CA (2.3 million, 0.9%, 3.5%), Minneapolis, MN (2.1 million, 0.5%, 3.3%), Orange County, CA (2.0 million, 1.0%, 2.4%), San Diego, CA (2.0 million, 1.3%, 3.4%), Nassau–Suffolk, NY (1.8 million, 0.7%, 12.3%), St. Louis, MO–IL (1.8 million, 0.6%, 3.1%), Baltimore, MD (1.7 million, 3.4%, 11.7%), Seattle–Bellevue–Everett, WA (1.7 million, 1.6%, 2.9%), Oakland, CA (1.7 million, 1.3%, 4.2%), Tampa–St. Petersburg–Clearwater, FL (1.6 million, 1.1%, 6.1%), Miami, FL (1.5 million, 0.6%, 22.8%), Denver, CO (1.5 million, 1.4%, 3.1%), Pittsburgh, PA (1.5 million, 0.9%, 3.9%), Cleveland–Lorain–Elyria, OH (1.5 million, 0.8%, 4.2%). We excluded the three MSAs with populations over 5 million: Los Angeles–Long Beach, CA (6.5 million, 1.5%, 3.8%), New York, NY (6.4 million, 1.4%, 21.2%), Chicago, IL (5.7 million, 0.6%, 8.4%).

injection [57]. Using these assumptions and estimates, we calculated the rate at which non-IDUs become IDUs and the rate at which IDUs enter ORT.

Disease Transmission. We incorporated HIV and HCV transmission from sexual partnerships and injection equipment sharing through risk-structured mass action. In each month, the number of sexual partnerships, using and not using condoms, and the number of injection equipment sharing partnerships, using and not using bleach, were calculated based on risk-group-specific average number of sexual and injection equipment sharing partners, condom rates, and bleach use rates [58,59,60,61,62]. We assumed preferential sexual mixing of IDUs with other IDUs (40% of IDU sexual partners were other IDUs) [54,63,64,65]. We assumed that the viral load reductions that occur during treatment for HIV and HCV resulted in reductions in infectivity. In the base case, regardless of how diagnosis occurred, we assumed that awareness of HIV-positive disease status resulted in an increase in condom use [63,66,67] and, among IDUs, a 20% reduction in needle sharing [68]. We assumed that awareness of HCV-positive disease status did not result in a reduction in needle sharing behavior [53,69,70,71]. We varied these assumptions in sensitivity analysis.

Screening Strategies

We assumed that individuals may learn of their HIV and/or HCV status through symptomatic case finding, an existing screening program, or a new screening intervention. We estimated baseline rates of diagnosis via existing screening programs through calibration to current rates of under-diagnosis of HIV and HCV among IDUs and non-IDUs (Appendix S1).

We considered two HIV and HCV screening technologies, conventional antibody testing and combined antibody and RNA testing. The HIV and HCV test sequence and confirmatory follow-up are based on those implemented in screening programs [72,73] and the CDC recommendations for suspected cases, respectively (Table S2) [2]. In the base case, we considered a 3rd generation HIV antibody test which we assumed identifies one-third of individuals infected in the past 3 months (acutely infected individuals); we considered HIV antibody tests with greater sensitivity in the acute infection period (such as a 4th generation HIV antibody and p24 antigen test) in sensitivity analysis. In scenarios with HIV RNA testing, individuals who did not test HIV antibody positive were subsequently tested for HIV RNA. The individuals screened are clients of an ORT program, so we assumed that 100% of individuals receive their test results. We considered several screening frequencies: once upon entry to ORT only; or upon entry to ORT and routinely thereafter, every 3, 6, or 12 months.

In the base case, we assumed 50% of individuals identified with acute HIV [74], individuals with a negative antibody test and a positive RNA test, and 40% of individuals identified with acute HCV would initiate treatment. The optimal duration of therapy

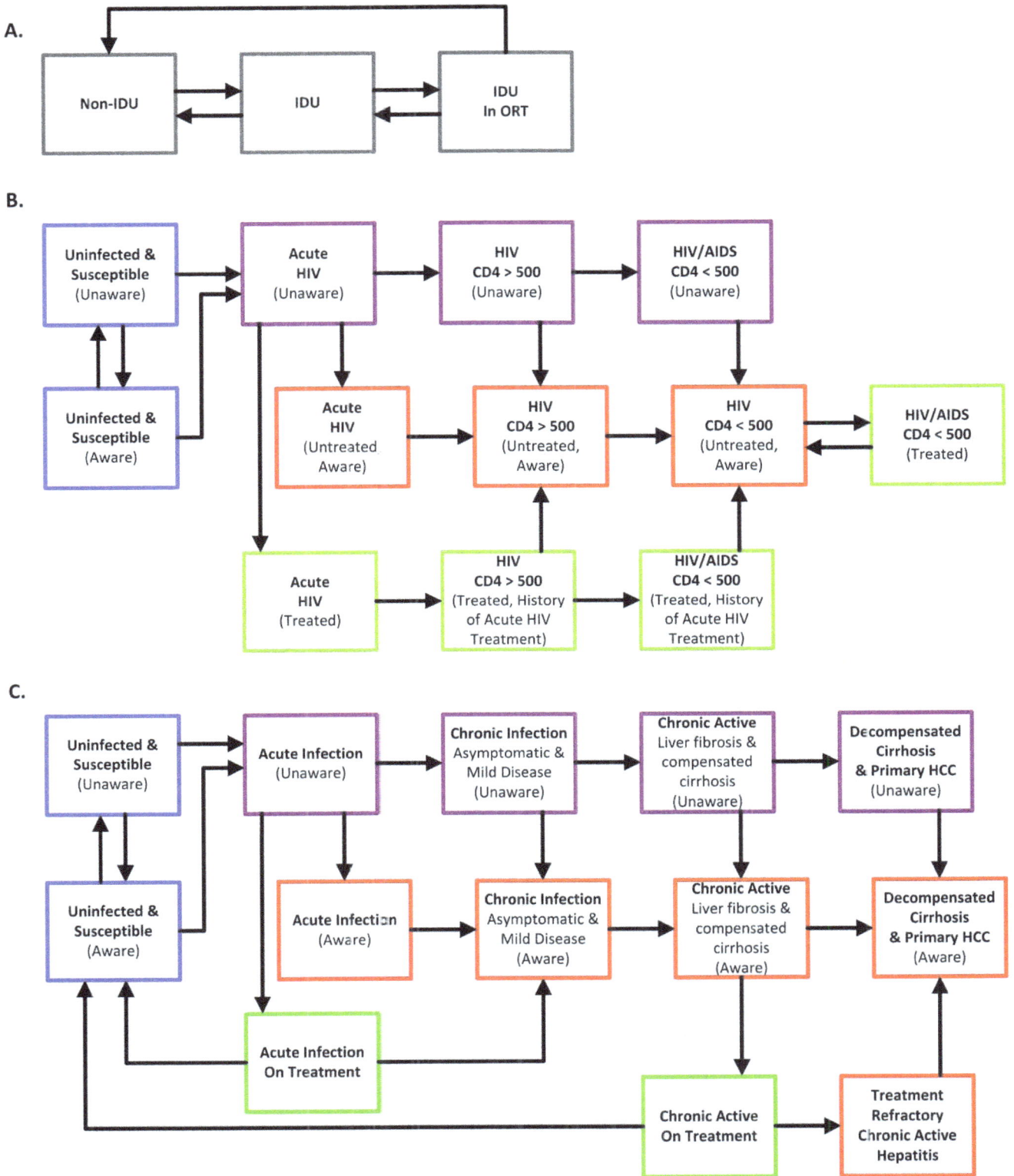

Figure 1. Model schematic. Each compartment is described by three characteristics: (A) risk group (IDU category), (B) HIV status, and (C) HCV status. In each cycle, individuals within any compartment may stay in the same compartment or may change in any or all of these dimensions. Rates of movement between levels of disease severity are conditional on the current state of the individual (including IDU status and presence of co-infection). Rates of movement between status of uninfected and infected are conditional on risk group, the number of infected individuals, and the sufficient contact rate.

for patients with acute HIV infection is unknown. We assumed that individuals who initiated ART during acute HIV infection continued ART after the acute phase even with a CD4 count >500 cells/mm^3 [75,76,77,78]. We assumed that ART reduces sexual infectivity by 90% and infectivity from injection transmission by 50% [79,80,81,82,83,84,85,86]. In the base case, we did not consider any change in the rate of HIV disease progression caused by ART initiation during acute or early HIV infection. We estimated the probability of sustained virologic response in patients who initiate PEG-IFN+RBV during acute HCV infection based on recent clinical trials [25,26,27,28,29,30,31,32]. Consistent with current evidence [28,87,88], we assumed that acute HCV treatment would be equally effective for IDUs in ORT and for non-IDUs.

Costs

Individuals accrued health care costs based on their health state each month and for transitions between states or events within a cycle such as screening and diagnosis. We expressed all costs in 2009 U.S. dollars using the U.S. GDP deflator [89].

Baseline costs. We estimated annual baseline health care expenditures for non-IDUs using age-specific averages for the U.S. population [90,91] and we increased this by $2,021 for HIV- and HCV-negative IDUs [92]. We estimated the annual cost of ORT to be $5,171 [93]. We estimated the cost of death for an IDU for causes other than HIV or HCV to be $8,350 based on Medicare reimbursement rates for an emergency room visit and hospitalization from drug overdose with major complications [94].

Disease-attributable HIV and HCV costs. We assumed that following diagnosis with HIV or HCV, all patients would have their disease staged and characterized to assist with treatment decisions; we assumed that this included assessment of viral load and genotyping and cost $500 and $438 per HIV and HCV diagnosis, respectively, based on the Medicare reimbursement schedule [94].

We used a recent modeling study to estimate the costs of HIV health states [95]. We assumed that asymptomatic HIV-infected individuals who are unaware of their disease incur no additional health care costs, while individuals with symptomatic disease incur additional costs regardless of whether their disease has been diagnosed. We assumed that the annual cost of ART is approximately $22,000 and the remainder of the HIV-associated health care cost is for disease monitoring, opportunistic infection prophylaxis, and other outpatient care [95]. We estimated the cost of health care in the last month of life with HIV to be $33,480 which is the cost of death from an opportunistic infection [95].

We used a prior cost-effectiveness analysis evaluating screening for HCV in the general population to inform our estimates of the HCV attributable costs [96]. We assumed that the weekly cost of PEG-IFN+RBV was $471 ($11,304 for 24-week course of treatment and $22,608 for a 48-week course of treatment) [97,98]. We estimated that combination therapy with a protease inhibitor cost an additional $1,100 per week which would add an average cost of $40,000 per patient. We assumed the incremental end-of-life costs associated with HCV to be the same as those accruing from non-HCV death.

Screening program costs. For screening costs, we used CDC estimates for pre- and post-test counseling and 2009 Medicare reimbursement rates for laboratory tests [73,94]. We assumed testing protocols as described by guidelines and in descriptions of practice [2,72,73,99] and assumed HIV and HCV antibody and RNA test costs based on the Medicare reimbursement schedule [94]. We assumed that 100% of screened

individuals would obtain their results and receive the appropriate post-test counseling [73].

Quality of Life

We assumed a baseline quality-of-life weight of 0.9 for healthy non-IDUs using age-specific values for the U.S. population and averaging based on the distribution of individual ages [100,101]. We estimated a baseline quality-of-life weight of 0.747 for IDUs after adjusting for the average age of the population in the model [102].

Additionally, we incorporated multiplicative quality-of-life weights for individuals with HIV [103,104,105,106] and HCV [107,108] based on their disease stage. Awareness of HIV and HCV status affects quality of life, so we included this in the model [109,110]. In addition, we included a decrement in quality of life associated with PEG-IFN+RBV(+/−PI) treatment [107].

Results

HIV and HCV Infections Averted

With no screening targeted to individuals in ORT (referred to as 'no screening'), we estimate that 7371 HIV infections and 25,704 HCV infections will occur over the next 20 years (discounted at 3% annually) in a population of 2.5 million with 26,100 IDUs entering ORT (2100 IDUs in ORT at any one time). Screening only for chronic HIV infection averted 13.8 to 27.6 HIV infections (depending on screening frequency) and, primarily through risk-reducing behavior changes associated with awareness of HIV-positive status, a very small number of HCV infections (Figure 2). Screening only for chronic HCV infection averted 18.0 to 20.0 HCV infections and 2.3 to 2.5 HIV infections. HIV infections were averted by HCV screening because all individuals newly diagnosed with one infection were screened for the other during follow-up; due to its relatively high prevalence (35%) and low rate of awareness (25%), HCV screening results in a large absolute number of diagnoses and, therefore, HIV tests.

Screening for HIV antibodies with increased frequency averted few incremental infections. For example, increasing screening frequency from annually to twice-annually averted only 3.3 additional HIV infections over 20 years. Incorporating HIV RNA testing to identify acute infections averted many more infections than increasing the frequency of HIV screening: for screening frequency of upon entry to ORT to every 3 months, including RNA detection averted 14.8 to 30.3 more HIV infections, respectively, than antibody screening alone. Across all screening strategies considered, approximately 52% of infections averted were averted in the non-IDU population. Identifying 1 IDU in ORT with chronic HIV with a CD4 count <500 cells/mm^3 and initiating ART averted 0.1 HIV infections over 20 years. Diagnosis during the acute phase averted more HIV infections than later diagnosis even if ART is not initiated: over 20 years, diagnosing 1 IDU in ORT with acute HIV infection averted 0.4 HIV infections if ART was not immediately initiated and 1.3 HIV infections if ART was immediately initiated.

Compared to screening for HCV antibodies annually, screening twice annually averted no additional HCV infections over 20 years. Including HCV viral RNA detection averted an additional 3.7 to 7.7 infections over 20 years compared to antibody screening alone for screening frequency of upon entry to ORT to every 3 months, respectively. Early identification and treatment of HCV averts few infections primarily because not all acutely infected individuals will progress to chronic infection and HCV re-infection is common, absent behavior change.

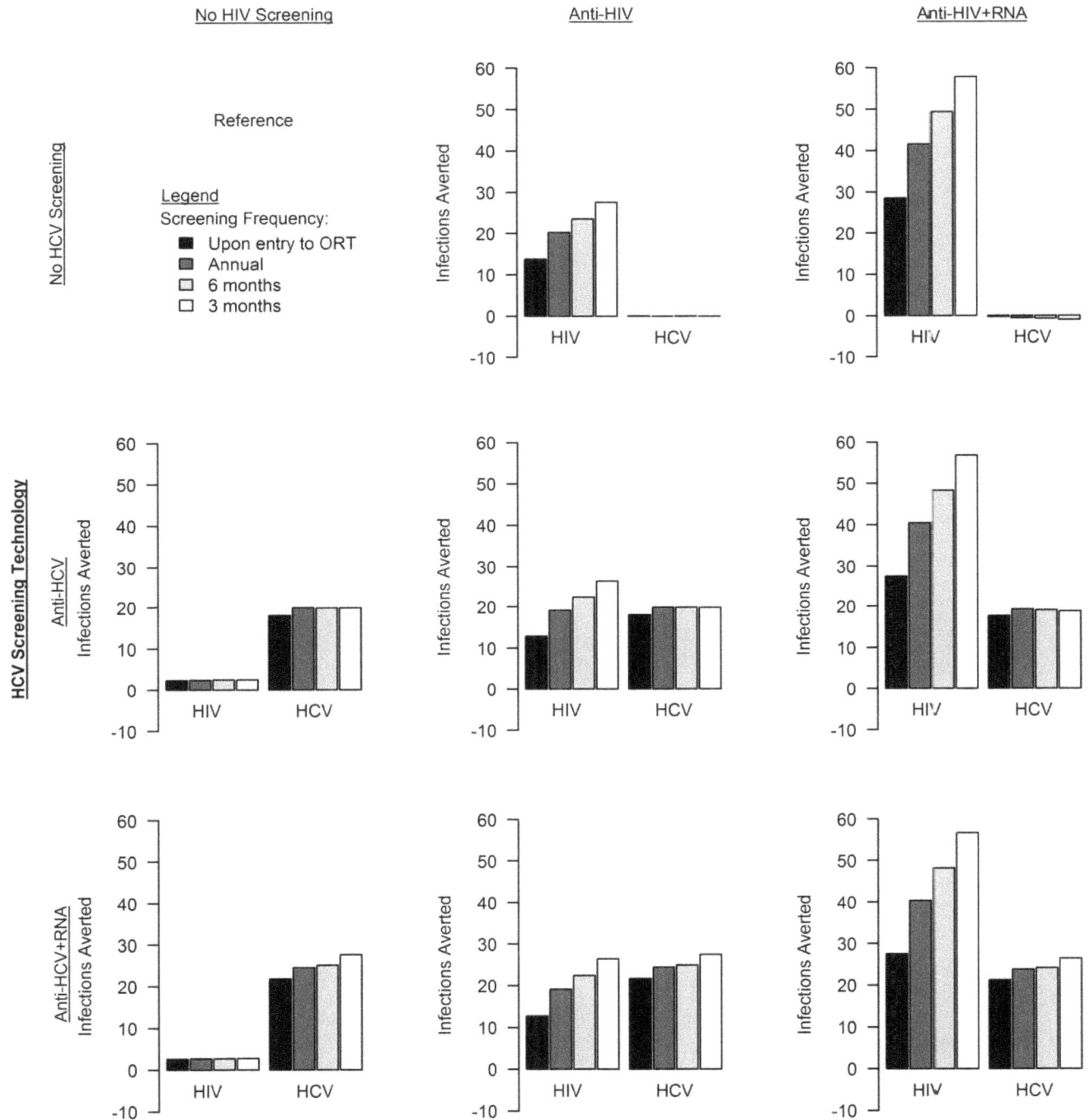

Figure 2. Estimated number of HIV and HCV infections averted for each screening strategy over a 20-year time horizon compared to a strategy of no screening of IDUs in ORT (discounted at 3% annually).

HIV and HCV Prevalence

Screening of IDUs in ORT for HIV and HCV prevents infections but has little effect on overall HIV and HCV prevalence because the number of people targeted through screening in ORT is small. Compared to no screening, the relative change in HIV prevalence in the total population in year 20 is 0.20% and 0.23% lower with annual and twice-annual HIV antibody testing,

respectively; whereas the relative change in HIV prevalence in year 20 is 0.43% and 0.51% lower with annual and twice-annual HIV antibody and RNA testing, respectively. In the IDU population, twice-annual screening for HIV antibody and RNA decreases HIV prevalence in year 20 by 1.1% (relative) compared to no screening. Across all strategies considered, the relative change in HCV prevalence in the total population in year 20 was

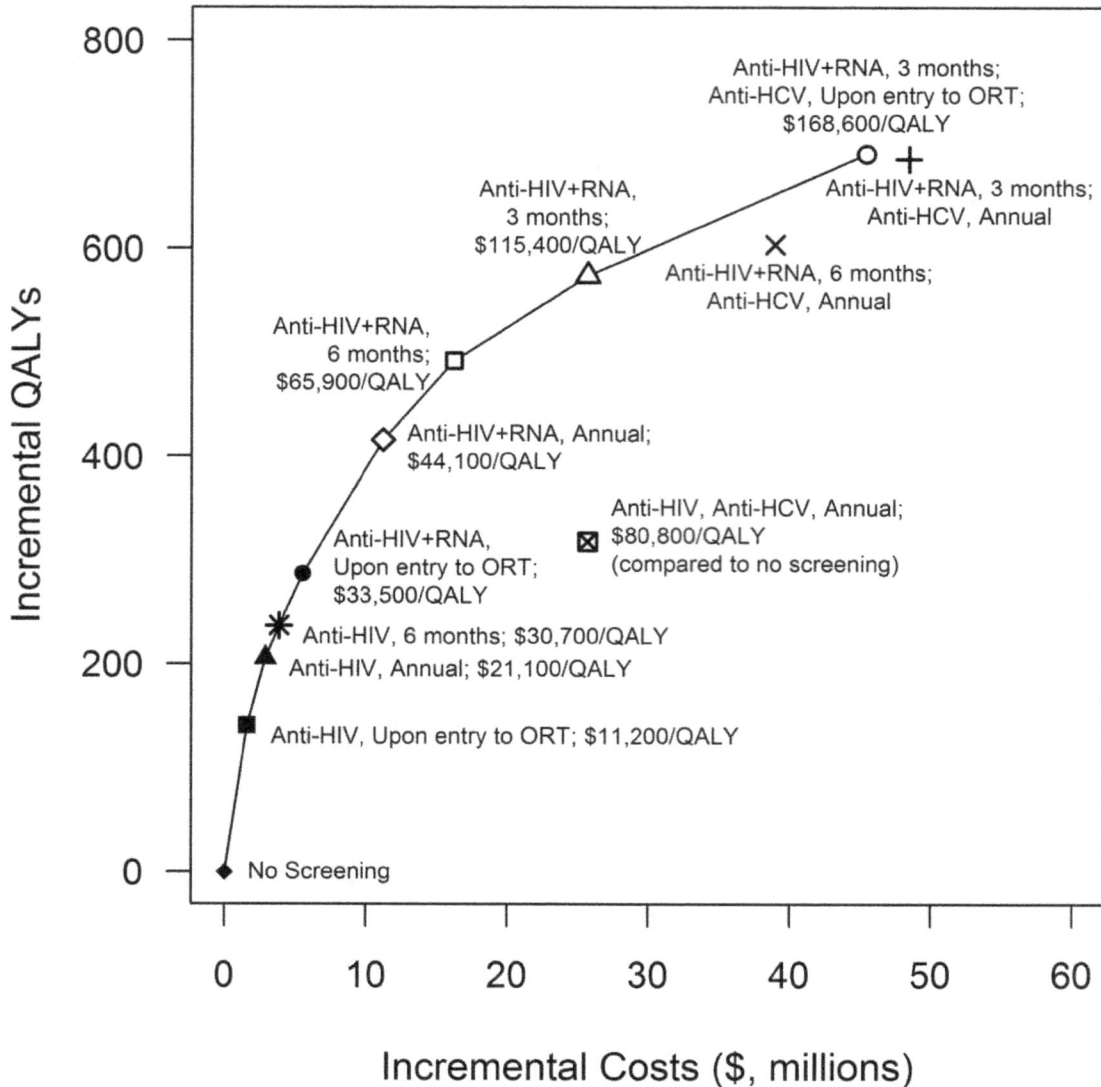

Figure 3. Cost-effectiveness plane presenting all non-dominated and selected dominated screening protocols and frequencies targeting injection drug users in ORT.

reduced no more than 0.32% compared to a strategy of no screening.

Cost Effectiveness

Following current guidelines of annual HIV and HCV antibody screening for all IDUs in ORT costs $35,100/LY gained and $80,800/QALY gained when compared to no screening of IDUs in ORT. However, this strategy costs more and provides fewer benefits than strategies that screen more frequently for HIV only (Figure 3).

Table 2 reports the incremental cost-effectiveness ratio (ICER) of each strategy compared to the next-best alternative for strategies on the efficient frontier; Table S3 shows results for all strategies. Results differed depending on the measure of benefit (LY gained or QALY gained), largely because of the decrease in quality of life associated with awareness of asymptomatic HIV or HCV infection. Screening every 6 months for HIV antibodies and RNA costs $65,900/QALY gained compared to screening annually. Screening every 3 months for HIV antibodies and

RNA costs $115,400/QALY gained. Further, including HCV antibody testing upon entry to ORT increases the ICER to $168,600/QALY. Screening every 6 months for HIV antibodies and RNA and for HCV antibodies upon entry to ORT costs $57,200/LY gained; further increasing the frequency of HCV antibody screening increases the cost to $71,400/LY gained. Screening every 3 months for HIV antibodies and RNA and annually for HCV antibodies costs $100,750/LY gained.

Sensitivity Analysis

We considered alternate-city scenarios by varying the number of IDUs, the fraction of IDUs in ORT and the HIV and HCV prevalence among IDUs. Varying the number of IDUs, the fraction of IDUs in ORT, and the prevalence of HCV among IDUs had little impact on the cost effectiveness of the screening strategies (Table S4). When we increased the proportion of IDUs in ORT to 40%, the ICER of screening for HIV antibodies and RNA every 6 months increased from $65,900/QALY gained to $100,600/QALY gained because high rates of ORT use lower the

Table 2. Base case outcomes and incremental cost-effectiveness ratios for non-dominated strategies in a representative city of 2.5 million individuals age 15–59 years, with 1.2% of the population IDU, and 6.5% and 35% prevalence of HIV and HCV among IDU, respectively.*

Screening Protocol	Screening Frequency**	HIV Infections Averted	HCV Infections Averted	Incremental Cost	Incremental LYs	Incremental QALYs	ICER ($/LY gained)	ICER ($/QALY gained)***
No screening****		Reference	Reference	Reference	Reference	Reference	Reference	Reference
Anti-HIV	Upon entry to ORT	13.78	0.01	1,580,365	169	141	9,365	11,191
Anti-HIV	Annual	20.22	0.00	2,874,166	245	206	16,938	20,075
Anti-HIV	6 months	23.55	0.02	3,832,733	281	237	26,436	30,713
Anti-HIV RNA	Upon entry to ORT	28.54	(0.37)	5,509,197	337	207	30,323	33,503
Anti-HIV+RNA	Annual	41.51	(0.60)	11,200,954	487	416	37,900	44,141
Anti-HIV+RNA	6 months	49.34	(0.75)	16,207,602	574	492	Dominated	65,883
Anti-HIV; Anti-HCV	Annual	19.10	19.85	25,652,696	731	318	Dominated	Dominated
Anti-HIV+RNA	3 months	57.82	(0.96)	25,664,563	668	574	Dominated	115,429
Anti-HIV+RNA; Anti-HCV	Annual Upon entry to ORT	40.57	17.33	30,938,150	930	533	44,532	Dominated
Anti-HIV+RNA; Anti-HCV	6 months Upon entry to ORT	48.42	17.17	35,936,712	1,017	609	57,192	Dominated
Anti-HIV+RNA; Anti-HCV	6 months Annual	48.26	19.06	38,956,858	1,060	604	71,399	Dominated
Anti-HIV+RNA; Anti-HCV	3 months Upon entry to ORT	56.90	16.96	45,390,578	1,111	691	Dominated	168,600
Anti-HIV+RNA; Anti-HCV	3 months Annual	56.75	18.86	48,410,723	1,154	686	100,749	Dominated
Anti-HIV+RNA; Anti-HCV	3 months 6 months	56.75	18.82	49,421,140	1,156	683	489,639	Dominated
Anti-HIV+RNA; Anti-HCV+RNA	3 months Annual	56.72	23.45	55,246,297	1,162	681	905,133	Dominated
Anti-HIV+RNA; Anti-HCV+RNA	3 months	56.71	26.47	64,329,321	1,170	689	1,220,703	Dominated

HIV – human immunodeficiency virus; HCV – hepatitis C virus; LYs – life years; QALYs – quality-adjusted life-years; ICER – incremental cost-effectiveness ratio; IDU – injection drug user.

*Outcomes for all strategies considered are shown in Table S3.

**Frequencies considered were: Upon entry to ORT; "Annual"= Upon entry to ORT and annually while in ORT; "6 months"= Upon entry to ORT and every 6 months while in ORT; "3 months"= Upon entry to ORT and every 3 months while in ORT.

***"Dominated" indicates that the strategy costs more and provides fewer benefits than another strategy or a combination of two strategies.

****This strategy consists of baseline case detection rates in the IDU and non-IDU populations and no screening targeted to individuals in ORT.

average HIV risk of the population (in the economic sense, ORT and HIV screening are partial substitutes). Our results were sensitive to HIV prevalence among IDUs. In low (3.5% of IDUs) and high (17% of IDUs) HIV-prevalence scenarios, screening for HIV antibodies and RNA every 6 months costs $107,000/QALY gained and $23,000/QALY gained, respectively. Results were not sensitive to the effectiveness of ORT or to the average time spent in ORT within realistic ranges (Table S5).

Results were robust to clinically relevant changes in the HIV natural history and ART effectiveness parameters, but sensitive to rates of HIV treatment initiation (Table S6). However, even with low uptake of ART (25%) among individuals identified with acute HIV infection, screening every 6 months for HIV antibodies and RNA cost $77,200/QALY gained. In general, our results were not sensitive to changing access to or effectiveness of HCV treatment (Table S7). We considered scenarios in which initiation of ART in individuals with CD4 counts >500 cell/mm^3 slowed HIV progression. These additional benefits increase the cost effectiveness of acute HIV screening strategies: screening every 6 months for HIV antibodies and RNA cost between $61,500 and $65,200/QALY gained depending of the reduction in progression rate (Table S6).

Results were sensitive to the length of time after infection until HIV is detectable (Table S8). As newer 4th generation HIV tests which combine sensitive HIV antibody technologies with p24 antigen tests become more widely available, fewer acute infections are identified by the addition of RNA testing to the screening protocol. If the window period of detection for the 4th generation HIV test is 1 month, screening every 6 months with a 4th generation test and RNA costs $116,000/QALY gained (compared to $65,900/QALY gained if the window is 2 months).

We also explored scenarios in which awareness of HCV status changed needle-sharing behavior. Assuming that awareness of HCV-positive status decreases needle-sharing by 5% substantially improved the cost-effectiveness of HCV screening. For example, screening every 6 months for HIV antibodies and RNA and for HCV antibodies upon entry to ORT costs $67,400/QALY gained. However, even with high rates of behavior change, screening for acute HCV infection always has very high ICERs (>$200,000 per QALY gained).

Assumptions relating to quality of life were important drivers in the difference between the results in terms of per LY gained and per QALY gained. However, varying the quality of life weights within clinically reasonable ranges that maintain the rank ordering of health states did not substantially change the conclusions, with one notable exception: the reduction in quality of life associated with HCV diagnosis. When we considered no reduction in quality of life associated with awareness of HCV-positive status in an asymptomatic individual, screening for HCV antibodies became increasingly attractive: screening for HIV antibodies and RNA annually and for HCV antibodies upon entry to ORT costs $44,200/QALY gained, screening for HIV antibodies and RNA every 6 months and for HCV antibodies upon entry to ORT costs $65,740/QALY gained, and screening for HIV antibodies and RNA every 6 months and for HCV antibodies annually costs $69,400/QALY gained (similar strategies in the base case analysis cost more than $100,000/QALY gained).

Discussion

Using a model which was calibrated to empirical data and expert estimates of trends if the status quo were continued, our analysis indicates that screening IDUs in ORT as frequently as every 6 months for HIV antibodies and RNA is likely to be a cost-effective means of reducing the spread of HIV among IDUs and non-IDUs. Although screening annually with antibodies to HIV and HCV is moderately cost effective relative to no screening, this strategy is less effective and more costly than strategies that include more frequent HIV screening. The cost effectiveness of HCV screening strategies improves when awareness of HCV-positive status is associated with a reduction in needle-sharing behavior and is not associated with a decrement in quality of life.

Initiation of treatment during the highly infectious acute period of HIV may be influential in reducing HIV transmission [9,14]. Our results demonstrate the importance of being able to distinguish between acute and chronic infections because it facilitates targeted treatment during the highly infectious acute phase. Thus, when 4th generation HIV tests are used, the preferred strategy is HIV antibody screening every 3 months (ICER of $38,000/QALY gained) and strategies that include HIV RNA testing have ICERs above $100,000/QALY gained. This tradeoff between more sensitive 4th generation HIV antibody and p24 antigen tests and the ability to distinguish between acute and chronic HIV infections has also been observed in other analyses comparing HIV RNA testing combined with 3rd or 4th generation HIV antibody tests [10]. As of 2012, ART is recommended for all HIV-infected individuals [78]. If, as a result, all patients initiate ART at diagnosis, distinguishing between acute and chronic infections will be less important.

Cost has been identified as a key factor preventing expanded access to acute HIV testing [111]. Pooling samples to reduce cost has been proposed and implemented in pilot projects of acute HIV testing [72,111,112,113]. Importantly, we find that twice-annual acute HIV screening costs less than $50,00/QALY gained even when each sample is tested individually at a cost of $51.25 per sample (the Medicare reimbursement level [94]), much higher than the average pooled cost per specimen of $3.53 reported elsewhere [72].

Initiation of PEG-IFN+RBV during acute and early HCV infection appears more likely to result in a sustained viral response than when treatment is initiated later in the course of disease [25,26,27,28,29]. However, our analysis indicates that relatively few HCV infections are averted per acute HCV infection treated because the lifetime risk of HCV infection remains very high among IDUs. Also, the prolonged asymptomatic phase of HCV infection results in a small present value of benefits to each treated patient from early intervention.

Recommendations for chronic HCV screening in high-risk individuals are a subject of debate [114]. The U.S. Preventive Services Task Force found the evidence supporting screening insufficient to make a recommendation [99] but the CDC and NIH recommend routine HCV screening of high-risk individuals [2,115]. How the recommendations will change with the availability of a more effective treatment for chronically infected genotype 1 patients is uncertain. While our analysis does not find acute HCV testing to be cost effective in any scenario, we do find that HCV antibody testing upon entry to ORT with subsequent treatment with PEG-IFN+RBV+PIs or PEG-IFN+RBV to have an ICER of just over $100,000/QALY gained when access to treatment is high. Further, the quality-of-life reduction associated with awareness of HCV-positive status was an important but highly uncertain parameter: with little to no quality-of-life reduction, HCV screening upon entry to ORT or annually is moderately cost effective. Additionally our results highlight the importance of behavior change, especially after HCV diagnosis, for achieving reduced HIV and HCV transmission, underscoring the need for effective counseling and access to clean needles and injection equipment.

Our findings are broadly consistent with prior studies of the cost effectiveness of HIV screening and treatment expansion [35,116,117] and screening for chronic HCV infection in IDUs [118,119,120,121]. We find, as have others [34,35,36,37], that HIV prevention strategies targeted to IDUs can substantially reduce the number of new HIV infections among non-IDUs. To our knowledge, no previous study has considered the cost effectiveness of routine screening for acute HIV infection in IDUs. Our results differ from the one study that considered the cost effectiveness of screening IDUs for acute/early HCV infection; that study found antibody screening every 6 months and initiation of treatment to be highly cost effective and potentially cost-saving [122]. However, that study assumed that 100% of identified cases among IDUs would be eligible for PEG-IFN+RBV treatment and did not include the possibility of re-infection, which is known to occur [123].

Our analysis has several limitations. Our 'representative city' does not perfectly represent the HIV-HCV co-epidemic in IDUs in any specific U.S. city. However, via sensitivity analysis of key 'city-specific' parameters we attempted to demonstrate the fairly wide generalizability of our model findings and to show how results change for cities with very high rates of ORT use or relatively low rates of HIV in IDUs. We only capture new infections among adults aged 15 to 59. Including older individuals would minimally impact the results as few new infections occur in persons over age 60. We did not include benefits from maternal transmissions averted or from contact tracing. Inclusion of these benefits may increase the cost effectiveness of screening. We did not consider screening for other diseases that also occur frequently in this population such as hepatitis B virus infection. We did not consider HIV screening technologies including rapid or oral tests, or the recently approved at-home HIV test. We did not include the risks of poor ART adherence resulting in drug-resistant HIV and the increase in costs associated with treating drug-resistant infections. We did not include many of the potential effects on behavior–either positive or negative–that might accrue from very frequent screening and counseling such as increased condom use or increases in serosorting [124,125,126]. Finally, we estimated the lifetime costs, LY, and QALYs for all individuals in the model at the end of the intervention horizon (20 years) based on their terminal health state using a model in which we did not continue the screening intervention and did not allow for any additional disease transmission. Although these two assumptions may have resulted in overestimations of the LYs and QALYs gained in this period, these estimates had little influence on the cost effectiveness of strategies.

Currently, testing for acute HIV is not widely available outside of pilot programs [9,72,111,127,128,129,130,131], and access to HIV and HCV counseling, testing, and treatment varies widely across drug treatment programs [132,133,134]. Fewer than 50% of IDUs receive the recommended annual testing for HIV and HCV [132,133,134]. For acute HIV screening to be effective, testing of samples, reporting of results, and initiation of treatment must occur quickly. Infrastructure changes and education of substance abuse workers and associated health professionals may be required [13,134,135]. Our analysis indicates that not testing IDUs in ORT frequently for acute and chronic HIV infection is a missed public health opportunity. Such screening could reduce the number of new HIV infections and would be cost effective.

Supporting Information

Figure S1 Results of calibration to total population and IDU rates of undiagnosed HIV (Figure S1a) and HCV (Figure S1b).

Figure S2 Results of calibration to prevalence of HIV in IDUs (Figure S2a) and the total population (Figure S2b) and calibration to prevalence of HCV in IDUs (Figure S2c) and the total population (Figure S2d).

Figure S3 Results of validation to total population HIV incidence (Figure S3a) and HCV incidence (Figure S3b).

Table S1 Base case parameter values and range for sensitivity analysis.

Table S2 Description of screening protocols.

Table S3 Base case results for all strategies considered.

Table S4 Sensitivity analysis on city-specific epidemic characteristics. Incremental cost-effectiveness ratio ($/QALY gained) for selected strategies on the efficient frontier compared to the next-best strategy.

Table S5 Sensitivity analysis on ORT effectiveness parameters. Incremental cost-effectiveness ratio ($/QALY gained) for selected strategies on the efficient frontier compared to the next-best strategy.

Table S6 Sensitivity analysis on HIV parameters. Incremental cost-effectiveness ratio ($/QALY gained) for selected strategies on the efficient frontier compared to the next-best strategy.

Table S7 Sensitivity analysis on HCV parameters. Incremental cost-effectiveness ratio ($/QALY gained) for selected strategies on the efficient frontier compared to the next-best strategy.

Table S8 Sensitivity analysis on the length of the HIV antibody test detection window. Incremental cost-effectiveness ratio ($/QALY gained) for selected strategies on the efficient frontier compared to the next-best strategy.

Appendix S1 Supplemental results and sensitivity analysis and supplemental model details.

Acknowledgments

The authors thank Steven Hurd for his assistance with computing resources.

Author Contributions

Conceived and designed the experiments: LEC GSZ DKO MLB. Performed the experiments: LEC. Analyzed the data: LEC GSZ MH EB DKO MLB. Contributed reagents/materials/analysis tools: LEC. Wrote the paper: LEC GSZ MLB. Model development: LEC. Editing and revising the manuscript: GSZ MH EB DKO MLB. Approved the final manuscript: LEC GSZ MH EB DKO MLB.

References

1. Centers for Disease Control and Prevention (CDC) (2008) Estimates of New HIV Infections in the United States.

2. (2002) Management of hepatitis C: 2002. NIH Consens State Sci Statements 19: 1–46.

3. Graham CS, Baden LR, Yu E, Mrus JM, Carnie J, et al. (2001) Influence of human immunodeficiency virus infection on the course of hepatitis C virus infection: a meta-analysis. Clin Infect Dis 33: 562–569.

4. Thein HH, Yi Q, Dore GJ, Krahn MD (2008) Natural history of hepatitis C virus infection in HIV-infected individuals and the impact of HIV in the era of highly active antiretroviral therapy: a meta-analysis. AIDS 22: 1979–1991.

5. Chen TY, Ding EL, Seage Iii GR, Kim AY (2009) Meta-analysis: increased mortality associated with hepatitis C in HIV-infected persons is unrelated to HIV disease progression. Clin Infect Dis 49: 1605–1615.

6. Thomas DL, Astemborski J, Rai RM, Anania FA, Schaeffer M, et al. (2000) The natural history of hepatitis C virus infection: host, viral, and environmental factors. JAMA 284: 450–456.

7. Maheshwari A, Ray S, Thuluvath PJ (2008) Acute hepatitis C. Lancet 372: 321–332.

8. Laguno M, Cifuentes C, Murillas J, Veloso S, Larrousse M, et al. (2009) Randomized trial comparing pegylated interferon alpha-2b versus pegylated interferon alpha-2a, both plus ribavirin, to treat chronic hepatitis C in human immunodeficiency virus patients. Hepatology 49: 22–31.

9. Pilcher CD, Eaton L, Kalichman S, Bisol C, de Souza Rda S (2006) Approaching "HIV elimination": interventions for acute HIV infection. Curr HIV/AIDS Rep 3: 160–168.

10. Long EF (2011) HIV screening via fourth-generation immunoassay or nucleic acid amplification test in the United States: a cost-effectiveness analysis. PLoS One 6: e27625.

11. Pilcher CD, Tien HC, Eron JJ Jr, Vernazza PL, Leu SY, et al. (2004) Brief but efficient: acute HIV infection and the sexual transmission of HIV. J Infect Dis 189: 1785–1792.

12. Prabhu VS, Hutchinson AB, Farnham PG, Sansom SL (2009) Sexually acquired HIV infections in the United States due to acute-phase HIV transmission: an update. AIDS 23: 1792–1794.

13. Kerndt PR, Dubrow R, Aynalem G, Mayer KH, Beckwith C, et al. (2009) Strategies used in the detection of acute/early HIV infections. The NIMH Multisite Acute HIV Infection Study: I. AIDS Behav 13: 1037–1045.

14. Pilcher CD, Eron JJ Jr, Galvin S, Gay C, Cohen MS (2004) Acute HIV revisited: new opportunities for treatment and prevention. J Clin Invest 113: 937–945.

15. Sterne JA, May M, Costagliola D, de Wolf F, Phillips AN, et al. (2009) Timing of initiation of antiretroviral therapy in AIDS-free HIV-1-infected patients: a collaborative analysis of 18 HIV cohort studies. Lancet 373: 1352–1363.

16. Emery S, Neuhaus JA, Phillips AN, Babiker A, Cohen CJ, et al. (2008) Major clinical outcomes in antiretroviral therapy (ART)-naive participants and in those not receiving ART at baseline in the SMART study. J Infect Dis 197: 1133–1144.

17. Lewden C, Chene G, Morlat P, Raffi F, Dupon M, et al. (2007) HIV-infected adults with a CD4 cell count greater than 500 cells/mm3 on long-term combination antiretroviral therapy reach same mortality rates as the general population. J Acquir Immune Defic Syndr 46: 72–77.

18. McHutchison JG, Lawitz EJ, Shiffman ML, Muir AJ, Galler GW, et al. (2009) Peginterferon alfa-2b or alfa-2a with ribavirin for treatment of hepatitis C infection. N Engl J Med 361: 580–593.

19. Hadziyannis SJ, Sette H Jr, Morgan TR, Balan V, Diago M, et al. (2004) Peginterferon-alpha2a and ribavirin combination therapy in chronic hepatitis C: a randomized study of treatment duration and ribavirin dose. Ann Intern Med 140: 346–355.

20. Torriani FJ, Rodriguez-Torres M, Rockstroh JK, Lissen E, Gonzalez-Garcia J, et al. (2004) Peginterferon Alfa-2a plus ribavirin for chronic hepatitis C virus infection in HIV-infected patients. N Engl J Med 351: 438–450.

21. Bacon BR, Gordon SC, Lawitz E, Marcellin P, Vierling JM, et al. (2011) Boceprevir for previously treated chronic HCV genotype 1 infection. N Engl J Med 364: 1207–1217.

22. Poordad F, McCone J Jr, Bacon BR, Bruno S, Manns MP, et al. (2011) Boceprevir for untreated chronic HCV genotype 1 infection. N Engl J Med 364: 1195–1206.

23. Chary A, Holodniy M (2010) Recent advances in hepatitis C virus treatment: review of HCV protease inhibitor clinical trials. Rev Recent Clin Trials 5: 158–173.

24. Liu S, Cipriano LE, Holodniy M, Owens DK, Goldhaber-Fiebert JD (2011) New Protease Inhibitors for the Treatment of Chronic Hepatitis C: A Cost-Effectiveness Analysis. Under review.

25. Alberti A, Boccato S, Vario A, Benvegnu L (2002) Therapy of acute hepatitis C. Hepatology 36: S195–200.

26. Licata A, Di Bona D, Schepis F, Shahied L, Craxi A, et al. (2003) When and how to treat acute hepatitis C? J Hepatol 39: 1056–1062.

27. Wiegand J, Deterding K, Cornberg M, Wedemeyer H (2008) Treatment of acute hepatitis C: the success of monotherapy with (pegylated) interferon alpha. J Antimicrob Chemother 62: 860–865.

28. Dore GJ, Hellard M, Matthews G, Grebely J, Haber PS, et al. (2009) Effective Treatment of Injecting Drug Users With Recently Acquired Hepatitis C Virus Infection. Gastroenterology.

29. Wiegand J, Buggisch P, Boecher W, Zeuzem S, Gelbmann CM, et al. (2006) Early monotherapy with pegylated interferon alpha-2b for acute hepatitis C infection: the HEP-NET acute-HCV-II study. Hepatology 43: 250–256.

30. Dominguez S, Ghosn J, Valantin MA, Schruniger A, Simon A, et al. (2006) Efficacy of early treatment of acute hepatitis C infection with pegylated interferon and ribavirin in HIV-infected patients. AIDS 20: 1157–1161.

31. Vogel M, Nattermann J, Baumgarten A, Klausen G, Bieniek B, et al. (2006) Pegylated interferon-alpha for the treatment of sexually transmitted acute hepatitis C in HIV-infected individuals. Antivir Ther 11: 1097–1101.

32. Gilleece YC, Browne RE, Asboe D, Atkins M, Mandalia S, et al. (2005) Transmission of hepatitis C virus among HIV-positive homosexual men and response to a 24-week course of pegylated interferon and ribavirin. J Acquir Immune Defic Syndr 40: 41–46.

33. Vogel M, Dominguez S, Bhagani S, Azwa A, Page E, et al. Treatment of acute HCV infection in HIV-positive patients: experience from a multicentre European cohort. Antivir Ther 15: 267–279.

34. Zaric GS, Barnett PG, Brandeau ML (2000) HIV transmission and the cost-effectiveness of methadone maintenance. Am J Public Health 90: 1100–1111.

35. Long EF, Brandeau ML, Galvin CM, Vinichenko T, Tole SP, et al. (2006) Effectiveness and cost-effectiveness of strategies to expand antiretroviral therapy in St. Petersburg, Russia. AIDS 20: 2207–2215.

36. Alistar SS, Owens DK, Brandeau ML (2011 (In Press)) Effectiveness and cost effectiveness of expanding harm reduction and antiretroviral therapy in a mixed HIV epidemic: An analysis for Ukraine. PLoS Medicine.

37. Barnett PG, Zaric GS, Brandeau ML (2001) The cost-effectiveness of buprenorphine maintenance therapy for opiate addiction in the United States. Addiction 96: 1267–1278.

38. Sorensen JL, Copeland AL (2000) Drug abuse treatment as an HIV prevention strategy: a review. Drug Alcohol Depend 59: 17–31.

39. Gibson DR, Flynn NM, McCarthy JJ (1999) Effectiveness of methadone treatment in reducing HIV risk behavior and HIV seroconversion among injecting drug users. AIDS 13: 1807–1818.

40. Connock M, Juarez-Garcia A, Jowett S, Frew E, Liu Z, et al. (2007) Methadone and buprenorphine for the management of opioid dependence: a systematic review and economic evaluation. Health Technol Assess 11: 1–171, iii-iv.

41. Lott DC, Strain EC, Brooner RK, Bigelow GE, Johnson RE (2006) HIV risk behaviors during pharmacologic treatment for opioid dependence: a comparison of levomethadyl acetate [corrected] buprenorphine, and methadone. J Subst Abuse Treat 31: 187–194.

42. Gold MR, Siegel JE, Russell LB, Weinstein MC, editors (1996) Cost-Effectiveness in Health and Medicine. New York: Oxford University Press.

43. Brady JE, Friedman SR, Cooper HL, Flom PL, Tempalski B, et al. (2008) Estimating the prevalence of injection drug users in the U.S. and in large U.S. metropolitan areas from 1992 to 2002. J Urban Health 85: 323–351.

44. Amon JJ, Garfein RS, Ahdieh-Grant L, Armstrong GL, Ouellet LJ, et al. (2008) Prevalence of hepatitis C virus infection among injection drug users in the United States, 1994–2004. Clin Infect Dis 46: 1852–1858.

45. McQuillan G, Kruszon-Moran D (2008) HIV Infection in the United States Household Population Aged 18–49 Years: Results from 1999–2006. Hyattsville, MD: Division of Health and Nutrition Examination Surveys, National Center for Health Statistics.

46. Armstrong GL, Wasley A, Simard EP, McQuillan GM, Kuhnert WL, et al. (2006) The prevalence of hepatitis C virus infection in the United States, 1999 through 2002. Ann Intern Med 144: 705–714.

47. Goedert JJ, Fung MW, Felton S, Battjes RJ, Engels EA (2001) Cause-specific mortality associated with HIV and HTLV-II infections among injecting drug users in the USA. AIDS 15: 1295–1302.

48. US. Census Bureau Population Division (September 2009) Resident Population Estimates for the 2000s: Monthly Postcensal Resident Population, by single year of age, sex, race, and Hispanic origin.

49. Arias E (2007) United States Life Tables, 2004. National Vital Statistics Reports, National Center for Health Statistics 56.

50. Degenhardt L, Hall W, Warner-Smith M (2006) Using cohort studies to estimate mortality among injecting drug users that is not attributable to AIDS. Sex Transm Infect 82 Suppl 3: iii56–63.

51. Zanis DA, Woody GE (1998) One-year mortality rates following methadone treatment discharge. Drug Alcohol Depend 52: 257–260.

52. Thiede H, Hagan H, Campbell JV, Strathdee SA, Bailey SL, et al. (2007) Prevalence and correlates of indirect sharing practices among young adult injection drug users in five U.S. cities. Drug Alcohol Depend 91 Suppl 1: S39–47.

53. Hagan H, Campbell J, Thiede H, Strathdee S, Ouellet L, et al. (2006) Self-reported hepatitis C virus antibody status and risk behavior in young injectors. Public Health Rep 121: 710–719.

54. Kapadia F, Latka MH, Hudson SM, Golub ET, Campbell JV, et al. (2007) Correlates of consistent condom use with main partners by partnership patterns among young adult male injection drug users from five US cities. Drug Alcohol Depend 91 Suppl 1: S56–63.

55. Kresina TF (2007) Medication assisted treatment of drug abuse and dependence: global availability and utilization. Recent Pat Antiinfect Drug Discov 2: 79–86.

56. Kimber J, Copeland L, Hickman M, Macleod J, McKenzie J, et al. (2010) Survival and cessation in injecting drug users: prospective observational study of outcomes and effect of opiate substitution treatment. BMJ 341: c3172.

57. Oviedo-Joekes E, Brissette S, Marsh DC, Lauzon P, Guh D, et al. (2009) Diacetylmorphine versus methadone for the treatment of opioid addiction. N Engl J Med 361: 777–786.

58. National Opinion Research Center General Social Surveys (GSS), 1972–2006. The National Data Program for the Sciences, University of Chicago.

59. Semaan S, Neumann MS, Hutchins K, D'Anna LH, Kamb ML (2010) Brief counseling for reducing sexual risk and bacterial STIs among drug users–results from project RESPECT. Drug Alcohol Depend 106: 7–15

60. Johnson RE, Chutuape MA, Strain EC, Walsh SL, Stitzer ML, et al. (2000) A comparison of levomethadyl acetate, buprenorphine, and methadone for opioid dependence. N Engl J Med 343: 1290–1297.

61. Sullivan LE, Moore BA, Chawarski MC, Pantalon MV, Barry D, et al. (2008) Buprenorphine/naloxone treatment in primary care is associated with decreased human immunodeficiency virus risk behaviors. J Subst Abuse Treat 35: 87–92.

62. Bayoumi AM, Zaric GS (2008) The cost-effectiveness of Vancouver's supervised injection facility. CMAJ 179: 1143–1151.

63. Marshall BD, Wood E, Zhang R, Tyndall MW, Montaner JS, et al. (2009) Condom use among injection drug users accessing a supervised injecting facility. Sex Transm Infect 85: 121–126.

64. Kapadia F, Latka MH, Wu Y, Strathdee SA, Mackesy-Amiti ME, et al. (2009) Longitudinal Determinants of Consistent Condom Use by Partner Type Among Young Injection Drug Users: The Role of Personal and Partner Characteristics. AIDS Behav.

65. Booth RE, Kwiatkowski CF, Chitwood DD (2000) Sex related HIV risk behaviors: differential risks among injection drug users, crack smokers, and injection drug users who smoke crack. Drug Alcohol Depend 58: 219–226.

66. Marks G, Crepaz N, Senterfitt JW, Janssen RS (2005) Meta-analysis of high-risk sexual behavior in persons aware and unaware they are infected with HIV in the United States: implications for HIV prevention programs. J Acquir Immune Defic Syndr 39: 446–453.

67. Weinhardt LS, Kelly JA, Brondino MJ, Rotheram-Borus MJ, Kirshenbaum SB, et al. (2004) HIV transmission risk behavior among men and women living with HIV in 4 cities in the United States. J Acquir Immune Defic Syndr 36: 1057–1066.

68. Brogly SB, Bruneau J, Lamothe F, Vincelette J, Franco EL (2002) HIV-positive notification and behavior changes in Montreal injection drug users. AIDS Educ Prev 14: 17–28.

69. Tsui JI, Vittinghoff E, Hahn JA, Evans JL, Davidson PJ, et al. (2009) Risk behaviors after hepatitis C virus seroconversion in young injection drug users in San Francisco. Drug Alcohol Depend 105: 160–163.

70. Ompad DC, Fuller CM, Vlahov D, Thomas D, Strathdee SA (2002) Lack of behavior change after disclosure of hepatitis C virus infection among young injection drug users in Baltimore, Maryland. Clin Infect Dis 35: 783–788.

71. Cox J, Morissette C, De P, Tremblay C, Allard R, et al. (2009) Access to sterile injecting equipment is more important than awareness of HCV status for injection risk behaviors among drug users. Subst Use Misuse 44: 548–568.

72. Pilcher CD, Fiscus SA, Nguyen TQ, Foust E, Wolf L, et al. (2005) Detection of acute infections during HIV testing in North Carolina. N Engl J Med 352: 1873–1883.

73. Farnham PG, Hutchinson AB, Sansom SL, Branson BM (2008) Comparing the costs of HIV screening strategies and technologies in health-care settings. Public Health Rep 123 Suppl 3: 51–62.

74. Juusola JL, Brandeau ML, Long EF, Owens DK, Bendavid E (2012) The cost-effectiveness of symptom-based testing and routine screening for acute HIV infection in men who have sex with men in the USA. AIDS 25: 1779–1787.

75. Office of the Medical Director (Updated January 2010) Diagnosis and Management of Acute HIV Infection. New York State Department of Health AIDS Institute. http://www.hivguidelines.org/clinical-guidelines/adults/diagnosis-and-management-of-acute-hiv-infection/.

76. Lundgren JD, Babiker A, El-Sadr W, Emery S, Grund B, et al. (2008) Inferior clinical outcome of the CD4+ cell count-guided antiretroviral treatment interruption strategy in the SMART study: role of CD4+ cell counts and HIV RNA levels during follow-up. J Infect Dis 197: 1145–1155.

77. El-Sadr WM, Lundgren JD, Neaton JD, Gordin F, Abrams D, et al. (2006) CD4+ count-guided interruption of antiretroviral treatment. N Engl J Med 355: 2283–2296.

78. Panel on Antiretroviral Guidelines for Adults and Adolescents (March 27, 2012) Guidelines for the use of antiretroviral agents in HIV-1-infected adults and adolescents. Available: http://www.aidsinfo.nih.gov/ContentFiles/AdultandAdolescentGL.pdf. Accessed: 2012 Jun 27.

79. Long EF, Brandeau ML, Owens DK (2009) Potential population health outcomes and expenditures of HIV vaccination strategies in the United States. Vaccine 27: 5402–5410.

80. Porco TC, Martin JN, Page-Shafer KA, Cheng A, Charlebois E, et al. (2004) Decline in HIV infectivity following the introduction of highly active antiretroviral therapy. AIDS 18: 81–88.

81. Granich RM, Gilks CF, Dye C, De Cock KM, Williams BG (2009) Universal voluntary HIV testing with immediate antiretroviral therapy as a strategy for elimination of HIV transmission: a mathematical model. Lancet 373: 48–57.

82. Del Romero J, Castilla J, Hernando V, Rodriguez C, Garcia S (2010) Combined antiretroviral treatment and heterosexual transmission of HIV-1: cross sectional and prospective cohort study. BMJ 340: c2205.

83. Castilla J, Del Romero J, Hernando V, Marincovich B, Garcia S, et al. (2005) Effectiveness of highly active antiretroviral therapy in reducing heterosexual transmission of HIV. J Acquir Immune Defic Syndr 40: 96–101.

84. Cohen MS, Chen YQ, McCauley M, Gamble T, Hosseinipour MC, et al. (2011) Prevention of HIV-1 infection with early antiretroviral therapy. N Engl J Med 365: 493–505.

85. Anglemyer A, Rutherford GW, Baggaley RC, Egger M, Siegfried N (2011) Antiretroviral therapy for prevention of HIV transmission in HIV-discordant couples. Cochrane Database Syst Rev: CD009153.

86. Donnell D, Baeten JM, Kiarie J, Thomas KK, Stevens W, et al. (2011) Heterosexual HIV-1 transmission after initiation of antiretroviral therapy: a prospective cohort analysis. Lancet 375: 2092–2098.

87. Bonkovsky HL, Tice AD, Yapp RG, Bodenheimer HC Jr, Monto A, et al. (2008) Efficacy and safety of peginterferon alfa-2a/ribavirin in methadone maintenance patients: randomized comparison of direct observed therapy and self-administration. Am J Gastroenterol 103: 2757–2765.

88. Van Thiel DH, Anantharaju A, Creech S (2003) Response to treatment of hepatitis C in individuals with a recent history of intravenous drug abuse. Am J Gastroenterol 98: 2281–2288.

89. Bureau of Economic Analysis U.S. Department of Commerce (2009) Implicit Price Deflators for Gross Domestic Product.

90. Meara E, White C, Cutler DM (2004) Trends in medical spending by age, 1963–2000. Health Aff (Millwood) 23: 176–183.

91. Hogan C, Lunney J, Gabel J, Lynn J (2001) Medicare beneficiaries' costs of care in the last year of life. Health Aff (Millwood) 20: 188–195.

92. Mark TL, Woody GE, Juday T, Kleber HD (2001) The economic costs of heroin addiction in the United States. Drug Alcohol Depend 61: 195–206.

93. Zarkin GA, Dunlap LJ, Homsi G (2004) The substance abuse services cost analysis program (SASCAP): a new method for estimating drug treatment services costs. Evaluation and Program Planning 27: 35–43.

94. Centers for Medicare & Medicaid Services (2009) Medicare Fee-for-Service Payment Schedule.

95. Schackman BR, Gebo KA, Walensky RP, Losina E, Muccio T, et al. (2006) The lifetime cost of current human immunodeficiency virus care in the United States. Med Care 44: 990–997.

96. Singer ME, Younossi ZM (2001) Cost effectiveness of screening for hepatitis C virus in asymptomatic, average-risk adults. Am J Med 111: 614–621.

97. Wong JB (2006) Hepatitis C: cost of illness and considerations for the economic evaluation of antiviral therapies. Pharmacoeconomics 24: 661–672.

98. Mitra D, Davis KL, Beam C, Medjedovic J, Rustgi V (2010) Treatment Patterns and Adherence among Patients with Chronic Hepatitis C Virus in a US Managed Care Population. Value Health 13(4): 479–86.

99. U.S. Preventive Services Task Force (2004) Screening for hepatitis C virus infection in adults: recommendation statement. Ann Intern Med 140: 462–464.

100. Nyman JA, Barleen NA, Dowd BE, Russell DW, Coons SJ, et al. (2007) Quality-of-life weights for the US population: self-reported health status and priority health conditions, by demographic characteristics. Med Care 45: 618–628.

101. Sullivan PW, Ghushchyan V (2006) Preference-Based EQ-5D index scores for chronic conditions in the United States. Med Decis Making 26: 410–420.

102. Dijkgraaf MG, van der Zanden BP, de Borgie CA, Blanken P, van Ree JM, et al. (2005) Cost utility analysis of co-prescribed heroin compared with methadone maintenance treatment in heroin addicts in two randomised trials. BMJ 330: 1297.

103. Tengs TO, Lin TH (2002) A meta-analysis of utility estimates for HIV/AIDS. Med Decis Making 22: 475–481.

104. Simpson KN, Luo MP, Chumney E, Sun E, Brun S, et al. (2004) Cost-effectiveness of lopinavir/ritonavir versus nelfinavir as the first-line highly active antiretroviral therapy regimen for HIV infection. HIV Clin Trials 5: 294–304.

105. Schackman BR, Goldie SJ, Freedberg KA, Losina E, Brazier J, et al. (2002) Comparison of health state utilities using community and patient preference weights derived from a survey of patients with HIV/AIDS. Med Decis Making 22: 27–38.

106. Kauf TL, Roskell N, Shearer A, Gazzard B, Mauskopf J, et al. (2008) A predictive model of health state utilities for HIV patients in the modern era of highly active antiretroviral therapy. Value Health 11: 1144–1153.

107. Thein HH, Krahn M, Kaldor JM, Dore GJ (2005) Estimation of utilities for chronic hepatitis C from SF-36 scores. Am J Gastroenterol 100: 643–651.

108. Cotler SJ, Patil R, McNutt RA, Speroff T, Banaad-Omiotek G, et al. (2001) Patients' values for health states associated with hepatitis C and physicians' estimates of those values. Am J Gastroenterol 96: 2730–2736.

109. Honiden S, Sundaram V, Nease RF, Holodniy M, Lazzeroni LC, et al. (2006) The effect of diagnosis with HIV infection on health-related quality of Life. Qual Life Res 15: 69–82.

110. Rodger AJ, Jolley D, Thompson SC, Lanigan A, Crofts N (1999) The impact of diagnosis of hepatitis C virus on quality of life. Hepatology 30: 1299–1301.

111. Kelly JA, Morin SF, Remien RH, Steward WT, Higgins JA, et al. (2009) Lessons learned about behavioral science and acute/early HIV infection. The NIMH Multisite Acute HIV Infection Study: V. AIDS Behav 13: 1068–1074.

112. Stekler J, Swenson PD, Wood RW, Handsfield HH, Golden MR (2005) Targeted screening for primary HIV infection through pooled HIV-RNA testing in men who have sex with men. AIDS 19: 1323–1325.

113. Pilcher CD, McPherson JT, Leone PA, Smurzynski M, Owen-O'Dowd J, et al. (2002) Real-time, universal screening for acute HIV infection in a routine HIV counseling and testing population. JAMA 288: 216–221.

114. Alter MJ (2005) Integrating risk history screening and HCV testing into clinical and public health settings. Am Fam Physician 72: 576, 579.

115. (1998) Recommendations for prevention and control of hepatitis C virus (HCV) infection and HCV-related chronic disease. Centers for Disease Control and Prevention. MMWR Recomm Rep 47: 1–39.

116. Sanders GD, Bayoumi AM, Sundaram V, Bilir SP, Neukermans CP, et al. (2005) Cost-effectiveness of screening for HIV in the era of highly active antiretroviral therapy. N Engl J Med 352: 570–585.

117. Paltiel AD, Walensky RP, Schackman BR, Seage GR 3rd, Mercincavage LM, et al. (2006) Expanded HIV screening in the United States: effect on clinical outcomes, HIV transmission, and costs. Ann Intern Med 145: 797–806.

118. Stein K, Dalziel K, Walker A, Jenkins B, Round A, et al. (2003) Screening for hepatitis C in genito-urinary medicine clinics: a cost utility analysis. J Hepatol 39: 814–825.

119. Stein K, Dalziel K, Walker A, Jenkins B, Round A, et al. (2004) Screening for Hepatitis C in injecting drug users: a cost utility analysis. J Public Health (Oxf) 26: 61–71.

120. Thompson Coon J, Castelnuovo E, Pitt M, Cramp M, Siebert U, et al. (2006) Case finding for hepatitis C in primary care: a cost utility analysis. Fam Pract 23: 393–406.

121. Sutton AJ, Edmunds WJ, Sweeting MJ, Gill ON (2008) The cost-effectiveness of screening and treatment for hepatitis C in prisons in England and Wales: a cost-utility analysis. J Viral Hepat 15: 797–808.

122. Tramarin A, Gennaro N, Compostella FA, Gallo C, Wendelaar Bonga LJ, et al. (2008) HCV screening to enable early treatment of hepatitis C: a mathematical model to analyse costs and outcomes in two populations. Curr Pharm Des 14: 1655–1660.

123. Grebely J, Conway B, Raffa JD, Lai C, Krajden M, et al. (2006) Hepatitis C virus reinfection in injection drug users. Hepatology 44: 1139–1145.

124. Burt RD, Thiede H, Hagan H (2009) Serosorting for hepatitis C status in the sharing of injection equipment among Seattle area injection drug users. Drug Alcohol Depend 105: 215–220.

125. Mizuno Y, Purcell DW, Latka MH, Metsch LR, Ding H, et al. (2010) Is sexual serosorting occurring among HIV-positive injection drug users? Comparison between those with HIV-positive partners only, HIV-negative partners only, and those with any partners of unknown status. AIDS Behav 14: 92–102.

126. Steward WT, Remien RH, Higgins JA, Dubrow R, Pinkerton SD, et al. (2009) Behavior change following diagnosis with acute/early HIV infection-a move to serosorting with other HIV-infected individuals. The NIMH Multisite Acute HIV Infection Study: III. AIDS Behav 13: 1054–1060.

127. Patel P, Mackellar D, Simmons P, Uniyal A, Gallagher K, et al. Detecting acute human immunodeficiency virus infection using 3 different screening immunoassays and nucleic acid amplification testing for human immunodeficiency virus RNA, 2006–2008. Arch Intern Med 170: 66–74.

128. Stekler JD, Swenson PD, Coombs RW, Dragavon J, Thomas KK, et al. (2009) HIV testing in a high-incidence population: is antibody testing alone good enough? Clin Infect Dis 49: 444–453.

129. Hightow-Weidman LB, Golin CE, Green K, Shaw EN, MacDonald PD, et al. (2009) Identifying people with acute HIV infection: demographic features, risk factors, and use of health care among individuals with AHI in North Carolina. AIDS Behav 13: 1075–1083.

130. Beckwith CG, Cornwall AH, Dubrow R, Chapin K, Ducharme R, et al. (2009) Identifying acute HIV infection in Rhode Island. Med Health R I 92: 231–233.

131. Dubrow R, Sikkema KJ, Mayer KH, Bruce RD, Julian P, et al. (2009) Diagnosis of acute HIV infection in Connecticut. Conn Med 73: 325–331.

132. Brown LS Jr, Kritz SA, Goldsmith RJ, Bini EJ, Rotrosen J, et al. (2006) Characteristics of substance abuse treatment programs providing services for HIV/AIDS, hepatitis C virus infection, and sexually transmitted infections: the National Drug Abuse Treatment Clinical Trials Network. J Subst Abuse Treat 30: 315–321.

133. Knudsen HK, Oser CB (2009) Availability of HIV-related health services in adolescent substance abuse treatment programs. AIDS Care 21: 1238–1246.

134. Strauss SM, Astone-Twerell JM, Munoz-Plaza C, Des Jarlais DC, Gwadz M, et al. (2006) Hepatitis C knowledge among staff in U.S. drug treatment programs. J Drug Educ 36: 141–158.

135. Remien RH, Higgins JA, Correale J, Bauermeister J, Dubrow R, et al. (2009) Lack of understanding of acute HIV infection among newly-infected persons-implications for prevention and public health: The NIMH Multisite Acute HIV Infection Study: II. AIDS Behav 13: 1046–1053.

136. Report of the workgroup on intravenous drug abuse (1988) Report of the Second Public Health Service AIDS Prevention and Control Conference. Public Health Rep 103 Suppl 1: 66–71.

137. Tempalski B, Lieb S, Cleland CM, Cooper H, Brady JE, et al. (2009) HIV prevalence rates among injection drug users in 96 large US metropolitan areas, 1992–2002. J Urban Health 86: 132–154.

138. Alary M, Joly JR, Vincelette J, Lavoie R, Turmel B, et al. (2005) Lack of evidence of sexual transmission of hepatitis C virus in a prospective cohort study of men who have sex with men. Am J Public Health 95: 502–505.

139. Rauch A, Rickenbach M, Weber R, Hirschel B, Tarr PE, et al. (2005) Unsafe sex and increased incidence of hepatitis C virus infection among HIV-infected men who have sex with men: the Swiss HIV Cohort Study. Clin Infect Dis 41: 395–402.

140. Stroffolini T, Lorenzoni U, Menniti-Ippolito F, Infantolino D, Chiaramonte M (2001) Hepatitis C virus infection in spouses: sexual transmission or common exposure to the same risk factors? Am J Gastroenterol 96: 3138–3141.

141. Vandelli C, Renzo F, Romano L, Tisminetzky S, De Palma M, et al. (2004) Lack of evidence of sexual transmission of hepatitis C among monogamous couples: results of a 10-year prospective follow-up study. Am J Gastroenterol 99: 855–859.

142. Kao JH, Liu CJ, Chen PJ, Chen W, Lai MY, et al. (2000) Low incidence of hepatitis C virus transmission between spouses: a prospective study. J Gastroenterol Hepatol 15: 391–395.

143. Sasase N, Kim SR, Kudo M, Kim KI, Taniguchi M, et al. (2010) Outcome and early viral dynamics with viral mutation in PEG-IFN/RBV therapy for chronic hepatitis in patients with high viral loads of serum HCV RNA genotype 1b. Intervirology 53: 49–54.

144. Ferenci P (2004) Predicting the therapeutic response in patients with chronic hepatitis C: the role of viral kinetic studies. J Antimicrob Chemother 53: 15–18.

145. Bailey SL, Ouellet LJ, Mackesy-Amiti ME, Golub ET, Hagan H, et al. (2007) Perceived risk, peer influences, and injection partner type predict receptive syringe sharing among young adult injection drug users in five U.S. cities. Drug Alcohol Depend 91 Suppl 1: S18–29.

146. Heller DI, Paone D, Siegler A, Karpati A (2009) The syringe gap: an assessment of sterile syringe need and acquisition among syringe exchange program participants in New York City. Harm Reduct J 6: 1.

147. (2000) Preventing blood-borne infections among injection drug users: A comprehensive approach. Academy for Educational Development.

148. Booth RE, Campbell BK, Mikulich-Gilbertson SK, C JT, Choi D, et al. (2010) Reducing HIV-Related Risk Behaviors Among Injection Drug Users in Residential Detoxification. AIDS Behav.

149. Beardsley M, Deren S, Tortu S, Goldstein MF, Ziek K, et al. (1999) Trends in injection risk behaviors in a sample of New York City injection drug users: 1992–1995. J Acquir Immune Defic Syndr Hum Retrovirol 20: 283–289.

150. Buchanan D, Tooze JA, Shaw S, Kinzly M, Heimer R, et al. (2006) Demographic, HIV risk behavior, and health status characteristics of "crack" cocaine injectors compared to other injection drug users in three New England cities. Drug Alcohol Depend 81: 221–229.

151. Longshore D, Annon J, Anglin MD (1998) Long-term trends in self-reported HIV risk behavior: injection drug users in Los Angeles, 1987 through 1995. J Acquir Immune Defic Syndr Hum Retrovirol 18: 64–72.

152. DeSimone J (2005) Needle exchange programs and drug infection behavior. J Policy Anal Manage 24: 559–577.

153. Latkin CA, Buchanan AS, Metsch LR, Knight K, Latka MH, et al. (2008) Predictors of sharing injection equipment by HIV-seropositive injection drug users. J Acquir Immune Defic Syndr 49: 447–450.

154. Burt RD, Hagan H, Garfein RS, Sabin K, Weinbaum C, et al. (2007) Trends in hepatitis B virus, hepatitis C virus, and human immunodeficiency virus prevalence, risk behaviors, and preventive measures among Seattle injection drug users aged 18–30 years, 1994–2004. J Urban Health 84: 436–454.

155. Centers for Disease Control and Prevention (2004) HIV Testing Survey, 2002. Atlanta: U.S. Deptmant of Health and Human Servies, Centers for Disease Control and Prevention. Available: http://www.cdc.gov/hiv/stats/hasrsupp.htm.

156. Weis SH, Leschek JD, Gary PW, MD (2003) HIV Era Occupational Exposures and Risks. AIDS and Other Manifestations of HIV Infection (Fourth Edition). San Diego: Academic Press. 811–838.

157. Kaplan EH, Heimer R (1992) A model-based estimate of HIV infectivity via needle sharing. J Acquir Immune Defic Syndr 5: 1116–1118.

158. Chung H, Kudo M, Kumada T, Katsushima S, Okano A, et al. (2003) Risk of HCV transmission after needlestick injury, and the efficacy of short-duration interferon administration to prevent HCV transmission to medical personnel. J Gastroenterol 38: 877–879.

159. Hamid SS, Farooqui B, Rizvi Q, Sultana T, Siddiqui AA (1999) Risk of transmission and features of hepatitis C after needlestick injuries. Infect Control Hosp Epidemiol 20: 63–64.

6

Pharmacological Treatment of Painful HIV-Associated Sensory Neuropathy: A Systematic Review and Meta-Analysis of Randomised Controlled Trials

Tudor J. C. Phillips[1]*, Catherine L. Cherry[2,3,4], Sarah Cox[5], Sarah J. Marshall[6], Andrew S. C. Rice[1]

1 Department of Anaesthetics, Pain Medicine and Intensive Care, Imperial College London, Chelsea and Westminster Hospital Campus, London, United Kingdom, 2 Centre for Virology, Burnet Institute, Melbourne, Australia, 3 Infectious Diseases Unit, Alfred Hospital, Melbourne, Australia, 4 Department of Medicine, Monash University, Melbourne, Australia, 5 Chelsea and Westminster NHS Foundation Trust, London, United Kingdom, 6 East Kent Hospitals University Foundation Trust and Pilgrims Hospices, Kent, United Kingdom

Abstract

Background: Significant pain from HIV-associated sensory neuropathy (HIV-SN) affects ~40% of HIV infected individuals treated with antiretroviral therapy (ART). The prevalence of HIV-SN has increased despite the more widespread use of ART. With the global HIV prevalence estimated at 33 million, and with infected individuals gaining increased access to ART, painful HIV-SN represents a large and expanding world health problem. There is an urgent need to develop effective pain management strategies for this condition.

Method and Findings: Objective: To evaluate the clinical effectiveness of analgesics in treating painful HIV-SN. Design: Systematic review and meta-analysis. Data sources: Medline, Cochrane central register of controlled trials, www.clinicaltrials.gov, www.controlled-trials.com and the reference lists of retrieved articles. Selection criteria: Prospective, double-blinded, randomised controlled trials (RCTs) investigating the pharmacological treatment of painful HIV-SN with sufficient quality assessed using a modified Jadad scoring method. Review methods: Four authors assessed the eligibility of articles for inclusion. Agreement of inclusion was reached by consensus and arbitration. Two authors conducted data extraction and analysis. Dichotomous outcome measures ($\geq$30% and $\geq$50% pain reduction) were sought from RCTs reporting interventions with statistically significant efficacies greater than placebo. These data were used to calculate RR and NNT values.

Results: Of 44 studies identified, 19 were RCTs. Of these, 14 fulfilled the inclusion criteria. Interventions demonstrating greater efficacy than placebo were smoked cannabis NNT 3.38 95%CI(1.38 to 4.10), topical capsaicin 8%, and recombinant human nerve growth factor (rhNGF). No superiority over placebo was reported in RCTs that examined amitriptyline (100mg/day), gabapentin (2.4g/day), pregabalin (1200mg/day), prosaptide (16mg/day), peptide-T (6mg/day), acetyl-L-carnitine (1g/day), mexilitine (600mg/day), lamotrigine (600mg/day) and topical capsaicin (0.075% q.d.s.).

Conclusions: Evidence of efficacy exists only for capsaicin 8%, smoked cannabis and rhNGF. However, rhNGF is clinically unavailable and smoked cannabis cannot be recommended as routine therapy. Evaluation of novel management strategies for painful HIV-SN is urgently needed.

Editor: Nitika Pant Pai, McGill University Health Center, Canada

Funding: The investigator TJCP was funded by a grant from The Derek Butler Trust (UK Reg Charity 1081995). The funders had no role in study design, data collection and analysis, decision to publish, or preparation of the manuscript.

Competing Interests: ASCR has received fees and associated expenses for research-related consultancy services contracted via Imperial College Consultants from Pfizer, Eisai, Solvay, Spinifex, Organon, Lectus Astellas, Alergan, GSK, NeuroGsx, Esteve and Daiichi Sankyo. ASCR is a member of the EU funded Innovative Medicines Initiative grant "Europain" in which a number of pharmaceutical companies are also participating: Astra-Zeneca, Esteve, Boehinger-Ingelheim, Pfizer, Eli Lilly, GlaxoSmithKline, Wyeth, UCB and Sanofi Aventis. ASCR has also received a research grant from Pfizer; CLC has had investigator initiated research grants from GlaxoSmithKline, Roche Australia and Zymes LLC; CLC is also on the advisory boards of Gilead Science and BMS Australia Virology, honoraria for both have been donated to charity. CLC undertakes consultancy work and is a principle investigator on two clinical studies for CNS Bio; TJCP, SM and SC have no financial interests that may be relevant to the submitted work.

* E-mail: a.rice@imperial.ac.uk

Introduction

HIV-associated distal sensory neuropathy (HIV-SN) is a frequently occurring neurological complication of HIV infection. HIV-SN prevalence has increased despite (or because of) the introduction of otherwise successful antiretroviral therapy [1]. HIV-SN is one of the most prevalent problems experienced by people receiving antiretroviral therapy and the associated pain has a major impact on quality of life in otherwise largely healthy individuals. HIV-SN is a distal symmetrical axonal, predominantly sensory polyneuropathy that affects the feet and less frequently the hands. HIV-SN is comprised of at least two clinically indistinguishable, and often coexisting, neuropathies: A distal sensory polyneuropathy associated with HIV disease itself (HIV-DSP), and a distal sensory polyneuropathy associated with antiretroviral treatment, Antiretroviral toxic neuropathy (HIV-ATN). HIV-DSP was recognised early in the HIV pandemic [2] and is associated with advanced HIV disease [1] [3]. HIV-ATN was initially observed following the introduction of particular nucleoside reverse transcriptase inhibitors (NRTI) – stavudine, didanosine and zalcitabine - the 'dNRTIs' [4–5]. The presence of sensory neuropathic symptoms in an ARV naïve patient is highly suggestive of HIV -DSP. Often only a temporal association between the onset of symptoms and the starting of a particular ARV agent gives the only hint as to aetiology, as in most other clinical respects the two are almost identical.

The introduction of combination antiretroviral therapy (cART) in the mid 1990s dramatically reduced the morbidity and mortality associated with HIV among patients who have access to treatment [6]. Life expectancy with HIV in well-resourced countries is now estimated to be up to two-thirds that of the general population [7–8]. While the incidence of most neurological complications of HIV has fallen with the introduction of effective therapy, rates of HIV-SN have been rising since the first effective antiretroviral drugs were developed [9]. Recent estimates of HIV-SN prevalence among cohorts with access to cART range from 20% [10] to >50% [11]. Importantly, the available evidence suggests that HIV-SN prevalence remains high among cART-treated patients, even in countries where known neurotoxic antiretroviral drugs such as stavudine are no longer commonly used. Depending on the population surveyed, HIV-SN, regardless of previous ARV exposure, has a prevalence of between 13% [12] and >50% [13–14] of HIV infected individuals, of whom 40% experience severe pain, $\geq 5/10$ Numeric Pain Rating Scale (NPRS), and 90% experiencing some pain, which can be severely debilitating [1]. In less well-resourced centres, use of stavudine, an inexpensive and effective antiretroviral, in first-line HIV treatment remains common despite the high risk of neurotoxicity [15].

Importantly two recent studies have emphasised the continued and growing global impact of HIV-SN. A large cross-sectional study of 598 HIV infected individuals in South Africa, reported that the frequency of symptomatic HIV-SN increases from 23% to 40% following exposure to ART therapy, with 60% being symptomatic if previously exposed to stavudine [16]. Another large cross-sectional study from the US studying 1539 HIV infected individuals has reported that 57%(881) demonstrated evidence of the presence of HIV-SN, with 38% of these individuals reporting pain [17].

Current estimates of global HIV prevalence stand at 33 million, with 2.7 new infections each year and more patients gaining access to cART [15]. With high rates of HIV-SN now reported globally, and up to 90% of affected patients experiencing potentially debilitating neuropathic pain, HIV-SN represents a large and potentially worsening source of global HIV-related morbidity. There is an urgent need to understand better the pathogenesis of HIV-SN, to identify risk factors, and identify and implement effective preventative and pain management strategies.

Evidence-based guidelines for the pharmacological management of neuropathic pain tend to focus on a "blanket" approach of recommending therapies across the spectrum of neuropathic pain, irrespective of the underlying condition [18–19]. Recent NICE guidance for the management of neuropathic pain in "non-specialist settings" have adopted this approach [20]. This may not be appropriate for HIV-SN for three main reasons. Firstly, neuropathic pain is a heterogeneous phenomenon, both within and across underlying conditions, and evidence obtained from the study of an analgesic in one condition cannot necessarily be applied to another [21–22]. Secondly, in high, middle and low income countries the pain associated with HIV-SN will usually be managed outside of specialist pain management clinics, so appropriate, disease specific guidance may be required. Finally, there are a number of randomised controlled trials (RCTs) conducted in HIV-SN, which were not identified in the NICE guidance. Therefore, we have conducted a systematic review and meta-analysis to elucidate the evidence base for pharmacological management of neuropathic pain in HIV-SN.

Methods

Eligibility, data sources and search strategy

In accordance with PRISMA [23], we sought to identify RCTs that included patients with painful HIV-SN and reported at least one clinically relevant pain outcome measure.

A systematic search, without language restrictions, was conducted on 20 June 2008, and a follow-up search on 22 February 2010, with the following databases: Medline (from 1966 to date searched), The Cochrane central register of controlled trials (Cochrane Library 2010, Issue 2), www.clinicaltrials.gov (a US registry of clinical trials) and www.controlled-trials.com (a meta-registry of controlled trials). Search terms used were: "HIV" "AIDS" "pain" "painful" "neuropathy" "neuropathic", in combination with "random" "randomised" and "double-blinded". Further trials were identified by hand searching the reference lists of identified trials and review articles, relevant NICE guidelines and Health Technology Assessment reports.

Study selection and risk of bias assessment

We excluded animal studies, reviews, letters, abstract-only trials, open-label trials, and trials that were not randomised. The identified RCTs then underwent independent quality assessment by four authors (TJCP, CLC, SC and ASCR) using a 7-point modified "Jadad" scoring system that assessed the presence and quality of double-blinding, randomisation, study size and reporting of withdrawal and drop outs [24–25]. RCTs with a score of less than five points and studies that enrolled fewer than five HIV-SN patients were excluded from the systematic review. Scoring discrepancies between authors were resolved through discussion and consensus; with final arbitration by ASCR.

Data extraction

Data were extracted from eligible RCTs by one author (TJCP). Data extracted included: year of publication; study design and duration; study sample population and characteristics; withdrawals; interventions; doses; pain and non-pain related primary and secondary outcome measures; and adverse events.

Where possible, dichotomous pain improvement outcome data were extracted from RCTs that reported efficacy superior to placebo. Intention to treat (ITT) responder rates for 30% and 50% pain relief were sought for the longest follow-up period reported in each study. If required, authors were contacted for missing or unreported data.

RCTs in which the primary pain outcome of a studied intervention did not show efficacy greater than placebo in the intention to treat population, were not included in subsequent analyses.

Statistical analysis

For each intervention the extracted dichotomous outcomes were used to calculate numbers needed to treat (NNT) by two authors (TJCP and ASCR), with 95% confidence intervals for 30% and 50% pain improvement responders. We originally planned to access heterogeneity according to the method of

Armitage & Berry [26], and visually [27] however as only three studies were used in the meta-analysis, this was felt to be inappropriate. Similarly, a sensitivity analysis was not performed, as there were insufficient data. All calculations were undertaken using Microsoft Excel 2007.

Results

We identified 44 potentially relevant articles (Figure 1). Twenty-five articles were excluded after screening identified these as being a review article, letter, open-label study, case report or other non-

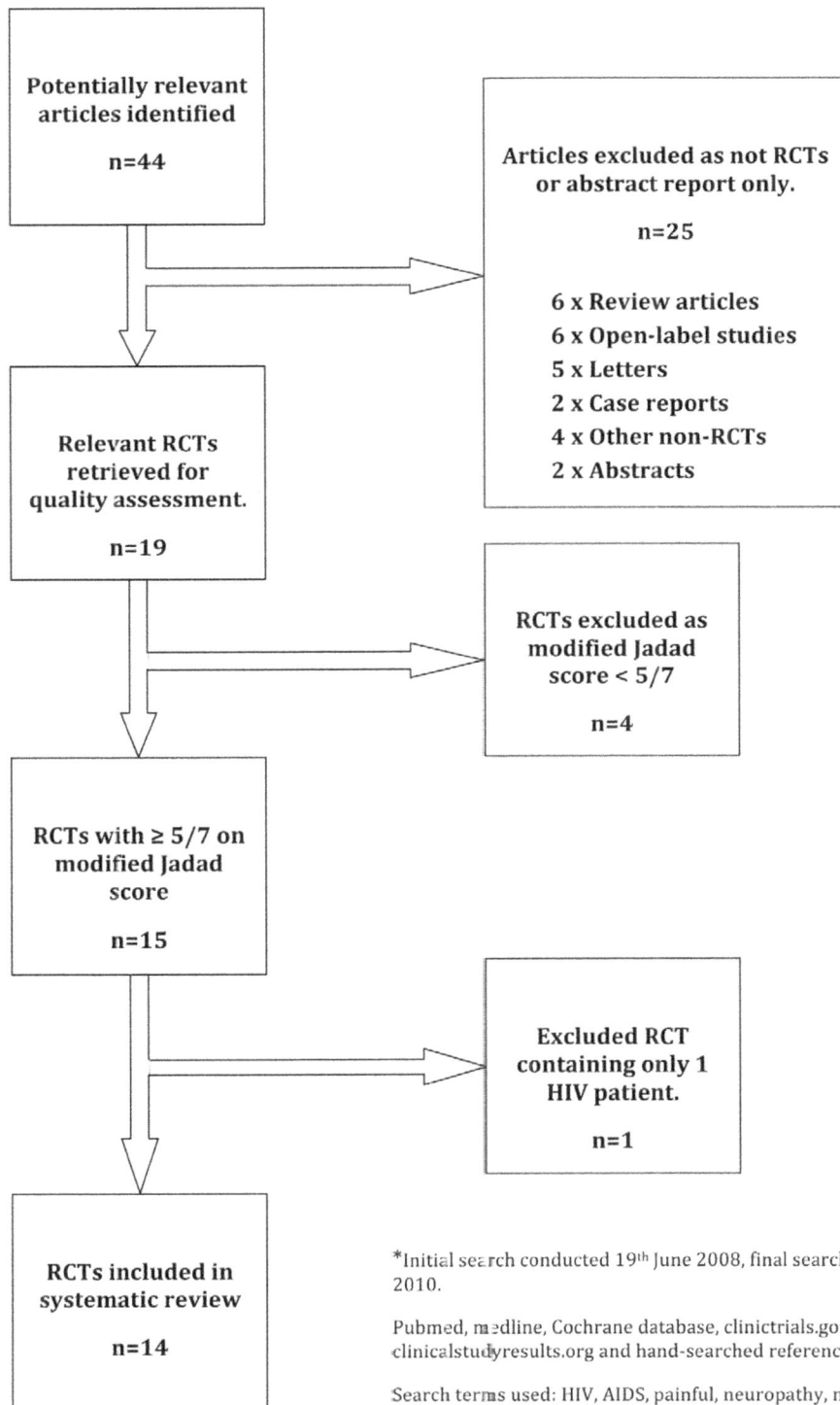

Figure 1. PRISMA flow diagram of included randomized controlled trials.

RCT study. The remaining 19 RCTs were retrieved and independently reviewed by four authors (TJCP, CLC, SC and ASCR). Four articles were excluded at this stage by scoring <5 out of 7-points with the modified Jadad score. A further RCT was excluded as having <5 HIV-SN patients enrolled. Details of these excluded RCTs, and therefore of interventions that must be regarded as not having been adequately tested, are shown in Table 1.

The remaining 14 RCTs were retained for further analysis (Table 2). Of the 14 trials retained for further analysis, 13 were of a parallel group design and one a cross-over design. All were placebo controlled with one using "active" placebo [28]. Data extraction was for the longest follow-up period reported by the article. In most cases this was to the end of the treatment phase, except for a study of a topical 8% capsaicin [28] that reported data for 12 weeks after a single treatment application.

In two studies [29] and [30] no reference to ITT analysis was made. In one of these RCTs studying topical capsaicin 0.075% efficacy [29] no primary outcome data were published, as it was reported that no superiority to placebo was seen. In a study of lamotrigine efficacy [31] only a per protocol (PP) population data

Table 1. Studies excluded from the analysis.

Reference	Treatment	Primary Reason for Exclusion
[37]	Acetyl-L-carnitine	Review
[61]	Acetyl-L-carnitine	Review
[43]	Cannabinoids	Review
[62]	Lamotrigine	Review
[63]	Antidepressants	Review
[64]	Herbal medicine	Review
[44]	8% capsaicin patch	Open-label
[45]	8% capsaicin patch	Abstract
[33]	Acetyl-L-carnitine	Open-label
[34]	Acetyl-L-carnitine	Open-label
[65]	Recombinant human NGF	Open-label
[66]	Flecainide	Open-label
[67]	5% lidocaine patch	Open-label
[68]	Acupuncture	Letter
[69]	Acupuncture	Letter
[70]	Acupuncture	Letter
[46]	Gabapentin	Letter
[47]	Gabapentin	Letter
[49]	Gabapentin	Case report
[71]	Prednisolone	Case report
[48]	Gabapentin	Abstract
[42]	Smoked cannabis	Other non-RCT
[35]	Acetyl-L-carnitine	Other non-RCT
[72]	Acupuncture	Other non-RCT
[32]	Acetyl-L-carnitine	Other non-RCT
[73]	5% lidocaine patch	Modified Jadad score <5
[74]	Mexiletine	Modified Jadad score <5
[75]	Memantine	Modified Jadad score <5
[76]	Nimodipine	Modified Jadad score <5
[52]	Lamotrigine	<5 patients enrolled

analysis was undertaken. This was reported to show no superiority over placebo; however no primary outcome data were reported.

Of the four trials that reported superiority of an intervention over placebo, three reported dichotomous pain outcome measures. Where possible we used responder rate data for ≥30% and ≥50% improvement in pain as measured using Visual Analogue Scale (VAS) or Numerical Pain Rating Scale (NPRS). These data were requested from the authors if they had not been reported.

Acetyl –L-carnitine

Whilst acetyl-L-carnitine has been the subject of six articles [32–37] in the treatment of painful HIV-SN, only one was an RCT [36] and eligible for inclusion. This was a parallel group trial of acetyl-L-carnitine (1000mg/day) and placebo intramuscular injections. In this RCT acetyl-L-carnitine, in an analysis of the PP population, showed a modest superiority to placebo. However an analysis of the ITT population did not show superiority to placebo: mean change in VAS (0–10cm)(SD) from baseline to the end of week 2: acetyl-L-carnitine −1.32 (1.84); placebo −0.61 (1.55) p = 0.07. Consequently we undertook no further analysis of this trial.

Amitriptyline and Mexilitine

Two trials [38] and [39] that were included studied the efficacy of amitriptyline. Both trials compared amitriptyline to placebo and another intervention. One RCT [38] examined efficacy of amitriptyline as part of a trial also assessing acupuncture treatment. However despite being described as a parallel group, placebo controlled RCT, its design was complex. Consequently the results of this trial are difficult to evaluate. In particular bias may have been introduced because of unconventional randomisation procedures and because true placebo controls were not used. Specifically, patients were allowed to 'opt-out' of being randomised to the amitriptyline arms of the trial based on personal preference. In addition, many participants included in the analysis of amitriptyline efficacy, had also received acupuncture or sham acupuncture, further complicating analysis. Ignoring the methodological concerns, amitriptyline demonstrated no superiority to placebo in the primary outcome measure. The mean change in Gracely pain scores from baseline to week 14 was −0.26 with amitriptyline (maximum dose 75mg/day) and −0.30 with placebo. The difference between amitriptyline and placebo was: 0.00 95%CI(−0.18 to 0.19) p = 0.99.

The second trial [39] compared amitriptyline, mexilitine and placebo. This trial was terminated early following an interim review of results. It was deemed by the trial monitoring board that further enrolment into the study was unlikely to detect significant differences in either amitriptyline or mexilitine arms compared to placebo. No superiority was reported in reducing mean Gracely pain scores (SD) from baseline to the end of treatment week 8 for: amitriptyline (maximum dose 100mg/day) −0.31 (0.31); mexilitine −0.23 (0.41); compared to placebo −0.20 (0.30).

Smoked Cannabis

The original literature search found four articles related to cannabinoid use and painful HIV-SN. Only two were RCTs [40–41]. The excluded articles included one clinical survey [42] and one review article [43].

One of these included articles [41] was a cross-over study that compared the efficacy of smoked cannabis (maximum tolerated dose 1 to 8% Δ-9-tetrahydrocannabinol q.d.s.) to placebo cigarettes in reducing subjects pain measured using the Descriptor Differential Scale (DDS). The DDS is a ratio scale (0 to 20) containing 24 words describing pain intensity and unpleasantness.

Table 2. Characteristics and results of included studies.

Reference	Participants recruited (completed)	Design and duration	Intervention (n = patient episodes)	Maximum dose studied	Primary Outcome	Data (ITT)	Superior to placebo?
Youle M et al 2007 [36]	90(76)	Parallel: 2 wks	Acetyl-L-carnitine 500 mg bd i.m. (n=43); placebo (n=47)	1000mg/day	VAS (0–10cm) change: baseline to wk 2.	ITT: Acetyl-L-carnitine: −1.32 (SD 1.84); placebo −0.61 (SD 1.55)(p=0.07)	No
Shlay JC et al 1998 [38]	136 (105)	Parallel: 14 wks	Amitriptyline (n=71); placebo (n=65)	75mg/day	GP score: change baseline to wk 14.	ITT with LOCF: Amitriptyline: −0.26; placebo: −0.30;difference 0.00 95%CI (−0.18 to 0.19)(p=0.99)	No
Paice JA et al 2000 [29]	26(14)	Parallel:4 wks.	Capsaicin 0.075% cream q.d.s. (n=15); placebo (n=11)	0.075% q.d.s.	NRS (0–10): change from baseline to wk 4.	No numeric data given. Stated no statistically significant difference between capsaicin 0.075% and placebo (p>0.05)	No
Simpson DM et al 2008 [28]	307(274)	Parallel: 12 wks follow-up.	Capsaicin 8% patch for 30min (n=72); 60min (n=78); 90min (n=75); placebo (capsaicin 0.04%) (n=82)	8% for 90min.	NPRS: % change baseline to wk 12.	ITT with LOCF: Capsaicin: −22.8 (SD 30.6); placebo −10.7 (SD 30.8); (p=0.0026)	Yes
Abrams DI et al 2007 [40]	55(50)	Parallel: 5 days	Smoked cannabis (n=27); placebo (n=28)	3.56% Δ-9- tetrahydrocannabinol t.d.s.	VAS: % change from baseline to day 5.	ITT: Cannabis: −34% (IQR −71 to −16); placebo −17% (IQR − 29 to 8) (p=0.03)	Yes
Ellis RJ et al 2009 [41]	34(27)	Crossover: 5 days, 2 wks washout, 5 days treatment.	Smoked cannabis (n=28); placebo (n=28)	Max tolerable: 1 to 8% Δ-9-tetrahydrocannabinol q.d.s.	DDS (0–20): median change from baseline to day 5.	Difference in DDS reduction cannabis vs placebo for PP: −3.3 p=0.016, no data for ITT: said to be 'similar' with p=0.020	Yes
Hahn K et al 2004 [30]	26(24)	Parallel: 4 wks treatment.	Gabapentin (n=15); placebo (n=11)	2400mg/day	VAS: median change: baseline to wk 4.	Gabapentin: −44.1; placebo: −29.8. Stated as being not statistically significant.	No
Simpson DM et al 2010 [50]	302(241)	Parallel: 14 wks treatment.	Pregabalin (n=151); placebo (n=151)	1200mg/day	NPRS: mean change: baseline to wk 14.	ITT: Pregabalin: −2.88; placebo −2.63 (p=0.39)	No
Simpson DM et al 2000 [51]	42(29)	Parallel: 14 wks treatment	Lamotrigine (n=20); placebo (n=22)	300mg/day	GP score: mean change: baseline to wk 14.	ITT with LOCF: Lamotrigine: −0.242 (SE 0.092); placebo: −0.183 (SE 0.087) (p=0.65)	No
Simpson et al 2003 [31]	227(172)	Parallel:12 wks treatment.	Lamotrigine (n=150); placebo (n=77)	600mg/day	GP score: change: baseline to wk 12.	PP: Lamotrigine vs placebo. No data given, stated no statistically significant difference seen in all or ARV stratum.	No
Keiburtz K et al 1998 [39]	145(104)	Parallel: 8 wks	Mexilitine (n=48); amitriptyline (n=47) placebo (n=50)	Mexilitine: 300mg/day Amitriptyline: 100mg/day	GP score: mean change: baseline to wk 8.	ITT: Amitriptyline: −0.31 (SD 0.31); mexilitine: −0.23 (SD 0.41); placebo −0.20 (SD 0.30) No p value given, stated no statistical significance	No
McArthur JC et al 2000 [53]	270(235)	Parallel:18 wks	Recombinant human NGF (n = 180); placebo (n = 90)	0.3μg/kg s.c. twice weekly	GP score: median change: baseline to wk 18.	ITT with LOCF: NGF 0.1μg/kg: −0.18 (−0.10 to −0.25)(p=0.05); NGF 0.3μg/kg: −0.21 (−0.14 to −0.29)(p=0.04); placebo: 0.06 (+0.01 to −0.14)	Yes
Simpson DM et al 1996 [54]	104(81)	Parallel: 12 wks	Peptide-T (n=40); placebo (n=41)* PP data	6mg/day intranasal	Modified GP score: mean change: baseline to wk 12.	PP: Peptide-T: −0.24 (±0.45); placebo −0.39 (±0.19) (p=0.32). ITT results not presented but stated showed the 'same pattern'.	No

GP - Gracely Pain Score, VAS – Visual Analogue Scale, ITT – Intention To Treat population, PP -Per Protocol population, NRS – Numerical Rating Scale, NPRS- Numerical Pain Rating Scale, DDS – Descriptor Differential Scale, LOCF - Last Observation Carried Forward.

Smoked cannabis was reported to be superior to placebo in reducing DDS from baseline to end of treatment day five in the PP population. The median difference between cannabis and placebo was −3.3 out of 20; p = 0.016. No data were reported for the ITT analysis, however the authors stated that the PP analysis was similar to the ITT analysis with p = 0.02. VAS data not reported by the authors, but was supplied on request, relating to cannabis and placebo subjects who reported a ≥30% (18/34 and 7/34 respectively) and ≥50% (13/34 and 4/34 respectively) improvement in pain intensity.

This trial reported a high proportion of inadvertent unblinding amongst subjects following dose titration with smoked cannabis cigarettes in the treatment arms, but not with placebo cigarettes.

A second study [40] compared smoked cannabis (3.56% Δ-9-tetrahydrocannabinol t.d.s.) to placebo cigarettes in a parallel group RCT. Smoked cannabis was shown to be superior to placebo in reducing pain from baseline to end of treatment day 5 in the ITT analysis: cannabis −34% (IQR −71 to −16), placebo −17% (IQR −29 to 8) p = 0.03. More subjects reported ≥30% VAS improvement with smoked cannabis compared to the placebo: 13/27 and 6/27 respectively.

Inclusion into the study required subjects to have had previous exposure to cannabis, with current users asked to discontinue prior to the study. Of note no attempt was made to assess unintentional unblinding during the course of the study, which may have been high due to subjects' previous experience with smoked cannabis.

Using the ITT analysis dichotomous VAS data from both trials, an NNT for smoked cannabis was calculated as 3.38 95%CI (2.19 to 7.50) (Table 3)

Topical Capsaicin

Four trials [44] [29] [28] and [45] were found that assessed topical capsaicin efficacy in painful HIV-SN. Two reports were excluded from further analysis; one was an open-label study [28] and the other has been reported in abstract form only [45]. Of the included trials, one [29] examined the efficacy of topical capsaicin 0.075% cream in a parallel group RCT. The authors stated that no superiority of capsaicin 0.075% over placebo in mean improvement in a numeric rating score (NRS) (0–10) was seen, however only graphical data were presented.

A second study [28] examined topical capsaicin 8%. Patients received either the 8% patch or an active placebo (capsaicin 0.04%) in a single application lasting either 30, 60 or 90 minutes.

Following this single application patients were followed-up for 12 weeks. Capsaicin 8% was found to be superior to placebo in the percentage reduction of the NPRS (SD) from baseline to week 2 to 12: 8% capsaicin: −22.8 (30.6); compared to placebo: −10.7 (30.8), (p = 0.0026). The study also reported responder rates as percentage of patients measured on the NPRS who experienced ≥30% mean reduction in pain: capsaicin 8%: 76/225; placebo (capsaicin 0.04%): 15/82; p = 0.0092. It is not possible to calculate an NNT that is strictly comparable to those calculated for other studies included in this review since the placebo control used here was not pharmacologically inactive. However, as an informative exercise using these data, and presuming that the control capsaicin 0.04% is a true placebo, an NNT of 6.46 95%CI(3.86–19.69) was calculated for treatment with capsaicin 8% patch.

Gabapentin

Only one retrieved report related to treatment of painful HIV-SN with gabapentin was an RCT. Four additional articles were excluded. Two were letters [46–47] one an abstract [48], and one a case series [49]. The included study [30] compared gabapentin (titrated to a maximum of 2400mg/day) to placebo in a parallel group RCT. At the longest treatment period assessed, no difference in efficacy was reported between gabapentin and placebo groups for the primary outcome measure, median change in VAS (0–100mm) baseline to end of week 4: gabapentin: −44.1, placebo: −29.8. No indication of variance or p value was documented.

It is noteworthy that this trial demonstrated an unusual placebo response. The placebo subjects' pain VAS baseline remained unchanged for the first two weeks, after which a stronger placebo response followed to week 4. This unusual placebo response may have contributed to the apparent superiority of gabapentin over placebo at week 2, which was not evident at week 4.

Pregabalin

One large multi-centre RCT [50] examined the efficacy of pregabalin, titrated over 2 weeks to a maximum tolerated dose up to 1200mg/day, in a multicentre, 14 week parallel group, placebo controlled RCT. No superiority of pregabalin over placebo in the primary pain outcome measure was reported: mean change in NPRS baseline to end of week 14: pregabalin −2.88; placebo −2.63, p = 0.39.

Table 3. Summary of RCTs which demonstrated treatment superior to placebo, for which Relative Risk and Number Needed to Treat values could be calculated.

	Active Treatment (maximum tested dose)	Number of patient Episodes	Benefit Efficacy on Treatment (≥30% improvement VAS	Efficacy on Placebo (≥30% improvement VAS)	RR (95% CI)	NNT (95% CI)
Smoked cannabis						
Abrams et al 2007 [40]	Smoked cannabis: 3.56% Δ-9-tetrahydrocannabinol	55 (50)	13/27	6/28	2.17 (0.97 to 4.86)	3.86 (1.98 to 71.11)
Ellis et al 2009 [41]	Smoked cannabis: 8% Δ-9-tetrahydro-cannabinol	68 (56)	18/34	7/34	2.57 (1.24 to 5.35)	3.09 (1.98 to 9.30)
Abrams et al [40]+Ellis et al [41]	Combined smoked cannabis studies	122 (106)	31/61	15/61	2.38 (1.38 to 4.10)	3.38 (2.19 to 7.50)

Lamotrigine

Three trials assessing the efficacy of lamotrigine in painful HIV-SN were identified [51,52] and [29,31]. One trial [52], enrolled only one painful HIV-SN patient (to the placebo control group) and was therefore excluded from further analysis. The included lamotrigine trials [51] and [31] were both conducted by the same group; with [51] being smaller and preceding [31]. The smaller study [51] did demonstrate some efficacy superior to placebo when the primary outcome for the PP population was analysed. However in the ITT analysis with 'last value carried forward' (LVCF), lamotrigine was not superior to placebo: improvement in mean Gracely pain score (SE): lamotrigine: -0.242 (0.009); placebo: -0.183 (0.087); (p = 0.65). The large number of drop-outs in the lamotrigine group (n = 11 of 20) compared to placebo (n = 3 of 22) suggest a narrow therapeutic index and make interpretation of the trial results difficult.

Similarly the larger trial [31], where participants were stratified according to previous exposure to neurotoxic ARVs, did not demonstrate a superiority of lamotrigine over placebo for the primary outcome measure (mean improvement in Gracely pain score) in the total cohort or in either stratum. However lamotrigine did show superiority to placebo in the neurotoxic ARV-exposed stratum in a secondary outcome measure, mean improvement in VAS (0–100mm) baseline to end of treatment: lamotrigine: -27.1; compared to placebo: -9.0; p = 0.003.

For each stratum the number of responders ($\geq 30\%$ improvement in VAS) were calculated from the published data. For the neurotoxic ARV stratum: lamotrigine 36/62, placebo 7/30 (p = 0.02) and for no exposure to neurotoxic ART: lamotrigine 46/88, placebo 21/47. As an informative exercise using these data the NNT for lamotrigine was calculated for each stratum, and for the overall trial. Subjects with exposure to neurotoxic ARVs: 2.88 95%CI(1.84 to 6.57); no exposure to neurotoxic ARVs: 13.17 95%CI(3.96 to -9.95) and for the unstratified population: 6.09 95%CI(3.51 to 23.08)(Not included in Table 3 as no superiority of lamotrigine over placebo was demonstrated for any primary endpoint).

NGF

One RCT [53] examined the efficacy of subcutaneous recombinant human Nerve Growth Factor (rhNGF) in the treatment of painful HIV-SN. This study assessed two doses (0.1 and 0.3μg/kg) given twice weekly compared with placebo for 18 weeks. rhNGF was superior to placebo for the primary outcome measure in the ITT analysis; median change of the Gracely pain score from baseline to end of week 18: rhNGF 0.1μg/kg: -0.18 (-0.10 to -0.25) p = 0.05, 0.3μg/kg: -0.21 (-0.14 to -0.29) p = 0.04, and placebo: 0.06 (+0.01 to -0.14).

No significant dose effect was reported and no differential effect was seen based on baseline stratification of subjects according to neurotoxic ARV drug exposure. As rhNGF was reported to be associated with myalgia, there may have been inadvertent breaking of the blinding.

Dichotomous data were requested from the authors however we were unable to calculate RR and NNT values for rhNGF from the data provided.

Prosaptide and Peptide –T

Two trials [54,55] examined the efficacy of the novel agents in placebo controlled parallel group RCTs. One [55] reported the use of subcutaneous prosaptide (maximum dose of 16mg/day) over 6 treatment weeks and did not report efficacy superior to placebo in the primary outcome measure; mean change in Gracely pain score baseline to week 6. The study was terminated after a planned interim futility analysis. Another trial [54] studied efficacy of intranasal peptide T (maximum dose 6mg/day), over 12 treatment weeks, but reported no superiority over placebo in the primary outcome measure; mean change in a modified Gracely pain score baseline to end of week 12.

Discussion

This systematic review found that RCT evidence of analgesic efficacy superior to placebo in the context of HIV-SN pain exists only for smoked cannabis, rhNGF and high dose (8%) topical capsaicin. Several other agents have been examined in high quality RCTs and found to be no more effective than placebo for managing HIV-SN pain in the doses examined, specifically acetyl-L carnitine (1g/day), amitriptyline (100mg/day), topical capsaicin 0.075%, gabapentin (2.4g/day), mexilitine (600mg/day), peptide – T (6mg/day), pregabalin(1200mg/day), lamotrigine (600mg/day) and prosaptide (16mg/day). Therefore, there is evidence that both of the first line therapies (pregabalin and amitriptyline) recommended in the NICE guidance for non-specialist management of neuropathic pain show no superiority to placebo in the management of pain in HIV-SN [20].

Of the pharmacological interventions shown to be effective for HIV-SN in RCTs, only topical capsaicin 8% is currently approved for marketing for neuropathic pain indications. In Europe 8% capsaicin has been approved for the treatment of peripheral neuropathic pain in non-diabetic adults, whilst the U.S. Food and Drug Administration (FDA) has approved its use only for the indication of post herpetic neuralgia. However, it should also be borne in mind that we located a preliminary report (conference abstract only and therefore excluded from the systematic review) of another parallel group RCT which included 494 patients with HIV-SN in which topical 8% capsaicin was compared to 0.04% topical capsaicin [45]. No analgesic superiority of 8% capsaicin over 0.04% was demonstrated. rhNGF therapy is not currently clinically available and both legal and mental health issues preclude routine recommendation of long term smoked cannabis for pain management [56].

This systematic review represents a comprehensive review of the literature relating to the pharmacological management of painful HIV-SN. It used a predefined protocol for the initial literature search, data extraction and analysis. There was also strict adherence to inclusion quality criteria as assessed by four independent authors using the modified Jadad score, a tool that assesses each study for potential bias as well as evaluating study power.

This systematic review was limited by the paucity of high quality RCTs examining pharmacological treatment of painful HIV-SN. Additionally the heterogeneity of the included studies design and size made evaluation and comparison of trials difficult. In particular, use of the Gracely pain scale (GPS) in five of the 15 included RCTs made evaluation and inter-study comparison complicated. The GPS is a log unit pain outcome measure that is not a frequently used measure outside trials of HIV-SN. In a recent consensus statement regarding core chronic pain outcome measures [57] it was not one of the recommended pain scales. Several of the studies utilising the Gracely pain score also included more validated secondary pain outcome measures such as either a VAS score or a NPRS. These were used here in preference to the Gracely pain score in the calculation of NNT and RR.

The Jadad tool has been validated and used widely to identify common and major sources of experimental bias in RCTs identified in systematic reviews. Nevertheless, whilst the use of the modified Jadad score improves the probability that only high quality RCTs were included in the systematic review, its use may conceivably have biased our systematic review in favour of more recently tested agents. The RCTs associated with these agents now routinely report the information required by the modified Jadad tool, because of the nature of the evolution of RCT methodology over the past few years.

Both of the RCTs that examined the efficacy of smoked cannabis, were of high quality, however the apparent marked superiority of smoked cannabis to placebo cigarettes should be tempered by the high proportion of potential unblinding measured in [41] (92% correctly guessing treatment allocation after treatment crossover), and its lack of measurement in [40] despite participants having all had previous experience of smoked cannabis. In a similar manner, the RCT investigating recombinant human NGF demonstrated a high degree of unblinding related to injection site myalgia, which when accounted for in a separate analysis reported a more attenuated treatment-related difference which consequently lost statistical significance.

Lamotrigine was the subject of two high quality RCTs. Both failed to show superiority over placebo in the primary pain outcome measure, improvement in the GPS in the ITT population. However, in the larger of the two RCTs, analysis of a secondary pain outcome measure, mean improvement in VAS, did demonstrate efficacy superior to placebo in the subpopulation of subjects who had been previously exposed to neurotoxic ARTs. If this stratum alone is examined an NNT of 2.88 is calculated.

Most of the included RCTs did not stratify subjects with painful HIV-SN according to their exposure to neurotoxic ARTs. This stratification was instrumental in demonstrating an efficacy of lamotrigine in neurotoxic ART exposed painful HIV-SN subjects. It is possible to speculate that a similar strategy of stratifying other RCTs might have elucidated other agents with sub-group efficacy, despite lack of observed analgesic efficacy in an unstratified painful HIV-SN subject population. Additionally, the included RCTs were not uniform in their approach to the use of concomitant analgesics; whilst most allowed continued use of drugs at stable doses, two elected to stop them [30] [58]. The use of such concomitant analgesics, and also the inclusion of participants with previously failed therapies, may conceivably have influenced the outcomes of these RCTs.

Gabapentin and pregabalin were the subject of two high quality RCTs in which neither agent was shown to be superior to placebo. This contrasts with the efficacy of these agents demonstrated in other peripheral neuropathic pain conditions [20] [59] [18,19]. However the gabapentin study was small, with only 30 patients randomised [30]. This finding may therefore represent a 'failed trial' rather than a true lack of efficacy.

Amitriptyline efficacy was examined in two large RCTs. The evaluation of one study [38] was made difficult by a complicated study design that may have not been truly randomised or placebo controlled. However the finding that amitriptyline did not display superior analgesic efficacy than placebo in the context of HIV-SN is supported by a similar finding a second, higher quality RCT [39]. Again, this finding directly contrasts with evidence of efficacy for tricyclic antidepressants in a range of other peripheral neuropathic pain conditions [20] [59] [19] [18].

Capsaicin 0.075% cream was the subject of a small RCT enrolling only 26 subjects. The authors stated that capsaicin 0.075% did not demonstrate statistically significant superiority to placebo in the primary pain outcome measure. However, outcome data were published only in a graphical representation of mean current pain scores from baseline to the end of treatment. From this graph there does appear to be a trend for capsaicin to be superior to placebo at this final time point measured at week 4.

However a high drop-out rate in both arms resulted in only 6/11 patients remaining in the capsaicin group, and only 8/15 in the placebo group. It is therefore difficult to determine from this study if capsaicin 0.075% was indeed without efficacy. This has two implications: the first being that capsaicin 0.075% might have some degree of clinically relevant efficacy in painful HIV-SN; and secondly, if capsaicin 0.075% is indeed efficacious, then the use of a similar concentration (capsaicin 0.04%) as an active placebo in the large capsaicin 8% patch RCT would change the design of this study from a placebo controlled to a superiority approach.

In the treatment of painful HIV-SN, the lack of efficacy compared with placebo of many agents with proven efficacy in other forms of neuropathic pain has implications in the understanding of neuropathic pain in general. These findings further support the hypothesis that neuropathic pain cannot be considered as a single symptom with a single pathogenesis [21,22]. A more mechanistic approach to the treatment of specific types of neuropathic pain is therefore warranted as has been established in trigeminal neuralgia and post herpetic neuralgia. Equally, caution should be exercised in the use of neuropathic pain treatment algorithms that do not consider these potential mechanistic differences, as their rationale may be fundamentally flawed.

The absence of studies examining the efficacy of opioid use in painful HIV-SN is notable and mandates additional research. Opioids have shown efficacy in other neuropathic pain conditions [18] [59] [19]. Furthermore, the efficacy of duloxetine in diabetic neuropathy, a condition that has similarities to HIV-SN, may suggest that it is worth investigating [20]. In addition, the efficacy of cannabis in HIV-SN would suggest that cannabinoids with an appropriate therapeutic index when delivered by a mechanism other than smoking might be worthy of investigation [56].

Conclusions

On the basis of current published evidence, topical capsaicin 8%, smoked cannabis and Nerve Growth Factor have evidence of efficacy in pain associated with HIV-SN. However this is potentially contentious, as a recent larger RCT, currently reported in abstract form only, has suggested this treatment is not superior to placebo [45]. Some commonly recommended analgesics, including opioids, have not been formally studied for the management of painful HIV-SN.

The current evidence base available for the treatment of painful HIV-SN is at odds with the recommendations made by NICE for neuropathic pain management in the non-specialist situation. This indicates the potential dangers of extrapolating efficacy from one neuropathic pain condition to another where efficacy has not been directly assessed. In particular amitriptyline, pregabalin, and gabapentin have been demonstrated to have no superiority to placebo in the treatment of painful HIV-SN.

With an estimated 33 million people living with HIV and more gaining access to ARV every day, the management of HIV-SN associated neuropathic pain is a problem of major global significance. There is an urgent need for the development of effective, evidence based analgesic strategies for this common condition. Gene microarrays have been used to identify novel drug targets [60]. Ongoing evaluation of both novel analgesics and existing untested strategies for HIV-SN is a clear research priority.

Author Contributions

Conceived and designed the experiments: ASCR. Performed the experiments: TP CC SC SJM ASCR. Analyzed the data: TP ASCR. Wrote the paper: TP CC SC ASCR.

References

1. Smyth K, Affandi JS, McArthur JC, Bowtell-Harris C, Mijch AM, et al. (2007) Prevalence of and risk factors for HIV-associated neuropathy in Melbourne, Australia 1993–2006. HIV Med 8: 367–373.

2. Lipkin WI, Parry G, Kiprov D, Abrams D (1985) Inflammatory neuropathy in homosexual men with lymphadenopathy. Neurology 35: 1479–1483.

3. Barohn R, Gronseth G, Leforce B, McVey A, McGuire A, et al. (1993) Peripheral nerve involvement in a large cohort of human immunodeficiency virus-infected individuals. Arch Neurol 50: 167–171.

4. Blum AS, Dal Pan GJ, Feinberg J, Raines C, Mayjo K, et al. (1996) Low-dose zalcitabine-related toxic neuropathy: frequency, natural history, and risk factors. Neurology 46: 999–1003.

5. Yarchoan R, Perno CF, Thomas RV, Klecker EW, Allain JF, et al. (1988) Phase I studies of 2',3'-dideoxycytidine in severe human immunodeficiency virus infection as a single agent and alternating with zidovudine (AZT). Lancet 1: 76–81.

6. Mocroft A, Ledergerber B, Katlama C, Kirk O Reiss P, et al. (2003) Decline in the AIDS and death rates in the EuroSIDA study: an observational study. Lancet 362: 22–29.

7. Antiretroviral Therapy Cohort Collaboration (2008) Life expectancy of individuals on combination antiretroviral therapy in high-income countries: a collaborative analysis of 14 cohort studies. Lancet 372 293–299.

8. Lohse N, Hansen AB, Pedersen G, Kronborg G Gerstoft J, et al. (2007) Survival of persons with and without HIV infection in Denmark, 1995–2005. Ann Intern Med 146: 87–95.

9. Bacellar H, Muñoz A, Miller EN, Cohen BA, Besley D, et al. (1994) Temporal trends in the incidence of HIV-1-related neurologic diseases Multicenter AIDS Cohort Study, 1985–1992. Neurology 44: 1892–1900.

10. Wright E, Brew B, Arayawichanont A, Robertson K, Samintharapanya K, et al. (2008) Neurologic disorders are prevalent in HIV-positive outpatients in the Asia-Pacific region. Neurology 71: 50–56.

11. Konchalard K, Wangphonpattanasiri K (2007) Clinical and electrophysiologic evaluation of peripheral neuropathy in a group of HIV-infected patients in Thailand. J Med Assoc Thai 90: 774–781.

12. Lichtenstein KA, Armon C, Baron A, Moorman AC, Wood KC, et al. (2005) Modification of the incidence of drug-associated symmetrical peripheral neuropathy by host and disease factors in the HIV outpatient study cohort. Clin Infect Dis 40: 148–157.

13. Morgello S, Estanislao L, Simpson D, Geraci A, DiRocco A, et al. (2004) HIV-associated distal sensory polyneuropathy in the era of highly active antiretroviral therapy: the Manhattan HIV Brain Bank. Arch Neurol 61: 546–551.

14. Simpson DM, Kitch D, Evans SR, McArthur JC, Asmuth DM, et al. (2006) HIV neuropathy natural history cohort study: assessment measures and risk factors. Neurology 66: 1679–1687.

15. UNAIDS JUNPOH (2009) AIDS epidemic update, December 2009. AIDS epidemic update, December 2009. www.unaids.org.

16. Maritz J, Benatar M, Dave JA, Harrison TB, Badri M, et al. (2010) HIV neuropathy in South Africans: frequency, characteristics, and risk factors. Muscle Nerve 41: 599–606.

17. Ellis RJ, Rosario D, Clifford DB, McArthur JC, Simpson D, et al. (2010) Continued high prevalence and adverse clinical impact of human immunodeficiency virus-associated sensory neuropathy in the era of combination antiretroviral therapy: the CHARTER Study. Arch Neurol 67: 552–558.

18. Finnerup NB, Sindrup SH, Jensen TS (2010) The evidence for pharmacological treatment of neuropathic pain. Pain 150: 573–581.

19. Dworkin RH, O'Connor AB, Backonja M, Farrar JT, Finnerup NB, et al. (2007) Pharmacologic management of neuropathic pain: evidence-based recommendations. Pain 132: 237–251.

20. Tan T, Barry P, Reken S, Baker M, Guideline Development Group (2010) Pharmacological management of neuropathic pain in non-specialist settings: summary of NICE guidance. BMJ 340: c1079.

21. Baron R, Tölle TR, Gockel U, Brosz M, Freynhagen R (2009) A cross-sectional cohort survey in 2100 patients with painful diabetic neuropathy and postherpetic neuralgia: Differences in demographic data and sensory symptoms. Pain 146: 34–40.

22. Scholz J, Mannion RJ, Hord DE, Griffin RS, Rawal B, et al. (2009) A novel tool for the assessment of pain: validation in low back pain. PLoS Med 6: e1000047.

23. Liberati A, Altman DG, Tetzlaff J, Mulrow C, Gøtzsche PC, et al. (2009) The PRISMA statement for reporting systematic reviews and meta-analyses of studies that evaluate health care interventions: explanation and elaboration. PLoS Med 6: e1000100.

24. Rice ASC, Lever IJ, Zarnegar R (2008) Cannabinoids and analgesia, with special reference to neuropathic pain. In: McQuay HJ, Kalso E, Moore RA, eds. Reviews and Meta-Analyses in Pain. Seattle: IASP Press. 233 p.

25. Jadad AR, Moore RA, Carroll D, Jenkinson C, Reynolds DJ, et al. (1996) Assessing the quality of reports of randomized clinical trials: is blinding necessary? Control Clin Trials 17: 1–12.

26. Armitage P, Berry G (1990) Statistical methods in medical research. Oxford: Blackwell Scientific Publications.

27. L'Abbé KA, Detsky AS, O'Rourke K (1987) Meta-analysis in clinical research. Ann Intern Med 107: 224–233.

28. Simpson DM, Brown S, Tobias J, NGX-4010 C107 Study Group (2008) Controlled trial of high-concentration capsaicin patch for treatment of painful HIV neuropathy. Neurology 70: 2305–2313.

29. Paice JA, Ferrans CE, Lashley FR, Shott S, Vizgirda V, et al. (2000) Topical capsaicin in the management of HIV-associated peripheral neuropathy. J Pain Symptom Manage 19: 45–52.

30. Hahn K, Arendt G, Braun JS, von Giesen HJ, Husstedt IW, et al. (2004) A placebo-controlled trial of gabapentin for painful HIV-associated sensory neuropathies. J Neurol 251: 1260–1266.

31. Simpson DM, McArthur JC, Olney R, Clifford D, So Y, et al. (2003) Lamotrigine for HIV-associated painful sensory neuropathies: a placebo-controlled trial. Neurology 60: 1508–1514.

32. Hart AM, Wilson AD, Montovani C, Smith C, Johnson M, et al. (2004) Acetyl-l-carnitine: a pathogenesis based treatment for HIV-associated antiretroviral toxic neuropathy. AIDS 18: 1549–1560.

33. Osio M, Muscia F, Zampini L, Nascimbene C, Maillard E, et al. (2006) Acetyl-l-carnitine in the treatment of painful antiretroviral toxic neuropathy in human immunodeficiency virus patients: an open label study. J Peripher Nerv Syst 11: 72–76.

34. Scarpini E, Sacilotto G, Baron P, Cusini M, Scarlato G (1997) Effect of acetyl-L-carnitine in the treatment of painful peripheral neuropathies in HIV+ patients. J Peripher Nerv Syst 2: 250–252.

35. Herzmann C, Johnson MA, Youle M (2005 Long-term effect of acetyl-L-carnitine for antiretroviral toxic neuropathy. HIV Clin Trials 6: 344–350.

36. Youle M, Osio M, ALCAR Study Group (2007) A double-blind, parallel-group, placebo-controlled, multicentre study of acetyl L-carnitine in the symptomatic treatment of antiretroviral toxic neuropathy in patients with HIV-1 infection. HIV Med 8: 241–250.

37. Chiechio S, Copani A, Gereau RW, Nicoletti F (2007) Acetyl-L-carnitine in neuropathic pain: experimental data. CNS Drugs 21 Suppl 1: 31–8; discussion 45–6.

38. Shlay JC, Chaloner K, Max MB, Flaws B, Reichelderfer P, et al. (1998) Acupuncture and amitriptyline for pain due to HIV-related peripheral neuropathy: a randomized controlled trial. Terry Beirn Community Programs for Clinical Research on AIDS. JAMA 280: 1590–1595.

39. Kieburtz K, Simpson D, Yiannoutsos C, Max MB, Hall CD, et al. (1998) A randomized trial of amitriptyline and mexiletine for painful neuropathy in HIV infection. AIDS Clinical Trial Group 242 Protocol Team. Neurology 51: 1682–1688.

40. Abrams DI, Jay CA, Shade SB, Vizoso H, Reda H, et al. (2007) Cannabis in painful HIV-associated sensory neuropathy: a randomized placebo-controlled trial. Neurology 68: 515–521.

41. Ellis RJ, Toperoff W, Vaida F, van den Brande G, Gonzales J, et al. (2009) Smoked medicinal cannabis for neuropathic pain in HIV: a randomized, crossover clinical trial. Neuropsychopharmacology 34: 672–680.

42. Woolridge E, Barton S, Samuel J, Osorio J, Dougherty A, et al. (2005) Cannabis use in HIV for pain and other medical symptoms. J Pain Symptom Manage 29: 358–367.

43. Beaulieu P, Ware M (2007) Reassessment of the role of cannabinoids in the management of pain. Curr Opin Anaesthesiol 20: 473–477.

44. Simpson DM, Estanislao L, Brown SJ, Sampson J (2008) An open-label pilot study of high-concentration capsaicin patch in painful HIV neuropathy. J Pain Symptom Manage 35: 299–306.

45. Clifford D, Simpson D, Brown S, Moyle G, Brew B, et al. (2010) A multicenter, randomized, double-blind, controlled study of NGX-4010 (Qutenza®), a high concentration capsaicin patch for the treatment of HIV-associated distal sensory polyneuropathy. 17th Conference on Retroviruses and Opportunistic Infections Feb 16–19th 2010 Abstract #411 – accessible at www.retroconference.org/2010/Abstracts/37371.htm.

46. Valdivelu N (1999) Neuropathic pain after anti-HIV gene therapy successfully treated with gabapentin. J Pain Symptom Manage. 1999 Mar;17(3): 155–6. 1999 Mar: 155–156.

47. Newshan G (1998) HIV neuropathy treated with gabapentin. (letter). AIDS 12: 219–221.

48. Gatti, Antonella; Jann, Stefano; Sandro, et al. (1998) Gabapentin in the Treatment of Distal Symmetric Axonopathy in HIV Infected Patients.[Abstract]. Neurology 50: A216.

49. La Spina I, Porazzi D, Maggiolo F, Bottura P Suter F (2001) Gabapentin in painful HIV-related neuropathy: a report of 19 patients, preliminary observations. Eur J Neurol 8: 71–75.

50. Simpson DM, Schifitto G, Clifford DB, Murphy TK, Durso-De Cruz E, et al. (2010) Pregabalin for painful HIV neuropathy: a randomized, double-blind, placebo-controlled trial. Neurology 74: 413–420.

51. Simpson DM, Olney R, McArthur JC, Khan A, Godbold J, et al. (2000) A placebo-controlled trial of lamotrigine for painful HIV-associated neuropathy. Neurology 54: 2115–2119.

52. Silver M, Blum D, Grainger J, Hammer AE, Quessy S (2007) Double-blind, placebo-controlled trial of lamotrigine in combination with other medications for neuropathic pain. J Pain Symptom Manage 34: 446–454.

53. McArthur JC, Yiannoutsos C, Simpson DM, Adornato BT, Singer EJ, et al. (2000) A phase II trial of nerve growth factor for sensory neuropathy associated

with HIV infection. AIDS Clinical Trials Group Team 291. Neurology 54: 1080–1088.

54. Simpson DM, Dorfman D, Olney RK, McKinley G, Dobkin J, et al. (1996) Peptide T in the treatment of painful distal neuropathy associated with AIDS: results of a placebo-controlled trial. The Peptide T Neuropathy Study Group. Neurology 47: 1254–1259.

55. Evans SR, Simpson DM, Kitch DW, King A, Clifford DB, et al. (2007) A randomized trial evaluating Prosaptide for HIV-associated sensory neuropathies: use of an electronic diary to record neuropathic pain. PLoS ONE 2: e551.

56. Rice AS (2008) Should cannabinoids be used as analgesics for neuropathic pain? Nat Clin Pract Neurol 4: 654–655.

57. Dworkin RH, Katz J, Gitlin MJ (2005) Placebo response in clinical trials of depression and its implications for research on chronic neuropathic pain. Neurology 65: S7–19.

58. Evans SR, Simpson DM, Kitch DW, King A, Clifford DB, et al. (2007) A randomized trial evaluating Prosaptide for HIV-associated sensory neuropathies: use of an electronic diary to record neuropathic pain. PLoS ONE 2: e551.

59. Hempenstall K, Nurmikko TJ, Johnson RW, A'Hern RP, Rice AS (2005) Analgesic therapy in postherpetic neuralgia: a quantitative systematic review. PLoS Med 2: e164.

60. Maratou K, Wallace VC, Hasnie FS, Okuse K, Hosseini R, et al. (2009) Comparison of dorsal root ganglion gene expression in rat models of traumatic and HIV-associated neuropathic pain. Eur J Pain 13: 387–398.

61. Youle M (2007) Acetyl-L-carnitine in HIV-associated antiretroviral toxic neuropathy. CNS Drugs 21 Suppl 1: 25–30; discussion 45–6.

62. Wiffen PJ, Rees J (2007) Lamotrigine for acute and chronic pain. Cochrane Database Syst Rev. pp CD006044.

63. Saarto T, Wiffen PJ (2007) Antidepressants for neuropathic pain. Cochrane Database Syst Rev. pp CD005454.

64. Liu JP, Manheimer E, Yang M (2005) Herbal medicines for treating HIV infection and AIDS. Cochrane Database Syst Rev. pp CD003937.

65. Schifitto G, Yiannoutsos C, Simpson DM, Adornato BT, Singer EJ, et al. (2001) Long-term treatment with recombinant nerve growth factor for HIV-associated sensory neuropathy. Neurology 57: 1313–1316.

66. von Gunten CF, Eappen S, Cleary JF, Taylor SG, Moots P, et al. (2007) Flecainide for the treatment of chronic neuropathic pain: a Phase II trial. Palliat Med 21: 667–672.

67. Dorfman D, Dalton A, Khan A, Markarian Y, Scarano A, et al. (1999) Treatment of painful distal sensory polyneuropathy in HIV-infected patients with a topical agent: results of an open-label trial of 5% lidocaine gel. AIDS 13: 1589–1590.

68. King SA (1999) Acupuncture and amitriptyline for HIV-related peripheral neuropathic pain. JAMA 281: 1271–1272.

69. Ulett GA (1999) Acupuncture and amitriptyline for HIV-related peripheral neuropathic pain. JAMA 281: 1270–1; author reply 1271–2.

70. Kaptchuk TJ (1999) Acupuncture and amitriptyline for HIV-related peripheral neuropathic pain. JAMA 281: 1270; author reply 1271–1270; author reply 1272.

71. Bradley WG, Verma A (1996) Painful vasculitic neuropathy in HIV-1 infection: relief of pain with prednisone therapy. Neurology 47: 1446–1451.

72. Phillips KD, Skelton WD, Hand GA (2004) Effect of acupuncture administered in a group setting on pain and subjective peripheral neuropathy in persons with human immunodeficiency virus disease. J Altern Complement Med 10: 449–455.

73. Estanislao L, Carter K, McArthur J, Olney R, Simpson D, Lidoderm-HIV Neuropathy Group (2004) A randomized controlled trial of 5% lidocaine gel for HIV-associated distal symmetric polyneuropathy. J Acquir Immune Defic Syndr 37: 1584–1586.

74. Kemper CA, Kent G, Burton S, Deresinski SC (1998) Mexiletine for HIV-infected patients with painful peripheral neuropathy: a double-blind, placebo-controlled, crossover treatment trial. J Acquir Immune Defic Syndr Hum Retrovirol 19: 367–372.

75. Schifitto G, Yiannoutsos CT, Simpson DM, Marra CM, Singer EJ, et al. (2006) A placebo-controlled study of memantine for the treatment of human immunodeficiency virus-associated sensory neuropathy. J Neurovirol 12: 328–331.

76. Navia BA, Dafni U, Simpson D, Tucker T, Singer E, et al. (1998) A phase I/II trial of nimodipine for HIV-related neurologic complications. Neurology 51: 221–228.

7

Effect of Genital Herpes on Cervicovaginal HIV Shedding in Women Co-Infected with HIV AND HSV-2 in Tanzania

Jim Todd[1]*, **Gabriele Riedner**[1,2], **Leonard Maboko**[2], **Michael Hoelscher**[3], **Helen A. Weiss**[1], **Eligius Lyamuya**[4], **David Mabey**[1], **Mary Rusizoka**[2], **Laurent Belec**[5,6], **Richard Hayes**[1]

1 Department of Population Health, London School of Hygiene & Tropical Medicine, London, United Kingdom, 2 National Institute for Medical Research - Mbeya Medical Research Programme, Mbeya, Tanzania, 3 Department of Infectious Diseases and Tropical Medicine, Klinikum, Ludwig-Maximilians-University, Munich, Germany, 4 Muhimbili University College of Health Sciences, Dar es Salaam, Tanzania, 5 Laboratoire de Microbiologie, hôpital Européen Georges Pompidou, Paris, France, 6 Faculté de Médecine Paris Descartes, Université Paris Descartes (Paris V), Paris, France

Abstract

Objectives: To compare the presence and quantity of cervicovaginal HIV among HIV seropositive women with clinical herpes, subclinical HSV-2 infection and without HSV-2 infection respectively; to evaluate the association between cervicovaginal HIV and HSV shedding; and identify factors associated with quantity of cervicovaginal HIV.

Design: Four groups of HIV seropositive adult female barworkers were identified and examined at three-monthly intervals between October 2000 and March 2003 in Mbeya, Tanzania: (1) 57 women at 70 clinic visits with clinical genital herpes; (2) 39 of the same women at 46 clinic visits when asymptomatic; (3) 55 HSV-2 seropositive women at 60 clinic visits who were never observed with herpetic lesions; (4) 18 HSV-2 seronegative women at 45 clinic visits. Associations of genital HIV shedding with HIV plasma viral load (PVL), herpetic lesions, HSV shedding and other factors were examined.

Results: Prevalence of detectable genital HIV RNA varied from 73% in HSV-2 seronegative women to 94% in women with herpetic lesions (geometric means 1634 vs 3339 copies/ml, p = 0.03). In paired specimens from HSV-2 positive women, genital HIV viral shedding was similar during symptomatic and asymptomatic visits. On multivariate regression, genital HIV RNA ($\log_{10}$ copies/mL) was closely associated with HIV PVL ($\beta = 0.51$ per $\log_{10}$ copies/ml increase, 95%CI:0.41–0.60, p<0.001) and HSV shedding ($\beta = 0.24$ per $\log_{10}$ copies/ml increase, 95% CI:0.16–0.32, p<0.001) but not the presence of herpetic lesions ($\beta = -0.10$, 95%CI:−0.28–0.08, p = 0.27).

Conclusions: HIV PVL and HSV shedding were more important determinants of genital HIV than the presence of herpetic lesions. These data support a role of HSV-2 infection in enhancing HIV transmissibility.

Editor: Rupert Kaul, University of Toronto, Canada

Funding: This work was supported by: European Commission, DGXII, INCO-DC, Grant nummber: ICA-CT-1998-10007; Wellcome Trust, Grant number: 060145/Z/00/A; and Department for International Development, Grant number: RD638. The funders had no role in study design, data collection and analysis, decision to publish, or preparation of the manuscript.

Competing Interests: The authors have declared that no competing interests exist.

* E-mail: jim.todd@lshtm.ac.uk

Introduction

Herpes simplex virus type-2 (HSV-2) infection is lifelong and a common cause of genital ulcers [1–3]. There is strong epidemiological evidence that HSV-2 infection increases the risk of HIV acquisition [4–6]. The potential effect of HSV-2 on HIV infectivity is also of interest. *In vitro* studies provide evidence of the effect of HSV-2 infection on HIV replication [7–9] and epidemiological studies link acute episodes of genital herpes to temporal increases in HIV plasma viral load [10]. A prospective study in Ugandan discordant couples has shown that the risk of HIV transmission is increased in the presence of genital ulcer disease when the plasma viral load exceeds 1,700 copies/mL [11]. Observational studies have shown an association between HSV-2 genital shedding and HIV genital shedding in some cases but not others [12–15]. Trials of HSV suppressive therapy in HIV positive women have shown varying impact on cervicovaginal HIV

shedding [16–22] while a trial of suppressive therapy delivered to the HIV positive partner in discordant couples found no effect on HIV transmission to their HIV negative partners [23].

The frequency of recurrent episodes of clinical herpes and of subclinical viral shedding varies both between individuals and over time within the same individual [24,25]. While research supports an association between HSV infection and HIV shedding, it is less clear whether any effect on HIV infectivity is restricted primarily to clinical episodes of genital herpes or if HIV transmission is also enhanced during asymptomatic HSV-2 infection [26]. This is particularly important since asymptomatic HSV shedding is observed to occur on up to 28% of days in infected individuals [27].

The objectives of this study were to compare the presence and quantity of cervicovaginal HIV in HIV seropositive women living in Mbeya Region, Tanzania with clinical episodes of herpes, subclinical HSV-2 infection and without HSV-2 respectively; to examine the association between genital shedding of HIV and HSV-2; and to investigate factors influencing the quantity of HIV genital shedding.

Methods

Subjects and Study Methods

As part of a study of the determinants of HIV super-infection in Mbeya Region, Tanzania, an open cohort of 600 female barworkers aged 18 to 35 years was established in late 2000. Study procedures have been described previously [28]. Briefly, behavioural and biological data were collected at baseline and during 3-monthly follow-up visits for up to 30 months. In this paper we present data collected from HIV infected participants between October 2000 and March 2003.

Laboratory Methods (for All Women)

Serological testing and plasma viral load. A diagnostic algorithm including two different enzyme-linked immunosorbent assays (HIV-Determine, Abott Laboratories, USA and Enzygnost HIV 1+2 plus, Behring, Germany) and a Western Blot assay (HIV Blot 2.2, Genelabs Diagnostics, Singapore) was used to determine HIV serostatus. Type-specific serological testing for HSV-2 was also performed by enzyme immune assay (Kalon Biological Ltd, Aldershot, UK). Syphilis testing was carried out using the Serodia *Treponema pallidum* particle agglutination assay (TPPA, Fujirebio Inc, Tokyo, Japan) and the rapid plasma reagin test (RPR, VD25, Murex Diagnostics Ltd, Cambridge, UK).

HIV-1 plasma viral load (PVL) was quantified by transcription polymerase chain reaction (PCR) (Versant 3.0 assay, Bayer diagnostics, Emeryville, California), with a detection threshold of 50 HIV-RNA copies/ml.

Genital ulcer specimens. A single dry swab was taken from genital ulcers and multiplex PCR (M-PCR) was used for the detection of *T pallidum*, *H ducreyi* and HSV [29]. Herpetic lesions were defined as ulcers or vesicles confirmed by M-PCR as positive for HSV.

Cervicovaginal specimens and vaginal swabs. Cervicovaginal secretions (CVS) were collected from all women at every study visit using standard vaginal lavage procedures [30], by washing with 5 ml of phosphate-buffered saline. After centrifugation, the cell-free supernatant and cell pellet were stored separately at -80°C until use. Real time PCR was used to quantify HIV-1 RNA in the acellular fraction and HIV-1 DNA in the cell pellet of genital secretions as previously described [31] using primers and probes synthesised by Eurogentec (Eurogentec SA, Seraing, Belgium). HSV DNA (Roche Molecular Diagnostics) was also quantified in the acellular fraction of secretions by real time PCR [32]. Detection thresholds were 250 copies/ml for HIV-1 RNA and HSV DNA, and 5 copies/10^6 cells for HIV-1 DNA. Cervicovaginal specimens were also tested for prostate specific antigen (PSA) using the VITROS immunodiagnostic product PSA reagent and calibrator packs on the automaton Ortho-Clinical Diagnostics VITROS Eci (Ortho-Clinical diagnostics, Issy Les Moulineaux, France), and for traces of haemoglobin using Multistix 8 SG strips (Bayer Diagnostics, Puteaux, France).

Vaginal swabs were tested for *Trichomonas vaginalis* by direct microscopy of a wet mount preparation and *Candida albicans* by wet mount preparation and gram stain.

Study Design for Shedding Sub-study

CVS specimens collected from HIV seropositive women at 3-monthly study visits were excluded from analyses if (i) the woman had a genital lesion of non-herpetic origin (12 specimens were excluded for confirmed syphilis and 7 specimens excluded for chancroid), (ii) there were traces of haemoglobin in the specimen or (iii) the specimen was positive for PSA. Specimens from (i) were excluded as HSV shedding may have been influenced by other ulcerative STIs, and those from (ii) and (iii) were excluded as any HIV-RNA or HIV-DNA found in the genital tract may not have been attributable to genital shedding from the woman. Specimens were categorised into four study groups according to the woman's HSV-2 serostatus and the presence or absence of confirmed herpetic genital lesions at the time of specimen collection. Women who experienced PCR-confirmed herpetic lesions at one or more study visits contributed to two study groups: Group 1 ("clinical herpes") included CVS specimens collected in the presence of herpetic lesions; Group 2 ("subclinical herpes"), included specimens taken from the same women at follow-up examinations at least 6 months after or 6 months before the visits at which herpetic lesions were detected. In Group 3 ("never lesions") a random sample of specimens were taken from HSV-2 seropositive women who never had herpetic genital lesions or a history of genital lesions at any of the study visits. Group 4 ("HSV-2 negative") was randomly chosen from specimens taken from women not infected with HSV-2.

Statistical Analyses

Differences between study groups in proportions of CVS specimens with HIV-1 (RNA and DNA) and HSV DNA above the detection threshold were tested using random effects logistic regression modelling to account for correlations within subjects. Analyses of quantity of genital viral shedding were restricted to specimens with viral loads above the threshold of detection. Logarithmic ($\log_{10}$) transformations were applied to plasma and genital viral loads for HIV and HSV-2 to obtain approximately normal distributions, geometric means (GM), and 95% confidence intervals (95%CI). Differences in mean viral loads between groups were assessed using a random effects linear regression model to account for correlations within subjects. Correlations between viral loads (plasma and genital) were assessed using Spearman's rank correlation coefficient.

The effect of genital herpetic lesions on HIV and HSV shedding was assessed by carrying out matched pair chi-squared tests on detection of virus, and a paired t-test on the quantity of shedding, for paired samples collected from the same women during clinical and subclinical phases of herpes, randomly selecting a single sample result if more than one eligible sample was available. Sample size calculations used the log scale for HIV shedding, assuming a within-women difference of 0.3 log copies/mL between episodes with herpetic lesions and those without herpetic lesions, and a standard deviation of 0.6 log copies/mL. With 60 women providing paired samples, the analysis had a 80% power to detect a difference of 0.3 as significant at the 5% level (which corresponds to a doubling of the HIV shedding in women with clinical lesions).

Initial analyses suggested that HSV shedding was a strong determinant of genital HIV shedding. We regrouped specimens of HSV-2 seropositive women in the subclinical and never lesions groups according to the presence of HSV shedding (asymptomatic HSV shedders) or absence of HSV shedding (HSV non-shedders). We then used random effects linear regression, accounting for multiple observations from the same individual, to examine the association of log-transformed HIV genital viral loads with HSV shedding status as well as other potential risk factors, including age, laboratory-diagnosed non-ulcerative sexually transmitted infections (STI), signs or symptoms of sexually transmitted diseases

(STD), enlarged lymph nodes and HIV plasma viral load. In this analysis, specimens with HIV or HSV genital viral load below the threshold of detection were assigned a value of half the threshold.

Analyses were performed using Stata 11.0 (Stata Corporation, Texas, USA). The study was approved by the national ethics review committee of the National Institute for Medical Research of the United Republic of Tanzania and the LSHTM Ethics Committee (Approval 668). It was conducted within the framework of the Mbeya Medical Research Programme. All participants provided written, informed consent to participate in the study.

Results

Characteristics of Participants

Analyses were based on 221 eligible CVS samples from 131 HIV seropositive women. The four study groups comprised 57 women at 70 study visits with clinically manifest genital herpes (Group 1), 39 of the same women at 46 study visits when they did not have visible ulcers (Group 2), 55 HSV-2 seropositive women at 60 study visits who were never observed with herpetic lesions (Group 3), and 18 women at 45 study visits who were HSV-2 seronegative (Group 4) (Table 1).

Thirty-five women contributed to both Groups 1 and 2; four other women in Group 2 were not sampled at the time of clinical herpes. Three women were HSV-2 seronegative (Group 4) and

later seroconverted, two with an episode of clinical herpes (Group 1) and one with no episode of clinical herpes (Group 3). Thirty-three women contributed more than one specimen to the same study group (up to 7 specimens from one HSV-2 seronegative woman).

Mean age was around 28 years for HSV-2 positive women and 25 years for HSV-2 negative women. Slightly higher proportions of women were using hormonal contraception among those who had never had lesions, and those who were HSV-2 negative, but this difference was not statistically significant (p = 0.35).

Geometric mean PVL was lowest (5,830 copies/ml) in samples from women uninfected with HSV-2 and highest (24,400 copies/ml) in samples from women with confirmed herpetic lesions. TPPA seropositivity, indicating past or current syphilis, was also lower in the HSV-2 uninfected group (p<0.001), and C Albicans was most common in the never lesions group (p = 0.08), but other STI or clinical signs of STD at the time of specimen collection did not differ significantly by study group (Table 1).

Genital Shedding of HIV and HSV by Study Group

The prevalence of detectable genital HIV RNA was lowest in the HSV-2 negative group (73%) and highest in the clinical herpes group (94%) (Table 1). The genital HIV RNA viral load in those with detectable virus showed a similar trend across the four groups, with the lowest quantity in the HSV-2 negative group

Table 1. Characteristics of participants and cervicovaginal viral shedding by study group.

Factor	Study group				
	Clinical herpes	Subclinical herpes	Never lesions	HSV-2 negative	
Women	**N = 57**	**N = 39**	**N = 55**	**N = 18**	**p-value[1]**
Age Mean (SD)	28.1 (4.20)	28.8 (4.13)	27.2 (4.27)	24.6 (4.34)	0.001 [2]
Hormonal contraceptive use	17 (30%)	8 (21%)	20 (36%)	7 (39%)	0.35
Specimens	N = 70	N = 46	N = 60	N = 45	
Plasma HIV-1 RNA					
Geo mean (95% CI)	24400 (16400–36300)	16300 (9900–26900)	10550 (6900–16100)	5830 (3540–9600)	<0.001[2]
Presence of STI (%)					
TV	9 (13%)	4 (9%)	8 (13%)	2 (4%)	0.49
CA	21 (30%)	9 (20%)	27 (45%)	16 (36%)	0.08
TPPA	32 (46%)	22 (48%)	33 (55%)	8 (18%)	<0.001
RPR	11 (16%)	5 (11%)	9 (15%)	2 (4%)	0.28
Warts	10 (14%)	9 (20%)	5 (8%)	3 (7%)	0.8
Cervicitis	9 (13%)	7 (15%)	9 (15%)	4 (9%)	0.88
Vaginal discharge	28 (40%)	21 (46%)	27 (45%)	28 (62%)	0.2
Lymphadenopathy	19 (27%)	8 (17%)	8 (13%)	6 (13%)	0.19
CVS HIV RNA	66 (94%)	41 (89%)	49 (82%)	33 (73%)	0.13
Geo mean[3] (95% CI)	3339 (2410–4626)	2460 (1653–3664)	1908 (1319–2758)	1634 (1096–2436)	0.025 [2]
CVS HIV DNA[4]	63 (100%)	43 (98%)	43 (90%)	43 (100%)	0.002
Geo mean[3] (95% CI)	252 (182–349)	152 (115–201)	141 (93–213)	143 (101–203)	0.025[2]
CVS HSV DNA	54 (77%)	9 (20%)	7 (12%)	–	<0.001
Geo mean[3] (95% CI)	4760 (2384–7613)	4336 (1245–15102)	1392 (288–6729)	–	0.37[2]

SD, standard deviation; STI, sexually transmitted infection; TV, *Trichomonas vaginalis*; CA, *Candida albicans*; TPPA, *Treponema pallidum* particle agglutination assay; RPR, rapid plasma reagin test; Geo mean, geometric mean in copies/ml (HIV RNA and HSV DNA) or copies/10^6 cells (HIV DNA); CVS, cervico-vagina lavage specimen.
[1]p-value from random effect logistic regression accounting for correlation within subjects.
[2]p-value from random effects linear model on log-transformed viral load accounting for correlation within subjects.
[3]Excluding data below the minimum detectable threshold.
[4]Missing values for 7 with clinical herpes, 2 with sub-clinical herpes, 12 with never lesions, and 2 HSV-2 negative.

(GM = 1634 copies per ml) and the highest in the clinical herpes group (GM = 3339 copies per ml) (p<0.025).

The prevalence of detectable genital HIV DNA also varied across study groups (p = 0.002). The pattern was less clear than for HIV RNA, but the highest viral load was seen in the clinical herpes group (GM = 252 copies per 10^6 cells) and the lowest in the never lesions group (GM = 141 copies per 10^6 cells) (Table 1).

All women with detectable genital HIV RNA also had detectable plasma HIV RNA. Among women with detectable genital HIV RNA, quantities of plasma and genital HIV RNA were significantly correlated (N = 189, Spearmans r = 0.49, p<0.001).

As expected, the prevalence of detectable genital HSV DNA varied substantially between the three study groups of HSV-2 positive women, with a much higher prevalence among women with clinical herpes (77%) than in the subclinical herpes (20%) and never lesions (12%) groups (p<0.001). HSV DNA viral load showed a similar, though non-significant trend (Table 1).

Of the 35 women who had specimens taken during clinical episodes of herpes and also at visits when they were asymptomatic, 30 (86%) had detectable HIV RNA on both occasions, while all 29 women with paired specimens analysed for HIV DNA were positive on both occasions. There was no evidence of a difference in the quantity of genital HIV shed between clinical and subclinical phases of herpes (Table 2). Although 23 (66%) of the 35 women had detectable genital HSV DNA during clinical herpes, only 7 (20%) had detectable HSV DNA during the subclinical phase (p<0.001), with 5 (14%) shedding on both occasions.

Association between Genital HIV Shedding and Genital HSV Shedding

To explore whether signs of clinical herpes or HSV-2 viral shedding were more important determinants of HIV shedding, we re-categorised the specimens into four new groups: clinical herpes, HSV-2 seropositive with detectable genital HSV DNA shedding (asymptomatic HSV shedders), HSV-2 seropositive without detectable genital HSV shedding (HSV non-shedders at that visit), and HSV-2 seronegative. In all four groups, the majority of specimens had detectable HIV RNA and HIV DNA, and the prevalence was highest in samples taken during clinical or subclinical shedding episodes (Table 3). Overall, the prevalence

and quantity of genital HIV-1 RNA and DNA shedding differed by sub-group (Table 3). Genital HIV-1 RNA and DNA viral loads were at least as high among asymptomatic HSV shedders as among specimens collected during episodes of clinical herpes. Similarly genital viral load was similar between HSV non-shedders and HSV-2 seronegative women.

Among specimens with HSV DNA shedding (with or without lesions), the genital viral loads of HIV RNA and HSV DNA were positively correlated (n = 86, r = 0.47, p<0.001). The correlation of genital HIV DNA and HSV DNA was weaker (n = 78, r = 0.24, p = 0.03), as was the correlation between plasma HIV RNA and genital HSV DNA (n = 78, r = 0.24, p = 0.03). A positive correlation between genital and plasma viral loads of HIV was seen in all women (Fig. 1 and Fig. 2). While the slopes of the regression lines were similar, the intercept was higher in the clinical herpes and HSV shedding groups indicating that, for any given PVL, the genital shedding of HIV was higher in those who were also shedding HSV-2.

Risk Factors for Genital HIV Shedding

Genital HIV RNA viral load increased with quantity of HIV PVL (p<0.001) and presence and quantity of genital HSV DNA (Table 4). Although the quantity of genital HIV RNA was higher in specimens from HSV-2 seropositive women (p = 0.009) and those with herpetic lesions (p = 0.002), the association with herpetic lesions was no longer statistically significant after adjusting for age, PVL and the quantity of genital HSV DNA (Table 4). The quantity of genital HIV RNA was unrelated to the presence of STI, signs or symptoms of other STD or enlarged lymph nodes (data not shown), or to the use of hormonal contraception.

Similarly, genital HIV DNA viral load increased with both HIV PVL (p<0.001) and genital HSV DNA viral load (Table 4). Although genital HIV DNA was more commonly detected in the presence of clinical herpes (p = 0.004), this association was no longer statistically after adjusting for age, PVL and the quantity of genital HSV DNA. The quantity of genital HIV DNA was unrelated to the presence of STI, signs or symptoms of other STD or enlarged lymph nodes (data not shown), or to the use of hormonal contraception.

Table 2. Cervicovaginal HIV-1 and HSV viral load in 35 women during the clinical and subclinical stages of herpes.

Viral shedding	N	Number (%) with detectable virus Geometric mean (95% CI)		p-value[1]	p-value[2]
		Clinical herpes	Subclinical herpes		
CVS HIV-1 RNA[3] Number (%)	35	31 (89%)	32 (91%)	0.56	
CVS HIV-1 RNA[3] Geometric mean (95% CI)	35	3137 (1914–5143)	2800 (1804–4345)		0.72
CVS HIV-1 DNA[3,4] Number (%)	29	29 (100%)	29 (100%)	1.0	
CVS HIV-1 DNA[3,4] Geometric mean (95% CI)	29	157 (90–221)	157 (110–221)		0.99
CVS HSV DNA[3] Number (%)	35	23 (66%)	7 (20%)	0.0003	
CVS HSV DNA[3] Geometric mean (95% CI)	35	3369 (1210–9380)	4236 (1351–13278)		0.24

Analyses restricted to women with samples in both the clinical and the subclinical groups.
[1]p-value from matched pairs chi-squared test.
[2]p-value from matched pairs t-test on logged values.
[3]Geometric mean in copies/ml (HIV RNA and HSV DNA) or copies/10^6 cells (HIV DNA), excluding data below the minimum detectable threshold at half the detectable level.
[4]Six women did not have HIV DNA samples tested (five with clinical herpes, and one with subclinical herpes) and are excluding from this comparison.

Table 3. Cervicovaginal HIV-1 RNA, HIV-1 DNA and HSV DNA viral load by HSV-2 group.

Genital viral Shedding	HSV-2 group				p-value[1]
	Clinical Herpes	Subclinical HSV shedders	Subclinical Non shedders	HSV-2 negative	
HIV-1 RNA	**N = 70**	**N = 16**	**N = 90**	**N = 45**	
Number (%)	66 (94%)	16 (100%)	74 (82%)	33 (73%)	0.11
Geo mean [2] (95% CI)	3339 (2410–4626)	4326 (2076–9012)	1840 (1392–2433)	1634 (1096–2436)	0.002
HIV-1 DNA	**N = 63**	**N = 15**	**N = 77**	**N = 43**	
Number (%)	63 (100%)	15 (100%)	71 (90%)	43 (100%)	0.04
Geo mean [2] (95% CI)	252 (182–349)	260 (131–517)	130 (100–203)	143 (101–203)	0.003
HSV DNA	**N = 70**	**N = 16**			
Number (%)	54 (77%)	16 (100%)	NA	NA	0.03
Geo mean [2] (95% CI)	4260 (2383–7613)	2637 (1064–6541)	NA	NA	0.4

IQR, interquartile range; CI, confidence interval.
[1]p-values from random effects logistic regression model, or random effects linear regression model.
[2]Geometric mean in copies/ml (HIV RNA and HSV DNA) or copies/10^6 cells (HIV DNA), excluding data below the minimum detectable threshold level.

Discussion

In this study we determined the frequency and quantity of cervicovaginal HIV and HSV using specimens collected from 131 HIV infected women who were followed up every three months for up to 30 months. The prevalence of detectable genital HSV DNA in asymptomatic HIV positive women was similar to studies from elsewhere in Africa [33] and, as in other studies, there was a strong correlation between genital and plasma HIV viral loads [15].

The main objective of our study was to determine whether genital shedding of HIV occurred more frequently in the presence of genital herpetic lesions. A strength of the study was the long follow-up period, providing an opportunity to observe women both during and between clinical episodes of herpes. Clinical herpes was associated with higher levels of genital HIV shedding, but only partially as there were episodes of herpetic ulceration where HSV genital shedding was not recorded, and conversely episodes of HSV genital shedding in asymptomatic women. In the multivariate analysis, we clearly saw that herpetic ulcers were not independently associated with genital shedding of HIV RNA (coefficient = −0.10, p = 0.27), whereas there remained a clear association between HSV genital shedding and genital shedding of HIV RNA (coefficient = +0.24, p<0.001), suggesting that this increase was related to the quantity of genital HSV and the HIV plasma viral load rather than to the presence or absence of

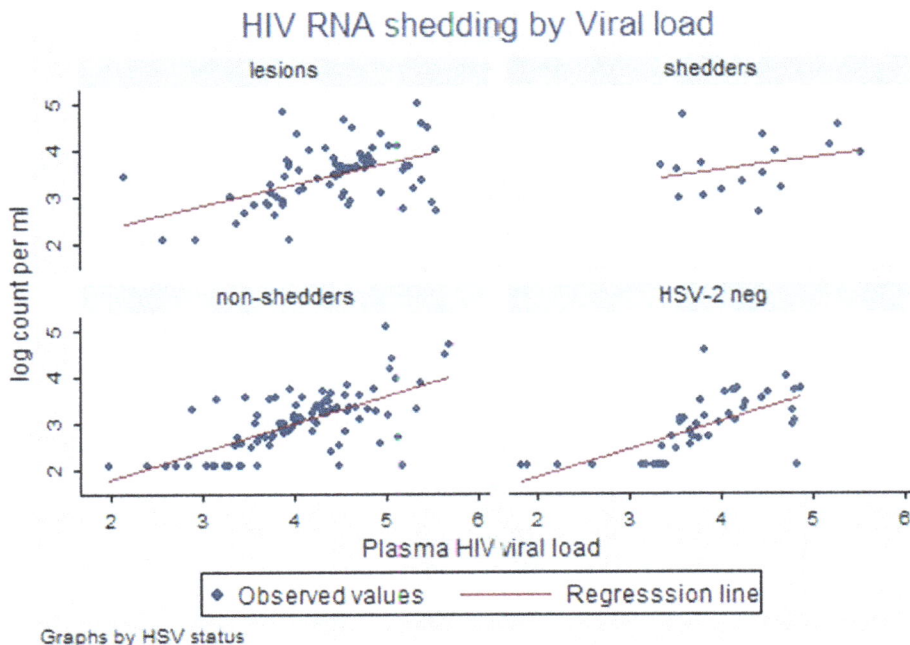

Figure 1. Relationship between HIV RNA genital shedding and HIV plasma viral load in women with herpetic lesions, asymptomatic women with and without HSV genital shedding and HSV-2 seronegative women.

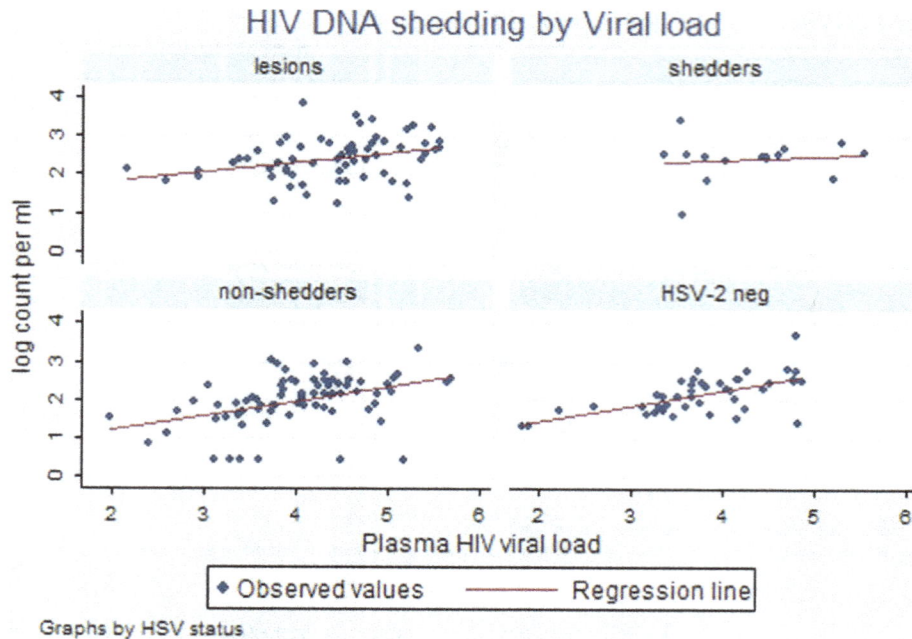

Figure 2. Relationship between HIV DNA genital shedding and HIV plasma viral load in women with herpetic lesions, asymptomatic women with and without HSV genital shedding and HSV-2 seronegative women.

herpetic lesions. In paired specimens taken from women with clinical herpes and from other study visits when they were asymptomatic, no difference was seen in HIV genital shedding at the two visits. When the original study groups were rearranged to examine the effect of genital HSV shedding, there was a clear difference in HIV genital shedding between HSV shedders and non-shedders, but no additional increase in HIV shedding in those with clinical herpes. Similarly, when risk factors for HIV genital shedding were examined in a multivariate regression analysis, the quantity of genital HIV RNA or DNA was significantly associated with HIV plasma viral load and HSV shedding, but after adjustment for these factors was not associated with clinical herpes.

Our findings are consistent with results from a study carried out in Bangui, Central African Republic, where among HIV positive women shedding HSV, there was a significant correlation between genital HIV RNA shedding and genital shedding of HSV [14]. A similar positive correlation between cervical HSV shedding and the quantities of cervical HIV-1 RNA and DNA was seen in a cross-sectional study of 200 women attending family-planning clinics in Mombasa, Kenya, and this was significant even after controlling for differences in CD4 count and plasma viral load [13]. Baseline data from a randomised controlled trial of herpes episodic treatment in Ghana and Central African Republic showed that, among 180 HSV-2/HIV-1 co-infected women, genital HIV RNA was detected more frequently and at higher median viral loads among women with genital HSV-2 infection (i.e. HSV-2 ulcers or HSV-2 in CVS) than women without any genital HSV-2 infection [34]. However, in a study of 214 Zimbabwean sex workers, genital HIV-1 RNA shedding increased with HIV plasma viral load but did not differ in women with or without HSV shedding, although the HSV shedding was not quantified [15]. A study in men and women in Thailand showed no association between the quantities of HIV shed and the presence of either HSV shedding or herpetic lesions [35].

The observational design of these studies limits inferences about causality, but stronger evidence concerning the effect of herpes on HIV infectivity comes from seven recently completed randomised controlled trials of herpes suppressive therapy. Four trials, using valacyclovir or high dose acyclovir (800 mg b.i.d.), found significant reductions in PVL as well as significant reductions in rectal and cervicovaginal HIV-1 RNA concentrations [16–19]. Trials of acyclovir 400 mg b.i.d have shown less effect. Two found no reduction in cervico-vaginal HIV-1 RNA detection [20,21], possibly attributable to sub-optimal adherence and the other found a reduction in frequency of cervico-vaginal HIV-1 RNA detection and plasma HIV-1 RNA load but no effect on viral load among those with detectable shedding [22]. Moreover, a trial of acyclovir (400 mg b.i.d.) delivered to the HIV positive partner in discordant couples ("Partners in Prevention") found no effect on HIV transmission to their HIV negative partners, although there was some evidence that acyclovir reduced risk of HIV-1 disease progression to either CD4 count below 200 cells/μL, use of ART or death (hazard ratio(HR) = 0.84, 95%CI 0.71–0.98) [36].

Our results are consistent with previous reports of an association between HSV-2 shedding and HIV PVL, and suggest that clinical and subclinical herpetic reactivations might increase genital HIV shedding not only through a direct viral interaction at the genital level, but also through their systemic effect on plasma HIV viral load [37]. In our study, HIV plasma viral load was the strongest determinant of HIV genital shedding, and higher plasma viral loads were observed in women with herpetic ulcers and asymptomatic herpes than in uninfected women.

In this study we used cervicovaginal specimens as a marker of genital shedding, and did not find evidence of increased HIV shedding in the presence of genital lesions. However, HIV shedding may also occur directly from a herpetic lesion, and we cannot exclude the possibility that overall HIV infectivity is increased in the presence of lesions, particularly as 64% of herpetic lesions seen in this study were found on the vulva [38]. The

Table 4. Association between cervicovaginal HIV-1 RNA and HIV-1 DNA viral load and potential risk factors.

Factors	No with characteristic	Age adjusted		Adjusted for age and other factors[1]	
		Coefficient (95% CI)	p-value	Coefficient (95% CI)	p-value
Genital HIV-RNA shedding		N = 221		N = 221	
Age group (years)			0.61		0.6
≤24	50	0		0	
25–29	101	+0.04 (−0.21, 0.30)		−0.06 (−0.24, 0.11)	
≥30	70	+0.03 (−0.25, 0.31)		−0.12 (−0.30, −0.07)	
Hormonal contraceptive use	84	−0.07 (−0.29, 0.14)	0.5	+0.05 (−0.10, 0.19)	0.54
Plasma HIV-1 RNA	All	+0.57 (0.48, 0.67)	<0.001	+0.51 (0.41, 0.60)	<0.001
HSV-2 seropositive	176	+0.37 (0.09, 0.65)	0.009	+0.65 (0.40, 0.91)	<0.001
Presence of herpetic lesions	70	+0.31 (0.12, 0.50)	0.002	−0.10 (−0.28, 0.08)	0.27
Genital HSV DNA shedding					
Any HSV DNA shedding [2]	70	+0.53 (0.34, 0.71)	<0.001	+0.04 (−0.22, 0.29)	0.77
Quantitative [3]	All	+0.13 (0.05, 0.22)	0.002	+0.24 (0.16, 0.32)	<0.001
Genital HIV-DNA shedding	No with characteristic	N = 198		N = 198	
Age group (years)			0.61		0.5
≤24	50	0		0	
25–29	101	+0.21 (−0.03, 0.46)		+0.20 (−0.00, 0.40)	
≥30	70	+0.13 (−0.14, 0.40)		+0.06 (−0.16, 0.27)	
Hormonal contraceptive use	84	−0.03 (−0.24, 0.18)	0.8	−0.01 (−0.16, 0.18)	0.9
Plasma HIV-1 RNA	All	+0.35 (0.25, 0.46)	<0.001	+0.33 (0.23, 0.44)	<0.001
HSV-2 seropositive	176	−0.09 (−0.37, 0.19)	0.5	+0.14 (−0.14, 0.43)	0.33
Presence of herpetic lesions	70	+0.26 (0.08, 0.44)	0.004	+0.11 (−0.09, 0.31)	0.29
Genital HSVDNA shedding					
Any HSV DNA shedding [2]	70	+0.31 (0.13, 0.49)	<0.001	+0.12 (−0.17, 0.40)	0.42
Quantitative [3]	All	+0.14 (0.06, 0.22)	<0.001	+0.15 (+0.06, 0.24)	<0.001

Linear coefficient on $\log_{10}$ scale; p-value from Wald test from a generalised least square random effects model.
[1]Adjusted for age, plasma viral load, quantitative cervico-vaginal shedding of HSV and HSV-2 seropositivity.
[2]Binary variable comparing samples from women with HSV DNA genital shedding and samples from women with no shedding.
[3]Quantitative analysis: Assessing the effect of a unit log increase in HSV DNA genital shedding. Women who were HSV-2 seronegative and women who were HSV-2 seropositive with undetectable HSV genital shedding were given a value of half the detectable threshold.

quantification of both the HIV shedding and the HSV shedding were taken from the dilution of the CVS supernatant, and these are dependent on the amount of vaginal fluid in the vaginal lavage.

Genital specimens from women with ulcers of other confirmed aetiology (*T pallidum* or *H ducreyi*) were excluded from this analysis, as were specimens with traces of blood or semen, although we cannot rule out the possibility that some HIV or HSV detected in CVS originated from infected sexual partners. Some CVS were collected from women with non-ulcerative STI, and this may have led to underestimation of the association between herpetic lesions and HIV shedding, as cervicovaginal secretion of HIV-1 has been associated with the presence of non-ulcerative STI such as gonorrhoea and Chlamydia and found to decrease after effective treatment [39–41]. However, in this study the presence of other STI was not associated with increased HIV shedding (data not shown), and all symptomatic participants were given treatment for all STI free-of-charge throughout the study.

Increased genital HIV-1 viral load has been shown to be associated with immunosuppression in some studies [14,41] but not others [42]. In our study, CD4 counts were not available, but most women had plasma HIV-1 RNA <30,000 copies/ml, and

few specimens were collected at a time when lymph nodes or other clinical signs or symptoms of HIV-related disease were present. Furthermore, the HSV type was not determined in this study and some of the detected HSV may have been HSV-1 rather than HSV-2.

In conclusion, this study adds to the accumulating evidence that HSV-2 infection increases genital shedding of HIV, and may therefore increase the infectivity of HIV infected individuals to their sexual partners. Our data suggest that the increase in HIV shedding is related to the quantity of HSV shedding rather than to the presence of clinical lesions of herpes. These findings emphasise the importance of developing and evaluating effective interventions to control herpes in populations where HSV-2 may account for a substantial proportion of HIV transmission.

Acknowledgments

We thank the women who participated in the study and the research team of the NIMR-Mbeya Medical Research Programme, and the Director and personnel in Mbeya Referral Hospital clinics and laboratories for making this study possible. We acknowledge the Medical officer in charge of Mbeya municipality, and the Tanzanian Minister of Health and Social

Welfare for their support. We thank Oliver Hoffmann, Karl-Heinz Herbinger, Britta Dechamps, Gudrun Schoen and Frowin Nichombe for their active support in Mbeya, and Heiner Grosskurth and Mar Pujades-Rodrigues for their support in London. We acknowledge the help of Dr Jerome Legoff in quantifying the HSV DNA in this study.

Author Contributions

Conceived and designed the experiments: GR MH DM RH LB. Performed the experiments: GR MR LM EL. Analyzed the data: GR JT HW RH. Contributed reagents/materials/analysis tools: LB ES EL MH. Wrote the paper: JT GR RH HW.

References

1. Limpakarnjanarat K, Mastro TD, Saisorn S, Uthaivoravit W, Kaewkungwal J, et al. (1999) HIV-1 and other sexually transmitted infections in a cohort of female sex workers in Chiang Rai, Thailand. Sex Transm Infect 75: 30–5.
2. Behets FM, Andriamiadana J, Randrianasolo D, Randriamanga R, Rasamilalao D, et al. (1999) Chancroid, primary syphilis, genital herpes, and lymphogranuloma venereum in Antananarivo, Madagascar. J Infect Dis 180: 1382–5.
3. Chen CY, Ballard RC, Beck-Sague CM, Dangor Y, Radebe F, et al. (2000) Human immunodeficiency virus infection and genital ulcer disease in South Africa: the herpetic connection. Sex Transm Dis 27: 21–9.
4. Wald A, Link K. (2002) Risk of human immunodeficiency virus infection in herpes simplex virus type 2-seropositive persons: a meta-analysis. J Infect Dis 185: 45–52.
5. del Mar Pujades Rodriguez M, Obasi A, Mosha F, Todd J, Brown D, et al. (2002) Herpes simplex virus type 2 infection increases HIV incidence: a prospective study in rural Tanzania. AIDS 16: 451–62.
6. Reynolds SJ, Risbud AR, Shepherd ME, Zenilman JM, Brookmeyer RS, et al. (2003) Recent herpes simplex virus type 2 infection and the risk of human immunodeficiency virus type 1 acquisition in India. J Infect Dis 187: 1513–21.
7. Mosca JD, Bednarik DP, Raj NB, Rosen CA, Sodroski JG, et al. (1987) Activation of human immunodeficiency virus by herpesvirus infection: identification of a region within the long terminal repeat that responds to a trans-acting factor encoded by herpes simplex virus 1. Proc Natl Acad Sci U S A 84: 7408–12.
8. Golden MP, Kim S, Hammer SM, Ladd EA, Schaffer PA, et al. (1992) Activation of human immunodeficiency virus by herpes simplex virus. J Infect Dis 166: 494–9.
9. Albrecht MA, DeLuca NA, Byrn RA, Schaffer PA, Hammer SM. (1989) The herpes simplex virus immediate-early protein, ICP4, is required to potentiate replication of human immunodeficiency virus in CD4+ lymphocytes. J Virol 63: 1861–8.
10. Mole L, Ripich S, Margolis D, Holodniy M. (1997) The impact of active herpes simplex virus infection on human immunodeficiency virus load. J Infect Dis 176: 766–70.
11. Gray RH, Wawer MJ, Brookmeyer R, Sewankambo NK, Serwadda D, et al. (2001) Probability of HIV-1 transmission per coital act in monogamous, heterosexual, HIV-1-discordant couples in Rakai, Uganda. Lancet 357: 1149–53.
12. Nagot N, Foulongne V, Becquart P, Mayaud P, Konate I, et al. (2005) Longitudinal assessment of HIV-1 and HSV-2 shedding in the genital tract of West African women. J Acquir Immune Defic Syndr 39: 632–634.
13. McClelland RS, Wang CC, Overbaugh J, Richardson BA, Corey L, et al. (2002). Association between cervical shedding of herpes simplex virus and HIV-1. AIDS 16: 2425–2430.
14. Mbopi-Keou FX, Gresenguet G, Mayaud P, Weiss HA, Gopal R, et al. (2000) Interactions between herpes simplex virus type 2 and human immunodeficiency virus type 1 infection in African women: opportunities for intervention. J Infect Dis 182: 1090–1096.
15. Cowan FF, Pascoe SJ, Barlow KL, Langhaug LF, Jaffar S, et al. (2006) Association of genital shedding of herpes simplex virus type 2 and HIV-1 among sex workers in rural Zimbabwe. AIDS 20: 261–267.
16. Nagot N, Ouédraogo A, Foulongne V, Konaté I, Weiss HA, et al. (2007) Reduction of HIV-1 RNA levels with therapy to suppress herpes simplex virus. N Engl J Med 356: 790–9.
17. Baeten JM, Strick LB, Lucchetti A, Whittington WL, Sanchez J, et al. (2008) Herpes simplex virus (HSV)-suppressive therapy decreases plasma and genital HIV-1 levels in HSV-2/HIV-1 coinfected women: a randomized, placebo-controlled, cross-over trial. J Infect Dis 198: 1804–8.
18. Dunne EF, Whitehead S, Sternberg M, Thepamnuay S, Leelawiwat W, et al. (2008) Suppressive Acyclovir Therapy Reduces HIV Cervicovaginal Shedding in HIV- and HSV-2-Infected Women, Chiang Rai, Thailand. J Acquir Immune Defic Syndr 49: 77–83.
19. Zuckerman RA, Lucchetti A, Whittington WL, Sanchez J, Coombs RW, et al. (2007) Herpes simplex virus (HSV) suppression with valacyclovir reduces rectal and blood plasma HIV-1 levels in HIV-1/HSV-2-seropositive men: a randomized, double-blind, placebo-controlled crossover trial. J Infect Dis 196: 1500–8.
20. Cowan FM, Pascoe SJ, Barlow KL, Langhaug LF, Jaffar S, et al. (2008) A randomised placebo-controlled trial to explore the effect of suppressive therapy with acyclovir on genital shedding of HIV-1 and herpes simplex virus type 2 among Zimbabwean sex workers. Sex Transm Infect 84: 548–53.
21. Tanton C, Weiss HA, Rusizoka M, Legoff J, Changalucha J, et al. (2010) Long-term impact of acyclovir suppressive therapy on genital and plasma HIV RNA in Tanzanian women: a randomised controlled trial. J Infect Dis 201: 1285–97.
22. Delany S, Mlaba N, Clayton T, Akpomiemie G, Capovilla A, et al. (2009) Impact of aciclovir on genital and plasma HIV-1 RNA in HSV-2/HIV-1 co-infected women: a randomized placebo-controlled trial in South Africa. AIDS 23: 461–9.
23. Celum C, Wald A, Lingappa JR, Magaret AS, Wang RS, et al. (2010) Acyclovir and transmission of HIV-1 from persons infected with HIV-1 and HSV-2. N Engl J Med 362: 427–39.
24. Zhu J, Koelle DM, Cao J, Vazquez J, Huang ML, et al. (2007) Virus-specific CD8+ T cells accumulate near sensory nerve endings in genital skin during subclinical HSV-2 reactivation. J Exp Med 204: 595–603.
25. Ashley RL, Wald A. (1999) Genital herpes: review of the epidemic and potential use of type-specific serology. Clin Microbiol Rev 12: 1–8.
26. Celum CL. The interaction between herpes simplex virus and human immunodeficiency virus. Herpes 2004;11 Suppl 1: 36A–45A.
27. Wald A, Corey L, Cone R, Hobson A, Davis G, et al. (1997) Frequent genital herpes simplex virus 2 shedding in immunocompetent women. Effect of acyclovir treatment. J Clin Inf 99: 1092–1097.
28. Riedner G, Rusizoka M, Hoffmann O, Nichombe F, Lyamuya E, et al. (2003) Baseline survey of sexually transmitted infections in a cohort of female bar workers in Mbeya Region, Tanzania. Sex Transm Infect 79: 382–7.
29. Orle KA, Gates CA, Martin DH, Body BA, Weiss JB. (1996) Simultaneous PCR detection of Haemophilus ducreyi, Treponema pallidum, and herpes simplex virus types 1 and 2 from genital ulcers. J Clin Microbiol 34: 49–54.
30. Belec L, Meillet D, Levy M, Georges A, Tevi-Benissan C, et al. (1995) Dilution assessment of cervicovaginal secretions obtained by vaginal washing for immunological assays. Clin Diagn Lab Immunol 2: 57–61.
31. Viard JP, Burgard M, Hubert JB, Aaron L, Rabian C, et al. (2004) Impact of 5 years of maximally successful highly active antiretroviral therapy on CD4 cell count and HIV-1 DNA level. AIDS 18: 45–9.
32. Espy MJ, Uhl JR, Mitchell PS, Thorvilson JN, Svien KA, et al. (2000) Diagnosis of herpes simplex virus infections in the clinical laboratory by LightCycler PCR. J Clin Microbiol 38: 795–9.
33. Mbopi Keou FX, Gresenguet G, Mayaud P, Weiss HA, Gopal R, et al. (1999) Genital herpes simplex virus type 2 shedding is increased in HIV-infected women in Africa. AIDS 13: 536–7.
34. LeGoff J, Weiss HA, Gresenguet G, Nzambi K, Frost E, et al. (2007) Cervicovaginal HIV-1 and herpes simplex virus type 2 shedding during genital ulcer disease episodes. AIDS. 21: 1569–78.
35. Chu K, Jiamton S, Pepin J, Cowan F, Mahakkanukrauh B, et al. (2006) Association between HSV-2 and HIV-1 viral load in semen, cervico-vaginal secretions and genital ulcers of Thai men and women. Int J STD AIDS 17: 681–6.
36. Lingappa JR, Baeten JM, Wald A, Hughes JP, Thomas KK, et al. (2010) Daily aciclovir for HIV-1 disease progression in people dually infected with HIV-1 and herpes simplex virus type 2: a randomised placebo-controlled trial. Lancet 375: 824–33.
37. Schacker T, Zeh J, Hu H, Shaughnessy M, Corey L. (2002) Changes in plasma human immunodeficiency virus type 1 RNA associated with herpes simplex virus reactivation and suppression. J Infect Dis 186: 1718–25.
38. Riedner G, Todd J, Rusizoka M, Mmbando D, Maboko L, et al. (2007) Possible reasons for an increase in the proportion of genital ulcers due to herpes simplex virus from a cohort of female bar workers in Tanzania. Sex Transm Infect 83: 91–6.
39. Ghys PD, Fransen K, Diallo MO, Ettiègne-Traoré V, Coulibaly IM, et al. (1997) The associations between cervicovaginal HIV shedding, sexually transmitted diseases and immunosuppression in female sex workers in Abidjan, Cote d'Ivoire. AIDS 11: F85–93.
40. Moss GB, Overbaugh J, Welch M, Reilly M, Bwayo J, et al. (1995) Human immunodeficiency virus DNA in urethral secretions in men: association with gonococcal urethritis and CD4 cell depletion. J Infect Dis 172: 1469–74.
41. Cohen MS, Hoffman IF, Royce RA, Kazembe P, Dyer JR, et al. (1997) Reduction of concentration of HIV-1 in semen after treatment of urethritis: implications for prevention of sexual transmission of HIV-1. AIDSCAP Malawi Research Group. Lancet 349: 1868–73.
42. Clemetson DB, Moss GB, Willerford DM, Hensel M, Emonyi W, et al. (1993) Detection of HIV DNA in cervical and vaginal secretions. Prevalence and correlates among women in Nairobi, Kenya. JAMA 269: 2860–4.

8

Risk Factors for HIV and Unprotected Anal Intercourse among Men Who Have Sex with Men (MSM) in Almaty, Kazakhstan

Mark Berry[1]*, Andrea L. Wirtz[1], Assel Janayeva[2], Valentina Ragoza[2], Assel Terlikbayeva[3], Bauyrzhan Amirov[3], Stefan Baral[1], Chris Beyrer[1]

1 Johns Hopkins Bloomberg School of Public Health, Department of Epidemiology, Baltimore, Maryland, United States of America, 2 Amulet Public Organization, Almaty, Kazakhstan, 3 Global Health Research Center of Central Asia, Almaty, Kazakhstan

Abstract

Introduction: Men who have sex with men (MSM) are at high risk for HIV infection. MSM in Central Asia, however, are not adequately studied to assess their risk of HIV transmission. Methods: This study used respondent driven sampling methods to recruit 400 MSM in Almaty, the largest city in Kazakhstan, into a cross-sectional study. Participation involved a one-time interviewer-administered questionnaire and rapid HIV screening test. Prevalence data were adjusted for respondent network size and recruitment patterns. Multivariate logistic regression was used to investigate the association between HIV and selected risk factors, and unprotected anal intercourse (UAI) and selected risk factors.

Results: After respondent driven sampling (RDS) weighted analysis, 20.2% of MSM were HIV-positive, and 69.0% had unprotected sex with at least one male partner in the last 12 months. Regression analysis showed that HIV infection was associated with unprotected receptive anal sex (AOR: 2.00; 95% CI: 1.04–3.84). Having unprotected anal intercourse with male partners, a measure of HIV risk behaviors, was associated with being single (AOR: 0.38; 95% CI: 0.23–0.64); very difficult access to lubricants (AOR: 11.08; 95% CI: 4.93–24.91); STI symptoms (AOR: 3.45; 95% CI: 1.42–8.40); transactional sex (AOR: 3.21; 95% CI: 1.66–6.22); and non-injection drug use (AOR: 3.10; 95% CI: 1.51–6.36).

Conclusions: This study found a high HIV prevalence among MSM in Almaty, and a population of MSM engaging in multiple high-risk behavior in Almaty. Greater access to HIV education and prevention interventions is needed to limit the HIV epidemic among MSM in Almaty.

Editor: Claire Thorne, UCL Institute of Child Health, University College London, United Kingdom

Funding: The study in this manuscript was funded by the Open Society Foundations (OSF) (URL: www.soros.org). OSF had no role in study design, data collection and analysis, decision to publish or preparation of the manuscript.

Competing Interests: The authors have declared that no competing interests exist.

* E-mail: mberry@jhsph.edu

Introduction

Studies conducted around the world consistently find that men who have sex with men (MSM) tend to be underserved, and have much higher risk of HIV acquisition than the heterosexual population, even in countries with generalized epidemics [1]. The disparity in HIV prevalence comparing MSM and the general population is found in many countries. A metanalysis of data from 38 countries found that MSM had a 19.3 times higher odds of HIV infection compared with the overall HIV prevalence [1]. The majority of data regarding the relative contribution of MSM to the HIV epidemic as a whole has been generated in high income countries, including the U.S., Australia, and Western European countries. However, there is now a significant body of evidence demonstrating that MSM are also at high risk for infection in low and middle income countries [1].

The Central Asian region has an expanding epidemic among injecting drug users, but much less is known about HIV among MSM [2]. Central Asia has one of the most glaring gaps of research on HIV and health risks among MSM [3]. Research has indicated that the HIV epidemic among countries in the former Soviet Union (which includes Central Asia) is escalating. This is mostly attributed to injecting drug use, and possibly partly in consequence to the social and economic upheaval caused by the disintegration of the Soviet Union [4,5], while sexual transmission has recently risen as a mode of transmission in several countries [2]. In fact, Central Asia and Eastern Europe have some of the most rapidly escalating HIV epidemics in the world [2]. Up to 75% of the HIV infections in the region are among people who inject drugs. The HIV prevalence in Kazakhstan among injection drug users (IDU) is 4%, based on sentinel surveillance, and some cities are seeing outbreaks of HIV among IDU [6]. Infections are rising in other groups, including female sex workers and their clients, migrants and prisoners [6]. Although injecting drug use likely contributes to the majority of HIV transmission in Central Asia [6], there is a need to monitor HIV prevalence and risk factors in other most at-risk populations.

Epidemiologic assessments of HIV among these at-risk populations, including the MSM population, have received growing government attention in Kazakhstan in recent years, though there remains a dearth of independent scientific investigations. The WHO and UNAIDS reported 27 cases of HIV among MSM in Kazakhstan, Central Asia's largest country and largest economy, from 2002 to 2006 [7]. One study in Kazakhstan found no HIV cases, but sampled only 100 MSM [1]. Sentinel surveillance has been conducted in Kazakhstan as well asa convenience sample study of 450 men, both of which that found very low HIV prevalence, but high levels of HIV risk behaviors and poor knowledge of how HIV is transmitted [8]. UNAIDS estimated a 1% HIV prevalence among MSM in Kazakhstan in 2007, but a much higher (10.8%) prevalence among MSM in neighboring Uzbekistan [2]. A meta-analysis from Caceres et al. found that MSM population prevalence and risk factors for HIV among MSM suggested that between 45 and 52% of MSM in Central Asia participated in high-risk sex (unprotected anal sex or commercial sex) in the previous year [3]. The lack of consistency in the results of these surveillance efforts indicates a need for rigorous sampling techniques to understand the level of risk behavior and HIV prevalence of MSM in Kazakhstan.

Many studies of MSM in low- and middle-income countries rely on convenience samples, such as those conducted in the streets or STI clinics. In these samples, high-risk sub-populations such as male sex workers and male-to-female transgenders may be overrepresented [9]. Probability sampling techniques allow researchers to draw conclusions about the general population under study.

The goal of this study was to measure the HIV risk factors and HIV prevalence among MSM in Almaty, Kazakhstan's economic capital and largest city. This information is needed to inform the type and size of prevention and advocacy responses. While HIV was the primary outcome of interest, we anticipated that the inception of the HIV epidemic among MSM may be recent in Kazakhstan and, therefore, the relationship between HIV and traditional risk factors may not follow the expected patterns, because HIV may not yet exist in some sexual networks. Therefore, we also studied the association between selected risk factors and unprotected anal intercourse (UAI) with a male partner in the last 12 months, as UAI is a good indicator of sexual risk.

Methods

Setting, participants and study design

This cross-sectional study recruited MSM (defined for the purposes of this study as any man reporting oral or anal intercourse with another man in the last 12 months), 18 years or older, who were residing in Almaty at the time of enrollment. An Almaty-based lesbian, gay, bisexual and transgender (LGBT) nongovernmental organization (NGO) provided experiential input to the design of the study and were responsible for participant recruitment and data collection.

Participants were recruited using respondent-driven sampling (RDS) methods [10]. RDS was selected over venue time sampling, as formative work identified too few (N = 2) venues for this approach to be feasible. RDS uses a peer-driven chain referral method, in which participants recruit a limited number of people from their social network. Traditional RDS methods are described in further details elsewhere [10]. Briefly, four "seeds," who are members of the target community, were recruited by the Almaty-based NGO after participating in formative research activities. Each seed initiated the chain referrals and were provided with two

coupons to recruit up to two MSM members from within the participant's social network. Each of those eligible recruits who complete the survey were, in turn, provided with two coupons to recruit MSM members of their social networks. Seeds and recruiters were paid the equivalent of $10 for participating in the study and $2.50 for each peer the participant recruited. Repeat participation was avoided by through eligibility assessment which asked if the potential participant had recently completed a survey for the implementing NGO and supported by staff recognition of duplicate participants. This process of referral continued until the sample size was reached; the sample size (400) of this study was calculated as the ability to detect a prevalence of unprotected anal intercourse of 25%, with adequate precision and a design effect of 2. RDS is a quasi-random sampling method, and analysts must statistically weight data for different probabilities of recruitment into the sample and for different patterns of social connections using a measure of network size and homophily (likeness) of recruiters to recruits for each variable of interest [11]. Ethical approval of the study was received from the Johns Hopkins Bloomberg School of Public Health Institutional Review Board and the Kazakhstan School of Public Health. Interviewers received oral consent from participants, to ensure their anonymity. The oral consent process was approved by both ethics committees. Interviewers recited the oral consent form, checked for understanding, and wrote his or her name on the form after receiving oral consent from participants.

Measures and data collection

Participants answered an interviewer-administered paper-based questionnaire with approximately 100 variables on the following domains: demographics; sexual behavior with male and female partners; alcohol and drug use history; HIV prevention and testing experiences; health conditions; and human rights contexts. The questionnaire was adapted from other questionnaires used for other sociobehavioral assessments of MSM [12]. HIV knowledge was assessed by the number of questions participants correctly answered. These four questions included: "What type of sex puts you most at risk for HIV infection?"; "What type of anal sex puts you most at risk for HIV infection?"; "Can you get HIV from using a needle to inject drugs?"; "What is the safest kind of lubricant for anal sex?" Transactional sex with another man was assessed by asking participants if they had given or received food, drugs, money, or other items of value in exchange for sex in the last 12 months. Condom and lubricant access were assessed through a likert scale with response options ranging from "very easy" to "very difficult."

A physician or nurse trained in HIV testing from the NGO assessed HIV-1 infection via fingerprick-acquired specimens collected and analyzed with Retrocheck HIV WB rapid immunochromatographic test (Qualpro Diagnostics, Goa, India), with 100% sensitivity and 99.8% sensitivity. Due to funding limitations, only one rapid test was performed; no confirmatory test was conducted and participants did not receive HIV results, due to the concern over false positive results. All participants were referred to the Almaty City AIDS Center for confirmatory testing. Sensitivity and specificity of the test was confirmed at the Johns Hopkins University serology laboratory.

All study activities were completed at the NGO study offices in Almaty. Study activities were carried out by NGO staff, from April to August 2010. Data was entered by NGO staff and stored on a secured, web-based application designed to support data capture for research studies. Data were cleaned and analyzed by a JHSPH researcher (MB).

Table 1. Crude and adjusted population* estimates of demographic and social characteristics of men who have sex with men (MSM) in Almaty, Kazakhstan (N = 400).

Variable	Sub category	Crude prevalence % (N)	Weighted prevalence % (95% CI)
Age			
	Less than 25 years	22.0 (88)	25.4 (16.9–34.5)
	25–27	26.0 (104)	29.9 (20.8–39.5)
	28–30	24.8 (99)	16.2 (10.6–22.0)
	Over 30	27.2 (109)	28.5 (2.0–38.4)
Marital status			
	Married	15.8 (63)	15.9 (9.7–22.9)
	Live with female partner	4.5 (17)	6.4 (1.8–13.6)
	Live with male partner	24.7 (98)	31.5 (21.4–40.8)
	Single	53.0 (209)	45.4 (36.2–54.9)
Income of more than 200,000 tenge ($1,348) per month		4.5 (18)	6.8 (1.7–14.2)
Had a regular place to live in last 12 months		82.0 (324)	88.6 (83.0–93.9)
Level of education completed			
	General secondary school	16.0 (64)	14.0 (7.8–20.5)
	Specialized secondary school	19.5 (79)	19.5 (12.0–28.9)
	Some university education	20.3 (81)	12.8 (7.6–18.9)
	University	36.0 (142)	47.1 (37.6–56.8)
Sexual orientation			
	Heterosexual	7.7 (31)	10.1 (4.4–17.4)
	Homosexual	64.5 (253)	55.0 (43.8–65.3)
	Bisexual	18.8 (75)	18.4 (12.1–25.5)
	Transgender	5.0 (20)	5.2 (1.4–11.6)
Disclosure of same sex attraction or practices		25.3 (100)	21.8 (12.7–30.7)
	Told non-MSM friends	10.6 (42)	5.4 (2.3–9.6)
	Told family	8.3 (33)	3.6 (1.4–6.4)
	Told health care provider	2.8 (11)	0.7 (0.2–1.3)

*Raw respondent driven sampling data were adjusted according to the network size and homophily.

Analysis

Risk factor outcomes: RDSAT statistical software (www.respondentdrivingsampling.org) was used to produce population estimates for behavioral and demographic variables by adjusting for network size and recruitment patterns. Initial analysis included: RDSAT-weighted prevalence of demographics and HIV risk factors. Regression modeling was performed in Stata/SE Version 11. Seeds were dropped from regression analyses, because they were not randomly recruited.

We constructed regression models to determine the association between HIV risk factors and two outcomes: HIV status and UAI with male partners in the last 12 months. Univariate and multivariate logistic regression was used to model the relationship between outcomes and exposures. We hypothesized a priori that age, social network size and education were the only confounders in the relationship between the risk factors and the outcomes, and only those variables were used in the multivariate model. No variables were dropped from the models regardless of statistical significance.

As a sensitivity analysis, we performed analyses in which the outcome was adjusted with weights exported from RDSAT, which is a technique typically used in RDS regression analyses [10,13]. However, while the prevalence estimates used the RDS weights, the regression analyses presented in this paper do not use weights, because sampling weights do not give correct standard errors in multivariate regressions [14], and there is debate among statisticians on whether RDS weights can be used in multivariate analysis [10,15]. Instead, we used network size as a confounder in the model to adjust for differences in recruitment due to differences in social network size (i.e. the number of MSM known by the participant), and assessed homophily in results to ensure that homophily did not greatly differ between outcome groups.

Results

Prevalence of demographic and risk behaviors

A total of 400 MSM participants were enrolled between April 2010 and August 2010, including the four seeds. All seeds were successful in recruiting other participants. All eligible participants agreed to participate in the interview and HIV screening, and 72.2% of the coupons distributed were returned by recruits seeking to participate. The median number of descendants per seed was 92 (range 83–129). Table 1 shows the adjusted and unadjusted

Table 2. Crude and adjusted population* estimates of HIV prevention practices of men who have sex with men (MSM) in Almaty, Kazakhstan (N = 400).

Variable	Sub category	Crude prevalence % (N)	Weighted prevalence % (95% CI)
Ever tested for HIV		36.0 (141)	33.2 (24.1–42.7)
Conversation with outreach/prevention worker, counselor on how to protect against HIV infection in last 12 months		24.8 (99)	7.6 (4.3–13.3)
Been to a doctor in last 12 months		32.0 (126)	23.1 (15.5–30.8)
Knew correct answer to four HIV questions**		3.2 (13)	3.4 (0.0–7.7)
	Knew anal sex is riskiest type of sex for HIV infection	39.9 (158)	34.4 (25.1–43.9)
	Knew that receptive anal sex is riskiest type of anal sex for HIV infection	11.1 (44)	7.2 (3.4–12.9)
	Knew needles can transmit HIV	44.2 (175)	51.5 (41.3–61.8)
	Knew that water/silicon-based lubricant is the safest lubricant	64.6 (256)	60.6 (50.3–71.1)
Ease of access to free condoms			
	Very easy	10.2 (39)	1.1 (0.6–1.9)
	Somewhat easy	9.5 (36)	4.3 (1.3–9.5)
	Somewhat difficult	12.8 (51)	7.3 (4.2–10.8)
	Very difficult	65.2 (260)	87.0 (81.2–91.6)
Ease of access to water/silicone-based lubricants			
	Very easy	18.0 (69)	17.5 (10.4–26.4)
	Somewhat easy	24.0 (95)	20.5 (13.2–28.6)
	Somewhat difficult	13.5 (53)	10.5 (6.0–15.1)
	Very difficult	30.2 (121)	38.1 (28.8–48.0)

*Raw respondent driven sampling data were adjusted according to the network size and homophily.
**Questions were: "What type of sex puts you most at risk for HIV infection?"; "What type of anal sex puts you most at risk for HIV infection?"; "Can you get HIV from using a needle to inject drugs?"; "What is the safest kind of lubricant for anal sex?".

demographic characteristics and table 2 shows access to HIV prevention among the sample of participants. The median age of participants was 28 years (range 18–60, IQR 25–31).More than 47% of participants completed university studies. About 55% self-identified as homosexual and 18.4% as bisexual, though only 21.8% had ever disclosed their sexual orientation to non-MSM friends, family members, or a health care provider. Only about one third of the participants had ever been tested for HIV, and 60% of those participants' last test was more than one year prior to the interview. None of those participants reported having tested positive in their previous HIV tests.

Table 3 displays results on prevalence and risk factors for HIV infection among MSM. HIV prevalence in this population is estimated to be 20.2%. These were unknown infections; of those participants testing positive for HIV infection, only 42.7% had ever been tested (CI: 19.3–65.0; unweighted prevalence: 45.3%) and all of those who received their result had been informed the result was negative. Regarding risk behavior, 82.5% of participants reported ever having anal sex without a condom, 69.0% had unprotected anal sex with at least one male partner in the last year, 3.9% had ever injected drugs (most commonly heroin, followed by opium), and 10.9% had used non-prescription and non-injection drugs in the last year. Also, 12.9% of men reported transactional sex (either providing or purchasing sex) in the last 12 months. Homophily between HIV-positives and HIV-negatives was fairly similar (0.07 and 0.44, respectively). The median social network size was 25 for both HIV-positive and HIV-negative participants. Homophily between participants who did and did not have UAI with a male partner in the last 12 months was very similar (0.16 and 0.05, respectively), while the median social network size was 80 and 20, respectively.

Risk factors for HIV and unprotected anal intercourse with male partners

Multivariate analysis showed that several risk factors were statistically significantly associated with HIV (table 4). Specifically, knowing the correct answer to four HIV questions was associated with HIV infection (adjusted odds ratio (AOR): 4.56; 95% CI: 1.41–14.78). Receptive UAI in the last 12 months was also associated with HIV infection (AOR: 2.00; 95% CI: 1.04–3.84). Having UAI with a male partner in the last 12 months (table 5) was associated with several factors, including: single marital status (AOR: 0.38; 95% CI: 0.23–0.63); having very difficult access to water- or silicon-based lubricants (AOR: 12.88; 95% CI: 5.65–29.34); self-reported STI symptoms in the last 12 months (AOR: 3.43; 95% CI: 1.41–8.35); transactional sex in the last 12 months (AOR: 3.18; 95% CI: 1.64–8.35); and using non-injection drugs (AOR: 3.10; 95% CI: 1.51–6.36). Further analysis of single marital status found that being single was significantly protective (AOR: 0.22; 95% CI: 0.14–0.36) against having had a main partner in the past 12 months.

Table 3. Crude and adjusted population* estimates of HIV risk behavior of men who have sex with men (MSM) in Almaty, Kazakhstan (N = 400).

Variable	Subcategory	Crude prevalence % (N)	Weighted prevalence % (95% CI)
HIV prevalence (by rapid screening test)		13.3 (53)	20.2 (10.6–29.8)
Circumcised		44.5 (177)	34.3 (26.0–43.2)
Binge drinking (five or more drinks in one session) in last 30 days		38.0 (152)	36.3 (26.6–46.0)
Sought partners on internet in last 12 months		38.2 (153)	16.4 (11.0–21.8)
Had concurrent sexual partnerships with at least two people in the last 12 months			
	Yes, male and female partners	16.5 (65.0)	19.3 (12.0–23.5)
	Yes, male partners only	24.0 (94.0)	9.9 (5.7–14.2)
Total number of anal or vaginal sex partners in last 12 months			
	1	25.0 (99)	44.3 (35.2–53.4)
	2–5	44.0 (174)	45.4 (35.8–54.4)
	6 or more	31.0 (122)	10.3 (6.5–13.7)
Number of main partners in the last 12 months (median 1, range 0–12)			
	0–1	83.1 (329)	93.2 (89.4–96.2)
	2 or more	16.9 (67)	6.8 (3.8–10.6)
Number of casual partners in the last 12 months (median 1.5, range 0–250)			
	0–1	50.0 (198)	69.4 (59.9–77.8)
	2 or more	50.0 (198)	30.6 (22.1–40.1)
Unprotected sex with female partners in the last 12 months		18.2 (72)	21.8 (13.3–30.3)
Unprotected sex with male partners in the last 12 months		71.6 (288)	69.0 (59.2–77.5)
Used noninjection drugs in last 12 months		20.5 (81)	10.9 (6.2–16.1)
Ever injected drugs		8.3 (33)	3.9 (1.9–6.1)
Ever had anal sex without a condom		87.5 (345)	82.5 (74.6–89.6)
Unprotected insertive anal sex in last 12 months		57.8 (232)	61.0 (52.6–70.4)
Unprotected receptive anal sex in last 12 months		39.0 (156)	55.5 (45.6–65.4)
STI symptoms in last 12 months		14.2 (55)	6.0 (3.0–9.7)
STI diagnosis in last 12 months		10.4 (41)	3.9 (1.9–6.9)
Transactional sex in the last 12 months		26.0 (100)	12.9 (7.9–19.4)

*Raw respondent driven sampling data were adjusted according to the network size and homophily.

Discussion

This study used respondent driven sampling to approximate a random sample of MSM in Almaty, Kazakhstan. The results found a high prevalence of HIV, high levels of risk factors for HIV infection, and low levels of access to health services and HIV prevention programs. In particular, MSM in Almaty tended to report low rates of HIV testing, which is a concern because being tested for HIV is proven to lower risk behavior, as well as provide the first step for entry into HIV care [16].

In multivariate analysis, HIV prevalence was strongly correlated with correctly knowing the answer to four questions about HIV infection, even after adjusting for education, age and social network size. The reason for this finding is uncertain. It could be that people who are exposed to education on risk factors for HIV tend to be people who are already engaged in risk behavior, and self-select for education on HIV. Approximately 40% of the men

who tested positive for HIV had previously been tested and, following HCT guidelines, should have received pre- and post-test counseling but may not have altered high risk sexual practices and may have seroconverted in the period between testing. People who are engaged in high-risk sexual networks may also be more likely to be exposed through these networks to the educational interventions existing in Almaty.

Receptive UAI was also associated with HIV infection. This is expected, because unprotected receptive anal sex has a transmission risk probability approximately 18 times higher than vaginal sex [17]. However, other factors that are traditionally associated with HIV infection, such as injecting drug use, not being circumcised, and transactional sex, were not statistically significantly associated with HIV infection in this population. The reasons for this lack of an association are unclear. The HIV epidemic among MSM in Almaty may be a recently developing epidemic, and HIV infections may still be contained within certain

Table 4. Univariate and multivariate* logistic regression on relationship between risk factors and HIV (N = 396).

Variable	Sub category	Univariate OR (95% CI)	P-value	Multivariate AOR (95% CI)	P-value
Education					
	No university education	1		1	
	Some university education	1.11 (0.62–1.99)	0.73	1.07 (0.59–1.96)	0.82
Age					
	Less than 25 years old	1		1	
	25–27 years old	1.05 (0.43–2.57)	0.91	1.11 (0.45–2.76)	0.82
	28–30 years old	1.56 (0.67–3.65)	0.30	1.62 (0.68–3.84)	0.27
	Over 30 years old	1.27 (0.54–2.99)	0.58	1.24 (0.52–3.00	0.63
Increasing personal network size		1.00 (1.00–1.00)	<0.01	1.00 (1.00–1.00)	<0.01
Increasing income		0.96 (0.78–1.18)	0.70	0.90 (0.71–1.15)	0.46
Marital status					
	Not single	1		1	
	Single	0.99 (0.56–1.77)	0.98	1.12 (0.60–2.09)	0.91
Access to condoms					
	Difficult or easier access to condoms	1		1	
	Very difficult access to free condoms	0.63 (0.35–1.14)	0.13	0.62 (0.34–1.15)	0.27
Access to lubricants					
	Difficult or easier access to lubricants	1		1	
	Very difficult access to lubricants	1.08 (0.58–2.02)	0.80	0.98 (0.51–1.86)	0.69
HIV knowledge**					
	Incorrect answer on at least one HIV question	1		1	
	Knows correct answer to all four HIV questions	4.36 (1.37–13.88)	0.01	4.56 (1.41–14.78)	0.02
Sexual orientation					
	Identifies as heterosexual or bisexual	1		1	
	Self-identifies as "gay/homosexual"	1.66 (0.87–3.17)	0.13	1.64 (0.86–3.15)	0.13
HIV testing					
	Never tested for HIV	1		1	
	Ever tested for HIV	1.59 (0.89–2.86)	0.12	1.51 (0.82–2.80)	0.20
Circumcised					
	No	1		1	
	Yes	0.92 (0.52–1.66)	0.79	0.99 (0.54–1.80)	0.79
STI symptoms					
	Did not report STI symptoms in last 12 months	1		1	
	STI symptoms last 12 months	0.90 (0.38–2.12)	0.81	0.91 (0.38–2.17)	0.81
Health care access					
	Not been to doctor in last 12 months	1	0.56	1	
	Been to doctor in last 12 months	0.82 (0.44–1.56)	0.56	0.77 (0.40–1.48)	0.56
Exchange sex					
	No transactional sex in last 12 months	1		1	
	Transactional sex in the last 12 months	0.85 (0.43–1.69)	0.64	0.86 (0.43–1.72)	0.46
HIV counseling					
	No HIV counseling recently	1		1	
	Met with HIV/STI counselor in last 12 months on male-male sex	1.50 (0.74–3.03)	0.26	1.50 (0.74–3.05)	0.56
Unprotected anal sex with any partner in the last 12 months					
	No	1		1	
	Yes	1.33 (0.64–2.76)	0.45	1.31 (0.63–2.74)	0.60

Table 4. Cont.

Variable	Sub category	Univariate OR (95% CI)	P-value	Multivariate AOR (95% CI)	P-value
Unprotected insertive anal sex in last 12 months					
	No	1		1	
	Yes	1.49 (0.81–2.74)	0.20	1.47 (0.80–2.70)	0.21
Unprotected receptive anal sex in last 12 months					
	No	1		1	
	Yes	1.94 (1.02–3.72)	0.04	2.00 (1.04–3.84)	0.04
Had concurrent sexual partnerships with at least two people in the last 12 months					
	Did not have concurrent partnerships	1		1	
	Male and female partners	0.38 (0.13–1.08)	0.07	0.36 (0.12–1.03)	0.08
	Male partners	0.72 (0.34–1.49)	0.37	0.62 (0.28–1.36)	0.23
Use of water- and silicon-based lube in last 12 months					
	Not always use lube during anal sex	1		1	
	Always use lube during anal sex	0.92 (0.50–1.69)	0.79	0.84 (0.44–1.58)	0.42
Binge drinking (five or more drinks in one session) in last 30 days					
	No binge drinking	1		1	
	At least one binge drinking	1.08 (0.59–1.94)	0.81	1.08 (0.60–1.96)	0.81
Noninjection drug use in last 12 months					
	Did not use noninjection drugs	1		1	
	Used noninjection drugs	0.77 (0.36–1.65)	0.50	0.81 (0.37–1.77)	0.44
Injection drug use					
	Never injected drugs	1		1	
	Ever injected drugs	1.85 (0.76–4.50)	0.18	1.98 (0.80–4.88)	0.15
Internet use to look for sexual partners in last 12 months					
	Did not use internet to look for partners	1		1	
	Used internet to look for partners	0.83 (0.45–1.53)	0.55	0.85 (0.46–1.56)	0.55

*Adjusted for age, educational level and social network size in the statistical model.
**Questions were: "What type of sex puts you most at risk for HIV infection?"; "What type of anal sex puts you most at risk for HIV infection?"; 'Can you get HIV from using a needle to inject drugs?"; "What is the safest kind of lubricant for anal sex?".

sexual networks, while HIV has not yet entered other sexual networks. As the epidemic matures and HIV has had time to spread into more sexual networks of MSM, we expect that the traditional risk factors that affect HIV transmission rates will become statistically significantly associated with HIV infection.

UAI was associated with several other risk factors. Being single (as opposed to married, divorced, or living with a male or female partner) was protective against unprotected anal intercourse. This could be because MSM who are in committed relationships may be having unprotected sex with their main partners, but single men were significantly less likely to have a main partner. There was a strong relationship between very difficult access to lubricants, and a statistically significant association with STI symptoms, trade sex (either giving or receiving favors or money in exchange for sex), and noninjection drug use. Characteristics like low access to lubricants, engaging in transactional sex and

noninjection drug use may be proxies for unmeasured variables, such as self-efficacy to use condoms and social support for safe sexual behavior. Given the association with non-injecting drugs observed here, as well as the growing body of evidence pointing to increased sexual risk practices and HIV infection associated with noninjecting drugs, such as methamphetamines [18], further prevention efforts should take drug use into consideration. Moreover, these findings indicate that there is a population of MSM in Almaty with multiple risk factors for HIV infection. While many of these men have not yet been infected, their behaviors indicate that they are at high risk for infection.

Results of the sensitivity analysis (not presented here) indicated that all the risk factors that were statistically significant in unweighted data remained statistically significant in the weighted analysis at p = 0.05. This is a cross-sectional study, and as such, cannot provide evidence of temporality between exposures and

Table 5. Univariate and multivariate* logistic regression on relationship between risk factors and unprotected anal intercourse with male partners in the last 12 months (N = 396).

Variable	Subcategory	Univariate OR (95% CI)	P-value	Multivariate AOR (95% CI)	P-value
Education					
	No university education	1		1	
	Some university education	0.77 (0.49–1.21)	0.26	0.77 (0.49–1.22)	0.27
Age					
	Less than 25 years old	1		1	
	25–27 years old	1.24 (0.67–2.30)	0.50	1.38 (0.73–2.60)	0.32
	28–30 years old	1.68 (0.87–3.21)	0.12	1.89 (0.97–3.69)	0.06
	Over 30 years old	1.26 (0.68–2.33)	0.46	1.55 (0.82–2.96)	0.18
Increasing personal network size		1.00 (1.00–1.00)	0.03	1.00 (1.00–1.00)	0.04
Increasing income		0.92 (0.78–1.08)	0.33	0.88 (0.73–1.06)	0.18
Marital status					
	Not single	1		1	
	Single	0.46 (0.29–0.74)	<0.01	0.38 (0.23–0.64)	<0.01
Access to condoms					
	Difficult or easier access to condoms	1		1	
	Very difficult access to free condoms	0.72 (0.45–1.16)	0.18	0.88 (0.53–1.46)	0.61
Access to lubricants					
	Difficult or easier access to lubricants	1		1	
	Very difficult access to lubricants	9.87 (4.43–21.99)	<0.01	11.08 (4.93–24.91)	<0.01
HIV knowledge**					
	Incorrect answer on at least one HIV question	1		1	
	Knows correct answer to all four HIV questions**	0.86 (0.26–2.88)	0.82	0.92 (0.27–3.18)	0.90
Sexual orientation					
	Identifies as heterosexual or bisexual	1		1	
	Self-identifies as "gay/homosexual"	0.66 (0.41–1.06)	0.09	0.63 (0.39–1.02)	0.06
HIV testing					
	Never tested for HIV	1		1	
	Ever tested for HIV	1.15 (0.72–1.82)	0.56	1.53 (0.69–1.95)	0.77
STI symptoms					
	Did not report STI symptoms in last 12 months	1		1	
	STI symptoms last 12 months	3.93 (1.63–9.47)	<0.01	3.45 (1.42–8.40)	<0.01
Health care access					
	Not been to doctor in last 12 months	1		1	
	Been to doctor in last 12 months	1.07 (0.67–1.72)	0.78	1.05 (0.64–1.71)	0.85
Exchange sex					
	No transactional sex in the last 12 months	1		1	
	Transactional sex in the last 12 months	3.67 (1.91–7.02)	<0.01	3.21 (1.66–6.22)	<0.01
HIV counseling					
	No HIV counseling recently	1		1	
	Met with HIV/STI counselor in last 12 months on male-male sex	0.84 (0.48–1.48)	0.55	0.62 (0.34–1.15)	0.13
Had concurrent sexual partnerships with at least two people in the last 12 months					
	Did not have concurrent partnerships	1		1	
	Male and female partners	0.82 (0.46–1.48)	0.52	0.90 (0.50–1.63)	0.74

Table 5. Cont.

Variable	Subcategory	Univariate OR (95% CI)	P-value	Multivariate AOR (95% CI)	P-value
	Male partners	0.50 (0.30–0.81)	<0.01	0.39 (0.23–0.66)	<0.01
Use of water- and silicon-based lube in last 12 months					
	Not always use lube during anal sex	1		1	
	Always use lube during anal sex	0.91 (0.56–1.47)	0.64	0.96 (0.57–1.59)	0.79
Binge drinking (five or more drinks in one session) in last 30 days					
	No binge drinking	1		1	
	At least one binge drinking occurrence	1.38 (0.87–2.19)	0.18	1.34 (0.84–2.15)	0.22
Noninjection drug use in last 12 months					
	Did not use noninjection drugs	1		1	
	Used noninjection drugs	3.33 (1.65–6.74)	<0.01	3.10 (1.51–6.36)	<0.02
Injection drug use					
	Never injected drugs	1		1	
	Ever injected drugs	2.30 (0.87–6.13)	0.09	2.03 (0.75–5.48)	0.19
Internet use to look for sexual partners in last 12 months					
	Did not use internet to look for partners	1		1	
	Used internet to look for partners	1.71 (1.06–2.74)	0.03	1.52 (0.93–2.48)	0.08

*Adjusted for age, educational level and social network size in the statistical model.
**Questions were: "What type of sex puts you most at risk for HIV infection?"; "What type of anal sex puts you most at risk for HIV infection?" "Can you get HIV from using a needle to inject drugs?"; "What is the safest kind of lubricant for anal sex?".

outcomes. However, there is a benefit from observing the prevalence of risk factors and associations between risk factors, regardless of temporality. Future studies would benefit from HIV screening in a longitudinal study of MSM, so that the relationship between risk factors and outcomes could be more precisely determined. As a pilot study, this assessment focused on sexual risk, and investigation into drug use among MSM, MSM partnerships, partner behaviors, and networks between MSM groups may be informative for future interventions.

Our enrolled 400 people, which is a modest sample size for an RDS study. This may have resulted in some associations that were due to chance, particularly when a variable had small cell sizes. For example, there was a statistically significant association between HIV knowledge and HIV infection, but only 3.3% of participants in the analysis knew the correct answer to all four questions. Finally, all respondent questionnaires are subject to information biases, such as recall bias and social desirability bias. However, these surveys were conducted anonymously and interviewers were trained in interviewing techniques, in order to minimize these biases.

There are few studies of MSM in Central Asia, and none in the body of peer-reviewed literature that report the use of probability-based sampling. Since RDS is peer-driven, it was able to access a large number of people who may not have otherwise been reached. This study provided one of the first rigorously sampled studies of MSM in Central Asia, which has historically been an understudied population. Furthermore, the involvement of a community-based organization to conduct research and access the most hidden and high risk populations should not be underestimated. An unusually high proportion of coupons were returned

by recruits seeking to participate, which may be partly due to the comfort MSM have with the NGO, and partly due to the fact that only 2 coupons were distributed to participants instead of the traditional 3. The fact participants displayed a variety of unexpected characteristics indicates this was not a biased sample, as would typically be observed with a venue-based sampling method. This study gives an accurate picture of the type and levels of HIV risk behaviors of the diverse population of MSM in Almaty, and their access to HIV prevention materials, so that public health workers can advocate for more HIV prevention interventions and plan effective interventions. In particular, these findings show that there is a group of MSM in Almaty that is engaging in multiple high-risk behaviors, and interventions such as MSM-friendly health care providers and testing sites are needed to prevent the spread of HIV within sexual networks.

Acknowledgments

The authors would like to thank the study participants; Homayoon Farzadegan and his laboratory, of Johns Hopkins School of Public Health; and Anne Brisson, Nabila El-Bassel and Tim Hunt of Columbia University.

Author Contributions

Conceived and designed the experiments: MB AW AJ VR AT BA SB CB. Performed the experiments: MB AW AJ VR AT BA SB CB. Analyzed the data: MB AW SB CB. Contributed reagents/materials/analysis tools: MB AW BA AT AJ VR CB SB. Wrote the paper: MB AW BA AT AJ VR CB SB.

References

1. Baral S, Sifakis F, Cleghorn F, Beyrer C (2007) Elevated risk for HIV infection among men who have sex with men in low- and middle-income countries 2000–2006: A systematic review. PLoS Med Dec;4(12):e339.

2. 2008 report on the global AIDS epidemic [Internet] (2008) Geneva, Switzerland: World Health Organization. Available: http://www.unaids.org/en/KnowledgeCentre/HIVData/GlobalReport/2008/2008_Global_report.asp.

3. Caceres C, Konda K, Pecheny M, Chatterjee A, Lyerla R (2006) Estimating the number of men who have sex with men in low and middle income countries. Sex Transm Infect Jun;82 Suppl 3:iii3–9.

4. Kelly JA, Amirkhanian YA (2003) The newest epidemic: A review of HIV/AIDS in central and eastern europe. Int J STD AIDS Jun;14(6):361–71.

5. Hamers FF, Downs AM (2003) HIV in central and eastern europe. Lancet Mar 22;361(9362):1035–44.

6. Thorne C, Ferencic N, Malyuta R, Mimica J, Niemiec T (2010) Central asia: Hotspot in the worldwide HIV epidemic. Lancet Infect Dis Jul;10(7):479–88.

7. EuroHIV (2007) HIV/AIDS surveillance in europe. end-year report 2006. Saint-Maurice: Institut de veille sanitaire. Report No.: 75.

8. Belguzhanova A KK (2007) In:Results of the sentinel surveillance survey among MSM. 2006 national conference on results of the sentinel surveillance in kazakhstan; April 9–10, 2007; Almaty, Kazakhstan.

9. Caceres CF, Konda K, Segura ER, Lyerla R (2008) Epidemiology of male same-sex behaviour and associated sexual health indicators in low- and middle-income countries: 2003–2007 estimates. Sex Transm Infect Aug;84 Suppl 1:i49–56.

10. Malekinejad M, Johnston LG, Kendall C, Kerr LR, Rifkin MR, et al. (2008) Using respondent-driven sampling methodology for HIV biological and behavioral surveillance in international settings: A systematic review. AIDS Behav Jul;12(4 Suppl):S105–30.

11. Salganik MJ (2006) Variance estimation, design effects, and sample size calculations for respondent-driven sampling. J Urban Health Nov;83(6 Suppl):i98–112.

12. Fay H, Baral SD, Trapence G, Motimedi F, Umar E, et al. Stigma, health care access, and HIV knowledge among men who have sex with men in malawi, namibia, and botswana. AIDS Behav 2011 Aug;15(6):1088–97.

13. Lane T, Raymond HF, Dladla S, Rasethe J, Struthers H, et al. High HIV prevalence among men who have sex with men in soweto, south africa: Results from the soweto men's study. AIDS Behav 2011 Apr;15(3):626–34.

14. Gelman A (2007) Struggles with survey weighting and regression modelling. Statistical Science 22(2):153–64.

15. Johnston LG, Malekinejad M, Kendall C, Iuppa IM, Rutherford GW (2008) Implementation challenges to using respondent-driven sampling methodology for HIV biological and behavioral surveillance: Field experiences in international settings. AIDS Behav. Jul;12(4 Suppl):S131–41.

16. Cambiano V, Rodger AJ, Phillips AN (2011) 'Test-and-treat': The end of the HIV epidemic? Curr Opin Infect Dis Feb;24(1):19–26.

17. Goodreau SM, Golden MR (2007) Biological and demographic causes of high HIV and sexually transmitted disease prevalence in men who have sex with men. Sex Transm Infect Oct;83(6):458–62.

18. Colfax G, Coates TJ, Husnik MJ, Huang Y, Buchbinder S, Koblin B, et al. (2005) Longitudinal patterns of methamphetamine, popper (amyl nitrite), and cocaine use and high-risk sexual behavior among a cohort of san francisco men who have sex with men. J Urban Health Mar;82(1 Suppl 1):i62–70.

9

Comparison of Audio Computer Assisted Self-Interview and Face-To-Face Interview Methods in Eliciting HIV-Related Risks among Men Who Have Sex with Men and Men Who Inject Drugs in Nigeria

Sylvia Adebajo[1]*, Otibho Obianwu[1], George Eluwa[1], Lung Vu[2], Ayo Oginni[1], Waimar Tun[3], Meredith Sheehy[4], Babatunde Ahonsi[1], Adebobola Bashorun[5], Omokhudu Idogho[6], Andrew Karlyn[7]

1 Population Council, Abuja, Nigeria, 2 Population Services International (PSI), Washington, DC, United States of America, 3 Population Council, Washington, DC, United States of America, 4 Population Council, New York, New York, United States of America, 5 Federal Ministry of Health, Abuja, Nigeria, 6 Society for Family Health, Abuja, Nigeria, 7 United States Agency for International Development (USAID), Washington, DC, United States of America

Abstract

Introduction: Face-to-face (FTF) interviews are the most frequently used means of obtaining information on sexual and drug injecting behaviours from men who have sex with men (MSM) and men who inject drugs (MWID). However, accurate information on these behaviours may be difficult to elicit because of sociocultural hostility towards these populations and the criminalization associated with these behaviours. Audio computer assisted self-interview (ACASI) is an interviewing technique that may mitigate social desirability bias in this context.

Methods: This study evaluated differences in the reporting of HIV-related risky behaviours by MSM and MWID using ACASI and FTF interviews. Between August and September 2010, 712 MSM and 328 MWID in Nigeria were randomized to either ACASI or FTF interview for completion of a behavioural survey that included questions on sensitive sexual and injecting risk behaviours. Data were analyzed separately for MSM and MWID. Logistic regression was run for each behaviour as a dependent variable to determine differences in reporting methods.

Results: MSM interviewed via ACASI reported significantly higher risky behaviours with both women (multiple female sexual partners 51% vs. 43%, p = 0.04; had unprotected anal sex with women 72% vs. 57%, p = 0.05) and men (multiple male sex partners 70% vs. 54%, p≤0.001) than through FTF. Additionally, they were more likely to self-identify as homosexual (AOR: 3.3, 95%CI:2.4–4.6) and report drug use in the past 12 months (AOR:40.0, 95%CI: 9.6–166.0). MWID interviewed with ACASI were more likely to report needle sharing (AOR:3.3, 95%CI:1.2–8.9) and re-use (AOR:2.2, 95%CI:1.2–3.9) in the past month and prior HIV testing (AOR:1.6, 95%CI 1.02–2.5).

Conclusion: The feasibility of using ACASI in studies and clinics targeting key populations in Nigeria must be explored to increase the likelihood of obtaining more accurate data on high risk behaviours to inform improved risk reduction strategies that reduce HIV transmission.

Editor: Anil Kumar, University of Missouri-Kansas City, United States of America

Funding: The study was funded by the UK Department for International Development (DFID) through the Enhancing Nigeria's Response to HIV/AIDS (ENR) program. The funders had no role in study design, data collection and analysis, decision to publish, or preparation of the manuscript. Find out more about DFID at https://www.gov.uk/government/organisations/department-for-international-development.

Competing Interests: The authors have declared that no competing interests exist.

* E-mail: sadebajo@popcouncil.org

Introduction

There is growing evidence that men who have sex with men (MSM) and men who inject drugs (MWID) in Nigeria are hyper-vulnerable to HIV infection [1–7] because of high levels of political, religious and cultural hostility as well as the criminalization of their behavior [4,8,9]. According to the two rounds of the Integrated Biological Behavioural Surveillance Survey (IBBSS) conducted in Nigeria in 2007 and 2010, the estimated HIV prevalence among MSM increased from 13.5% in 2007 to 17.2%

in 2010 and among PWID, HIV prevalence decreased from 5.2% in 2007 to 4.2% in 2010 [1,2]. The surveys also revealed low self-perceived risk, significant levels of risky sexual and injecting practices and poor health-seeking behaviours among MSM and MWID in Nigeria [1,2].

Unbiased measurements of socially sensitive behaviours are necessary to accurately study sensitive behaviours that may determine acquisition and transmission of sexually transmitted infections (STIs) including HIV [10,11]. In some populations, an audio computer-based technology that enables respondents to self-administer questionnaires in complete privacy, such as the audio computer assisted self-interview (ACASI), has succeeded in eliciting unbiased responses for socially sensitive behaviours [10,12,13]. Studies comparing responses from clinician interviews and ACASI of self-reports of socially sensitive behaviours revealed that ACASI responses were more complete for socially sensitive behaviours like admitting to having same-gender sex partners and illicit drug use, group sex, rape, commercial sex than face-to-face (FTF) interviews [14–18]. Advantages of ACASI formatted surveys include consistency in the way questions are asked thus, maximizing standardization; limiting handling of data forms, protecting participant confidentiality and direct data capturing thereby, decreasing staff effort and enhancing data quality [10,12,16,19,20].

The ACASI technology is ideal for research with key populations such as MSM and people who inject drugs (PWID) for reliable and frank reporting of sensitive behaviours. However there is limited testing of the instrument in low resource settings such as Nigeria [12,13,15,21–23]. We evaluated differences in the reporting of risky HIV-related behaviours among MSM and MWID using ACASI and FTF. The hypothesis was that MSM and MWID interviewed by ACASI method would be more likely to report sensitive HIV-risk behaviours compared to those interviewed FTF.

Methods

Study sites

This study was conducted at three Men's Health Network, Nigeria (MHNN) clinics in Abuja, located in north central Nigeria, and Lagos and Ibadan, both located in southwest Nigeria. MHNN provides HIV prevention services including behaviour change communications, HIV counselling and testing (HCT), syndromic management of STIs, and condom and lubricant distribution to key male populations (MSM and MWID) and their male and female sex partners.

Study populations and sampling strategy

MSM were defined as men aged 18 years and above who reported sexual activity (oral or anal) with another man at least once in the 12 months preceding the survey. MWID were defined as men aged 18 years and older who injected drugs recreationally at least once in the last 12 months. Participants were recruited through respondent-driven sampling (RDS), an adaptation of snowball or chain referral sampling typically used to recruit hard-to-reach populations where peers recruit their peers into the study [24,25]. Recruitment of MSM and MWID spanned six weeks from August to September, 2010.

Ethics statement

Due to the sensitive nature of the study, special precautions were taken in conducting the study to maximize the safety and confidentiality of participants. Ethical approval was obtained from the Institutional Review Boards of the Nigerian Institute for Medical Research, Nigeria and the Population Council, New York. Participation in the study was voluntary and did not in any way compromise participants' access to services offered by the Men's Health Network, Nigeria (MHNN). Written informed consent was obtained from all participants prior to conducting all study procedures. Participants were able to receive laboratory tests for STIs (syphilis, gonorrhoea, chlamydia, HBV, and HCV) free-of-charge if they desired. They were also compensated NGN500 for participating in the first visit of this study and an additional NGN500 at their follow-up visit for each additional eligible peer

they successfully recruited into the study. The total amount of compensation was between NGN 1,000 (USD 6.60) and NGN 2,000 (USD 13.30) depending on the number of peers each participant was able to recruit.

Data collection

Behavioural data were collected by the administration of face to face (FTF) interviews and by ACASI. The questionnaire was available in both English and Pidgin English in both interview modes. Participants were randomized to either the ACASI or FTF interview arm for completion of the behavioural survey. Randomization was determined by a set of random numbers generated from Random Allocation Software [26]. ACASI interviews were conducted in private cubicles with the use of laptops and headphones. Each respondent was given a short orientation to familiarize them with the system and to ensure respondent's comfort with the laptop, mouse, and the format of the questionnaire. Survey questions for both arms of the study were identical, and participants had the option of not answering any question. At the end of the ACASI interview, a random 10% of participants were selected to answer a short exit survey assessing participants' experience using ACASI and their opinions about future use of ACASI. The survey lasted for about 30 minutes in the FTF method and 40 minutes in the ACASI method.

Variables of Interest

To test the study hypothesis, a set of sensitive sexual and injecting risk behaviours was selected based on literature review. For MSM, the following indicators were selected: 1) sexual identity; 2) having multiple sex partners in the past two months; 3) having anal sex with women in the past two months; 4) having unprotected anal sex with men and women at last sex; 5) injecting drugs; 6) having STI symptoms in the past 12 months; 7) using drugs in the past 12 months; and 8) ever testing for HIV. For MWID, the following questions were selected: 1) having multiple sex partners; 2) having unprotected sex at last sex; 3) having casual sex partners, including commercial sex in past two months; 4) age at first injecting drugs; 5) years of injecting drug; 6) sharing of needles and syringes; 7) STI symptoms in the past 12 months; and 8) ever testing for HIV. To elicit STI symptoms, respondents were asked if they had experienced any pain, itching, ulcer/sore or discharge from the penis or anal region in the past 12 months.

Statistical Analyses

Data were analyzed separately for MSM and MWID using STATA software version 11. MSM data were pooled across the 3 sites to provide sufficient statistical power. To determine whether the randomization was successful, demographic characteristics including age (age = 0.41), education (p = 0.26) and employment status (p = 0.07) were compared between the two groups. Descriptive analysis was conducted to describe the sample characteristics. For bivariate analysis we used chi-squared test to determine differences in reporting for categorical variables and t-test to determine differences in reporting for continuous variables by interview mode. Logistic regression model was run for each sensitive behaviour as a dependent variable to determine if ACASI elicited significantly different responses from FTF while controlling for age, education, HIV status, and study sites. The influence of age and socio-economic status (using education and study sites as proxies at the individual and structural levels respectively) on reporting of health outcomes is well documented [27,28]. Odds ratios, confidence intervals and p-values are reported. The level of significance was determined at $p < 0.05$.

Results

Characteristics of the study population

For recruitment of MSM in Abuja, five of seven seeds actively recruited with a maximum of eleven waves of recruitment and an average of six waves for each active seed In Ibadan, three of four seeds actively recruited with a maximum of eight recruitment waves and an average of seven waves while in Lagos all three seeds were active with a maximum of 14 waves of recruitment and an average of six waves.

A total of 712 MSM and 328 MWID were recruited. Median age was 23 years and 40 years, respectively (Table 1). A large proportion of MSM (65%) and MWID (45%) had completed at least secondary level education and about a third of both MSM and MWID were unemployed. Among the MSM, 42% self-identified as homosexual and 87% had had anal sex with a man in the past twelve months.

Reporting of sensitive information by interview mode

Men who have sex with men. Table 2 compares the reports of sexual behaviours by participants using ACASI and FTF interviewing techniques. Interestingly, a significantly higher proportion of respondents in the ACASI group compared with the FTF group reported being married or cohabiting with a woman (15% vs. 11%; p≤0.0001) or cohabiting with a man (26% vs. 15%; p≤0.0001) (data not shown). Similarly, a higher proportion of respondents in the ACASI group reported having more than one female sex partner in the past two months compared to those in the FTF group (51% vs. 43%; p = 0.04). In the ACASI group, a significantly higher proportion of respondents reported anal sex with women in the past two months prior to the survey (72% vs. 21%; p≤0.001), unprotected anal sex with women (72% vs. 57%; p = 0.05), being paid for sex in the past six months (54% vs. 46%; p = 0.05), having two or more male sex partners in the past two months compared to FTF (70% vs. 54%; p≤0.001), and reporting drug use in the last 12 months (6% vs. 1%; p<0.001) compared to those in the FTF group. The use of cocaine (5% vs 1%; p≤0.001), heroine (2% vs 1%; p≤0.001) and marijuana (21% vs. 12%; p≤0.001) in the past 12 months was higher among those interviewed via ACASI compared to FTF. However, there was no difference between the ACASI and FTF groups for unprotected anal sex with a male partner at last sexual intercourse (42% vs. 45%; p>0.05) and self-report of ever testing for HIV (58% vs. 52%; p = 0.12).

Men who inject drugs. Among MWID, the median age of first injection was lower among those interviewed via ACASI compared to FTF (28 years vs. 30 years; p = <0.01). For injecting risk behaviours, there was higher reporting of sharing (13% vs. 5%; p<0.05) and reusing needles by the same individual (40% vs. 27%; p = 0.03) among those interviewed via ACASI than FTF. Although, a higher proportion of MWID in the FTF reported being married or cohabiting with a woman compared with the ACASI (47% vs. 33%; p = 0.02) (data not shown), however, there were no significant differences between the ACASI and FTF groups in their reports of the number of female sex partners (18% vs. 17%; p = 0.9), unprotected sex at last sex (18% vs. 15%; p = 0.6) and injecting drugs in the past month (76% vs. 76%; p = 0.9).

Likelihood of reporting sensitive behaviours

Table 2 reports the results of the multivariate analysis of the two interview modes. MSM interviewed by ACASI were more likely to self-identity as homosexual (AOR:3.3, 95% CI:2.4–4.6), to report multiple female partners (AOR:1.4, 95% CI:1.1–1.9); multiple male partners (AOR: 2.1, 95% CI: 1.5–2.8); anal sex with women (AOR:13.1, 95% CI: 7.9–21.7); and unprotected anal sex with women (AOR:2.1, 95% CI:1.1–4.1). Additionally, MSM in the ACASI arm were more likely to report STI symptoms in the last 12 months (AOR: 2.9, 95% CI: 2.1–4.1) and to use drugs in the past 12 months (AOR: 40.0, 95% CI: 9.6–166.0).

Among MWID, those interviewed by ACASI were more likely to report needle sharing in the past month (AOR:3.3, 95% CI: 1.2–8.9), reusing of their own needles (AOR:2.2, 95% CI:1.2–3.9), and ever testing for HIV (AOR:1.6, 95% CI:1.02–2.5) (Table 3).

Acceptability of ACASI

About 76% of respondents reported that they were interviewed via FTF in a behavioural survey at least once in the past. Nonetheless, more than 80% (Table 4) felt comfortable using the ACASI interview method and found it not difficult to use. On a scale of 1–5 (with 1 representing do not like the ACASI at all and 5 liking it very much), over two-thirds of respondents liked the ACASI method very much. Almost half of the respondents (47%) liked the ACASI because of privacy and 31% liked it because it was clearer (by being able to both read and listen to the questions). Nearly all respondents (97%) would like to use ACASI in the future if given a choice. On average, the ACASI method took

Table 1. Demographic characteristics of the study population.

Variables	MSM (n = 712) % (n)	MWID (n = 328) % (n)
Age		
(median & range)	23 (18–52)	40 (18–50)
Education		
Primary or less	6.5 (46)	26.8 (88)
Secondary	64.9 (462)	44.8 (147)
Tertiary	28.7 (204)	28.4 (93)
Unemployment	33.4 (238)	34.5 (113)
Being HIV positive	22.6 (150)	1.8 (6)
Self-reported homosexual identity	42.0 (275)	n/a
Had anal sex with a man in the past 2 months	86.7 (617)	n/a
Injected drug in the past month	7.7 (55)	75.7 (237)

Table 2. Multivariate analysis for reported HIV risks by interview modes among MSM.

Variables	FTF (N = 372) % (n)	ACASI (N = 342) % (n)	p-value	AOR (95% CI)
Self-reported homosexual identity	29.1 (103)	57.1 (172)	≤0.001	3.3 (2.4–4.6)***
Had multiple female sex partner in the past two month	43.0 (159)	50.6 (173)	0.04	1.4 (1.1–1.9)*
Had multiple male sex partner past two months	54.1 (200)	70.0 (239)	≤0.001	2.1 (1.5–2.8)***
Had anal sex with women in past two month	21.3 (60)	71.6 (121)	≤0.001	13.1 (7.9–21.7)***
Had unprotected anal sex with men at last sex	45.1 (167)	41.5 (142)	0.33	0.9 (0.7–1.2)
Had unprotected anal sex with women at last sex	57.1 (36)	71.7 (86)	0.05	2.1 (1.1–4.1)*
Had STI symptoms in the past 12 months	20.5 (76)	42.7 (146)	≤0.00	2.9 (2.1–4.1)***
Ever tested for HIV	52.2 (191)	57.9 (198)	0.12	1.2 (0.8–1.6)
Injected drug past 12 months	0.6 (2)	16.0 (53)	0.00	40.0 (9.6–166.0)***
Used cocaine in past 12 months	1.4 (5%)	4.7 (16)	≤0.001	
Used heroine in past 12 months	0.8 (3)	2.3 (8)	≤0.001	
Used marijuana in past 12 months	11.6 (43)	21.4 (73)	≤0.001	

Note: AOR = Adjusted odds ratio, CI = confidence interval,
*: significant at $p<.05$,
**: significant at $p<.01$,
***: significant at $p<.001$.
Age, education, HIV status, and study sites were adjusted for in the regression models looking at likelihood of reporting HIV risks by interview method (reference FTF).

about 10 minutes longer than the FTF method (40 minutes vs. 30 minutes).

Discussion

This is the first study to evaluate self-reports of sexual risk behaviours among MSM and MWID in Nigeria using ACASI and FTF. We observed some important findings. First, MSM interviewed via ACASI were more likely to self-identify as homosexual or gay and report significantly higher levels of engagement in sexual risk behaviours with both women and men for the following indicators: multiple male and female sexual partnerships and unprotected anal sex with women. Second, MSM respondents in the ACASI group reported significantly

higher use of psychoactive drugs, highlighting drug use among MSM. Third, MWID were more likely to report sharing needles and reporting younger age at injection debut via ACASI than FTF. Fourth, the study showed high levels of acceptability and preference for ACASI among respondents because of privacy and ease of use. These findings have important implications for HIV research and programming in Nigeria. Furthermore, the higher levels of bisexuality and risky sexual behaviors reported by ACASI respondents in this study and elsewhere [6,7,29,30] highlights the urgent need for MSM interventions in Nigeria to incorporate information on safer sex with both male and female sex partners.

The study also identified significantly higher reporting of gay or homosexual identity, cohabiting with a male partner and engaging in HIV-related risks with ACASI. This highlights the challenges

Table 3. Reported HIV risks by interview modes among MWID (N = 328).

Variables	FTT (N = 166) % (n)	ACASI (N = 162) % (n)	χ2 or t (p-value)	OR (95% CI)
Had multiple female sex partners in past 2 months	17.5 (29)	16.7 (27)	0.04 (0.85)	1.0 (0.5–1.7)
Had unprotected sex at last sex	17.5 (29)	15.4 (25)	0.2 (0.61)	0.9 (0.5–1.6)
Had casual sex partners in past 2 months	7.9 (5)	26.4 (14)	7.2 (0.03)	3.7 (1.2–11.4)*
Age first injected drugs [mean (std.)][a]	30.1 (0.5)	27.6 (0.7)	3.0 (0.003)	0.96 (0.93–0.99)*
Number of years injecting drugs [mean (std.)][a]	8.4 (0.5)	7.9 (0.6)	0.7 (0.49)	1.0 (0.95–1.02)
Injected drugs in the past month	75.8 (122)	75.7 (115)	0.00 (0.98)	1.0 (0.6–1.7)
Shared needle/syringes in the past month	4.9 (6)	13.3 (15)	5.1 (0.02)	3.3 (1.2–8.9)*
Used your own needle and syringes over again	26.6 (91)	40.0 (46)	4.8 (0.03)	2.2 (1.2–3.9)**
Had STI symptoms in the past 12 months	4.8 (8)	11.1 (18)	4.4 (0.04)	2.4 (1.02–5.8)*
Ever tested for HIV	47.2 (76)	36.0 (58)	4.1 (0.04)	1.6 (1.02–2.5)*

Note: AOR = adjusted odds ratio, CI = confidence interval,
*: significant at $p<.05$,
**: significant at $p<.01$.
Age, education, and HIV status were adjusted for in the regression models looking at reported HIV risks among ACASI method vs. FTF interview method.
[a]significant levels were determined using t-test comparing 2 continuous variables.

Table 4. Experience and preference regarding the use of ACASI (N = 94).

	% (n)
How often you use computer?	
Everyday/almost everyday	42.5 (40)
Once/twice a week	23.4 (22)
Once/twice a month	19.2 (18)
Almost never	14.9 (14)
How comfortable were you using the ACASI?	
Very comfortable	80.9 (76)
Comfortable	18.1 (17)
Uncomfortable	1.1 (1)
How difficult in using the ACASI?	
Very difficult	3.2 (3)
Somewhat difficult	12.8 (12)
Not at all	84.0 (79)
How did you rate the ACASI?*	
1	3.2 (3)
2	2.1 (2)
3	12.8 (12)
4	13.8 (13)
5	68.1 (64)
What did you like most about using computer?	
More fun	17.0 (16)
More private	46.8 (44)
Clearer because I can read and listen to the questions	30.9 (29)
Nothing	5.3 (5)
Have you done a FTF interview before?	
Yes	75.5 (71)
No	24.5 (23)
Which type of interview did you like?	
ACASI	64.5 (49)
FTF	9.2 (7)
Both equally	26.3 (20)
Would like to use computer in the future to answer questions	
Yes	96.8 (90)
No	3.2 (3)

Note: *1 = did not like it at all, 5 = liked it very much.

that researchers may face in obtaining accurate estimates of HIV-related risks with standard behavioural surveys administered via FTF, including the Integrated Biological and Behavioral Surveillance Survey (IBBSS). Compared to the IBBSS, more MSM respondents interviewed via ACASI reported having experienced STI symptoms in the past 12 months (43% vs. 15%), had two or more male partners (70% vs. 50%) and did not use condom at last sex with men (67% vs. 50%) and female sex workers (72% vs. 35%). In addition, health care providers serving key populations may also encounter challenges in identifying risky behaviours to guide adequate counselling and the development of appropriate risk reduction plans. Another significant finding of this study was the higher reporting of drug use among MSM. MSM interviewed with the ACASI were forty times more likely to report drug use than those interviewed with FTF. This indicates that drug use

among MSM may be much higher than is often reported. In addition, because drug use is associated with higher sexual-risk taking, deeper knowledge of this risk factor among MSM is required to better inform the design of effective comprehensive interventions.

The acceptability and preference of ACASI by MSM and MWID is high, indicating the feasibility of ACASI use in future surveys. Privacy and ease of use are possible factors that contribute to the higher reporting of risk behaviours among both MSM and MWID. Qualitative studies in Zimbabwe [31] and in the United States [14] reported that the perceived privacy and confidentiality of ACASI are reasons behind more accurate reporting of sensitive behaviours. The acceptability of ACASI has also been found to be high even among respondents with low levels of computer literacy in resource limited settings [31].

The findings of this study demonstrate that efforts and resources must be geared towards using ACASI in future surveys to elicit more accurate behavioural information to guide evidence-based HIV prevention programming. Furthermore, obtaining accurate estimates of HIV-related risks is important for measuring the effectiveness of interventions and modelling optimal packages for HIV preventions.

Limitations

This study has some limitations. We did not assess the reporting of HIV-related risk behaviour using both methods on the same individuals hence, we were unable to assess the validity and consistency of each interview method. However, given that the assessment was part of a larger cross-sectional survey that assessed HIV and STI prevalence and risks, randomization of respondents into two study arms was the most feasible option.

Conclusion

This is the first study to compare self-reports of HIV risk behaviours among MSM and MWID in Nigeria using ACASI and FTF interview modes. The significantly higher reporting of risk behaviours of ACASI respondents suggests that risks of MSM and

MWID may be underestimated in traditional FTF surveys. As accurate reporting of HIV-risk behaviours is important for HIV programming, research and allocation of resources, ACASI or CASI is highly recommended in both clinical and research settings to reduce social desirability bias. This may be of particular importance in surveys among key populations who engage in behaviours that are stigmatized and often illegal.

Acknowledgments

We acknowledge the immense contributions of the study participants. Special thanks go to Jean Njab, Sandra Johnson, Emeka Nwachukwu, Apera Iorwakwagh, Oliver Anene, Dennis Akpona, Segun Sangowawa, Akin Toyose, Folasade Ogunsola, Issa Kawu, Aderemi Azeez and the entire ACASI Study Team. The findings and recommendations of this study are those of the authors and do not necessarily reflect the views of the funder.

Consent: Obtained for all participants

Author Contributions

Conceived and designed the experiments: SA AK LV WT MS OI. Performed the experiments: SA LV WT MS AB. Analyzed the data: LV AO. Wrote the paper: OO GE SA LV AO BA.

References

1. FMOH (2007) Integrated Biological and Behavioral Surveillance Survey (IBBSS). Abuja, Nigeria.
2. FMOH (2010) Integrated Biological and Behavioral Surveillance Survey (IBBSS). Abuja, Nigeria.
3. Merrigan M, Azeez A, Afolabi B, Chabikuli ON, Onyekwena O, et al. (2011) HIV prevalence and risk behaviours among men having sex with men in Nigeria. Sex Transm Infect. 87(1):65–70.
4. Allman D, Adebajo S, Myers T, Odumuye O, Ogunsola S (2007) Challenges for the sexual health and social acceptance of men who have sex with men in Nigeria. Culture, health & sexuality 9(2):153–68.
5. Vu L, Andrinopoulos K, Tun W, Adebajo S (2013) High levels of unprotected anal intercourse and never testing for HIV among men who have sex with men (MSM) in Nigeria: A call for targeted and novel approaches to HIV prevention among MSM. AIDS and Behavior. In Press.
6. Sheehy M, Tun W, Vu L, Adebajo S, Obianwu O, et al. (2013) High levels of bisexual behavior and factors associated with bisexual behavior among men having sex with men (MSM) in Nigeria. AIDS Care 6:6.
7. Vu L, Adebajo S, Tun W, Sheehy M, Karlyn A, et al. (2013) High HIV prevalence among men who have sex with men in Nigeria: implications for combination prevention. Journal of Acquired Immune Deficiency Syndrome 63(2):221–7.
8. ENR (2010) Prevalence of STIs among MSM and IDUs and Validation of ACASI in Abuja, Lagos and Ibadan. Abuja: Population Council.
9. Adebajo SB, Eluwa G, Allman D, Myers T, Ahonsi B (2012) Prevalence of internalized homophobia and HIV associated risks among men who have sex with men in Nigeria. African Journal of Reproductive Health 2012 16(4): 21–28.
10. Ghanem KG, Hutton HE, Zenilman JM, Zimba R, Erbelding EJ (2005) Audio computer assisted self interview and face to face interview modes in assessing response bias among STD clinic patients. Sex Transm Infect. 81:421–5.
11. Gregson S, Zhuwau T, Ndlovu J, Nyamukapa CA. (2002) Methods to reduce social desirability bias in sex surveys in low-development settings: experience in Zimbabwe. Sex Transm Dis 29:568–75.
12. Turner CF, Ku L, Rogers SM, Lindberg LD, Pleck JH, et al. (1998) Adolescent sexual behaviour, drug use, and violence: increased reporting with computer survey technology. Science 280:867–73.
13. Johnson AM, Copas AJ, Erens B, Mandalia S, Fenton K, et al. (2001) Effect of computer-assisted self-interviews on reporting of sexual HIV risk behaviours in a general population sample: a methodological experiment. AIDS 15:111–5.
14. Torrone EA, Thomas JC, Maman S, Pettifor EA, Kaufman JS, et al. (2010) Risk behavior disclosure during HIV test counseling. AIDS patient care and STDs 24:9.
15. Kurth AE, Martin DP, Golden MR, Weiss NS, Heagerty PJ, et al. (2004) A comparison between audio computer-assisted self-interviews and clinician interviews for obtaining the sexual history. Sex Trans Dis 31:719–26.
16. van der Elst H, Okuku HS, Nakamya P, Muhaari A, Davies A, et al. (2009) Is Audio Computer-Assisted Self-Interview (ACASI) useful in risk behaviour assessment of female and male sex workers, Mombasa, Kenya? PLoS ONE 4(5).
17. Mensch BS, Hewett PC, Erulkar AS (2003) The reporting of sensitive behaviour among adolescents: a methodological experiment in Kenya. Demography 40:247–68.
18. Hewett PC, Mensch BS, Erulkar AS (2004) Consistency in the reporting of sexual behaviour by adolescent girls in Kenya: a comparison of interviewing methods. Sex Trans Inf. 80 (Suppl II):ii43–ii8.
19. Jaya, Hindin MJ, Ahmed S (2008) Differences in young people's reports of sexual behaviors according to interview methodology: a randomized trial in India. Am J Public Health 98:169–74.
20. Aday LA, Cornelius LA (2006) Designing and conducting health surveys: a comprehensive guide. San Francisco Jossey-Bass.
21. Kissinger P, Rice J, Farley T, Trim S, Jewitt K, et al. (1999) Application of computer-assisted interviews to sexual behaviour research. Am J Epidemiol. 149:950–54.
22. Des Jarlais D, Paone D, Milliken J, Turner CF, Miller H, et al. (1999) Audiocomputer interviewing to measure risk behaviour for HIV among injection drug users: a quasi-randomised trial. Lancet 353 (9165):1657–61.
23. Williams ML, Freeman RC, Bowen AM, Zhao Z, Elwood WN, et al. (2000) A comparison of the reliability of self-reported drug use and sexual behaviours using computer-assisted versus face-to-face interviewing. AIDS Educ Prev. 12:199–213.
24. Salganik M (2006) Variance estimation, design effects and sample size calculations for respondent driven sampling. Journal of Urban Health 83(6suppl):i98–112.
25. Heckthorn DD (1997) Respondent-driven sampling: A new approach to the study of hidden populations. Social Problems 44:174–99.
26. Saghaei M (2004) Random Allocation Software. 1.0 ed. Isfahan, Iran.
27. Hallman K (2004). Disadvantage and unsafe sexual Behaviors among young women and men in South Africa. NY: Population Council.
28. WHO (2009) Environment and Health Risks: The influence and effects of social inequalities: report of an expert group meeting Bonn, Germany.
29. Vu L, Adebajo S, Tun W, Sheehy M, Karlyn A, et al. (2013) High HIV prevalence among men who have sex with men in Nigeria: implications for combination prevention. Journal of acquired immune deficiency syndromes 63(2):221–7.
30. Beyrer C, Trapence G, Motimedi F, Umar E, Lipinge S, et al. (2010) Bisexual concurrency, bisexual partnerships, and HIV among Southern African men who have sex with men. Sex Transm Infect. 86(4):323–7.
31. Langhaug LF, Cheung YB, Pascoe SJ, Chirawu P, Woelk G, et al. (2011) How you ask really matters: randomized comparison of four sexual behavior questionnaire delivery modes in Zimbabwean youth. Sex Transm Infect. 87:165–73.

10

Can Interferon-Gamma or Interferon-Gamma-Induced-Protein-10 Differentiate Tuberculosis Infection and Disease in Children of High Endemic Areas?

Mohammed Ahmed Yassin[1,2], Roberta Petrucci[1], Kefyalew Taye Garie[2], Gregory Harper[1], Isabel Arbide[3], Melkamsew Aschalew[4], Yared Merid[4], Zelalem Kebede[2], Amin Ahmed Bawazir[1], Nabil Mohamed Abuamer[1], Luis Eduardo Cuevas[1]*

1 Liverpool School of Tropical Medicine, Liverpool, United Kingdom, **2** Faculty of Medicine, University of Hawassa, Awassa, Ethiopia, **3** Bushulo Major Health Centre, Awassa, Ethiopia, **4** Southern Region Health Bureau, Awassa, Ethiopia

Abstract

Background: Diagnosis of childhood tuberculosis (TB) is difficult in high TB burden settings. Interferon-gamma-induced protein 10 (IP10) has been suggested as a marker of TB infection and disease, but its ability to differentiate the two conditions remains uncertain.

Objectives: To describe Interferon-gamma (INFγ) and IP10 expression in children with TB infection and disease and controls to assess their potential to differentiate latent and active TB.

Methods: This was a cross sectional study of 322 1–15 years old children with symptoms of TB (28 *confirmed*, 136 *probable* and 131 *unlikely* TB), 335 children in contact with adults with pulmonary TB and 156 community controls in Southern Ethiopia. The Tuberculin Skin Test (TST) and Quantiferon-In-Tube (QFT-IT) were performed. INFγ and IP10 were measured in plasma supernatants.

Results and Interpretation: Children with *confirmed* and *probable* TB and *contacts* were more likely to have TST+ (78.6%, 59.3% and 54.1%, respectively) than children with *unlikely* TB (28.7%) and controls (12.8%) (p<0.001). Children with *confirmed* TB (59.3%) and *contacts* (44.7%) were more likely to have INFγ+ than children with *probable* (37.6%) or *unlikely* TB (28.1%) and controls (13.1%) (p<0.001). IP10 concentrations were higher in INFγ+ children independently of TST (p<0.001). There was no difference between IP10 concentrations of children with *confirmed* TB and *contacts* (p = 0.8) and children with and without HIV (p>0.1). INFγ and IP10 can identify children with TB infection and disease, but cannot differentiate between the two conditions. HIV status did not affect the expression of IP10.

Editor: Laura Ellen Via, National Institute of Allergy and Infectious Disease, United States of America

Funding: This study was funded by a research grant awarded by the Thrasher Foundation, United States of America. The funders had no role in study design, data collection and analysis, decision to publish, or preparation of the manuscript.

* E-mail: lcuevas@liv.ac.uk

Introduction

One of the most significant barriers for the appropriate management of Tuberculosis (TB) is the lack of suitable diagnostic tests. This problem is especially critical in settings where facilities are limited and other infections with overlapping clinical presentation are highly prevalent. Childhood TB presentation differs from adult TB as children experience more extra-pulmonary TB (EPTB) and lung involvement is frequently disseminated and without cavitations. Young children are unable to expectorate sputum and the specimens collected, such as gastric aspirates, are often paucibacillary and sometimes contain test inhibitors. Most diagnostics for TB thus perform poorly in children [1,2] and new tests or markers to diagnose TB in children are needed.

Interferon-gamma (INFγ) release assays (IGRAs) were developed in the last decade and are reported to have comparable sensitivity and higher specificity than the Tuberculin Skin Test (TST) to identify latent TB infections (LTBI). Their performance however is less reliable in young children and in patients co-infected with the Human Immunodeficiency Virus (HIV) [3,4,5]. These assays are frequently used by clinicians to support a diagnosis of symptomatic TB [3,6,7], even though they cannot distinguish between LTBI and symptomatic disease. IGRAS are also increasingly used in high TB incidence settings, despite the limited information of their performance in these locations [8,9,10].

INFγ-induced protein 10 (IP10, also known as Chemokine (C-X-C motif) ligand 10 or CXCL10) is another biomarker recently reported to identify LTBI, which, when combined with IGRAS is said to increase the sensitivity of the assays [10]. IP10 expression is putatively less affected by HIV [11] and young age [12,13] and it is said to have potential to differentiate between LTBI and symptomatic infections [12,14].

We have thus conducted a study in Southern Ethiopia to describe INFγ and IP10 concentrations of children presenting with symptoms compatible with TB, asymptomatic children in contact with adults with smear-positive pulmonary TB (PTB) and asymptomatic community controls to explore whether INFγ or IP10 can distinguish between symptomatic and asymptomatic infections in a high TB burden setting and assess whether these markers could be used to support the diagnosis of children with symptoms of TB.

Materials and Methods

This was a cross sectional study of 1 to 15 year old children with symptoms suggestive of TB, children in contact with adults with smear-positive PTB and community controls without known contact with TB. The study was based in Awassa, in the Southern Region of Ethiopia, which has a population of over 15 million.

Children with symptoms of TB (called *symptomatics*) were enrolled consecutively at three health service providers (Awassa Health Centre, Bushullo Major Health Centre and University of Hawassa referral hospital). These included consecutive children with cough or fever for more than 2 weeks, night sweats, anorexia, weight loss, failure to thrive or non-specific symptoms in the presence of a history of contact with an adult with PTB. Children were invited to participate at the time of presentation to the clinic. All children underwent a clinical examination, chest X-rays, TST, three sputum or gastric lavage examinations and fine needle aspiration if enlarged lymph nodes were detected. All specimens were examined using light smear microscopy and culture on Lowenstein Jensen media and children were classified as having *confirmed* (positive smear microscopy or culture), *probable* (negative smear microscopy and culture, clinical and radiological findings consistent with TB, no improvement after a full course of antibiotics and the clinician initiating anti-TB treatment) or *unlikely* TB (children with alternative diagnosis or clinical improvement after a course of broad spectrum antibiotics).

In addition, *contact* children 1–15 year old residing with adults with smear-positive PTB (called *contacts*) were enrolled by identifying adults attending the same study centres with a history of cough for more than 2 weeks duration who had sputum smear-positive PTB. Once a smear-positive adult had been identified, study investigators inquired whether they had children at home and visited the households if the family resided within a 20 km radius from Awassa. All children living under a single roof who shared meal times with the adult were invited to participate after obtaining informed parental consent, unless they had previously received treatment for TB. All children who shared meals at home with the index cases were included, regardless of the duration of contact.

Community *controls* were defined as children residing in the community who did not have a known contact with adults with PTB. *Controls* were selected from Awassa and surrounding *kebeles*, which are the smallest administrative units of Ethiopia and comprise at least five hundred families or 3,500 to 5,000 inhabitants. A list of all villages and *kebeles* located within a 20 Km radius from Awassa was constructed. Controls were enrolled from villages adjacent to the villages where contacts resided. We enrolled more controls from rural villages than from urban areas as the risk of TB transmission from casual contact could be higher among urban residents. Households within a village were selected by spinning a pen in a street somewhere between the centre and the edge of the village and children were enrolled after obtaining informed parental consent. Households were excluded if the parent indicated the family had been in

contact with an adult with cough for more than 2 weeks duration in the previous 2 years or if a family member had received treatment for TB. All children were applied a TST using 2 units of Purified Protein Derivate (PPD, RT 23, Statens Serum Institute, Copenhagen, Denmark) using the Mantoux method and indurations were measured using the palpation method 48 to 72 hours later. TST results were graded as negative (<5 mm), intermediate (≥5 and <10 mm) and positive (≥10 mm). Any child with signs and symptoms suggestive of TB was investigated for disease activity and treated. *Contact* children <6 years old were offered INH prophylaxis for 6 months independently of their TST result, following Ethiopian TB Control Programme guidelines.

INFγ and IP10 concentrations were assayed using commercially available Enzyme Linked Immunoassay (ELISA) kits. INFγ was measured using the QuantiFERON-TB Gold In-Tube (QFT-IT) test (Cellestis, Victoria, Australia). Blood samples for QFT-IT were collected in 3 tubes, one containing the *Mycobacterium tuberculosis* ESAT-6, CFP10 and TB7-7 antigens; one with non-specific mytogen (phytohemoagglutinin) to serve as positive control and one blank tube (nil) to serve as negative control. The three tubes were incubated at 37° for 16–24 hours. Supernatant plasma was harvested after centrifugation to separate the blood cells and stored at −70°C. INFγ was measured using the manufacturer's ELISA in a Bio-Rad Plate reader (Model n 550) and read at 450 nm. IGRAs were classified as positive, negative or indeterminate using the manufacturer's software. IP10 concentrations were measured in the same supernatant using a Human IP10 ELISA Construction Kit (Antigenix America Inc, New York, NY). HIV infections were established using two blood-based ELISA methods.

Means and standard deviations (SD) or medians and interquartile ranges (IQR) were used to describe continuous variables. Parametric tests and non parametric tests were used to compare means and medians. The proportion of children in each study category with positive/negative tests compared using Chi-Square and Fisher's exact tests (if expected values were less than<5) and the agreement between TST and INFγ was described using Kappa statistics. IP10 concentrations were described using boxplots stratified by TST and INFγ concordance. The sample size calculations took into account the feasibility to visit about 200 households (of index cases) within the available time and resources and that each household had an average of two children <5 years old and it was expected that 200 children with signs and sypmtoms of TB would attend the health services. It was expected that 50% of the participants would be TST positive and 70% and 30%, of TST-positive children would be INF-γ positive and negative, respectively. It was also assumed that 30% and 70% of TST-negative children would be INF-γ positive and negative, respectively. This sample size would allow estimating the proportion of children with positive and negative INF-γ results by study group with a precision of ±7%. Sample size calculation for the comparison of quantitative data (i.e. differences in IP-10 concentrations by study group) would have required prior information of the dispersion of IP-10 concentrations to estimate standard deviations or medians. As this information was not available, this study should be considered "exploratory", as it might not have enough power for the differences reported. The ability of IP10 to discriminate between children with and without TB infection or disease was evaluated using Receiver Operating Characteristic (ROC) curves using Prism 5 software (GraphPad PRISM, version 5). ROC curves were constructed with children with *confirmed* TB and controls and *contact* children with TST+/INFγ+ and *controls*. Only *controls* with TST-/INFγ- results were included in the ROC analysis to select children unlikely to have TB infection. The area under the curve (AUC) for both *confirmed* and *contact* children were compared to ascertain whether IP10 could discriminate between the two conditions. Statistical tests were considered significant if p values were <0.05.

The study protocol was approved by the Health Bureau of the Southern Region and the Research Ethics Committees of the Liverpool School of Tropical Medicine, Hawassa University and the Sciences and Technology Commission of Ethiopia. The study protocol was registered in the clinicatrials.gov clinical trials register (registration number NCT00456469)

Results

Eight hundred thirteen, 322 *symptomatic*, 335 *contact* and 156 *control* children were enrolled. The flow chart of the three groups is described in Figure 1. Twenty eight (3.7%) of 322 *symptomatic* children had *confirmed*, 136 (42.2%) *probable* and 131 (40.7%) *unlikely* TB and 27 were excluded because a definitive diagnosis was not reached or the child left the hospital before completing the investigations. The 335 *contact* children were recruited from 125 adult index cases who had "scanty" (18, 5.5%), "+" (188, 57%), "++" (109, 33%) or "+++" (15, 4.5%) smear microscopy grades in their sputum smear examination. In five *contacts* the smear result of the adult was not recorded. The median contact duration was 10 hours per week (range of 1 to 41 hours). The characteristics of the participants are shown in Table 1. Children with *probable* TB were more likely to be male (67.6%), while children in the other groups had similar proportions of males and females. Children had similar median age with symptomatic and control children having a median age of 6 years and contacts having a median of 8 years. Although the proportion of children reporting to have received BCG was similar across the groups, BCG scars were found less frequently in children with *confirmed* and *probable* TB (p<0.001). HIV was positive in none of the children with *confirmed* TB, 14 (10.9%) children with *probable* and 8 (6.5%) *unlikely* TB cases, 27 (8.2%) *contacts* and 3 (1.9%) *controls* (p = 0.005). The number of residents per household was higher among children with *symptoms*

of TB than among *contacts* and *controls* (means 8, 7.1 and 6.4 persons, respectively, p = 0.003). A significantly high proportion of children had lost one or both parents, with *symptomatic* and *contact* children being more likely to have lost a parent than *controls* (p = 0.01).

TST and INFγ results are shown in table 2. Children with *confirmed* and *probable* TB and *contacts* were more likely to have positive TST (TST+) (78.6%, 59.3% and 54.1%, respectively) than children with *unlikely* TB (28.7%) and *controls* (12.8%) (p<0.001). A high proportion of children had indeterminate INFγ tests, with children with *probable* and *unlikely* TB having a higher proportion of indeterminates than children with *confirmed* TB, *contacts* and *controls*. This problem was mostly due to failure of the positive control tube and was not associated with HIV infection (26/52 (50%) in HIV positive, compared to 256/641 (40%) in HIV-negative children, p = 0.2).

Children with *confirmed* TB (59.3%) and *contacts* (44.7%) were also more likely to have positive INFγ (INFγ+) than children with *probable* (37.6%) or *unlikely* TB (28.1%) and *controls* (13.1%) (p<0.001). Twenty two (78.6%) children with *confirmed*, 73 (53.7%) with *probable* and 68 (52%) with *unlikely* TB, 209 (62.4%) *contacts* and 114 (73.1%) *controls* had paired TST and IFNγ results after exclusion of intermediate TST and indeterminate INFγ tests. Concordance between INFγ and TST varied across the groups. Children with *confirmed* and *probable* TB and *contacts* were more likely to have concordant positive TST and INFγ (15 (68.2%) of 22, 38 (52.1%) of 73 and 87 (41.6%) of 209, respectively), while children with *unlikely* TB and *controls* were more likely to have concordant negative TST and INFγ (29 (42.6%) of 68 and 86 (75.4%) of 114, respectively). Discordant TST+/INFγ− results were more frequent among children with *probable* TB (20.5%) and *contacts* (18.7%) and discordant TST−/INFγ− results were more frequent among children with *unlikely* TB (22.1%) and *controls* (11.5%). Agreement between TST and IFNγ tests varied from 81% (k = 0.49) in children with *confirmed* TB, 73% (k = 0.40) in *probable* TB and 66% (k = 0.23) in *unlikely* TB, 70% (k = 0.39) in *contacts* and 81% (k = 0.24) in *controls*.

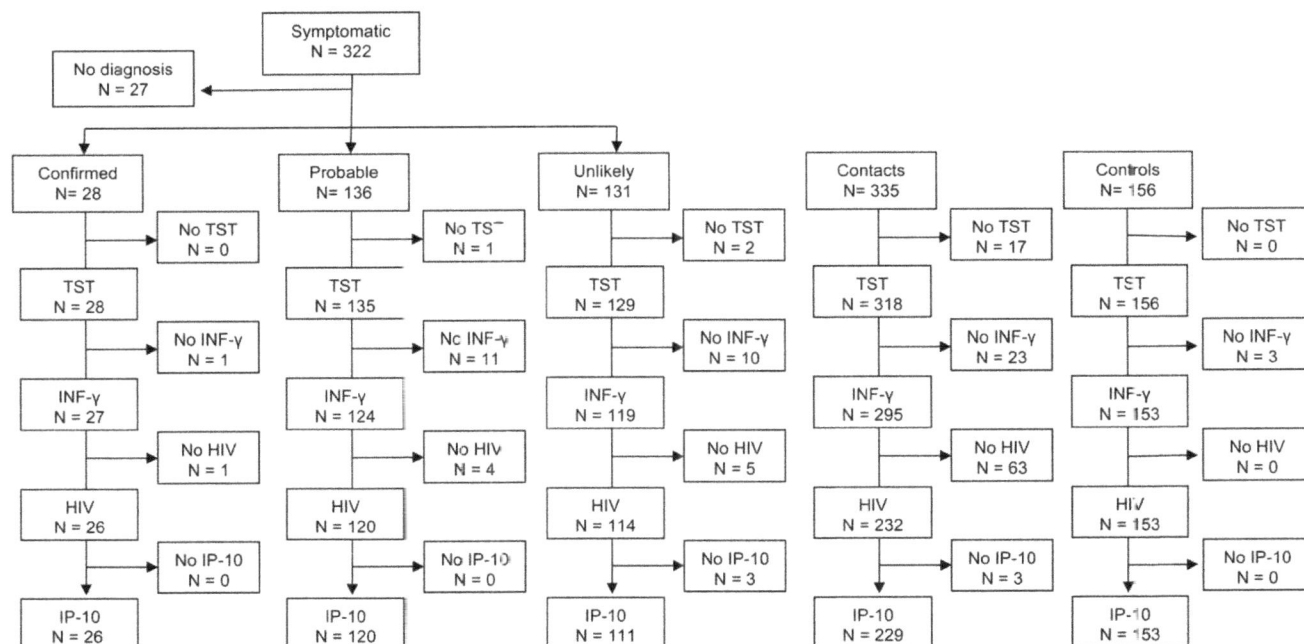

Figure 1. Flow chart of study participants.

Table 1. Characteristics of the study children.

Variables	Symptomatic cases N = 295					
	Confirmed TB N = 28	Probable TB N = 136	Unlikely TB N = 131	Contacts N = 335	Controls N = 156	p
Male/Female (% Male)	13/15 (46.4)	92/44 (67.6)	67/64 (51.1)	168/166 (50.3)	79/77 (50.6)	
Median age (years)	8	5	7	8	6	<0.001
Range	1–15	1–15	1–15	1–15	1–15	
Received BCG	14 (63.6)	69 (63.3)	82 (70.7)	249 (74.3)	120 (76.9)	0.01
BCG scar present (%)	7 (25)	35 (25.7)	51 (38.9)	174 (51.9)	93 (59.6)	<0.001
Mean (SD) BCG scar (mm)	7.4 (3.2)	5.3 (1.8)	5.5 (2.1)	4.7 (2.4)	5.4 (2.5)	<0.001
Range	4–13	2–9	2–10	1–13	2–13	
HIV status, Pos/tested (%Pos)	0/27 (0)	14/114 (10.9)	8/116 (6.5)	27/231 (8.2)	3/153 (1.9)	0.005
Mean (SD) residents/household	8.3 (7.5)	8.9 (8.3)	7.2 (6.3)	7.1 (2.6)	6.4 (2.4)	0.002
Illiterate Father, N (%)	17 (70.8)	63 (55.8)	55 (48.7)	112 (38.6)	87 (60.4)	<0.001
Mother, N (%)	21 (84)	97 (77.6)	87 (68.5)	170 (52.3)	123 (78.8)	<0.001
Alive Father, N (%)	24 (85.7)	113 (83.1)	113 (86.3)	293 (88.3)	144 (92.3)	0.2
Mother, N (%)	25 (89.3)	124 (92.5)	128 (98.5)	325 (97.6)	156 (100)	<0.001
Both parents, N (%)	23 (82.1)	109 (81.3)	112 (80)	293 (88)	144 (92.3)	0.01

IP10 concentrations are shown in Figure 2. Stimulated concentrations were much higher than non-stimulated concentrations in all groups (p<0.001). Non-stimulated concentrations were highest in children with *confirmed* TB and lowest in *controls* (medians 1606 and 386 pg/ml). Stimulated concentrations were higher in children with *confirmed* TB and *contacts* (7812 and 5616 pg/ml, respectively) than in children with *probable* and *unlikely* TB (3680 and 2532 pg/ml, respectively, Kruskal-Wallis, p = 0.02). The difference of stimulated minus non-stimulated concentrations are shown in Table 3 by TST and INFγ results and study group. Among patients with positive TST, *symptomatic* and *contact* children had higher IP10 concentrations than *controls* (p = 0.03 and p<0.001, respectively). Among children with negative TST, children with *confirmed* TB and *contacts* had higher IP10 concentrations than *controls* (p = 0.02 and p = 0.001, respectively. There was no difference in the IP10 concentrations across study groups among children with INFγ− results, while *contact* children with INFγ+ results had the highest IP10 concentrations, followed by *symptomatic* and *control* children. Median (IQR) IP10 concentrations (stimulated minus non-stimulated) are shown in Figure 3 by TST and INFγ concordance. Children with concordant TST+/INFγ+ had higher IP10 concentrations than children with TST−/INFγ− results in all study groups. Children with *confirmed* TB had high IP10 concentrations independently of the TST or INFγ result including two of the three children who had TST−/INFγ− results. In contrast, most *controls* had low IP10 concentrations with the exception of children with TST+/INFγ+ results, who had high IP10 concentrations (p = 0.04). Children with HIV had similar

Table 2. TST and INFγ results and concordance among the tests by study group.

Variables	Symptomatic cases N = 295				
	Confirmed TB N = 28 (%)	Probable TB N = 136 (%)	Unlikely TB N = 131 (%)	Contacts N = 335 (%)	Controls N = 156 (%)
TST					
Positive	22 (78.6)	80 (59.3)	37 (28.7)	172 (54.1)	20 (12.8)
Intermediate	0	10 (7.4)	9 (7)	48 (15.1)	15 (9.6)
Negative	6 (21.4)	45 (33.3)	83 (64.3)	98 (30.8)	121 (77.6)
INFγ					
Positive	16 (59.3)	47 (37.6)	34 (28.1)	139 (44.7)	20 (13.1)
Indeterminate	5 (18.5)	47 (37.6)	44 (36.4)	52 (16.7)	25 (16.3)
Negative	6 (22.2)	31 (24.8)	43 (35.5)	120 (38.6)	108 (70.6)
TST/INFγ concordance					
TST+/INFγ+	15 (68.2)	38 (52.1)	14 (20.6)	87 (41.6)	6 (5.3)
TST+/INFγ−	3 (13.6)	15 (20.5)	10 (14.7)	39 (18.7)	10 (8.8)
TST−/INFγ+	1 (4.5)	5 (6.8)	15 (22.1)	24 (11.5)	12 (10.5)
TST−/INFγ−	3 (13.6)	15 (20.5)	29 (42.6)	59 (28.2)	86 (75.4)

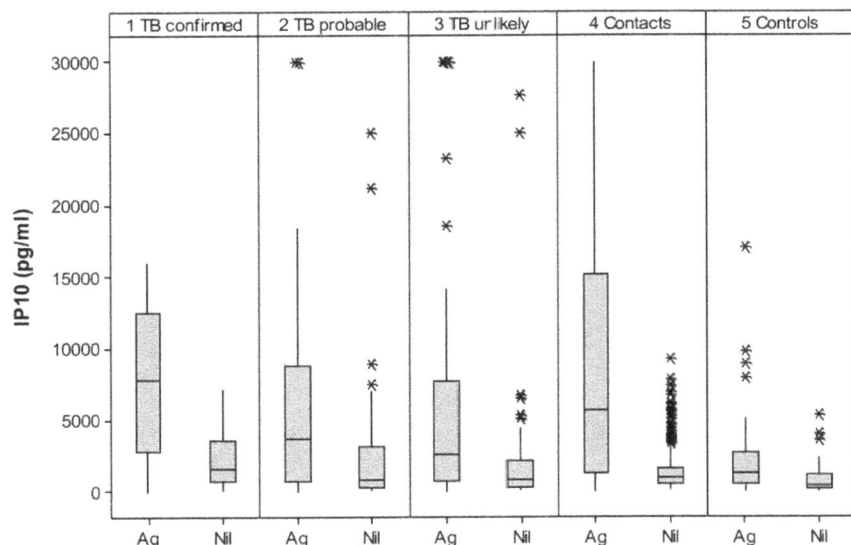

Figure 2. IP10 (pg/ml) concentrations in stimulated (Ag) and non-stimulated (Nil) samples by study group. Box plots describe medians, interquantile values and range. Asterisks depict outliers

IP10 concentrations than children without HIV across all study groups (p>0.1) as shown in Figure 4.

IP10 concentrations of children with *confirmed* TB (N = 22, median IP10 7774 pg/ml) and *contacts* with TST+ and/or INFγ+ (N = 148, median IP10 12490 pg/ml) where compared against *controls* with TST− and INFγ− (N = 86, median IP10 704 pg/ml) to construct the ROC curves, as shown in Figure 5. The ROC curves for both *confirmed* and *contact* children had the same shape, with cut-off points for best performance being 3128 pg/ml (sensitivity 81.8%, 95%CI = 59.7–94.8, specificity 96.5% 95%CI 90.1–99.3 and area under the curve (AUC) of 0.37%, 95%CI 0.75–0.99) for *confirmed* TB and 3022 pg/ml (sensitivity 77%, 95%CI 69.4–83.5%, specificity 96.5%, 95%CI 90.14–99.3%, and an AUC of 0.87, 95%CI 0.82–0.92) for *contacts*.

Discussion

Despite significant research efforts and technological breakthroughs to develop new diagnostics for TB [15], current diagnostic tests have lower sensitivity in children than in adults [1,2]. New diagnostics are needed to identify children with TB and to differentiate between latent and active TB in high incidence settings with limited resources.

Despite a large body of evidence of the performance characteristics of IGRAs for the diagnosis of LTBI and the identification of individuals infected during TB outbreaks in low TB incidence settings [6,16,17,18,19], there is a small number of studies assessing the IGRAS performance and their utility in high incidence countries [20,21,22]. The data presented here therefore represents a rare opportunity to compare TST, INFγ and IP10 in children with different degrees of exposure to infection and certainty of diagnosis residing in a high TB burden setting.

An important difference to reports from industrialized countries was the high proportion of QFT-IT tests with indeterminate results. Other studies from Africa have reported high rates of indeterminate results [23], and the reason for this high frequency remains unexplained. Our team has conducted similar studies in Nigeria [24], Nepal [8] and Yemen, took care to re-stock tests frequently and used high altitude control tubes provided by the manufacturer. Most indeterminate results however were due to failure of the positive control and further studies are needed to explore whether this was due to a loss of test integrity or an unidentified background morbidity such as parasitic, bacterial or viral infections [25]. The interpretation of the data is also hampered by the lack of reference standards for LTBI. The data however confirms that INFγ, as TST, are more likely to be

Table 3. Medians and interquantile ranges of IP10 concentrations (stimulated minus non-stimulated, in pg/ml) according to the TST and INFγ results by study group.

	TST			INFγ		
	Positive	**Intermediate**	**Negative**	**Positive**	**Indeterminate**	**Negative**
TB confirmed	5116 (2092–9624)	-	6788 (1672–11344)	8848 (4296–11414)	1672 (56–2092)	4560 (8–7496)
TB probable	2592 (64–8272)	768 (0–7424)	512 (84–3348)	7254 (3360–10548)	84 (0–604)	288 (140–4548)
TB unlikely	2404 (326–8868)	2903 (692–8688)	674 (54–2558)	7594 (3328–12028)	548 (0–2208)	674 (120–1372)
Contacts	9304 (708–14536)	6078 (476–17632)	1486 (308–5544)	13800 (11128–17728)	348 (20–1932)	770 (196–3224)
Controls	528 (72–1392)	1124 (40–2320)	704 (116–1932)	1784 (364–2562)	180 (0–1184)	684 (144–1792)

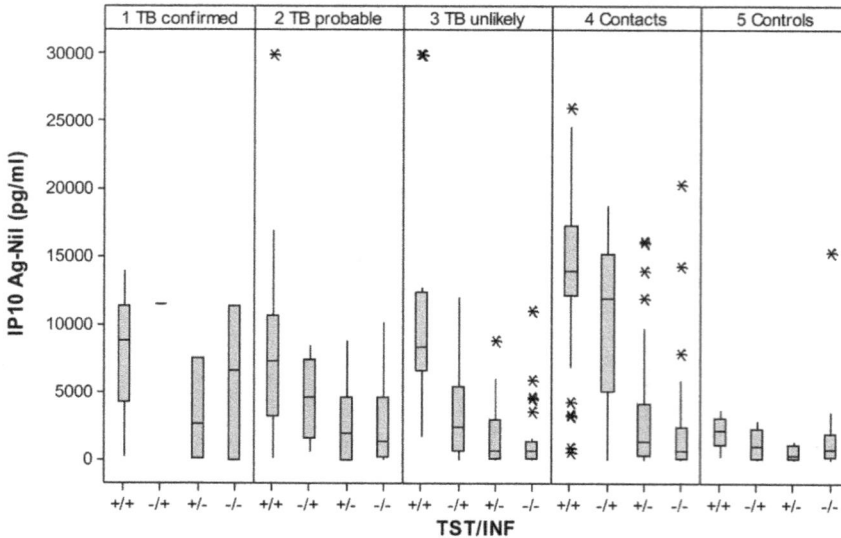

Figure 3. IP10 concentrations (stimulated minus non-stimulated) by TST and INFγ results and study group. Box plots describe medians, interquantile values and range. Asterisks depict outliers.

positive in children with *contact* or *confirmed* TB than in *controls*. Neither INFγ nor TST differentiate between active and latent infections and thus their diagnostic value is restricted to the confirmation of a history of infection [3,19,26]. Given that a number of children had discrepant INFγ/TST results, cost and logistic constrains aside, the use of both TST and INFγ would identify a higher number of children with evidence of infection than a single test alone.

This study also describes IP10 concentrations of children at different risk of infection, and how these concentrations vary with TST, INFγ and HIV. IP10 is a cytokine expressed in response to IFNγ stimulation by cell types involved in delayed-type hypersensitivity [27], including lymphocytes, monocytes, endothelial cells and fibroblasts and is a chemo-attractant to monocytes and activated Th1 lymphocytes [28], promoting selective enhancement of Th1 responses and increasing IFN-γ

gene expression [29]. Recent studies have reported that IP10 expression is enhanced in individuals with active TB [30,31] and latent infection [12,13,32] and that combined with INFγ could increase the sensitivity of the IGRAS [9,12]. Although some reports have suggested that this marker could differentiate between active and latent infection [14,33], not all studies have replicated these observations [10,14].

IP-10 concentrations were higher among children with *confirmed* TB and *contacts*, with the highest concentrations observed in *contact* children, which is in agreement with recently recent reports from low incidence settings [12,14]. IP10 concentrations were generally higher among children with INFγ+ results and there was no difference in the median concentrations of children with and without HIV infection. This latter characteristic could have practical applications, increasing the sensitivity of INFγ based tests in areas of high HIV prevalence.

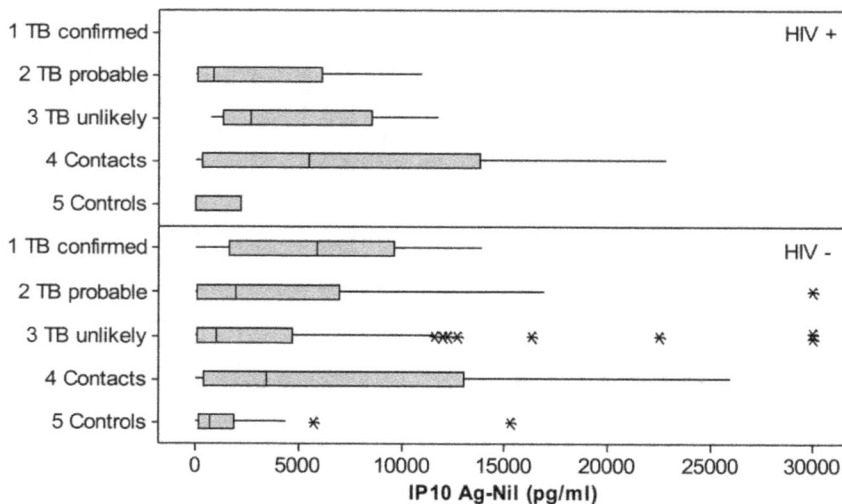

Figure 4. IP10 concentrations (stimulated minus non-stimulated) by HIV status and study group. Box plots describe medians, interquantile values and range. Asterisks depict outliers.

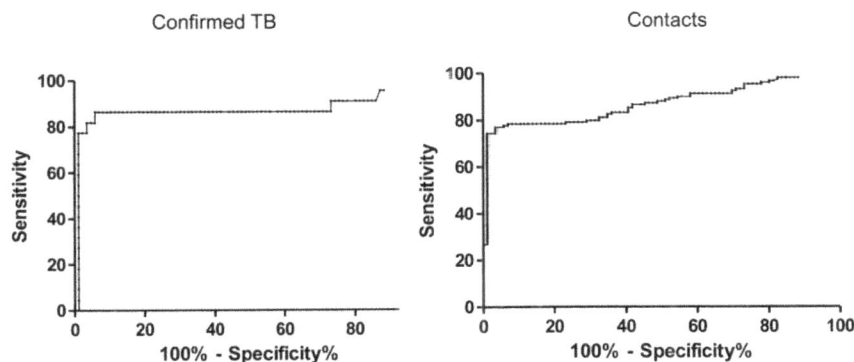

Figure 5. Receiver Operating Characteristic (ROC) curve of IP10 in children with *confirmed* TB and *contacts*, when compared to community *controls* with TST- and INFγ results.

Interestingly, non-stimulated IP10 concentrations were higher in children with *confirmed* TB, resulting in a smaller difference between stimulated and non-stimulated concentrations. Although non-specific IP10 increases have been described in acute and chronic diseases other than TB [34,35,36,37], these findings suggest that IP10 expression may vary during the course of disease progression, maybe with higher expression during the primary stages of granuloma formation, which involves the recruitment of monocytes and Th1 gammadelta T-cells [38] and lower expression in the presence of progressive unchecked infections, in the presence of immunosuppression, as described for INFγ.

The ROC curve analysis however suggested that the cut offs with best test performance to differentiate children with *confirmed* TB and *controls* was similar to the cut offs to differentiate *contacts* and *controls*, with similar AUC. Thus, similar to INFγ and TST, IP10 differentiated between infected and non-infected children but is unable to differentiate between latent and active TB. Data from children residing in a high burden areas is scarce and the sensitivity of 81.8% obtained is lower than reported from Indian adults [10] in Chennai (92.5%, 95%CI: 88.6%–96.4%), which also reported a lower specificity (48%). Ruhwald et. al. [39] selected a cut off of 673 pg/ml for Danish adolescents and adults and Lighter et. al [12] selected a cut off of 732 pg/ml for USA children. Applying Ruhwald et. al., cut off to Ethiopia would increase the sensitivity to 86% and reduce the specificity to 48%, which is similar to those reported by Kabeer et al in India, suggesting that there is more agreement of test performance across settings than suggested by these reports.

This study therefore describes INFγ and IP10 expression in children at different risk of infection and disease in a country with a high incidence of TB. Children with *probable* TB had different tests results patterns than children with *confirmed* TB as the former

had more TST but less INFγ positive results, thus reflecting the heterogeneity of this group and underscoring the importance of using clear reporting group categories based on the certainty of diagnosis to facilitate the interpretation of data.

Our findings therefore demonstrate that both INFγ and IP10 identify children with latent and active TB. IP10 is less affected by the presence of HIV co-infection than INFγ and has the potential to increase the sensitivity of the IGRAS when used in combination with INFγ. INFγ, IP10 and TST however are unable to differentiate between latent and active disease.

Longitudinal studies to describe the natural variation of these markers over time and their ability to identify children with latent infections at risk of disease progression or children at risk of poor treatment response after initiation of anti-TB therapy are needed. However, given the high cost of the IGRAS and the high proportion of indeterminate results obtained, control programmes should refrain from incorporating these tests until clear advantages over the TST are demonstrated.

Acknowledgments

We are grateful for the Southern Region Health Bureau's support for this study and the research assistants (Girum Asnake, Habiba Jemal, Tadesse Mamo and Koratu) and laboratory technicians (Tesfaye Tusuna and Kedir Yesuf) who collected the data. Our thanks go to all children and parents participating in the study.

Author Contributions

Conceived and designed the experiments: YM LC. Performed the experiments: YM GH AB NA. Analyzed the data: RP YM LC. Contributed reagents/materials/analysis tools: YM. Wrote the paper: YM LC RP. Coordinated field work and data processing: IA KG MA ZK.

References

1. Zar HJ, Hanslo D, Apolles P, Swingler G, Hussey G (2005) Induced sputum versus gastric lavage for microbiological confirmation of pulmonary tuberculosis in infants and young children: a prospective study. Lancet 365: 130–134.

2. Marais BJ, Pai M (2007) Recent advances in the diagnosis of childhood tuberculosis. Arch Dis Child 92: 446–452.

3. Wallis RS, Pai M, Menzies D, Doherty TM, Walzl G, et al. (2010) Biomarkers and diagnostics for tuberculosis: progress, needs, and translation into practice. Lancet 375: 1920–1937.

4. Bamford AR, Crook AM, Clark JE, Naderri Z, Dixon G, et al. (2010) Comparison of interferon-{gamma} release assays and tuberculin skin test in predicting active tuberculosis (TB) in children in the UK: a paediatric TB network study. Arch Dis Child 95: 180–186.

5. Detjen AK, Keil T, Roll S, Hauer B, Mauch H, et al. (2007) Interferon-gamma release assays improve the diagnosis of tuberculosis and nontuberculous

mycobacterial disease in children in a country with a low incidence of tuberculosis. Clin Infect Dis 45: 322–328.

6. Menzies D, Pai M, Comstock G (2007) Meta-analysis: new tests for the diagnosis of latent tuberculosis infection: areas of uncertainty and recommendations for research. Ann Intern Med 146: 340–354.

7. Zar HJ, Connell TG, Nicol M (2010) Diagnosis of pulmonary tuberculosis in children: new advances. Expert Rev Anti Infect Ther 8: 277–288.

8. Petrucci R, Abu Amer N, Gurgel RQ, Sherchand JB, Doria L, et al. (2008) Interferon gamma, interferon-gamma-induced-protein 10, and tuberculin responses of children at high risk of tuberculosis infection. Pediatr Infect Dis J 27: 1073–1077.

9. Ruhwald M, Petersen J, Kofoed K, Nakaoka H, Cuevas LE, et al. (2008) Improving T-cell assays for the diagnosis of latent TB infection: potential of a diagnostic test based on IP-10. PLoS One 3: e2358.

10. Syed Ahamed Kabeer B, Raman B, Thomas A, Perumal V, Raja A (2010) Role of QuantiFERON-TB gold, interferon gamma inducible protein-10 and tuberculin skin test in active tuberculosis diagnosis. PLoS One 5: e9051.
11. Juffermans NP, Verbon A, van Deventer SJ, van Deutekom H, Belisle JT, et al. (1999) Elevated chemokine concentrations in sera of human immunodeficiency virus (HIV)-seropositive and HIV-seronegative patients with tuberculosis: a possible role for mycobacterial lipoarabinomannan. Infect Immun 67: 4295–4297.
12. Lighter J, Rigaud M, Huie M, Peng CH, Pollack H (2009) Chemokine IP-10: an adjunct marker for latent tuberculosis infection in children. Int J Tuberc Lung Dis 13: 731–736.
13. Ruhwald M, Ravn P (2009) Biomarkers of latent TB infection. Expert Rev Respir Med 3: 387–401.
14. Whittaker E, Gordon A, Kampmann B (2008) Is IP-10 a better biomarker for active and latent tuberculosis in children than IFNgamma? PLoS One 3: e3901.
15. Boehme CC, Nabeta P, Hillemann D, Nicol MP, Shenai S, et al. (2010) Rapid molecular detection of tuberculosis and rifampin resistance. N Engl J Med 363: 1005–1015.
16. Ewer K, Deeks J, Alvarez L, Bryant G, Waller S, et al. (2003) Comparison of T-cell-based assay with tuberculin skin test for diagnosis of Mycobacterium tuberculosis infection in a school tuberculosis outbreak. Lancet 361: 1168–1173.
17. Higuchi K, Kondo S, Wada M, Hayashi S, Ootsuka G, et al. (2009) Contact investigation in a primary school using a whole blood interferon-gamma assay. J Infect 58: 352–357.
18. Pai M, Kalantri S, Dheda K (2006) New tools and emerging technologies for the diagnosis of tuberculosis: part I. Latent tuberculosis. Expert Rev Mol Diagn 6: 413–422.
19. Chang KC, Leung CC (2010) Systematic review of interferon-gamma release assays in tuberculosis: focus on likelihood ratios. Thorax 65: 271–276.
20. Dheda K, van Zyl Smit R, Badri M, Pai M (2009) T-cell interferon-gamma release assays for the rapid immunodiagnosis of tuberculosis: clinical utility in high-burden vs. low-burden settings. Curr Opin Pulm Med 15: 188–200.
21. Barth RE, Mudrikova T, Hoepelman AI (2008) Interferon-gamma release assays (IGRAs) in high-endemic settings: could they play a role in optimizing global TB diagnostics? Evaluating the possibilities of using IGRAs to diagnose active TB in a rural African setting. Int J Infect Dis 12: e1–6.
22. Hill PC, Jackson-Sillah DJ, Fox A, Brookes RH, de Jong BC, et al. (2008) Incidence of tuberculosis and the predictive value of ELISPOT and Mantoux tests in Gambian case contacts. PLoS One 3: e1379.
23. Seshadri C, Uiso LO, Ostermann J, Diefenthal H, Shao HJ, et al. (2008) Low sensitivity of T-cell based detection of tuberculosis among HIV co-infected Tanzanian in-patients. East Afr Med J 85: 442–449.
24. Nakaoka H, Lawson L, Squire SB, Coulter B, Ravn P, et al. (2006) Risk for tuberculosis among children. Emerg Infect Dis 12: 1383–1388.
25. Shanaube K, De Haas P, Schaap A, Moyo M, Kosloff B, et al. (2010) Intra-assay reliability and robustness of QuantiFERON(R)-TB Gold In-Tube test in Zambia. Int J Tuberc Lung Dis 14: 828–833.
26. Bianchi L, Galli L, Moriondo M, Veneruso G, Becciolini L, et al. (2009) Interferon-gamma release assay improves the diagnosis of tuberculosis in children. Pediatr Infect Dis J 28: 510–514.
27. Kaplan G, Luster AD, Hancock G, Cohn ZA (1987) The expression of a gamma interferon-induced protein (IP-10) in delayed immune responses in human skin. J Exp Med 166: 1098–1108.
28. Farber JM (1997) Mig and IP-10: CXC chemokines that target lymphocytes. J Leukoc Biol 61: 246–257.
29. Moser B, Loetscher P (2001) Lymphocyte traffic control by chemokines. Nat Immunol 2: 123–128.
30. Ruhwald M, Bjerregaard-Andersen M, Rabna P, Kofoed K, Eugen-Olsen J, et al. (2007) CXCL10/IP-10 release is induced by incubation of whole blood from tuberculosis patients with ESAT-6, CFP10 and TB7.7. Microbes Infect 9: 806–812.
31. Azzurri A, Sow OY, Amedei A, Bah B, Diallo S, et al. (2005) IFN-gamma-inducible protein 10 and pentraxin 3 plasma levels are tools for monitoring inflammation and disease activity in Mycobacterium tuberculosis infection. Microbes Infect 7: 1–8.
32. Ruhwald M, Bjerregaard-Andersen M, Rabna P, Eugen-Olsen J, Ravn P (2009) IP-10, MCP-1, MCP-2, MCP-3, and IL-1RA hold promise as biomarkers for infection with M. tuberculosis in a whole blood based T-cell assay. BMC Res Notes 2: 19.
33. Dheda K, Van-Zyl Smit RN, Sechi LA, Badri M, Meldau R, et al. (2009) Clinical diagnostic utility of IP-10 and LAM antigen levels for the diagnosis of tuberculous pleural effusions in a high burden setting. PLoS One 4: e4689.
34. Korpi-Steiner NL, Bates ME, Lee WM, Hall DJ, Bertics PJ (2006) Human rhinovirus induces robust IP-10 release by monocytic cells, which is independent of viral replication but linked to type I interferon receptor ligation and STAT1 activation. J Leukoc Biol 80: 1364–1374.
35. Dhillon NK, Peng F, Ransohoff RM, Buch S (2007) PDGF synergistically enhances IFN-gamma-induced expression of CXCL10 in blood-derived macrophages: implications for HIV dementia. J Immunol 179: 2722–2730.
36. Jain V, Armah HB, Tongren JE, Ned RM, Wilson NO, et al. (2008) Plasma IP-10, apoptotic and angiogenic factors associated with fatal cerebral malaria in India. Malar J 7: 83.
37. Antonelli A, Ferri C, Fallahi P, Ferrari SM, Sebastiani M, et al. (2008) High values of CXCL10 serum levels in mixed cryoglobulinemia associated with hepatitis C infection. Am J Gastroenterol 103: 2488–2494.
38. Ferrero E, Biswas P, Vettoretto K, Ferrarini M, Uguccioni M, et al. (2003) Macrophages exposed to Mycobacterium tuberculosis release chemokines able to recruit selected leucocyte subpopulations: focus on gammadelta cells. Immunology 108: 365–374.
39. Ruhwald M, Bodmer T, Maier C, Jepsen M, Haaland MB, et al. (2008) Evaluating the potential of IP-10 and MCP-2 as biomarkers for the diagnosis of tuberculosis. Eur Respir J 32: 1607–1615.

11

The Risk and Timing of Tuberculosis Diagnosed in Smear-Negative TB Suspects: A 12 Month Cohort Study in Harare, Zimbabwe

Munyaradzi Dimairo[1], Peter MacPherson[2]*, Tsitsi Bandason[1], Abbas Zezai[1], Shungu S. Munyati[1], Anthony E. Butterworth[3], Stanley Mungofa[4], Simba Rusikaniko[5], Katherine Fielding[6], Peter R Mason[1], Elizabeth L. Corbett[3]

1 Biomedical Research and Training Institute, Harare, Zimbabwe 2 Wellcome Trust Tropical Centre, University of Liverpool, Liverpool, United Kingdom, 3 Clinical Research Unit, London School of Hygiene and Tropical Medicine, London, United Kingdom, 4 Harare City Health, Harare, Zimbabwe, 5 University of Zimbabwe College of Health Sciences, Harare, Zimbabwe, 6 Infectious Disease Epidemiology Unit, London School of Hygiene and Tropical Medicine, London, United Kingdom

Abstract

Background: Cases of smear-negative TB have increased dramatically in high prevalence HIV settings and pose considerable diagnostic and management challenges.

Methods and Findings: Between February 2006 and July 2007, a cohort study nested within a cluster-randomised trial of community-based case finding strategies for TB in Harare, Zimbabwe was undertaken. Participants who had negative sputum smears and remained symptomatic of TB were follow-up for one year with standardised investigations including HIV testing, repeat sputum smears, TB culture and chest radiography. Defaulters were actively traced to the community. The objectives were to investigate the incidence and risk factors for TB. TB was diagnosed in 218 (18.2%) participants, of which 39.4% was bacteriologically confirmed. Most cases (84.2%) were diagnosed within 3 months, but TB incidence remained high thereafter (111.3 per 1000 person-years, 95% CI: 86.6 to 146.3). HIV prevalence was 63.3%, and HIV-infected individuals had a 3.5-fold higher risk of tuberculosis than HIV-negative individuals.

Conclusion: We found that diagnosis of TB was insensitive and slow, even with early radiography and culture. Until more sensitive and rapid diagnostic tests become widely available, a much more proactive and integrated approach towards prompt initiation of ART, ideally from within TB clinics and without waiting for TB to be excluded, is needed to minimise the risk and consequences of diagnostic delay.

Editor: Philip Campbell Hill, MRC Laboratories, Gambia

Funding: ELC receives funding from the Wellcome Trust, UK. PM is funded by the Wellcome Trust Clinical PhD programme at the University of Liverpool. The funders had no role in study design, data collection and analysis, decision to publish, or preparation of the manuscript.

Competing Interests: The authors have declared that no competing interests exist.

* E-mail: p.macpherson@liv.ac.uk

Introduction

Southern Africa has experienced steeply rising TB incidence rates driven by the HIV epidemic, and now carries over three-quarters of the global burden of HIV-positive TB cases [1,2]. In many high HIV prevalence countries the most striking increase has been in smear-negative TB cases [1].

In resource poor settings, smear-negative TB is difficult to diagnose and also difficult to exclude, especially in HIV-infected patients [3,4]. Case series and post-mortem studies have shown the diagnosis of smear-negative TB to be highly specific [5]. However, the mounting evidence of low sensitivity of smear microscopy [6] and the high mortality, loss to follow-up and rate at which clinical deterioration occurs during diagnostic work up of HIV-positive smear negative TB suspects [7,8] prompted a recent change in international management guidelines. In 2007, new guidelines [9] for use in settings with generalised HIV epidemics promoted diagnostic HIV testing of TB suspects, earlier use of radiography,

increased access to sputum culture, a lower threshold for starting TB treatment in HIV-infected patients, and greater recognition of the symptoms of extra-pulmonary and disseminated TB (such as rapid weight loss and night sweats) in addition to chronic cough. For ambulant patients, a routine trial of broad-spectrum antibiotics in TB suspects was not recommended under these guidelines, but the need to exercise "clinical judgement" before starting TB treatment was retained.

We applied a standardised diagnostic protocol that predated but shared several key features of the new WHO guidelines, including early use of culture and chest radiography to a cohort of smear-negative TB suspects identified through a community-based intervention in Harare, Zimbabwe, who were then followed up for one year with active tracing of defaulters. The aims of the study were to investigate whether or not TB suspects had a high incidence of being diagnosed with TB in the year following initial work-up, suggesting missed diagnosis, and to investigate the role of routine culture in the diagnosis of smear-negative TB. Access to antiretroviral therapy (ART) was through the public health care system in Harare.

Methods

This was a cohort study nested within a cluster randomised trial investigating two strategies (household enquiry vs. self-referral to a mobile community clinic) of community-based intensified case finding for TB in an urban community with a high prevalence of TB and HIV infection (DETECTB) [10].

Ethical Approval

Ethical approval was obtained from the Medical Research Council of Zimbabwe, the Biomedical and Research and Training Institute, Harare and the London School of Hygiene and Tropical Medicine. Written informed consent was obtained from all participants. All participants were offered diagnostic HIV testing and counselling, with referral for assessment for ART if positive. Unreported HIV results taken for study purposes were held under a dedicated HIV test number, and only linked with other data through a computer programme that merged files and immediately dropped all personal identifiers, thus maintaining confidentiality.

Study Setting and Population

Forty-six neighbourhood clusters in Western Harare, Zimbabwe, were provided with 6-monthly outreach access to TB microscopy at community-level as part of a cluster-randomised trial. The cohort reported here was drawn from participants in the cluster-randomised trial and who were recruited between February 2006 and June 2007. Inclusion criteria for the nested cohort study were: age 16 year or older; underwent outreach screening for TB in the community; had two negative sputum smears (morning and spot specimens); had ongoing symptoms of: cough; or weight-loss; night sweats; or a history of haemoptysis within the last year; and returned to take up our offer of follow-up investigations at the study clinic situated in a TB and HIV treatment facility.

Initial Assessment for TB and HIV Testing

On first presentation at the TB and HIV clinic, initial assessment included recording of TB symptoms chest radiography, repeat morning and spot sputum smears and TB culture; and treatment with seven days of broad-spectrum antibiotics (amoxicillin). Participants with radiological features strongly suggestive of TB (including pleural or pericardial effusion) were referred for immediate TB treatment [9].

Additionally, on first assessment, all participants were asked to consent to provide an HIV specimen for study purposes and were advised to have diagnostic HIV testing and counselling (HTC), provided initially through routine testing and counselling services, and later through diagnostic HIV testing within the study clinic. HIV-positive participants were prescribed cotrimoxazole prophylaxis and referred to the adjacent public ART clinic where initiation criteria were CD4 count of ≤ 200 cells/ul, or a WHO stage 4 illness. From May 2006 all participants accepting diagnostic HTC also had blood taken for CD4 count. Participants who declined diagnostic HIV testing were asked for consent to provide a specimen for HIV testing for study purposes.

Follow-up Procedures

Follow-up review for participants who were clinically stable was undertaken at the TB and HIV clinic 1, 8 and 12 months after initial assessment. Participants were advised to attend for unscheduled assessment and management if they became unwell. During follow-up assessments, participants underwent repeat assessment of symptoms and submitted further samples for sputum smear and TB culture. Chest x-ray was repeated if the participant was coughing. Participants with positive smears or cultures, with symptoms that did not respond to antibiotics, or with radiological signs of TB were referred for TB treatment. Participants who did not return for scheduled visits were followed-up at their home address.

Participants started on TB treatment were followed up at 1,8 and 12 months after commencing TB treatment. The 8 months review was chosen to allow assessment of TB treatment outcomes.

Case Definitions for Diagnosis of TB

A confirmed TB case was defined as a positive smear (including scanty positive) or one or more positive cultures for *M. tuberculosis*. Smear- and culture-negative TB was defined by a clinical or radiological illness consistent with TB that did not respond to broad-spectrum antibiotics but did respond to one month of anti-tuberculosis treatment, or where TB treatment was started independently by an outside provider. Participants were classified as lost-to-follow-up if they did not attend for review (scheduled or unscheduled) during the study period and could not be traced.

Laboratory Methods

Microbiology work was undertaken at the Biomedical and Research Training Institute, Harare, Zimbabwe. Smears were made from concentrated decontaminated (4% NaOH) specimens and read by fluorescence microscopy after staining with auramine-O. Positives were confirmed with Ziehl-Neelsen staining. Culture used Lowenstein-Jensen (LJ) slopes. Species were classified as *M.tuberculosis* or non-tuberculous mycobacteria according to colony morphology, microscopic cording, ability to grow on PNB-containing LJ media, and growth at 45°C, 37°C and room temperature. From 2008, MBP84 lateral flow assays for rapid species identification were also used.

Diagnostic HIV testing was offered with pre-and post test counselling (parallel testing with Determine™ HIV-1/2, Abbott Japan, Inverness Medical Japan, Tokyo, Japan and Uni-Gold Recombigen®, Trinity Biotech, Dublin, Ireland); unreported study HIV tests used serial testing (Abbott Determine™ with all positives and 10% of negatives confirmed by Uni-Gold Recombigen®) or oral mucosal transudate from participants not willing to provide serum, tested using Vironostika® Uni- form II (BioMérieux, Marcy l'Etoile, France).

Statistical Analysis

We investigated TB free survival time from first clinical assessment to the earliest of last clinical review date, date of TB diagnosis or date of death. Incidence rates for outcomes were calculated using the Poisson distribution. Eight confirmed TB cases had missing data for date of TB diagnosis and so multiple imputation using chained equations, taking into account potential clustering, was used in these cases [11].

Baseline characteristics of participants were expressed as proportions and compared by HIV status using Fisher's exact test. We used Cox proportional hazard regression to assess the association of sex, age, weight, CD4 count and previous TB treatment with TB free survival, stratified by HIV status. Knowledge of HIV-status was not included due to high collinearity with unknown CD4 count category. Plots of Schoenfeld residuals were inspected to ensure the validity of the proportional hazards assumptions.

Data management and analysis was conducted using EpiInfo 2003 (CDC, Atlanta) and STATA 10.1 (College Station, Texas, USA).

Results

Baseline characteristics and follow-up

Between February 21, 2006 and June 6 2007, 5731 adults participated in the cluster-randomised parent study, and had two negative sputum smears. All participants in the parent study were provided with a clinic appointment card that could be used to obtain further investigations if smears were negative: 1,234 (21.5%) took up this opportunity and so form the starting cohort of this study (Figure 1). Thirty-nine (3.2%) participants were excluded from this analysis: 15 (1.2%) had missing baseline information and 24 (1.9%) did not attend any subsequent review after their initial appointment, leaving 1195 participants who were smear-negative TB suspects in this analysis (Figure 1). During the 12-month study period, 170 (14.2%) cohort participants were lost to follow-up. As reported separately, mortality rates were high with 97 participants dying without a diagnosis of TB and a further 42 participants dying after TB was diagnosed giving a total of 139 (11.6%) deaths during the study period (122.3 per 1000 person-years (95% CI: 104.4 to 144.3).

A total of 1143 participants underwent HIV testing with a further 52 (4.4%) refusing. Among participants who tested HIV-positive, 494 (68.3%) accepted diagnostic HIV testing and counselling (HTC) and 229 (31.7%) declined HTC but gave samples for unreported study testing. HIV prevalence was 63.3%. Baseline characteristics of HIV-positive and HIV-negative participants are shown in Table 1. HIV-positive participants were more likely than HIV-negative participants to be female (p = 0.019), and to have previously been treated for TB (p<0.001). They were also more highly symptomatic, with breathlessness at rest the only one of 12 considered symptoms that was not significantly more prevalent than in HIV-negative participants. Median CD4 count (limited to those accepting diagnostic HTC after May 2006: see Methods) was 149 (IQR 69 to 255) cells/ul: only 15.3% of counts were above 350 cells/ul, with a further 21.7% between 200 and 350 cells/ul.

TB cases diagnosed during follow-up

From the 1195 participants, 218 (18.2%) TB cases were diagnosed in 1051.2 person-years of follow-up (Table 2). Eighty-six (39.4%) had confirmed TB and 127 (58.3%) were smear- and culture-negative. Five (2.3%) participants were treated for TB without clinical response, so failing to meet study case-definitions. HIV prevalence was 83.5% (95% CI: 77.8 to 88.2%) in participants diagnosed with TB.

Early (within 3 months) TB diagnoses

TB free survival stratified by HIV status is shown in Figure 2. The majority of TB cases (139, 63.8%) were identified in the early period (0–3 months), and so are likely to represent prevalent disease at cohort entry. One hundred and seventeen (84.2%) of the participants diagnosed between 0 to 3 months were HIV-positive. HIV-stratified TB incidence within the first 3 months was 705.9 (95% CI: 580.8 to 860.2) and 205.0 (95% CI: 123.9 to 364.2) per 1000 person-years for HIV-positive and- negative participants respectively.

Late (3 to 12 months) TB diagnoses

Between 3 and 12 months of follow-up, a further 79/218 (36.2%) TB cases were diagnosed. Incidence rates for this time

period were 111.3 per 1000 person-years (95% CI: 86.6 to 146.3) in HIV-positive participants and 31.3 per 1000 person years (95% CI: 19.7 to 53.1) in HIV negative participants.

Bacteriologically confirmed disease was diagnosed more frequently amongst participants diagnosed with TB within the first 3 months (60/139; 43.2%) compared with participants diagnosed in the subsequent 9 months of follow-up (26/79; 32.9%; p = 0.151).

HIV Positive Participants

51/117 (43.6%) had bacteriologically confirmed TB diagnosed within the first 3 months compared to only 16/65 (36.8%) in the subsequent 9 months (odds ratio (OR) = 2.4, 95% CI: 1.2 to 4.6; p = 0.016) in HIV positives individuals.

HIV Negatives Participants

8/21 (38.1%) had bacteriologically confirmed TB diagnosed within the first 3 months compared to 9/13 (69.2%) in the subsequent 9 months (OR = 0.3, 95% CI: 0.1 to 1.2; p = 0.157) in HIV negatives participants.

Delay in Diagnosis of TB

Median delay in diagnosis of bacteriologically confirmed and smear- and culture-negative disease TB was 2.0 (IQR: 1.2 to 3.4) months and 2.3 (1.5 to 5.4) months, respectively. HIV-negative participants had a longer delay in diagnosis of bacteriologically confirmed TB (3.1 months, IQR: 2.0 to 5.5) than HIV-positive (1.9 months, IQR: 1.1 to 3.0; p = 0.04), but similar delay to diagnosis of smear- and culture-negative TB (HIV-positive = 2.3 months IQR: 1.5 to 6.0; HIV-negative = 2.3 months IQR: 1.6 to 2.8; p = 0.61).

Risk Factors for TB Diagnosis

HIV infection was the predominant risk factor for TB diagnosis, with TB incidence 3.5 times higher in HIV-positive participants (incidence 311.6 per 1000 person years, 95% CI: 266.7 to 364.9) compared to HIV-negative participants (incidence 81.8 per 1000 person-years, 95% CI: 58.3 to 118.2).

In univariable analysis among HIV-positive participants (Table 3), low weight (hazard ratio (HR): 2.11, 95% CI: 1.19 to 3.74) and CD4 count between 50 and 100 cells/ul (HR: 1.68, 95% CI: 1.08 to 2.62) were associated with an increased hazard of incident TB, while female sex showed a reduced hazard of TB (HR: 0.71, 95% CI: 0.50 to 1.01). These associations remained on multivariable analysis. On adjusted analysis there was an association between trend towards low CD4 count (p_t = 0.024), low weight (p_t = 0.026) and TB diagnosis. Among HIV-negative participants (Table 4), factors associated with a TB diagnosis in both univariable and multivariable analysis were a history of past TB treatment (adjusted hazard ratio (aHR): 2.18, 95% CI: 1.04 to 4.57), and older age (aHR: 2.07 [95% CI 0.88–4.89] for 35–45 years, 2.47 [95% CI: 1.22 to 5.02] for >45 years compared with <35 years).

Outcomes of TB Treatment

Two hundred and fourteen of 218 participants diagnosed with TB were started on TB treatment (4 were lost to follow-up in the interim) and followed for treatment outcomes. Ten participants defaulted from TB treatment and 10 were transferred out. Treatment completion rates were 69.6% (126/182) for HIV-positive and 75.0% (24/32) for HIV-negative participants, with case-fatality rates higher among HIV-positive (21.5%: 39 deaths on treatment) than HIV-negative (9.4%: 3 deaths, p<0.001) participants.

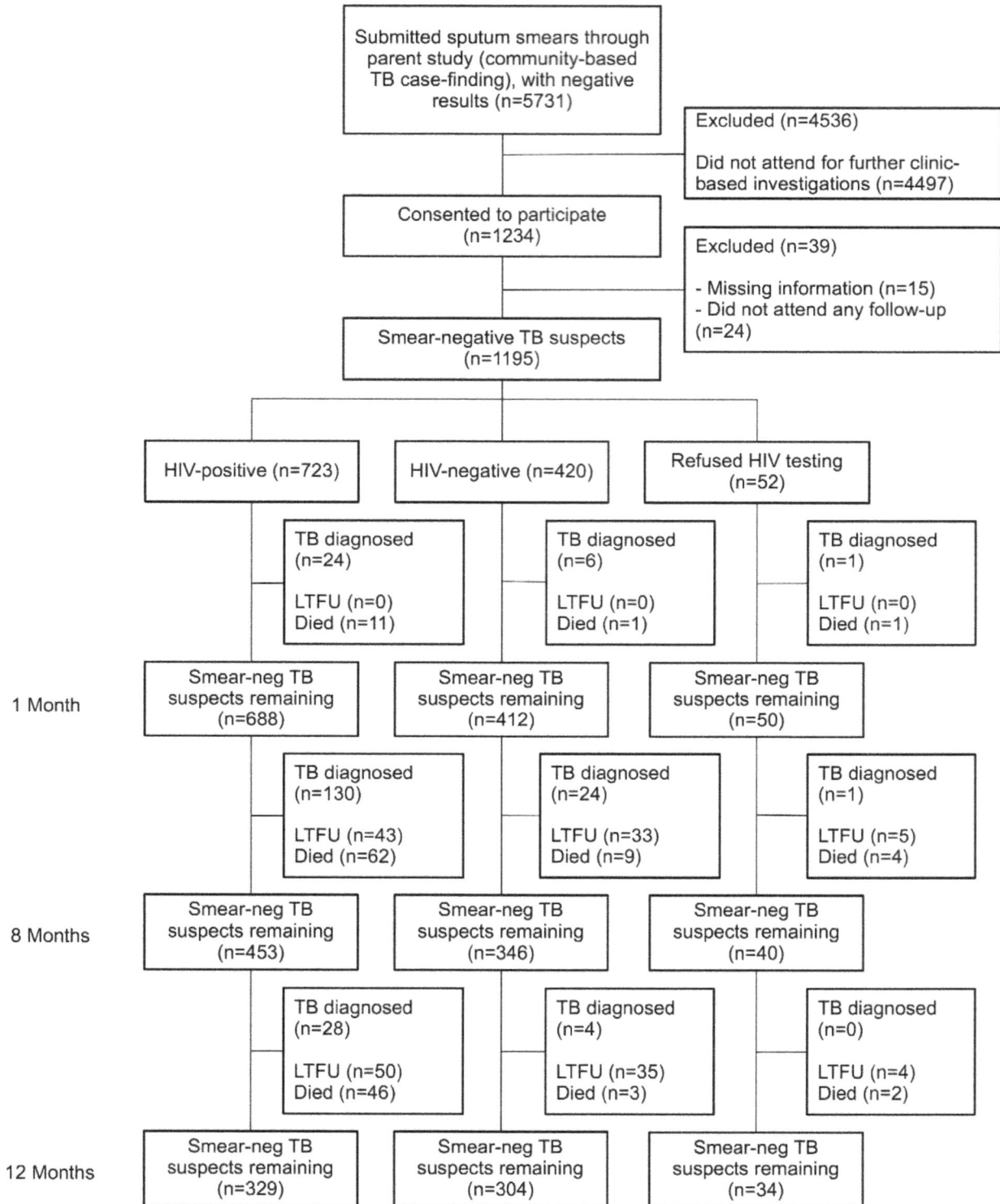

Figure 1. Cohort Flowchart. Diagnostic outcomes of smear negative TB suspects. LTFU: Lost to follow-up before TB diagnosis or in participant without TB diagnosed.

Uptake of ART

Although 494 (68.3%) of the HIV-positive participants accepted diagnostic HTC and were referred for ART, only 106 (20.9% of those referred and 14.7% of all HIV positive participants) were started on ART during the 12-month follow-up. 145 (37.0%) of patients with known CD4 counts did not meet the ART initiation criteria (CD4 count of ≤200 cells/ul or WHO stage 4 illness), and limited availability of ART in the Zimbabwean public health care system was also a major constraint. Median time between TB diagnosis and ART

Table 1. Baseline characteristics and symptoms of smear-negative TB suspects by HIV status.

Characteristic	Scoring	HIV+ (%)	HIV− (%)	P
Total*		**723 (63.3)**	**420 (36.8)**	
Sex	Female	470 (65.0)	243 (57.9)	0.019
	Male	253 (35.0)	177 (42.1)	
Age (years)	Median (IQR)	36 (30.0 to 42.0)	39 (30.0 to 54.0)	
	<25	60 (8.3)	47 (11.2)	
	25–34	261 (36.1)	111 (26.4)	<0.001
	35–45	264 (36.5)	95 (22.6)	
	>45	138 (19.1)	167 (39.8)	
CD4 count (cells/ul) (391 patients)	Median (IQR)	149 (69 to 255)	-	
	0–≤50	78 (19.9)	-	
	50–≤100	60 (15.3)	-	
	100–≤200	108 (27.6)	-	
	200–≤350	85 (21.7)	-	
	>350	60 (15.3)		
Previous TB treatment	Yes	138 (19.1)	35 (8.3)	<0.001
Chest x-ray: attending clinician classification	Normal	219 (30.8)	167 (39.8)	<0.001
	Typical of TB	27 (3.7)	7 (1.7)	
	Atypical abnormality, but consistent with TB	275 (38.0)	93 (22.1)	
	Suggests an alternative (non-TB) diagnosis	18 (2.5)	18 (4.3)	
	Not done	184 (25.5)	135 (32.1)	
Symptoms				
Cough greater than 3 weeks	Yes	543 (75.1)	263 (52.6)	<0.001
Sputum	Yes	401 (55.5)	168 (40.0)	<0.001
Purulent sputum	Yes	313 (43.3)	123 (29.3)	<0.001
Blood in sputum	Yes	145 (20.1)	37 (8.8)	<0.001
Duration with TB symptoms (weeks)	Median (IQR)	11.5 (4.0 to 20.0)	12 (4.0 to 24.0)	–
Chest pain	Yes	332 (45.9)	155 (36.9)	<0.001
Pleuritic painful cough	Yes	208 (28.8)	100 (23.8)	<0.001
Exertional dyspnoea	Yes	400 (55.3)	184 (43.8)	<0.001
Dyspnoea at rest	Yes	92 (12.7)	38 (9.0)	0.066
Night sweats	Yes	447 (61.8)	228 (54.3)	0.015
Change sheets or bedclothes due to sweats	Yes	326 (45.1)	127 (30.2)	<0.001
Recent weight loss	Yes	557 (77.0)	231 (55.0)	<0.001
Respiratory rate>20 breaths per minute	Yes	403 (55.7)	217 (51.6)	0.174

*HIV status not known for 52 (4.4%) participants.
IQR: Interquartile range, HIV+: HIV positive, HIV−: HIV negative

initiation was 2.7 months (IQR: 1.1–7.1) and between study enrolment and ART initiation in those in whom TB was not diagnosed was 3.0 (IQR; 2.0 to 4.3) months.

Discussion

The main finding from this large cohort of smear-negative TB suspects is the high incidence of TB diagnoses throughout 12 months of follow-up, for both HIV-positive and HIV-negative participants. HIV infection increased the risk of TB substantially in both early (within 3 months) and later periods.

In this cohort low weight and CD4 counts below 200 cells/ul were the main risk factors for subsequent diagnosis of HIV-related TB, while older age and past history of TB treatment were risk

factors for HIV-negative TB. Past TB was a strong risk factor for recurrent disease in HIV-negative, but not HIV-positive, participants. This difference probably reflects the high susceptibility to rapid progression following re-infection with *M.tuberculosis* in HIV-positive individuals [12,13].

TB was confirmed microbiologically in only 39.4% of TB cases, despite routine solid media culture for all TB suspects. With advanced HIV disease, sputum smears are more likely to be negative [14] and chest radiography may be normal [15]. Other studies from high HIV prevalence settings using combined clinical and bacteriological case-definitions and not restricted to smear-negative suspects have reported between 10% and 45% of patients as culture-negative [16–18]. The high rates of late diagnoses and low rates of culture-confirmed TB implies that diagnosing smear-negative TB

Table 2. TB cases diagnosed during study period.

TB case definition	Total* (n = 218)	HIV+ (n = 182)	HIV− (n = 34)
	n (% of cases)	n (%)	n (%)
Bacteriology confirmed[†]	86 (39.4)	67 (36.8)	17 (50.0)
Time to diagnosis			
0 to 3 months:	60 (69.8)	51 (76.1)	8 (47.1)
>3 to 12 months:	26 (30.2)	16 (23.9)	9 (52.9)
Smear- and culture-negative[‡]	127 (58.3)	110 (60.4)	17 (50.0)
Type of diagnosis			
Chest x-ray abnormal:	115 (90.6)	101 (91.8)	14 (82.4)
Clinical:	12 (9.4)	9 (8.2)	3 (17.6)
Time to diagnosis:			
0 to 3 months	76 (59.8)	63 (57.3)	13 (76.5)
>3 to 12 months	51 (40.2)	47 (42.7)	4 (23.5)
Case definition not met[§]	5 (2.3)	5 (2.7)	0 (0.0)

*2 patients with TB declined HIV testing, both with smear- and culture-negative disease.
[†]83 Pulmonary TB, 3 pleural TB.
[‡]105 Pulmonary TB, 9 pleural TB, 4 miliary, 6 other extra-pulmonary TB (ETB), 1 combined ETB and PTB, 2 not classified.
[§]Treated for TB but case definitions were not met due to lack of response to treatment (4 pulmonary TB, 1 pleural TB).
HIV+: HIV positive, HIV−: HIV negative.

remains problematic even with access to culture and early radiography [9].

We cannot distinguish between three explanations for the high TB incidence in the later period: a) that culture failed to detect true smear-negative TB initially, or b) misdiagnosis of other (non-TB) conditions as TB, or c) a high incidence of new TB during follow-up. But, given the consistent autopsy findings that disseminated TB is frequently missed in HIV-infected patients

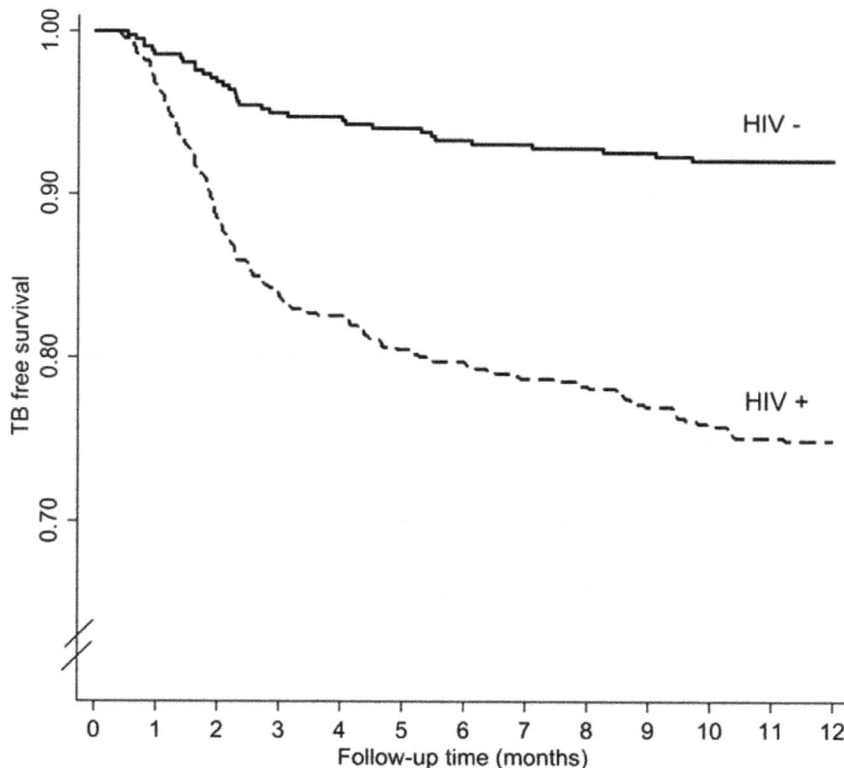

Figure 2. TB free survival stratified by HIV status. Kaplan-Meier estimates showing TB-free survival of cohort members stratified by HIV status.

Table 3. Univariable and multivariable analysis of risk factors associated with TB diagnosis in HIV-positive participants.

	TB cases/PYFU	Unadjusted HR (95% CI)	P-Value	Adjusted HR (95% CI)	P-Value
Overall (0–12 months)	182/584.1				
Sex					
Male	74/186.4	1.0		1.00	
Female	108/397.7	0.71 (0.50 to 1.01)	0.058	0.66 (0.47 to 0.94)	0.020
Age (years)					
<25	18/49.0	1.0		1.00	
25–34	68/213.6	0.85 (0.51 to 1.41)		0.94 (0.57 to 1.55)	
35–45	69/207.3	0.89 (0.54 to 1.47)		0.98 (0.56 to 1.71)	
>45	27/114.2	0.65 (0.32 to 1.32)	0.611	0.73 (0.32 to 1.64)	0.733
Weight (kg)					
0–49	47/98.4	2.11 (1.19 to 3.74)		2.05 (1.08 to 3.87)	
50–59	79/241.5	1.49 (0.83 to 2.66)		1.35 (0.73 to 2.52)	
60–69	40/168.6	1.13 (0.65 to 1.26)		1.08 (0.62 to 1.87)	
>70	16/75.6	1.00	0.008	1.00	0.026
CD4 count (cells/ul)					
<50	20/45.6	1.41 (0.82 to 2.43)		1.18 (0.69 to 2.01)	
50–<100	33/88.6	1.68 (1.08 to 2.62)		1.66 (1.04 to 2.64)	
100–<200	31/132.2	1.53 (0.90 to 2.59)		1.43 (0.82 to 2.48)	
≥200	77/259.6	1.0	0.091*	1.00	0.024*
Unknown	150/473.0	1.19 (0.80 to 1.79)		1.05 (0.68 to 1.62)	
Previous TB treatment					
No	150 (473.0)	1.0			
Yes	32 (111.1)	0.92 (0.59 to 1.42)	0.709		
HIV status known†					
No	51/214.5	1.0			
Yes	131/369.6	1.48 (1.04 to 2.12)	0.065		

*Test for Trend.
†Not included in multivariate model due to collinearity with CD4 count unknown category.
HR: hazard ratio; PYFU: person years follow-up; CI: confidence interval.

[19] and that response to TB treatment was documented in all but a few of our cases, we assume that delayed diagnosis of prevalent TB was the main contributor.

TB culture is the current international standard for diagnosis of smear-negative TB [20]. In low-prevalence HIV settings, TB culture on solid medium is highly sensitive (80–85%) and specific (98%) [21], although growth is slow (up to six weeks) and laboratory intensive [22]. In high prevalence HIV settings, sensitivity may be reduced [23], while the rapid pace at which HIV-related TB progresses makes waiting for culture results clinically inappropriate [7]. Liquid culture systems with early growth indicators provide more rapid and sensitive growth and could reduce diagnostic delay [3]. Other sensitive rapid diagnostics have shown great promise when evaluated against culture [24] but also need be evaluated against culture-negative disease, as the diagnostic barriers to management of TB suspects will not be completely resolved until rapid diagnostic methods with sensitivity approaching 100% become widely available [22].

By 12 months one quarter of our HIV-positive smear-negative TB suspects had been diagnosed with TB, highlighting the challenge that suspected HIV-related TB presents in the context of ART scale-up. Our finding that, rather than having disease

excluded, participants continued to be diagnosed with TB at high incidence throughout follow-up supports a move towards starting ART promptly without allowing TB investigations to cause undue delay [25].

In this cohort, uptake of ART was extremely low and delayed despite low CD4 counts in most participants accepting diagnostic HIV testing. This in part reflects the unique limitations of public sector HIV care in Zimbabwe at the time, but other African ART programmes also report long delays between registration and ART initiation [26].

Based on these results, we suggest two revisions to the current recommended management of TB suspects. Firstly, lowering the threshold for TB treatment in HIV-infected TB suspects who do not have access to immediate ART. This would move away from the current recommendations of not starting TB treatment unless TB is considered likely towards prompt initiation of TB treatment within a few weeks of presentation as a TB suspect where there are still any clinical signs or symptoms consistent with TB. Inevitably this will mean more patients started on TB treatment, with some negative consequences: the specificity of the diagnosis of smear-negative TB would be reduced. More patients would also be subjected to the considerable costs and inconvenience of unnecessary TB treatment.

Table 4. Univariable and multivariable analysis of risk factors associated with TB diagnosis in HIV-negative participants.

	TB cases/PYFU	Unadjusted HR (95% CI)	P Value	Adjusted HR (95% CI)	P Value
Overall (0–12 months)	34/415.4				
Sex					
Male	16/169.3	1.00		1.00	
Female	18/246.0	0.79 (0.51 to 1.23)	0.301	0.82 (0.52 to 1.30)	0.403
Age (years)					
<25–34	7/159.6‡	1.00		1.00	
35–45	9/94.1	2.18 (0.92 to 5.13)		2.07 (0.88 to 4.89)	
>45	18/161.6	2.56 (1.25 to 5.24)	0.033	2.47 (1.22 to 5.02)	0.040
Weight (kg)					
0–59	19/167.5	2.45 (0.91 to 6.54)			
60–69	10/135.6	1.61 (0.53 to 4.89)			
>70	5/112.3	1.00	0.184		
Previous TB treatment					
No	28/381.3	1.00		1.00	
Yes	6/34.1	2.42 (1.12 to 5.24)	0.024	2.18 (1.04 to 4.57)	0.039

‡Age groups <25 and 25–34 combined.
HR: hazard ratio; PYFU: person years follow-up; CI: confidence interval.

In many respects the preferable second alternative is prompt and early initiation of ART that would serve both a therapeutic purpose while also providing the means to rapidly confirm or exclude TB without leaving patients in the dangerous therapeutic limbo of having neither their confirmed HIV nor their possible TB treated. HIV is easy to diagnose, and ART "unmasks" TB [8]. Furthermore, a strategy of early ART initiation would ensure TB suspects are enrolled in structured follow-up where deterioration of symptoms can be promptly identified and managed. A recent randomised control trial has highlighted the benefit of early ART initiation for TB patients [27]. Our proposed strategy will increase the incidence of immune reconstitution inflammatory syndrome (IRIS) related to TB [28], especially in patients with advanced immunosupression [8,29], but the risk of death from unmasking IRIS is low and likely to be considerably lower than the risk of death during prolonged clinical observation before ART initiation [30]. Although mortality may be lowered with this strategy, an increase in IRIS-related morbidity may be anticipated. This strategy could improve integration of TB and HIV services, and the CD4 count profile reported here suggests that ART initiation is warranted on CD4 count criteria in all but a small minority of HIV-infected TB suspects.

Uptake of ART by HIV-positive TB patients can be as low as 20% even in well-resourced ART programmes [31] unless careful attention is paid to avoiding the high costs incurred by multiple visits to different clinics [32]. This same phenomenon is likely to apply to TB suspects as well, whereby patients with limited resources are effectively forced to choose to invest either in continued TB investigations or in ART access [32,33].

There were a number of limitations to this study. Firstly, as this cohort was drawn from participants in the parent cluster-randomised trial who self-presented for clinic assessment, there may be some differences from individuals in the general community and parent study who did not present for assessment. However, the large cohort number and the provision of a transport voucher to provide costs to access the clinic went some way towards mitigating this. As discussed, we cannot distinguish

new incident disease from delayed diagnosis of prevalent disease. Clinic nurses undertaking assessment for TB were not blinded to participant's HIV status and this may have influenced their decision to commence TB treatment.

Over half of diagnoses were not bacteriologically confirmed, and so may have been incorrect despite documented treatment response. Our conclusions concerning culture may be less applicable to liquid than solid culture. Radiographs were read by attending clinicians, with no attempt beyond a weekly radiological meeting to monitor accuracy of interpretation, which is known to be highly subjective. Attempts were made to minimise bias in commencement of TB treatment by having explicit criteria for initial of TB treatment. Loss to follow-up was 14.2% in this cohort and it is possible that some of those who were lost to follow up in fact had TB, or died. In cohorts of HIV-positive individuals, mortality rates among those classified as lost to follow up are known to be as high as 50% [34]. A relatively low proportion of participants in this study were diagnosed clinically and this may reflect the use of TB cultures and chest radiology. Despite these limitations, our findings have important implications for the clinical management of smear-negative TB suspects in resource-limited settings.

Conclusions

In conclusion, management of HIV-positive smear-negative TB suspects remains unsatisfactory when based upon early culture and radiology and routine HIV care services. Unless careful attention is paid to ensuring integrated and timely access to ART, patients may find themselves caught between programmes with signs and symptoms that are insufficient to prompt a clinical decision to start TB treatment, but are sufficient to delay acceptance into ART clinics. Integrated HIV and TB management to prioritise early initiation of ART, with all TB and HIV components ideally managed by the same clinic, may have more impact on the unsatisfactory scenario reported here and the current focus on improving diagnostic accuracy.

Acknowledgments

We thank the staff of Harare City Health, and all participants for their cooperation.

References

1. World Health Organization (2009) Global Tuberculosis Control 2009.
2. Corbett EL, Marston B, Churchyard GJ, De Cock KM (2006) Tuberculosis in sub-Saharan Africa: opportunities, challenges, and change in the era of antiretroviral treatment. Lancet 367: 926–937.
3. Colebunders R, Bastian I (2000) A review of the diagnosis and treatment of smear-negative pulmonary tuberculosis. Int J Tuberc Lung Dis 4: 97–107.
4. Harries AD, Maher D, Nunn P (1998) An approach to the problems of diagnosing and treating adult smear-negative pulmonary tuberculosis in high-HIV-prevalence settings in sub-Saharan Africa. Bull World Health Organ 76: 651–662.
5. Martinson NA, Karstaedt A, Venter WD, Omar T, King P, et al. (2007) Causes of death in hospitalized adults with a premortem diagnosis of tuberculosis: an autopsy study. AIDS 21: 2043–2050.
6. Getahun H, Harrington M, O'Brien R, Nunn P (2007) Diagnosis of smear-negative pulmonary tuberculosis in people with HIV infection or AIDS in resource-constrained settings: informing urgent policy changes. Lancet 369: 2042–2049.
7. Lawn SD, Myer L, Bekker LG, Wood R (2006) Burden of tuberculosis in an antiretroviral treatment programme in sub-Saharan Africa: impact on treatment outcomes and implications for tuberculosis control. AIDS 20: 1605–1612.
8. Lawn SD, Wilkinson RJ, Lipman MC, Wood R (2008) Immune reconstitution and "unmasking" of tuberculosis during antiretroviral therapy. Am J Respir Crit Care Med 177: 680–685.
9. World Health Organization (2007) Improving the diagnosis and treatment of smear-negative pulmonary and extra-pulmonary tuberculosis among adults and adolescents: Recommendations for HIV-prevalent and resource-constrained settings.
10. Corbett EL (2009) Protocol 06PRT/3449: A cluster randomised trial of two intensified tuberculosis care-finding strategies in an urban community severely affected by HIV (DETECTB) (ISRCTN 84352452). Lancet Available from http://www.thelancet.com/journals/lancet/misc/protocol/protocolreviews. Accessed 2010 Feb 6.
11. Carlin JB, Galati JC, Royston P (2008) A new framework for managing and analyzing multiply imputed data in Stata. Stata Journal 8: 49.
12. Crampin AC, Mwaungulu JN, Mwaungulu FD, Mwafulirwa DT, Munthali K, et al. (2009) Recurrent TB: relapse or reinfection? The effect of HIV in a general population cohort in Malawi. AIDS. In press.
13. Sonnenberg P, Glynn JR, Fielding K, Murray J, Godfrey-Faussett P, et al. (2005) How soon after infection with HIV does the risk of tuberculosis start to increase? A retrospective cohort study in South African gold miners. J Infect Dis 191: 150–158.
14. Harries AD, Parry C, Nyongonya Mbewe L, Graham SM, Daley HM, et al. (1997) The pattern of tuberculosis in Queen Elizabeth Central Hospital, Blantyre, Malawi: 1986–1995. Int J Tuberc Lung Dis 1: 346–351.
15. Dawson R, Masuka P, Edwards DJ, Bateman ED, Bekker LG, et al. (2010) Chest radiograph reading and recording system: evaluation for tuberculosis screening in patients with advanced HIV. Int J Tuberc Lung Dis 14: 52–58.
16. Apers L, Wijarajah C, Mutsvangwa J, Chigara N, Mason P, et al. (2004) Accuracy of routine diagnosis of pulmonary tuberculosis in an area of high HIV prevalence. Int J Tuberc Lung Dis 8: 945–951.
17. Munyati SS, Dhoba T, Makanza ED, Mungofa S, Wellingtor M, et al. (2005) Chronic cough in primary health care attendees, Harare, Zimbabwe: diagnosis and impact of HIV infection. Clin Infect Dis 40: 1818–1827.
18. Mutetwa R, Boehme C, Dimairo M, Bandason T, Munyati SS, et al. (2009) Diagnostic accuracy of commercial urinary lipoarabinomannan detection in African tuberculosis suspects and patients. Int J Tuberc Lung Dis 13: 1253–1259.
19. Lucas SB, Hounnou A, Peacock C, Beaumel A, Djomand G, et al. (1993) The mortality and pathology of HIV infection in a west African city. AIDS 7: 1569–1579.
20. Hopewell PC, Pai M, Maher D, Uplekar M, Raviglione MC (2006) International standards for tuberculosis care. Lancet Infect Dis 6: 710–725.
21. Morgan MA, Horstmeier CD, DeYoung DR, Roberts GD (1983) Comparison of a radiometric method (BACTEC) and conventional culture media for recovery of mycobacteria from smear-negative specimens. J Clin Microbiol 18: 384–388.
22. Reid MJA, Shah NS (2009) Approaches to tuberculosis screening and diagnosis in people with HIV in resource-limited settings. Lancet Infect Dis 9: 173–184.
23. Johnson JL, Vjecha MJ, Okwera A, Hatanga E, Byekwaso F, et al. (1998) Impact of human immunodeficiency virus type-1 infection or the initial bacteriologic and radiographic manifestations of pulmonary tuberculosis in Uganda. Int J Tuberc Lung Dis 2: 397–404.
24. Foundation for innovative new diagnostics (2009) Rapid scale up of integrated molecular diagnostic laboratories. Available: http://www.finddiagnostics.org/export/sites/default/resource-centre/presentations/stop_tb_forum_mar09/rapid_scale_up_rio_molecular_2.pdf. Accessed 2010 Feb 8.
25. Harries AD, Zachariah R, Lawn SD (2009) Providing HIV care for co-infected tuberculosis patients: a perspective from sub-Saharan Africa. Int J Tuberc Lung Dis 13: 6–16.
26. Lawn SD, Myer L, Orrell C, Bekker LG, Wood R (2005) Early mortality among adults accessing a community-based antiretroviral service in South Africa: implications for programme design. AIDS 19: 2141–2148.
27. Abdool Karim SS, Naidoo K, Grobler A, Padayatchi N, Baxter C, et al. (2010) Timing of initiation of antiretroviral drugs during tuberculosis therapy. N Engl J Med 362: 697–706.
28. Meintjes G, Rabie H, Wilkinson RJ, Cotton MF (2009) Tuberculosis-associated Immune Reconstitution Inflammatory Syndrome and Unmasking of Tuberculosis by Antiretroviral Therapy. Clin Chest Med 30: 797–810.
29. Meintjes G, Lawn SD, Scano F, Maartens G, French MA, et al. (2008) Tuberculosis-associated immune reconstitution inflammatory syndrome: case definitions for use in resource-limited settings. Lancet Infect Dis 8: 516–523.
30. Murdoch DM, Venter WD, Feldman C, Van R e A (2008) Incidence and risk factors for the immune reconstitution inflammatory syndrome in HIV patients in South Africa: a prospective study. AIDS 22: 601–610.
31. Zachariah R, Teck R, Ascurra O, Gomani P, Manzi M, et al. (2005) Can we get more HIV-positive tuberculosis patients on antiretroviral treatment in a rural district of Malawi? Int J Tuberc Lung Dis 9: 238–247.
32. Zachariah R, Harries AD, Manzi M, Gomani P, Teck R, et al. (2006) Acceptance of anti-retroviral therapy among patients infected with HIV and tuberculosis in rural Malawi is low and associated with cost of transport. PLoS ONE 1: e121.
33. Zachariah R, Van Engelgem I, Massaquoi M, Kocho-la L, Manzi M, et al. (2008) Payment for antiretroviral drugs is associated with a higher rate of patients lost to follow-up than those offered free-of-charge therapy in Nairobi, Kenya. Trans R Soc Trop Med Hyg 102: 288–293.
34. Yu JK, Chen SC, Wang KY, Chang CS, Makombe SD, et al. (2007) True outcomes for patients on antiretroviral therapy who are "lost to follow-up" in Malawi. Bull World Health Organ 85: 550–554.

Author Contributions

Conceived and designed the experiments: AZ SM AB SM SR KF PRM ELC. Performed the experiments: AZ AB ELC. Analyzed the data: MD PM TB KF ELC. Contributed reagents/materials/analysis tools: AZ SM SM SR PRM. Wrote the paper: MD PM AB KF ELC.

12

Uptake of Community-Based HIV Testing during a Multi-Disease Health Campaign in Rural Uganda

Gabriel Chamie[1,2,3]*, **Dalsone Kwarisiima**[2,3,4], **Tamara D. Clark**[1,2,3], **Jane Kabami**[2,3], **Vivek Jain**[1,2,3], **Elvin Geng**[1,2,3], **Laura B. Balzer**[3,5], **Maya L. Petersen**[3,5], **Harsha Thirumurthy**[3,6], **Edwin D. Charlebois**[2,3,7], **Moses R. Kamya**[2,3,8], **Diane V. Havlir**[1,2,3]

1 HIV/AIDS Division, Department of Medicine, San Francisco General Hospital, University of California San Francisco, San Francisco, United States of America, 2 Makerere University-University of California San Francisco (MU-UCSF) Research Collaboration, Uganda, 3 The Sustainable East Africa Research in Community Health (SEARCH) Consortium, 4 Mulago-Mbarara Joint AIDS Program, Kampala and Mbarara, Uganda, 5 School of Public Health, University of California, Berkeley, United States of America, 6 Gillings School of Global Public Health, University of North Carolina at Chapel Hill, United States of America, 7 Center for AIDS Prevention Studies, Department of Medicine, University of California San Francisco, San Francisco, United States of America, 8 Department of Medicine, School of Medicine, Makerere University College of Health Sciences, Kampala, Uganda

Abstract

Background: The high burden of undiagnosed HIV in sub-Saharan Africa is a major obstacle for HIV prevention and treatment. Multi-disease, community health campaigns (CHCs) offering HIV testing are a successful approach to rapidly increase HIV testing rates and identify undiagnosed HIV. However, a greater understanding of population-level uptake is needed to maximize effectiveness of this approach.

Methods: After community sensitization and a census, a five-day campaign was performed in May 2012 in a rural Ugandan community. The census enumerated all residents, capturing demographics, household location, and fingerprint biometrics. The CHC included point-of-care screening for HIV, malaria, TB, hypertension and diabetes. Residents who attended vs. did not attend the CHC were compared to determine predictors of participation.

Results: Over 12 days, 18 census workers enumerated 6,343 residents. 501 additional residents were identified at the campaign, for a total community population of 6,844. 4,323 (63%) residents and 556 non-residents attended the campaign. HIV tests were performed in 4,795/4,879 (98.3%) participants; 1,836 (38%) reported no prior HIV testing. Of 2674 adults tested, 257 (10%) were HIV-infected; 125/257 (49%) reported newly diagnosed HIV. In unadjusted analyses, adult resident campaign non-participation was associated with male sex (62% male vs. 67% female participation, p = 0.003), younger median age (27 years in non-participants vs. 32 in participants; p<0.001), and marital status (48% single vs. 71% married/widowed/divorced participation; p<0.001). In multivariate analysis, single adults were significantly less likely to attend the campaign than non-single adults (relative risk [RR]: 0.63 [95% CI: 0.53–0.74]; p<0.001), and adults at home vs. not home during census activities were significantly more likely to attend the campaign (RR: 1.20 [95% CI: 1.13–1.28]; p<0.001).

Conclusions: CHCs provide a rapid approach to testing a majority of residents for HIV in rural African settings. However, complementary strategies are still needed to engage young, single adults and achieve universal testing.

Editor: Barbara Ensoli, Istituto Superiore di Sanità, Italy

Funding: Sources of Funding – The National Institutes of Health/National Institute of Allergy and Infectious Diseases (grant 3P30AI027763-19S1 to DVH). Maya Petersen is a recipient of a Doris Duke Clinical Scientist Development Award. The funders had no role in study design, data collection and analysis, decision to publish, or preparation of the manuscript.

* E-mail: Gabriel.chamie@ucsf.edu

Introduction

The high burden of undiagnosed HIV represents a major obstacle to implementation of HIV prevention and antiretroviral treatment (ART) strategies in sub-Saharan Africa. Late HIV diagnosis translates into missed opportunities for HIV prevention and delayed antiretroviral treatment resulting in increased HIV-related morbidity and mortality, and ongoing HIV transmission. In Uganda, less than 25% of HIV-infected persons are estimated

to be aware of their status, and among 15–49 year olds one-third of women and over half of men have never tested for HIV [1,2].

Health facility-based approaches to HIV testing in rural Africa are limited by several factors: cost of patient travel and waiting time when accessing centralized services, stigma, lack of awareness of HIV risk, and the minimal or non-specific symptoms experienced by many patients early in HIV disease [3,4,5]. Provider-initiated voluntary counseling and testing succeeds in reaching clinic patients who might not otherwise seek testing, but is dependent on a person seeking medical care [6,7]. As a consequence, late presentations to HIV care are common. In a recent study, the median CD4 count at HIV diagnosis in an urban Ugandan hospital was <250 cells/µL [8].

Community health campaigns (CHC) that offer rapid HIV testing can close the "gap" between those who know and those who do not know their HIV status. CHCs aim to achieve universal testing across a community by removing significant barriers to HIV testing in a high-throughput format. CHCs offer HIV testing within broader service delivery (such as hypertension screening for adults and deworming of young children), thereby normalizing HIV testing as routine health care. CHCs also decentralize testing locations to minimize travel costs and waiting time, and actively mobilize community members to attend regardless of perceived risk. As a consequence, CHCs have succeeded in identifying large populations of persons reporting no prior testing, and in diagnosing HIV early [9,10].

We have previously demonstrated high uptake of community-wide HIV testing with CHCs in rural Uganda [9]. In the present study, we implemented a census followed by a repeat five-day, high-throughput HIV testing and referral campaign in order to better understand barriers to CHC participation for residents of a rural Ugandan community. This information is critical as CHC approaches are scaled up to maximize their impact and to develop complementary testing strategies for nonparticipants.

Methods

In May 2011, a multi-disease community health campaign (CHC) was conducted in a rural community, Kakyerere parish, in Mbarara District southwestern Uganda, with the results previously described [9]. In April and May 2012, an augmented study was conducted in the same parish, and included community sensitization, a baseline community census (to accurately measure participation rates and study reasons for non-participation), and a multi-disease CHC. We sought to understand predictors of participation in a CHC, a public-health approach to universal HIV testing.

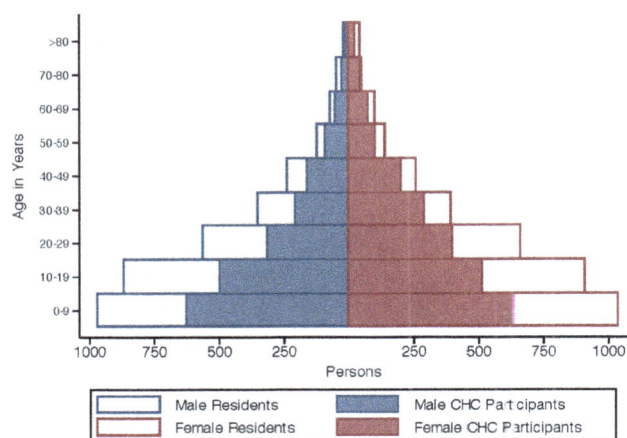

Figure 1. Population distribution of Kakyerere parish as determined from a twelve-day study census (open blue and red bars), and Community Health Campaign participation over five days among residents (solid blue and red bars), by age and sex.

Community sensitization

In an effort to maximize campaign uptake, regional and village political leaders implemented community sensitization activities one month before the campaign. Routine meetings were held between the investigators and the village leaders to answer questions raised by community members and to emphasize that the campaign services were available to all community residents regardless of HIV status, age, sex, or prior engagement in clinical care. Sensitization activities included announcements at local places of worship and at village gatherings as chosen by village leaders (including weddings and funerals), and distribution of colorful posters and flyers describing the campaign services provided written in both English and Runyankole (the local language). Campaign services were also described during household visits in the baseline census.

In addition, as low adult male participation was observed in the 2011 CHC (with men making up 34% of adult participants), efforts were made to increase male participation in the 2012 CHC [9]. After soliciting ideas from village leaders to increase male participation, a targeted incentive of a free T-shirt was introduced for each adult male participant upon campaign completion. The T-shirt incentive for men was also promoted during the community sensitization activities.

Baseline Census

In April 2012 a census was performed to enumerate the baseline population as the last national census in Uganda occurred in 2002. With the help of local leaders, census workers enumerated and collected basic demographics (age, sex, marital status and occupation) on all household members. Information on household members not present during a census visit was obtained from the head of household or other adults. Workers recorded household locations using handheld global positioning system (GPS) devices (Etrex Legend H Navigator, Garmin) and fingerprint biometric measurements (U.are.u 4500, Digital Persona) on all persons home during the census.

2012 Community Health Campaign

The campaign occurred over five days in May 2012 at four sites across the community. Well-known public gathering sites (a market place, a government council headquarters, and two primary schools) were chosen by the village leaders and investigators based on their convenience for villagers and to minimize transport costs and distance traveled reaching the campaigns. The campaign offered point-of-care (POC) HIV, hypertension and diabetes screening, tuberculosis (TB) symptom screening for all, and malaria testing for participants with self-reported fever, as previously described [9]. All participants screening HIV antibody positive underwent confirmatory testing with a POC rapid testing algorithm, followed by POC CD4+ T cell count testing (PIMA, Inverness Medical) [9]. They then received on-site post-test counseling, and were given an appointment to the local health center for HIV treatment. Finger-prick diagnostics eliminated the need for phlebotomy at the campaign.

Statistical Methods

Residence in Kakyerere parish was defined by enumeration in the census. Self-report during the campaign questionnaire was also accepted to define parish residence, but only if the participant could name a household member identified in the census. Fingerprint biometric measures were used to verify resident identity upon campaign registration; if fingerprinting failed, name-based matching was used. The prevalence of each disease was estimated with the sample proportion, where the number of participants tested for each disease served as the denominator. Unadjusted analyses of variables affecting CHC attendance among adults residents were based on Pearson's Chi-squared test for proportions, Student's t-test for means and the Wilcoxon rank sum test for medians. For a set of *a priori* specified characteristics (sex, single marital status and in-person contact at the census), adjusted analyses were based on targeted minimum loss-based estimation (TMLE) [11]. Specifically, TMLE was used to estimate the relative risk of each variable of interest, after controlling for the other factors and age continuously. Unlike standard logistic regression, TMLE avoids parametric modeling assumptions and yields marginal (unconditional) estimates.

Ethics statement

Verbal consent was obtained for all participants in order to maintain anonymity during HIV testing at the community health campaign, as written consent would have been the only name-linked identifier between a participant and his/her HIV test result. Campaign uptake was linked to the census data by a digital fingerprint biometric alone. Children from 13–17 years could provide verbal consent if a parent/guardian was not present, consistent with Uganda MOH policy [12]. Children <13 years could not participate without an assenting parent/guardian present. Verbal consent was documented by study staff for each study participant during the census and at entry into the campaign, and linked to an anonymous study identification number. The Makerere University School of Medicine Research and Ethics Committee, the Ugandan National Council on Science and Technology, and the UCSF Committee on Human Research approved the consent procedures and the study.

Results

Census

Over 12 days in April 2012, 18 census workers enumerated 6,343 parish residents (29 residents/day per worker). Based on population projections from the 2002 Ugandan Census, there were an estimated 6,400 Kakyerere parish residents in 2012 [13]. 4,247 (67%) residents were at home during the census, and 2,096

residents (33%) were enumerated but not at home. Of 4,247 residents at home during the census, 4,071 (96%) provided fingerprint biometric measures, and 176 (4%) declined. 3,149 (50%) of residents enumerated in the census were adults (>18 years), of whom 1,714 (54%) were female. Adults were home during census visits more often than children (2345/3149 [74%] vs. 1902/3194 [60%], respectively). Among adults, women were more likely to be home during census visits than men (1396/1714 [81%] vs. 949/1435 [66%]; p<0.001), and the median age was greater among residents at home (32 [IQR: 24–45] years) than residents not at home (25 [IQR: 20–38] years; p<0.001). Married, widowed and divorced/separated adults were also more likely to be home than single adults (1850/2262 [82%] vs. 493/880 [56%], respectively; p<0.001). During the health campaign, 501 persons not enumerated in the census reported residence in the community and could name a specific household member from the census, for a total parish population of 6,844 people.

Community Health Campaign

In five days, 4,879 people participated in the health campaign for an average of 976 participants/day. 4,282 (63%) of 6,844 community residents participated (see Figure 1), and 597/4,879 (12%) participants were non-residents from neighboring communities. Overall, 55% (2,687/4,879) of participants were adults, and 1,249 (46%) adult participants were men (see Figure 2). HIV tests were performed in 4,795/4,879 (98.3%) participants, of whom 1,836 (38%) reported no prior HIV testing. Of 257 HIV-infected adults, 125 (49%) reported newly diagnosed HIV. Median CD4 count among newly diagnosed adults was 436 cells/μL and 90 (72%) had a CD4 cell count >350 cells/μL. Among HIV-infected adults, 199/257 (77%) had at least one of four TB symptoms recommended by the WHO for intensified TB case finding [14]. Among HIV-uninfected adults, 318/2,417 (13%) reported cough for >2 weeks. 1,234/4,879 (25%) of CHC participants reported fever, and 51 (4%) tested positive for malaria by RDT. The prevalence of hypertension and diabetes among adult participants was 18% and 2%, respectively. Screening results are shown in Table 1. Among adult residents participating in the campaign, 1,071/2,204 (51%) reported attending our CHC held in the same community in May 2011. The final campaign day was at the local

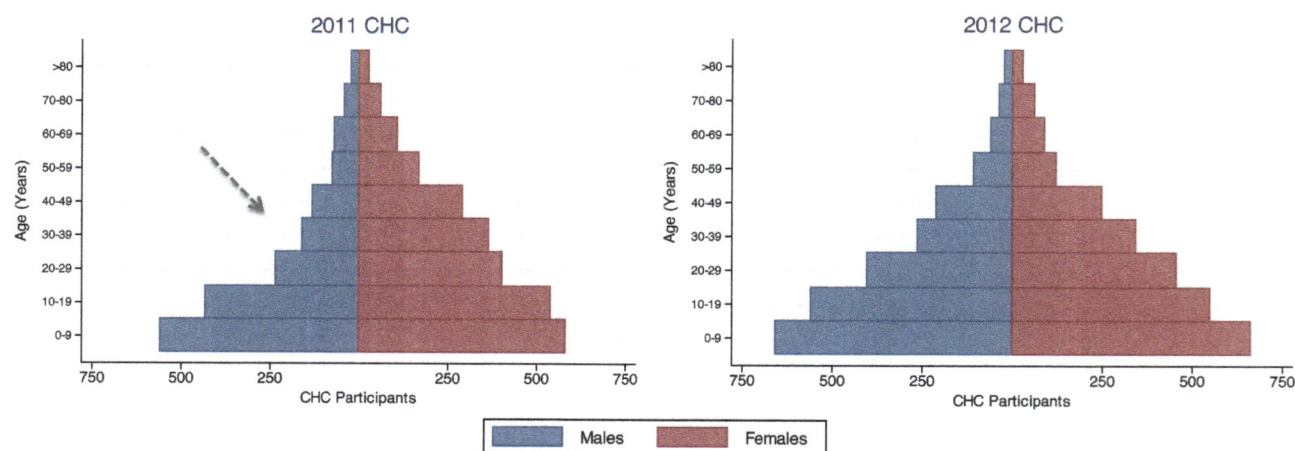

Figure 2. Change in male and female participation from a 2011 to a 2012 community health campaign (CHC) in Kakyerere parish, a rural Ugandan community. Shown are the age and sex distribution of CHC participants, including non-residents of the community, by year. The dashed arrow indicates the low proportion of adult male participants in the 2011 CHC.

Table 1. Screening results by disease during a five-day Community Health Campaign in Kakyerere parish, Uganda.

Community Health Campaign Participants N = 4,879	Number of participants screening positive	%
HIV (N = 4,795 tested)		
Children (<18 years) (N = 2,121)	12	1%
Adult (>18 years) (N = 2,674)	257	10%
Median CD4 count, adults (N = 210)	426 cells/μL	IQR: 306–613
New diagnoses in HIV-infected adults (N = 257)	125	49%
Median CD4 in newly diagnosed adults (N = 101)	436 cells/μL	IQR: 306–617
TB symptoms, adults (N = 2,674 screened)		
HIV-uninfected (N = 2,417)		
Cough >2 weeks	318	13%
HIV-infected (N = 257)		
Current cough	89	35%
Fever	81	32%
Weight loss	83	32%
Night sweats	125	49%
Any of above 4 symptoms	199	77%
Malaria (N = 4,879 screened for fever)		
Self-reported fever	1234	25%
Confirmed malaria, if febrile	51	4%
Age <10 years (N = 341)	27	8%
Age >10 years (N = 893)	24	3%
Hypertension, adults (N = 2,687 screened)		
Systolic>140 or diastolic>90 mmHg, or prior self-reported diagnosis	483	18%
Diabetes, adults (N = 2,672 screened)		
Adults with positive screening test	63	2%
New adult diagnoses	18	29%
Smoking (self-report)		
Men (N = 1246 screened)	393	32%
Women (N = 1437 screened)	152	11%

trading center on a weekend market day. A significantly greater proportion of adults attending the trading center site compared to the other three campaign sites, were male (55% vs. 44%; p<0.001), single (26% at trading center vs. 20% at other sites; p = 0.001), and younger (median age: 30 vs. 34 years; p<0.001).

Predictors of campaign participation

Of 6,844 community residents, 4,282 (63%) residents participated and 2,562 (37%) residents did not participate in the campaign. Adult residents were more likely to participate than children (2,204/3,446 [64%] vs. 2,078/3,398 [61%], respectively; unadjusted p = 0.017). In unadjusted analyses, adult participants compared to non-participants were more likely to be female (1222/1843 [66%] women vs. 982/1,603 [61%] men participated; p = 0.002), older (median age: 32 [IQR: 24–45] years in participants vs. 27 [22–38] in non-participants; p<0.001), non-single (70% of married/widowed/divorced vs. 48% single adults participated; p<0.001), farmers (75% of farmers vs. 51% of non-farmers participated; p<0.001) and to have been home during the census (70% adults at home vs. 34% not at home participated; p<0.001). Figure 3 shows the proportion of each sex and age group that attended the campaign. The average distance from

household to nearest campaign site was not significantly different in campaign participants (1.14 km) vs. non-participants (1.08 km; p = 0.87). Campaign participation by the head of household was significantly associated with campaign participation by other household members (68% [2,041/3,516] participation if household head participated vs. 41% [695/1,680] participation if household head did not participate; p<0.001).

After multivariate adjustment with TMLE, the estimated probability of attending the campaign was significantly lower among single compared to non-single adults (RR: 0.63; p<0.001 after adjusting for sex, being home during the census and age), and among adults who were not at home vs. at home during the census (adjusting for sex, single marital status, and age, RR: 0.83; p<0.001), whereas sex was no longer significantly associated with participation (Table 2).

Discussion

Our findings demonstrate the continued yield of multi-disease, community health campaign (CHC)-based HIV testing in identifying persons with no prior testing and with undiagnosed HIV infection in a community with year-round access to facility-based testing. Using rigorous methods to define community

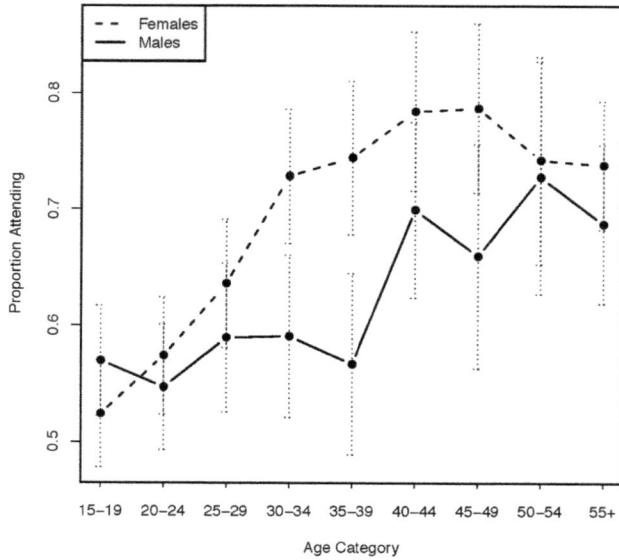

Figure 3. Proportion of residents attending the 2012 community health campaign (CHC) according to sex and age group among residents ≥15 years old. The dashed vertical lines indicate 95% confidence intervals.

residence, including a baseline census with fingerprint biometric measurements for identification, we found that young, single adults were significantly less likely than older, non-single adults to access HIV-testing via CHCs, suggesting that novel testing approaches are needed to reach this high-risk group.

Multi-disease CHCs have been successfully implemented in Uganda and Kenya and represent an effective and rapid strategy for scale-up of HIV testing services in rural, resource-limited settings [9,10]. Although several modalities for non-facility based testing have been successfully implemented in rural Africa, including home-based testing (HBT) and mobile testing vans, CHCs offer the advantages of acting as a platform for multi-disease testing and rapid scale-up to population coverage in a period of days. With point-of-care CD4 count testing and co-location of HIV clinic staff at the CHC, the early cascade of HIV care (testing, counseling and disease staging) can be performed in a single encounter taking less than three hours. Multi-disease service provision may also encourage repeat HIV testing or testing on a regular basis, which is likely to be a necessary part of any "test and treat" approach, and indeed we found that half of the campaign participants reported HIV testing at a CHC held one year prior.

However, our findings also suggest that complementary approaches will be needed to achieve universal HIV testing across

a population. By understanding how uptake varies with testing strategy, non-facility based testing strategies may be optimized to achieve universal testing coverage. Factors found to decrease uptake of home-based HIV testing (HBT) have varied considerably depending on the population studied, and include older age (>25 years) [4], as well as young adulthood [15], having a concurrent partnership at the time of HBT [4], lack of participation by the male head of household [16], single marital status, higher educational attainment [17], and high (>30%) prior rates of HIV testing in a community [18]. In our study population several factors were associated with lower testing uptake, notably younger age and single marital status. How these factors influence testing at CHCs remains unknown and multiple causal pathways are likely at play. For example, increased testing uptake with older age may be due to interest in the non-communicable disease screening offered at CHCs, whereas increased uptake among persons whose head of household participated in testing suggests that social networks influence CHC participation.

Low HIV testing uptake among young adults is a particularly important challenge due to the high HIV risk they face as they enter adulthood, and the enormous opportunity for HIV prevention among African youth. Despite the high risk of HIV faced by young adults, their testing rates are among the lowest of any demographic, particularly among young men, [19,20,21] and neither CHCs nor home-based testing approaches are immune to this [15]. A better understanding of the reasons for low HIV testing uptake among young, single adults and their perception of HIV risk is needed, and could inform novel approaches to reaching young adults and adolescents. Lower engagement by young adults in HIV prevention activities is not limited to HIV testing. Trials of HIV prevention interventions, such as pre-exposure prophylaxis with oral tenofovir-containing regimens have also found lower adherence as measured by drug levels among young women (age <25 years) and unmarried women in sub-Saharan Africa, further highlighting the challenges in HIV prevention interventions among young adults [22]. In spite of this challenge, community (non-facility) based HIV testing approaches such as CHCs have achieved higher testing uptake among young adults than health facility based testing and represent an opportunity to engage young adults in their communities for HIV prevention messaging and interventions. The relatively higher rate of young adult testing in the CHC seen at the marketplace also suggests that selecting testing sites with optimal convenience for young, working adults may increase testing uptake, and merits further exploration.

Despite lower rates of participation by young adults, adult male CHC participation was increased in the 2012 campaign to nearly half of adult participants (see Figure 2). Through a process of soliciting village leader input for a specific barrier to CHC uptake, incentives may have played a significant role in increasing male

Table 2. Results from the unadjusted and adjusted analyses of the *a priori*-specified variables of interest on the relative risk (RR) of CHC attendance.

Variable	Unadjusted RR	95% CI	p-value	Adjusted RR	95% CI	p-value
Male	0.92	0.89–0.98	0.002	0.99	0.94–1.04	0.76
Single	0.68	0.63–0.73	<0.001	0.63	0.53–0.74	<0.001
Contacted during census	1.33	1.25–1.41	<0.001	1.20	1.13–1.28	<0.001

The reference groups were female, married/widowed/divorced/separated and not-contacted, respectively. The adjusted analyses (TMLE) controlled for the other factors and age continuously.

CHC participation, as has been described in a mobile testing approach in South Africa [23]. Several factors may have contributed to increased male participation in 2012 as well, such as increased familiarity with the campaign from the 2011 CHC, and inclusion of a marketplace as a campaign site. Lower HIV testing rates among men compared to women has been well described in a variety of settings, [9,10,21,24] and likely contributes to lower rates of ART uptake in men [25,26]. CHCs, incorporating input from local leadership, multi-disease services and simple incentives, offer a means of rapidly increasing adult male HIV testing uptake and reaching populations that might otherwise "fall through the cracks" of facility-based testing.

Our study has several limitations. The campaign was designed to accommodate 1,000 persons per day, and was limited to five days. The additional testing yield of having more campaign days, particularly among young, single adults, remains unknown. In addition, on the only campaign day occurring on a weekend, we observed a significantly younger median age and a greater proportion of single and male adults than the other four campaign days. This suggests that the lower participation rates of young, single adults may have been due in part to conflicts with their work schedules rather than lack of interest. The incentive used, a free T-shirt for adult males, was chosen by this community's leadership, and might not be effective or feasible in a different setting. Finally, our finding that being home during the census was significantly associated with campaign participation may reflect migration patterns, with persons not available during the census at higher likelihood of being away from home during the campaign days, rather than a mobilizing effect of the census. Despite these limitations, our data provide a rigorous evaluation of uptake of HIV testing using a CHC approach in a rural Ugandan community.

Conclusions

In light of the increasing number of effective biomedical options for HIV prevention among both HIV-infected and uninfected persons, and increased access to antiretroviral therapy in sub-Saharan Africa, the opportunities for reducing HIV-associated morbidity and mortality and dramatically reducing HIV transmission are greater than ever, but depend on knowing one's HIV status. Achieving universal HIV testing across large populations will likely require several complementary testing approaches. Multi-disease community health campaigns provide a rapid means of jump-starting this process, and will serve as the engine driving universal HIV testing in the SEARCH "test and treat" cluster randomized-control trial we are conducting in East Africa, comparing universal HIV testing with antiretroviral therapy (ART) start at any CD4+ T cell count vs. CD4-guided ART start.

Acknowledgments

We thank the residents of Kakyerere Parish, Mbarara District, Uganda, for their generous participation in our study. We also thank the village local councilors from Kakyerere Parish, the staff of the Bwizibwera Level IV Health Centre, Mbarara and the Mulago-Mbarara Joint AIDS Programme (MMJAP) for their assistance, and the Uganda Ministry of Health for the donation of HIV rapid test kits and male condoms for use in this health campaign.

Author Contributions

Conceived and designed the experiments: GC DK TC JK VJ EG LB MP HT EC MK DH. Performed the experiments: GC DK TC JK VJ EC MK DH. Analyzed the data: GC LB MP EC DH. Wrote the paper: GC DH. Interpretation and editing of this manuscript: GC DK TC JK VJ EG LB MP HT EC MK DH.

References

1. World Health Organization (WHO), UNAIDS and UNICEF (2009) "Towards Universal Access: Scaling up priority HIV/AIDS interventions in the health sector: progress report 2009".
2. Uganda Ministry of Health and ICF International (2012) 2011 Uganda AIDS Indicator Survey: Key Findings. Calverton, Maryland, USA: MOH and ICF International.
3. Cherutich P, Kaiser R, Galbraith J, Williamson J, Shiraishi RW, et al. (2012) Lack of knowledge of HIV status a major barrier to HIV prevention, care and treatment efforts in Kenya: results from a nationally representative study. PLoS ONE 7: e36797.
4. Helleringer S, Kohler HP, Frimpong JA, Mkandawire J (2009) Increasing uptake of HIV testing and counseling among the poorest in sub-Saharan countries through home-based service provision. Journal of acquired immune deficiency syndromes 51: 185–193.
5. Mulogo EM, Abdulaziz AS, Guerra R, Baine SO (2011) Facility and home based HIV Counseling and Testing: a comparative analysis of uptake of services by rural communities in southwestern Uganda. BMC health services research 11: 54.
6. Creek TL, Ntumy R, Seipone K, Smith M, Mogodi M, et al (2007) Successful introduction of routine opt-out HIV testing in antenatal care in Botswana. Journal of acquired immune deficiency syndromes 45: 102–107.
7. Dalal S, Lee CW, Farirai T, Schilsky A, Goldman T, et al (2011) Provider-initiated HIV testing and counseling: increased uptake in two public community health centers in South Africa and implications for scale-up. PLoS ONE 6: e27293.
8. Wanyenze RK, Kamya MR, Fatch R, Mayanja-Kizza H, Baveewo S, et al. (2011) Missed opportunities for HIV testing and late-stage diagnosis among HIV-infected patients in Uganda. PLoS ONE 6: e21794.
9. Chamie G, Kwarisiima D, Clark TD, Kabami J, Jain V, et al. (2012) Leveraging rapid community-based HIV testing campaigns for non-communicable diseases in rural Uganda. PLoS ONE 7: e43400.
10. Lugada E, Millar D, Haskew J, Grabowsky M, Garg N, et al. (2010) Rapid Implementation of an Integrated Large-Scale HIV Counseling and Testing, Malaria, and Diarrhea Prevention Campaign in Rural Kenya. PLoS ONE 5: e12435.
11. Bembom O, Petersen ML, Rhee SY, Fessel WJ, Sinisi SE, et al. (2009) Biomarker discovery using targeted maximum-likelihood estimation: application to the treatment of antiretroviral-resistant HIV infection. Statistics in Medicine 28: 152–172.
12. Uganda Ministry of Health (2005) Uganda national policy guidelines for HIV voluntary counselling and testing. Kampala: Ministry of Health.
13. Uganda Bureau of Statistics: Population Projections 2008–2012. December, 2008.
14. WHO Guidelines for intensified tuberculosis case-finding and isoniazid preventive therapy for people living with HIV in resource-constrained settings (2010) Department of HIV/AIDS, Stop TB Department.
15. Lugada E, Levin J, Abang B, Mermin J, Mugalanzi E, et al. (2010) Comparison of home and clinic-based HIV testing among household members of persons taking antiretroviral therapy in Uganda: results from a randomized trial. Journal of acquired immune deficiency syndromes 55: 245–252.
16. Kranzer K, McGrath N, Saul J, Crampin AC, Jahn A, et al. (2008) Individual, household and community factors associated with HIV test refusal in rural Malawi. Tropical medicine & international health: TM & IH 13: 1341–1350.
17. Matovu JK, Kigozi G, Nalugoda F, Wabwire-Mangen F, Gray RH (2002) The Rakai Project counselling programme experience. Tropical medicine & international health: TM & IH 7: 1064–1067.
18. Sabapathy K, Van den Bergh R, Fidler S, Hayes R, Ford N (2012) Uptake of home-based voluntary HIV testing in sub-Saharan Africa: a systematic review and meta-analysis. PLoS Med 9: e1001351.
19. UNICEF & UNAIDS (2011) "Opportunity in Crisis: Preventing HIV from early adolescence to young adulthood".
20. Ferrand RA, Munaiwa L, Matsekete J, Bandason T, Nathoo K, et al. (2010) Undiagnosed HIV infection among adolescents seeking primary health care in Zimbabwe. Clinical infectious diseases: an official publication of the Infectious Diseases Society of America 51: 844–851.
21. Ramirez-Avila L, Nixon K, Noubary F, Giddy J, Losina E, et al. (2012) Routine HIV testing in adolescents and young adults presenting to an outpatient clinic in Durban, South Africa. PLoS ONE 7: e45507.
22. Marrazzo J, Ramjee G, Nair G, Palanee T, Mkhize B, et al. (2013) Pre-exposure Prophylaxis for HIV in Women: Daily Oral Tenofovir, Oral Tenofovir/Emtricitabine, or Vaginal Tenofovir Gel in the VOICE Study (MTN 003). Abstract 26LB, Conference on Retroviruses and Opportunistic Infections (CROI), Atlanta, GA, March 4; 2013; Atlanta, GA.

23. Kranzer K, Govindasamy D, van Schaik N, Thebus E, Davies N, et al. (2012) Incentivized recruitment of a population sample to a mobile HIV testing service increases the yield of newly diagnosed cases, including those in need of antiretroviral therapy. HIV Med 13: 132–137.

24. Venkatesh KK, Madiba P, De Bruyn G, Lurie MN, Coates TJ, et al. (2011) Who gets tested for HIV in a South African urban township? Implications for test and treat and gender-based prevention interventions. Journal of acquired immune deficiency syndromes 56: 151–165.

25. Braitstein P, Boulle A, Nash D, Brinkhof MW, Dabis F, et al. (2008) Gender and the use of antiretroviral treatment in resource-constrained settings: findings from a multicenter collaboration. Journal of women's health 17: 47–55.

26. Muula AS, Ngulube TJ, Siziya S, Makupe CM, Umar E, et al. (2007) Gender distribution of adult patients on highly active antiretroviral therapy (HAART) in Southern Africa: a systematic review. BMC Public Health 7: 63.

13

HIV Incidence Remains High in KwaZulu-Natal, South Africa: Evidence from Three Districts

Annaléne Nel[1], Zonke Mabude[2,8], Jenni Smit[2,8], Philip Kotze[3], Derek Arbuckle[4], Jian Wu[5], Neliëtte van Niekerk[6], Janneke van de Wijgert[7]*

1 International Partnership for Microbicides, Silver Spring, Maryland United States of America, **2** MatCH, Department of Obstetrics and Gynecology, University of the Witwatersrand Durban, KwaZulu-Natal, South Africa, **3** Qhakaza Mbokodo Research Clinic, Ladysmith, KwaZulu-Natal, South Africa, **4** PHIVA Project, Pinetown, KwaZulu-Natal, South Africa, **5** JW Consulting, Hurstville Grove, New South Wales, Australia, **6** International Partnership for Microbicides, Paarl, Western Cape, South Africa, **7** Academic Medical Center of the University of Amsterdam and Amsterdam Institute for Global Health and Development, Amsterdam, The Netherlands, **8** International Partnership for Microbicides, Paarl, Western Cape, South Africa

Abstract

Background: HIV prevalence and incidence among sexually active women in peri-urban areas of Ladysmith, Edendale, and Pinetown, KwaZulu-Natal, South Africa, were assessed between October 2007 and February 2010 in preparation for vaginal microbicide trials.

Methodology/Principal Findings: Sexually active women 18–35 years, not known to be HIV-positive or pregnant were tested cross-sectionally to determine HIV and pregnancy prevalence (798 in Ladysmith, 1,084 in Edendale, and 891 in Pinetown). Out of these, approximately 300 confirmed non-pregnant, HIV-negative women were subsequently enrolled at each clinical research center (CRC) in a 12-month cohort study with quarterly study visits. Women in the cohort studies were required to use a condom plus a hormonal contraceptive method. HIV prevalence rates in the baseline cross-sectional surveys were high: 42% in Ladysmith, 46% in Edendale and 41% in Pinetown. Around 90% of study participants at each CRC reported one sex partner in the last 3 months, but only 14–30% stated that they were sure that none of their sex partners were HIV-positive. HIV incidence rates based on seroconversions over 12 months were 14.8/100 person-years (PY) (95% CI 9.7, 19.8) in Ladysmith, 6.3/100 PY (95% CI 3.2, 9.4) in Edendale, and 7.2/100 PY (95% CI 3.7, 10.7) in Pinetown. The 12-month pregnancy incidence rates (in the context of high reported contraceptive use) were: 5.7/100 PY (95% CI 2.6, 8.7) in Ladysmith, 3.1/100 PY (95% CI 0.9, 5.2) in Edendale and 6.3/100 PY (95% CI 3.0, 9.6) in Pinetown.

Conclusions/Significance: HIV prevalence and incidence remain high in peri-urban areas of KwaZulu-Natal.

Editor: Ruanne V. Barnabas, University of Washington, United States of America

Funding: No current external funding sources for this study.

Competing Interests: Jian Wu is a consultant (JW consulting is a one person business) and was paid to conduct the statistical analyses for this paper.

* E-mail: j.vandewijgert@amc-cpcd.org

Introduction

The South African province of KwaZulu-Natal is experiencing one of the worst HIV epidemics worldwide. The epidemic has been described as hyperendemic, generalized and mature, with HIV prevalence rates in the general population of over 15% [1–5]. Data from the Department of Health antenatal surveys and the Human Sciences Research Council (HSRC) cross-sectional population-based household surveys have shown a stabilization of prevalence rates since 2005 [3–5]. HIV prevalence is expected to increase in the context of a mature epidemic with increasing access to antiretroviral therapy because people living with HIV will survive longer [6,7]. Therefore, HIV incidence data are increasingly important because only data on new HIV infections will provide insight into ongoing transmission dynamics [6,7].

KwaZulu-Natal is divided into 11 districts. The HIV epidemics in two of these districts have been extensively studied: the urban district of eThekwini (Durban Metropolitan Area and surrounding area) and the rural district of uMkhanyakude (where the Africa Centre of the University of KwaZulu-Natal is located) [8–11]. Recent studies in these districts found HIV incidence rates of 6.4/100 person-years (PY) among urban women and 6.5/100 PY among rural women aged 14–30 years [8] and 3.6/100 PY among rural women aged 15–55 years [11]. Our research was conducted in eThekwini district (in the small town of Pinetown, about 16 km west of Durban) and in two under-researched districts of KwaZulu-Natal: Ladysmith, the capital city of the uThukela district, and Edendale (near Pietermaritzburg) in the uMgungundlovu district. All three study areas can be characterized as peri-urban. According to the 2009 and 2010 antenatal surveys, the HIV prevalence rates in pregnant women in eThekwini, uThukela, and uMgungundlovu districts were 41.4/41.1%, 46.4/36.7%, and 40.9/42.3%, respectively [3,4].

We conducted HIV prevalence and incidence studies in sexually active women in the above-mentioned peri-urban areas of KwaZulu-Natal to better understand how many and where new HIV infections are occurring and to assess the feasibility of undertaking vaginal microbicide trials for HIV prevention in these populations.

Methods

Study design and populations

In preparation for future vaginal microbicide trials for HIV prevention in KwaZulu-Natal, cross-sectional studies (targeting 800–1,000 women each) were conducted at three clinical research centers (CRC) to determine HIV prevalence and to identify HIV-negative, non-pregnant women for enrollment in subsequent cohort studies (targeting 300 women each). The main aim of the cohort studies was to determine HIV incidence in seroconversions per 100 PY. The CRCs were located in Ladysmith, Edendale, and Pinetown. Each CRC established a Community Advisory Group (CAG) to provide community input in study procedures and to assist the researchers with community education and mobilization. CRC staff, with the assistance of CAG members, organized meetings in public spaces (at public meetings, in shopping centers and in waiting areas of clinics), where the study was presented. Women who expressed an interest in study participation were then invited to visit the CRC for screening and possible enrollment. In addition, door-to-door or family visits were conducted by study staff. While the recruitment strategies were CRC-specific, the same study procedures were followed at each CRC from the moment women were screened for study participation.

Women were eligible for the cross-sectional studies if they were 18–35 years, not HIV-positive or pregnant by self-report, not breastfeeding, and sexually active (defined as at least one penetrative vaginal coital act per month for the previous three months). Women who tested HIV- and pregnancy-negative in the cross-sectional studies, still met the entry criteria described above, and met additional entry criteria for the cohort studies, were subsequently offered enrollment into the cohort studies. These additional entry criteria included using a condom plus a hormonal (oral or injectable) contraceptive method [12], not injecting non-therapeutic drugs, not participating in other studies, not suffering from specified chronic diseases or allergies, refraining from anal sex and planning to stay in the study area for the duration of the study. Follow-up visits were scheduled at 3, 6, 9 and 12 months.

At all study visits, women were interviewed regarding demographics, sexual behavior, vaginal hygiene practices, and medical history; and received HIV risk reduction and contraceptive counseling, condoms, and syndromic management of sexually transmitted infections (STI) free of charge [13]. Confirmed HIV-positive women were referred for HIV care, and pregnant women were referred for antenatal care. HIV-positive and pregnant women enrolled in the cohort studies could continue study participation if so desired. The study was approved by two ethical review committees in South Africa: the University of Witwatersrand Human Research Ethics Committee and Pharma-Ethics. Formal support for the study was also obtained from provincial, district, hospital and clinical authorities, and from local community leaders. Written informed consent was obtained from all study participants.

Laboratory testing

An HIV testing algorithm was used to determine the presence of prevalent and incident HIV infections. Women were first tested by OraQuick ADVANCE Rapid HIV-1/2 Antibody Test using oral swabs (OraSure Technologies Inc., Bethlehem, PA, USA) or by Uni-Gold Recombigen HIV test using blood (Trinity Biotech, Bray, Wicklow, Ireland). When this first HIV test was positive, blood samples were tested by Determine HIV-1/2 rapid test (Inverness Medical Professional Diagnostics, Princeton, NJ, USA), and by enzyme-linked immunosorbant assay (ELISA) if a tiebreaker was needed. Blood samples from women who were confirmed HIV-positive were also tested by BED assay (Calypte Biomedical Corporation, Portland, OR, USA) according to the manufacturer's instructions. A specimen with a final normalized optical density value of less than or equal to 0.8 was considered to be from a participant who was infected less than 155 days before [14]. Urine samples from each participant were tested for pregnancy using an hCG pregnancy test.

Data Analysis and Statistics

Case report forms were processed using the DataFax data management system (Clinical DataFax Systems Inc., Hamilton, Ontario, Canada) and analyzed using SAS version 9.2 (SAS Institute, Cary, NC, USA). Descriptive statistics were used to summarize baseline demographic, behavioral and clinical characteristics. Categorical variables were expressed as percentages, and continuous data as medians with inter-quartile ranges.

Incidence rates in the cohort studies were calculated based on a Poisson distribution with PY at risk in the denominator. A person's time at risk began at the enrollment visit and ended at the last study visit attended (usually the Month 12 visit) or when HIV infection or pregnancy occurred. HIV infection and pregnancy were assumed to have occurred at the mid-point between the last available negative test and first positive test. A woman who reached an HIV endpoint was no longer considered at risk for HIV but was still considered at risk for pregnancy, and vice versa. HIV incidence rates and 95% confidence intervals based on BED results in the cross-sectional studies were calculated using the formula, and accompanying spreadsheet, provided by McWalter and Welte [15,16]. Inputs in the formula include the total number of HIV-positive and HIV-negative individuals in the sample, the number of HIV-positive individuals who also tested positive on the BED assay, the BED window period, and an estimated BED false-recent rate (FRR). A recent study in KwaZulu-Natal found a local FRR of 1.7% [17] and a study in Zimbabwe a window period of 187 days (instead of the 155 days that are specified in the package insert) [18]. Two BED adjustments were therefore made: one using a window period of 155 days and a FRR of 1.7%, and another one using a window period of 187 days and a false recent rate of 1.7%. Incidence estimates are expressed as an incidence rate (number of new HIV infections per 100 PY).

Age-adjusted and multivariable logistic regression models were used to assess predictors of prevalent HIV infection and pregnancy, with p-values from the Wilcoxon-Mann-Whitney test for continuous variables and the Chi-square and Fisher's exact tests for categorical variables. Age-adjusted Cox proportional hazards regression models were used to assess predictors of HIV seroconversion and incident pregnancy.

Results

Disposition

Women were enrolled in the cross-sectional studies between 2007 and 2009 as follows: 798 women in Ladysmith, 1,084 women in Edendale, and 891 women in Pinetown. The Ladysmith and Edendale CRCs subsequently enrolled 300 women in their cohort studies and the Pinetown CRC 297 women, accumulating 223, 254, and 223 PY respectively. In Ladysmith, 129 of 300 (43%) participants completed all scheduled visits; 53 women withdrew early from the cohort study, 32 were lost to follow-up, and none died. In Edendale, 210 of 300 (70%) participants completed all scheduled visits; 6 women withdrew early from the cohort study,

Table 1. Characteristics of Cross-sectional Study Participants.

Characteristic n (%)	Ladysmith N = 798	Edendale N = 1,084	Pinetown N = 891
Age in years (median; range)	24 (18–35)	24 (18–35)	23 (18–35)
Race: Black African	792 (99.2)	1,081 (99.7)	890 (99.9)
Marital status			
Single	723 (90.6)	988 (91.1)	799 (89.7)
Married/or living together	75 (9.4)	90 (8.3)	91 (10.2)
Separated/divorced/widowed	0	6 (0.6)	1 (0.1)
Education			
No school	2 (0.3)	5 (0.5)	3 (0.3)
Some/completed primary school	26 (3.3)	40 (3.6)	81 (9.1)
Some/completed high school	651 (81.6)	1,002 (92.5)	743 (84.3)
Some/completed tertiary school	119 (14.9)	36 (3.3)	55 (6.2)
Source of income[1]			
Formal/informal work	193 (24.2)	56 (5.2)	123 (13.8)
Government grants	321 (40.2)	639 (59.1)	509 (57.2)
Husband/partner	95 (11.9)	25 (2.3)	78 (8.8)
Other	471 (59.0)	397 (36.7)	234 (26.3)
Average monthly income			
0-R500	542 (67.9)	1034 (95.7)	772 (86.6)
>R500	256 (32.1)	47 (4.3)	119 (13.4)
Male sex partners in last 3 months			
1	718 (90.0)	998 (92.1)	780 (87.5)
2 or more	80 (10.0)	86 (7.9)	111 (12.5)
Male sex partners in last 7 days			
0	152 (19.9)	215 (19.9)	135 (15.2)
1	608 (79.5)	859 (79.3)	750 (84.4)
2 or more	5 (0.7)	9 (0.8)	4 (0.4)
Condom used during last sex act	374 (46.9)	577 (53.2)	550 (62.0)
Condom use in last 7 day[2]			
Always	228 (35.5)	404 (42.2)	322 (42.2)
Inconsistent	197 (30.7)	137 (14.3)	182 (23.9)
Never	217 (33.8)	416 (43.5)	259 (33.9)
Any chance that any current sex partner is HIV-positive			
Yes	210 (26.3)	178 (16.7)	182 (20.5)
No	235 (29.5)	187 (17.5)	125 (14.1)
Don't know	352 (44.2)	702 (65.8)	579 (65.3)
Ever had anal sex	4 (0.5)	28 (2.6)	3 (0.3)
Ever had oral sex	115 (14.4)	169 (15.6)	145 (16.3)
Ever vaginal cleansing before or after sex	8 (1.0)	20 (1.8)	67 (7.6)
Ever vaginal drying before or after sex	1 (0.1)	16 (1.5)	37 (4.1)
Self assessment of HIV risk[3]			
No/low risk	392 (51.4)	449 (42.2)	407 (50.1)
Moderate risk	58 (7.6)	188 (17.7)	20 (2.5)
High risk	312 (40.9)	426 (40.1)	385 (47.4)
Reported genital symptom at baseline[4]	34 (4.3)	15 (1.4)	27 (3.0)

[1]Multiple responses allowed.
[2]Women who reported any sexual intercourse in the last 7 days only.
[3]Women who said 'don't know' were excluded.
[4]Includes lower abdominal pain, genital discharge, odor, ulcers sores, itching or swelling, burning pain on urination.

Table 2. Age-adjusted Determinants of Prevalent HIV Infection in the Cross-Sectional Studies[1].

Determinant	Ladysmith (N = 798)		Edendale (N = 1,084)		Pinetown (N = 891)	
	% HIV+	Age-adjusted OR (95% CI)	% HIV+	Age-adjusted OR (95% CI)	% HIV+	Age-adjusted OR (95% CI)
Marital status:						
Married/living together	48.0	0.8 (0.5, 1.3)	60.0	1.0 (0.6, 1.5)	53.3	1.2 (0.8, 2.0)
Single, separated or divorced (reference)	41.4		44.8		39.9	
Highest level of education achieved:						
Some/completed primary education	50.0	2.9 (1.2, 7.4)	70.0	9.1 (2.9, 28.9)	54.3	6.2 (2.5, 15.1)
Some/completed high school	45.3	3.0 (1.9, 4.9)	46.2	4.3 (1.7, 10.7)	41.8	3.7 (1.7, 8.1)
Some/completed tertiary education (reference)	21.8		16.7		14.8	
Source of income:						
Formal/informal work (reference)	53.9		48.2		44.2	
Government grants	36.4	0.6 (0.4, 0.9)	52.1	1.2 (0.7, 2.1)	46.8	1.1 (0.7, 1.7)
Husband/Other	39.4	0.9 (0.6, 1.3)	35.9	1.0 (0.5, 1.8)	30.7	0.9 (0.5, 1.4)
Average monthly income[5]						
0-R500 (reference)	40.2		45.8		42.5	
>R500	45.7	0.8 (0.6, 1.1)	51.1	1.1 (0.6, 2.0)	33.3	0.5 (0.3, 0.8)
Number of sex partners in last 3 months						
1 (reference)	40.7		46.3		40.1	
More than 1	53.8	1.9 (1.2, 3.2)	43.0	1.2 (0.7, 1.9)	49.5	1.7 (1.1, 2.6)
Condom use in last 7 days						
Always (reference)	27.2		32.4		32.5	
Inconsistent	50.3	2.5 (1.7, 3.8)	58.1	2.6 (1.7, 4.0)	48.6	1.9 (1.3, 2.8)
Never	47.5	2.1 (1.4, 3.1)	56.7	2.4 (1.8, 3.3)	50.8	1.8 (1.3. 2.6)
Ever had oral sex[2]						
Yes	43.5	1.0 (0.7, 1.6)	43.8	1.0 (0.7, 1.4)	41.7	1.1 (0.7, 1.5)
No (reference)	41.7		46.4		41.2	
Self assessment of HIV risk						
No/low risk (reference)	24.7		25.2		26.8	
Moderate risk	53.4	3.6 (2.0, 6.4)	58.3	3.8 (2.6, 5.6)	60.0	3.0 (1.2, 7.7)
High risk	58.7	4.1 (3.0, 5.8)	61.5	3.9 (2.9, 5.3)	53.3	2.9 (2.1, 3.9)
Any chance that any current sex partner is HIV+						
Yes	51.0	3.2 (2.1, 4.9)	62.4	4.7 (2.9, 7.8)	51.1	2.6 (1.6, 4.3)
No (reference)	23.4		20.9		27.2	
Don't know	49.1	3.0 (2.0, 4.3)	48.2	3.1 (2.0, 4.6)	41.6	1.8 (1.2, 2.8)
Reported genital symptom at baseline						
Yes	55.9	1.9 (0.9, 4.0)	46.7	1.1 (0.4, 3.2)	70.4	4.2 (1.7, 10.2)
No (reference)	41.4		46.1		40.4	

[1]Each row represents one bivariable model including age and the predictor of interest.
[2]Anal sex, vaginal cleansing and vaginal drying were too infrequently reported to be assessed as a predictor of HIV prevalence (see Table 1).

24 were lost to follow-up, and none died. In Pinetown, 167 of 297 (56%) participants completed all scheduled visits; 5 women withdrew early from the cohort study, 74 were lost to follow-up, and none died.

Demographic and behavioral characteristics

In the cross-sectional studies, the median age of study participants was 23 or 24 years (Table 1). Almost all participants were black African, and more than 80% at each CRC was single, had only one sexual partner in the last 3 months, and had at least some high school education. About half of the participants (47–62%) had used a condom during their last sex act, while only 14–30% was sure that they did not currently have a sex partner who was HIV-positive. Anal sex was rarely reported at each CRC (<3%), but oral sex was more common (14–16%). Women in Pinetown were more likely to report cleansing or drying the vagina before or after sex (8% and 4%, respectively) than women in Ladysmith and Edendale. Less than 4% of all women reported a genital symptom. At each CRC, demographic and sexual behavior characteristics of cohort study participants at enrollment were

Table 3. Determinants of Prevalent HIV Infection in the Cross-Sectional Studies – Multivariable Models.

Determinant	Ladysmith (N = 798)	Edendale (N = 1,084)	Pinetown (N = 891)
	Adjusted OR (95% CI)	Adjusted OR (95% CI)	Adjusted OR (95% CI)
Age (year)	1.12 (1.07, 1.17)	1.16 (1.12, 1.20)	1.13 (1.09, 1.18)
Highest level of education achieved:			
Some/completed primary education	1.87 (0.59, 5.94)	12.77 (2.93, 55.66)	4.57 (1.50, 13.95)
Some/completed high school	1.92 (1.09, 3.40)	6.72 (2.02, 22.40)	3.21 (1.21, 8.53)
Some/completed tertiary education (reference)			
Average monthly income			
0-R500 (reference)			
>R500	0.90 (0.59, 1.37)	1.46 (0.62, 3.41)	0.45 (0.26, 0.76)
Number of sex partners in last 3 months			
1 (reference)			
More than 1	1.95 (1.09, 3.50)	1.02 (0.58, 1.79)	1.27 (0.76, 2.12)
Condom use in last 7 days			
Always (reference)			
Inconsistent	1.89 (1.16, 3.07)	2.27 (1.39, 3.72)	1.24 (0.71, 2.16)
Never	1.27 (0.78, 2.06)	1.40 (0.96, 2.03)	1.07 (0.65, 1.76)
Self assessment of HIV risk			
No/low risk (reference)			
Moderate risk	2.72 (1.35, 5.46)	3.54 (2.29, 5.47)	2.29 (0.65, 8.04)
High risk	3.16 (2.10, 4.75)	3.15 (2.12, 4.67)	2.12 (1.32, 3.40)
Any chance that any current sex partner is HIV+			
Yes	2.61 (1.55, 4.40)	2.90 (1.62, 5.21)	2.58 (1.33, 5.03)
Don't know	2.36 (1.48, 3.78)	2.34 (1.46, 3.76)	1.56 (0.89, 2.72)
No (reference)			

similar to cross-sectional participants. However, fewer women in the cohort than in cross-sectional studies felt that they were at high risk for HIV (25% vs. 41% in Ladysmith, 22% vs. 40% in Edendale, and 31% vs. 47% in Pinetown). Furthermore, women enrolled in the cohort in Edendale reported more condom use during the last sex act than those enrolled in the cross-sectional study (69% vs. 53%).

Condom use dynamics

More than 80% of women at all three CRCs reported that they themselves, or they and their partner together, decided about condom use (data not shown). About one third of women (28% in Ladysmith, 16% in Edendale, and 39% in Pinetown) reported to have refused sex in the last 7 days due to lack of a condom. The most common reasons for using a condom were 'to protect myself from HIV' (49% in Ladysmith, 74% in Edendale, and 70% in Pinetown), followed by 'to prevent pregnancy' (41% in Ladysmith, 66% in Edendale, and 52% in Pinetown), and 'to protect myself from STIs' (29% in Ladysmith, 38% in Edendale, and 58% in Pinetown). Protecting sexual partners from HIV or STIs was less often mentioned in Ladysmith and Edendale, and rarely mentioned in Pinetown (data not shown). The most common reason for not using a condom was partner refusal (40% in Ladysmith, 28% in Edendale, and 33% in Pinetown).

HIV prevalence

HIV prevalence was higher than 40% at all three CRCs: 42.0% (95% CI 38.5, 45.5) in Ladysmith, 46.1% in Edendale (95% CI

43.1, 49.1), and 41.3% (95% CI 38.0, 44.6) in Pinetown. Factors positively associated with prevalent HIV infection at all three CRCs in age-adjusted and multivariable models were: age, lower educational level, self-assessment of HIV risk as moderate or high (compared to no or low risk), and suspected positive or unknown HIV serostatus of a current sexual partner; no or inconsistent condom use was associated with HIV infection in all age-adjusted models but not in all multivariable models (Tables 2 and 3). Having an income below 500 Rand per month, having more than one sex partner in the last 3 months, and the presence of genital symptoms at baseline were only associated with prevalent HIV in Pinetown (Tables 2 and 3). Being married or living together and oral sex were not associated with prevalent HIV.

HIV incidence

Overall HIV incidence rates based on seroconversions during the 12-month follow-up period in the cohort studies were 14.8/ 100 PY (95% CI 9.7, 19.8) in Ladysmith, 6.3/100 PY (95% CI 3.2, 9.4) in Edendale, and 7.2/100 PY (95% CI 3.7, 10.7) in Pinetown (Table 3). No clear trends in incidence rates over time could be discerned (Figure 1). Statistically significant predictors of HIV seroconversion were not identified, most likely due to limited statistical power, with the following exceptions: reporting 3 or more sex partners in the last 3 months (compared to 1 or 2 sex partners), and reporting genital symptoms at baseline, were associated with HIV seroconversion in Edendale (data not shown). The adjusted HIV incidence rates estimated by cross-sectional BED testing are shown in Table 4.

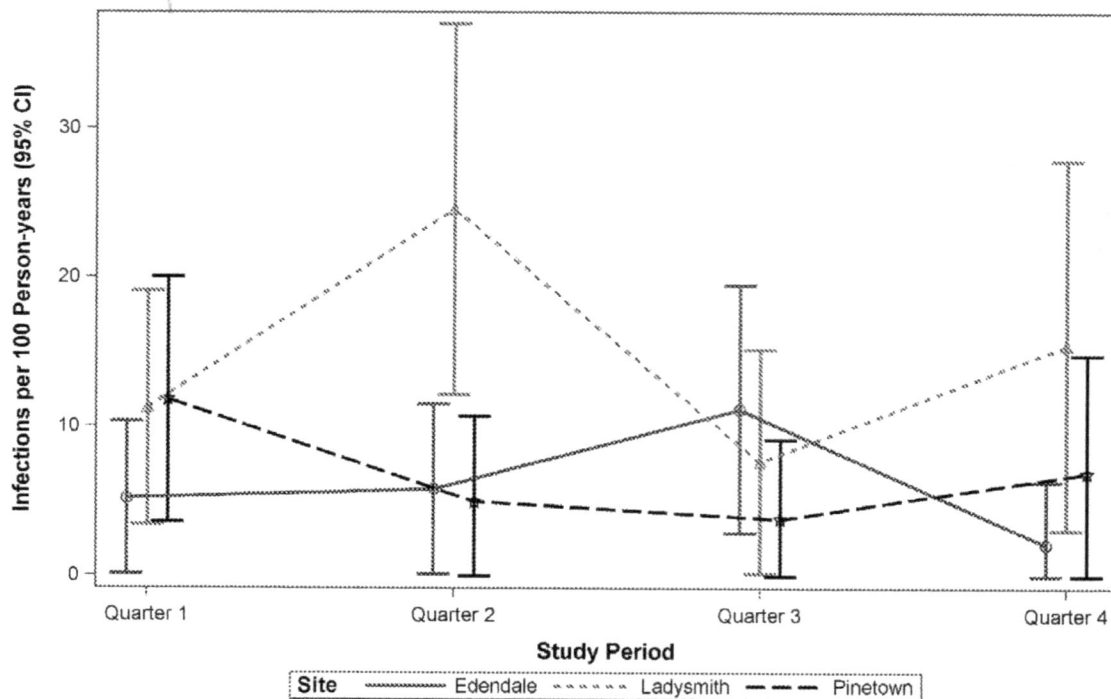

Figure 1. HIV incidence in the prospective cohort studies. Women enrolled in the 12-month cohort studies visited the CRC at 3, 6, 9, and 12 months after enrollment for HIV testing. HIV incidence rates were calculated based on a Poisson distribution with PY at risk in the denominator. They are expressed as number of cases per 100 PY with 95% confidence intervals. HIV infection was assumed to have occurred at the mid-point between the last available negative test and first positive test.

Pregnancy prevalence and incidence

The pregnancy prevalence rates in the cross-sectional studies were low at all three CRCs in accordance with the recruitment strategy (only women reporting not to be pregnant were eligible for study participation): 2.6% (95% CI 1.6, 4.0) in Ladysmith, 4.1% (95% CI 3.0, 5.4) in Edendale, and 1.5% (95% CI 0.8, 2.5) in Pinetown. Pregnancy was associated with inconsistent condom use (age-adjusted OR 3.5, 95% CI 1.1, 11.4) and self-reported genital symptoms (age-adjusted OR 4.2, 95% CI 1.2, 15.2) in Ladysmith, and with 'never used condoms' (age-adjusted OR 4.1 (95% CI 1.8, 9.7) and self-reported moderate or high HIV risk (age-adjusted OR 3.7 (95% CI 1.5, 9.6) and 3.8 (95% CI 1.7, 8.8), respectively) in Edendale. In the cohort studies, overall pregnancy incidence for the 12-month period was 5.7 (95% CI 2.6, 8.7) in Ladysmith, 3.1 (95% CI 0.9, 5.2) in Edendale, and 6.3 (95% CI

3.0, 9.6) in Pinetown. Again, no trends were observed over time (Figure 2).

Discussion

Our data confirm that HIV prevalence and incidence continue to be high in sexually active women aged 18–35 years living in peri-urban areas of KwaZulu-Natal. Our prevalence rates are similar to those reported in the 2009 and 2010 national antenatal surveys but higher than those reported in the 2008 HSRC population-based household survey (26% for women and men combined and for all districts of KwaZulu-Natal combined) [3–5]. The latter is most likely due to the fact that the HIV prevalence is higher in South African women than in men; unfortunately, only aggregate data were reported [5]. Compared to women aged 20–

Table 4. HIV and Pregnancy Incidence Rates in the Prospective Cohort Studies.

	Ladysmith	Edendale	Pinetown
HIV incidence after 12 months	14.8 (9.7, 19.8)	6.3 (3.2, 9.4)	7.2 (3.7, 10.7)
HIV incidence in first 6 months	17.4 (10.3, 24.5)	5.5 (1.7, 9.3)	8.6 (3.5, 13.7)
HIV incidence in second 6 months	11.0 (4.2, 17.8)	7.3 (2.3, 12.4)	5.2 (0.6, 9.8)
HIV incidence BED adjusted (155 days; 1.7%) [17]	15.0 (10.1, 19.9)	10.2 (6.8, 13.7)	11.6 (7.6, 15.7)
HIV incidence BED adjusted (187 days; 1.7%) [17,18]	12.5 (8.4, 16.6)	8.5 (5.6, 11.4)	9.7 (6.3, 13.0)
Pregnancy incidence after 12 months	5.7 (2.6, 8.7)	3.1 (0.9, 5.2)	6.3 (3.0, 9.6)
Pregnancy incidence in first 6 months	7.4 (2.8, 12.0)	2.0 (0, 4.4)	7.0 (2.4, 11.6)
Pregnancy incidence in second 6 months	3.2 (0, 6.7)	4.4 (0.5, 8.3)	5.3 (0.7, 9.9)

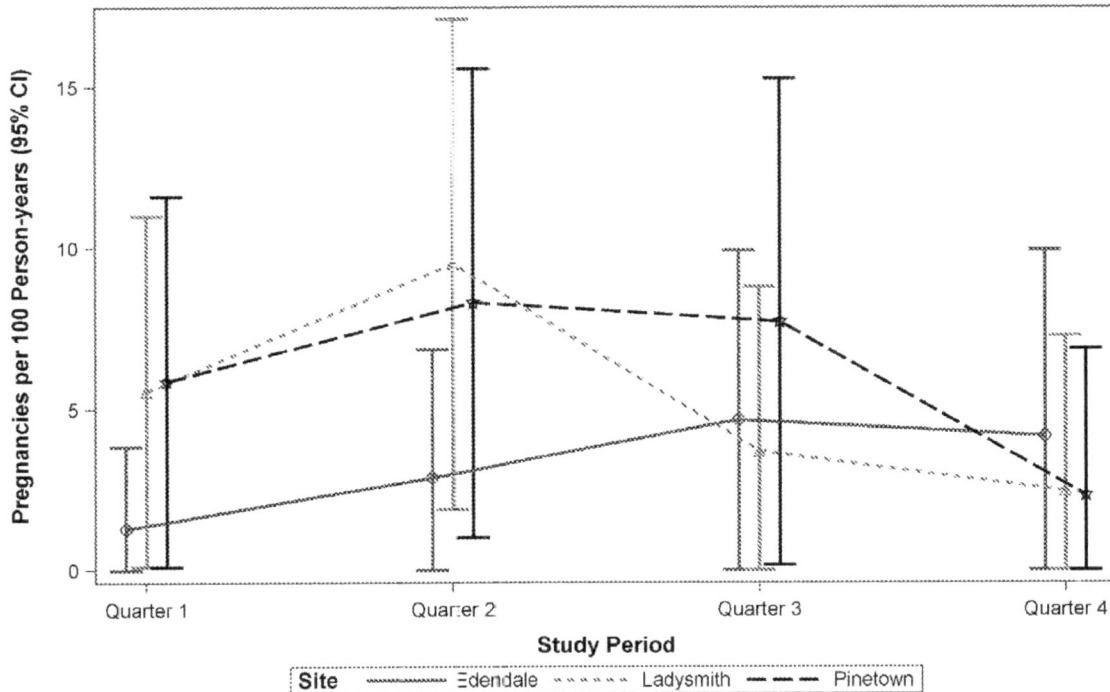

Figure 2. Pregnancy incidence in the prospective cohort studies. Urine pregnancy tests were done at each study visit (screening, enrollment, and 3, 6, 9, and 12 months after enrollment in the cohort study). If test result was positive, the participant was to continue on study for follow-up per protocol. Estimated date of conception and estimated due date were to be recorded. If possible, follow-up was to continue for pregnancy outcome. Contraceptive counseling was provided and condoms were dispensed at each study visit.

34 participating in the HSRC survey, a higher proportion of our study participants reported having had 2 or more partners in the last 3 months (8–13% versus 4%) and a slightly lower proportion reported condom use during the last sex act (47–62% versus 67%) [5].

Our HIV incidence rates of 6.3 to 14.8 per 100 PY suggest that HIV transmission is still rampant in KwaZulu-Natal. Our incidence rates for Edendale (6.3/100 PY; uMgungundlovu district) and Pinetown (7.2/100 PY; eThekwini district) fall within the range of rates recently reported for urban and rural women in eThekwini and uMkhanyakude districts (6.4/100 PY among urban women and 6.5/100 PY among rural women aged 14–30 years [7] and 3.6/100 PY among rural women aged 15–55 [10]). Our incidence rate for Ladysmith (14.8/100 PY; uThukela district), however, was substantially higher than any of these rates and we were not able to identify any reported incidence rates for Ladysmith or uThukela district to compare ours to. The higher incidence rate in Ladysmith cannot be explained by a higher HIV prevalence. HIV prevalence in uThukela district was slightly higher than in the other districts in 2009 but fell with almost 10% to a relatively low level of 37% in 2010 [3,4]. We also found hardly any significant differences in demographics (age, education and marital status) and sexual behavior between the three study populations. A higher proportion of women in Ladysmith had an average monthly income higher than R500 than in the other two study areas (32% versus 4 and 13%) but income was not associated with HIV seroconversion. Data on male circumcision, alcohol use, the presence of laboratory-confirmed sexually transmitted infections, and migration were not collected; temporary migration to other urban areas (such as Johannesburg and Durban) for work may fuel the HIV epidemic in Ladysmith more than in the other districts. Furthermore, HIV incidence was particularly high in the

second quarter of the study, which is when recruitment in more remote rural areas of uThukela district was initiated. This population had not previously had access to high quality HIV counseling and testing services.

As expected, HIV incidence rates based on the adjusted BED-CEIA results were higher than those based on seroconversions per 100 PY for the two sites with lower HIV incidence (Edendale and Pinetown; Table 4) [17,18]. However, the confidence intervals overlap substantially for all three study sites.

While HIV incidence at the three study sites seems sufficiently high for implementation of HIV microbicide efficacy trials, retention rates would have to be improved (currently 43–70%) and pregnancy incidence would have to be reduced. Women in our studies were required to use a condom and a hormonal method of contraception but the high pregnancy incidence rates indicate that these methods were not used correctly and consistently.

A few limitations of our data should be noted. The eligibility criteria for study participation may have limited generalizability of our results. The HIV prevalence rates apply only to young, sexually active women who were not known to be HIV-infected or pregnant, and who agreed to be tested regularly for HIV. The total number of seroconversions in each prospective cohort study were low (16–33 cases) and the 95% confidence intervals were therefore wide. The low retention rates of our cohort studies (43–70%) may have biased our HIV incidence estimates based on seroconversions. We do not have any indications that the women who left the cohort studies early were at higher or lower risk of HIV acquisition than the women who remained in the study but we cannot be certain. The 95% confidence intervals of the cross-sectional BED-based HIV incidence estimates were also wide. Furthermore, we did not measure local false-recent rates or window periods and could therefore not adjust our BED estimates as recommended by WHO [19].

In conclusion, HIV prevalence and incidence remain very high in sexually active women living in peri-urban areas of KwaZulu-Natal. HIV prevention interventions in these populations should be strengthened.

Acknowledgments

The authors gratefully acknowledge the study teams at the CRCs in Ladysmith, Edendale, and Pinetown and the study team at the International Partnership for Microbicides, in particular Dr. Mercy Kamupira (Clinical Safety Physician) and Karen Bester (Project Manager). The authors would also like to thank Dr. Sarah Braunstein for conducting preliminary data analyses.

Author Contributions

Conceived and designed the experiments: AN JvdW. Performed the experiments: AN ZM JS PK DA. Analyzed the data: JW JvdW NvN. Wrote the paper: JvdW. Critically reviewed the manuscript: AN JvdW ZM JS PK DA NvN.

References

1. UNAIDS (2010) UNAIDS report on the global AIDS epidemic 2010. Geneva: UNAIDS. Available: http://www.unaids.org/globalreport/global_report.htm. Accessed 2012 March 16.
2. Pettifor AE, Rees HV, Kleinschmidt I, Steffenson AE, McPhail C, et al. (2005) Young people's sexual health in South Africa: HIV prevalence and sexual behaviors from a nationally representative household survey. AIDS 19: 1525–1534.
3. Department of Health (2010) National antenatal sentinel HIV and syphilis prevalence survey, 2009, South Africa. Pretoria: National Department of Health.
4. Department of Health (2011) The 2010 national antenatal sentinel HIV and syphilis prevalence survey in South Africa. Pretoria: National Department of Health.
5. South African national HIV prevalence, incidence, behavior and communication survey, 2008, South Africa. Cape Town: HSRC Press, 2009.
6. Ghys PD, Kufa E, George MV (2006) Measuring trends in prevalence and incidence of HIV infection in countries with generalized epidemics. Sex Transm Infect 82(Suppl 1): i52–56.
7. Braunstein S, van de Wijgert J, Nash D (2009) HIV incidence in sub-Saharan Africa: a review of available data with implications for surveillance and prevention planning. AIDS Reviews 11: 140–156.
8. Adool Karim Q, Kharsany A, Frohlich JA, Werner L, Mashego M, et al. (2011) Stabilizing HIV prevalence masks high HIV incidence rates amongst rural and urban women in KwaZulu-Natal, South Africa. Intern J Epidemiol 40: 922–930.
9. Abdool Karim Q, Abdool Karim SS, Frohlich JA, Grobler AC, Baxter C, et al. (2010) Effectiveness and safety of tenofovir gel, an antiretroviral microbicide, for the prevention of HIV infection in women. Science 329: 1168–1174.
10. Welz T, Hosegood V, Jaffar S, Bätzing-Feigenbaum J, Herbst K, et al. (2007) Continued very high HIV prevalence in rural KwaZulu-Natal. South Africa: a population-based longitudinal study.
11. Tanser F, Bärnighausen T, Hund L, Garnett GP, McGrath N, et al. (2011) Effect of concurrent sexual partnerships on rare of new HIV infections in a high prevalence, rural South African population: a cohort study. Lancet 378: 247–255.
12. WHO Department of Reproductive Health (2010) Medical Eligibility Criteria for Contraceptive Use, 4th edition. Geneva: WHO. Available: http://www.who.int/reproductivehealth/publications/family_planning/9789241563888/en/index.html. Accessed 2012 March 16.
13. National Department of Health, South Africa (2008) First line comprehensive management and control of sexually transmitted infections (STIs): protocol for the management of a person with a sexually transmitted infection according to the Essential Drug List. Pretoria: National Department of Health.
14. Parekh BS, Kennedy MS, Dobbs T, Pau CP, Byers R, et al. (2002) Quantitative detection of increasing HIV type 1 antibodies after seroconversion: a simple assay for detecting recent HIV infection and estimating incidence. AIDS Res Hum Retroviruses 18: 295–307.
15. McWalter TA, Welte A (2009) Relating recent infection prevalence to incidence with a sub-population of assay non-progressors. J Math Biol 60: 687–710.
16. Formula spreadsheet. Aavailable: http://www.sacema.com/page/assay-based-incidence-estimation. Accessed 2012 March 16.
17. Bärnighausen T, Wallrauch C, Welte A, McWalter TA, Mbizana N, et al. (2008) HIV incidence in rural South Africa: comparison of estimates from longitudinal surveillance and cross-sectional cBED assay testing. PLoS ONE 3: e3640.
18. Hargrove JW, Humphrey JH, Mutasa K, Parekh BS, McDougal JS, et al. (2008) Improved HIV-1 incidence estimates using the BED capture enzyme immunoassay. AIDS 22: 511–518.
19. UNAIDS/WHO (2011) When and how to use assays for recent infection to estimate HIV incidence at a population level. Geneva: UNAIDS/WHO.

14

Rising Population Cost for Treating People Living with HIV in the UK, 1997-2013

Sundhiya Mandalia[1,2,3], Roshni Mandalia[1], Gary Lo[1,3], Tim Chadborn[4], Peter Sharott[5], Mike Youle[1,6], Jane Anderson[7], Guy Baily[8], Ray Brettle[9], Martin Fisher[10], Mark Gompels[11], George Kinghorn[12], Margaret Johnson[6], Brendan McCarron[13], Anton Pozniak[3], Alan Tang[14], John Walsh[15], David White[16], Ian Williams[17], Brian Gazzard[1,2,3], Eduard J. Beck[1,3,18]*, for the NPMS-HHC Steering Group

1 NPMS-HHC Coordinating and Analytic Centre, London, United Kingdom, 2 Imperial College, London, United Kingdom, 3 Chelsea and Westminster Hospital, London, United Kingdom, 4 Health Protection Agency, London, United Kingdom, 5 London Specialised Commissioning Group, London Procurement Programme, London, United Kingdom, 6 Royal Free Hospital, London, United Kingdom, 7 Homerton University Hospital NHS Foundation Trust, London, United Kingdom 8 London and Barts Hospitals, London, United Kingdom, 9 Edinburgh General Hospital, Edinburgh, United Kingdom, 10 Royal County Sussex Hospital, Brighton, United Kingdom, 11 Southmead Hospital, Bristol, United Kingdom, 12 Royal Hallamshire Hospital, Sheffield, United Kingdom, 13 James Cook University Hospital, Middlesborough, United Kingdom, 14 Royal Berkshire Hospital, Berkshire, United Kingdom, 15 St. Mary's Hospital, London, United Kingdom, 16 Birmingham Heartlands Hospital, Birmingham, United Kingdom, 17 Mortimer Market Centre, London, United Kingdom, 18 London School of Hygiene & Tropical Medicine, London, United Kingdom

Abstract

Background: The number of people living with HIV (PLHIV) is increasing in the UK. This study estimated the annual population cost of providing HIV services in the UK, 1997–2006 and projected them 2007–2013.

Methods: Annual cost of HIV treatment for PLHIV by stage of HIV infection and type of ART was calculated (UK pounds, 2006 prices). Population costs were derived by multiplying the number of PLHIV by their annual cost for 1997–2006 and projected 2007–2013.

Results: Average annual treatment costs across all stages of HIV infection ranged from £17,034 in 1997 to £18,087 in 2006 for PLHIV on mono-therapy and from £27,649 in 1997 to £32,322 in 2006 for those on quadruple-or-more ART. The number of PLHIV using NHS services rose from 16,075 to 52,083 in 2006 and was projected to increase to 78,370 by 2013. Annual population cost rose from £104 million in 1997 to £483 million in 2006, with a projected annual cost between £721 and £758 million by 2013. When including community care costs, costs increased from £164 million in 1997, to £583 million in 2006 and between £1,019 and £1,065 million in 2013.

Conclusions: Increased number of PLHIV using NHS services resulted in rising UK population costs. Population costs are expected to continue to increase, partly due to PLHIV's longer survival on ART and the relative lack of success of HIV preventing programs. Where possible, the cost of HIV treatment and care needs to be reduced without reducing the quality of services, and prevention programs need to become more effective. While high income countries are struggling to meet these increasing costs, middle- and lower-income countries with larger epidemics are likely to find it even more difficult to meet these increasing demands, given that they have fewer resources.

Editor: Rupert Kaul, University of Toronto, Canada

Funding: During 2008/2009, the NPMS-HHC was financially supported through a non-restrictive grant from Tibotec, with no influence on the independence of the Steering Group and its editorial policy. The funders had no role in study design, data collection and analysis, decision to publish, or preparation of the manuscript.

Competing Interests: During 2008/2009, the NPMS-HHC was financially supported through a non-restrictive grant from Tibotec, with no influence on the independence of the Steering Group and its editorial policy.

* E-mail: becke@unaids.org

Introduction

The UK has the fastest growing HIV epidemic in Western Europe [1]. The number of PLHIV alive and using NHS services have increased, partly due to more effective ART regimens resulting in their longer survival [2], partly due to uninfected people continuing to be infected with HIV either in the UK or abroad [3]. This combination has resulted in increasing number of PLHIV using NHS services [4] which is likely to have resulted in increased population costs for HIV treatment and care. The aim

of this study was to estimate the treatment and care costs for PLHIV in the UK population by stage of HIV infection and type of ART between 1997 and 2006 and project costs for 2007–2013.

Methods

The National Prospective Monitoring System on the use, cost and outcome of HIV service provision in UK hospitals - HIV Health-economics Collaboration (NPMS-HHC) monitors prospectively the effectiveness, efficiency, equity and acceptability of treatment and care in participating HIV units since 1996. Using an agreed minimum dataset, standardized data are routinely collected in clinics and transferred to the NPMS-HHC Coordinating and Analytic Centre, ensuring both patient and clinic confidentiality. The data analyses are performed both at clinic and aggregate levels. The clinic specific analyses remain confidential, while aggregate analyses become public documents [5,6].

Use and Cost of Hospital Services

Information on the use of hospital inpatient (IP), outpatient (OP), and dayward (DW) services between 1st January 1997 and 31st December 2006, was obtained from 14 hospitals participating in this analysis. The mean number of IP days, OP and DW visits per patient-year (PPY) by stage of HIV infection - asymptomatic, symptomatic non-AIDS or AIDS - were calculated per patient-year from 1997 to 2006. The methods used for calculating the mean use of hospital services per patient year (PPY) were similar to those employed in our previous studies [2,7,8].

The denominator consisted of the total duration of follow up for all patients during a calendar year, from when they were first seen during that year till the end of the year if still alive, or when they died, or if they were lost to follow up, which ever came first. Numerators were calculated by summing the use of IP, OP or DW services and annual mean use of services PPY were calculated using the following formula:

$$M = \frac{\sum\limits_{i=1}^{n} \sum\limits_{j=1}^{k} S_{ij}}{\sum\limits_{i=1}^{n} \sum\limits_{j=1}^{k} (t_{ij} - t_{i(j-1)})} \times 365$$

Where: n = total number of individuals;
k = day of censoring;
S_{ij} = use of service of individual i at jth day;
t_{ij} = number of days since diagnosis of stage of HIV infection of individual i and remaining within the same stage;
M = mean of services S per patient-year by stage of HIV infection.

Annual cost PPY estimates for HIV-service provision for individual PLHIV by stage of infection were produced by linking mean number of IP days, OP visits and DW visits with their respective unit costs (2006 prices). The unit cost estimates for an average IP day was £475, average OP visit was £94 and £384 for a DW visit [9]. Costs were in UK pounds at 2006 prices.

Unit Costs of Antiretroviral Therapy

Average costs for treatment regimens were based on London Specialised Commissioning Group prices of each licensed antiretroviral (ARV) drug. Average annual cost, including 17.5% value added tax (VAT), were calculated for different antiretroviral therapy (ART) regimens - mono-, dual-, triple- or quadruple-or-more therapy - and stratified by stages of HIV infection: asymptomatic, symptomatic non-AIDS or AIDS.

Overall Cost of Services by Stage of HIV Infection and Type of Antiretroviral Therapy

The costs for different ART by stage of HIV infection were added to the cost for IP, OP and DW services for each of the clinical stages; costs of 'other' drugs and tests and procedures performed [9], were added to obtain the total direct costs for

treatment and care for PLHIV by stage of HIV infection and type of ART. The primary analysis was from a public service perspective focused on hospital costs [10], while annual population cost-estimates were also presented including community care costs [9] as indicated.

PLHIV Using NHS Services by Type of Antiretroviral Therapy

The annual number of PLHIV by stage of HIV infection using NHS services by type of ART prescribed, were obtained from the Health Protection Agency (HPA). Not all of these data sets were complete; for some PLHIV their stage of HIV infection was known but the type of ART prescribed was unknown. These individuals were proportionally distributed across the respective ART strata, ensuring that the proportion of subjects represented in each category remained unchanged. Secondly, HPA figures indicated that no subjects had been prescribed quadruple-or-more therapy in 1997 and 1998, which was unlikely and probably due to incorrect reporting during those calendar years. For these years linear least squares regression analysis [11] was used to estimate the number of PLHIV likely to have been prescribed quadruple- or-more therapy.

UK HIV Population Cost Estimate

To obtain the population cost estimates, the total annual treatment and care costs for a PLHIV by stage of HIV infection and type of ART were multiplied by the number of PLHIV within those categories for each year. Costs were then added across stages of HIV and types of ART regimens to obtain a total population cost by year, while community care costs were also included for population estimates [9].

UK HIV Population and Cost Projection

Projections were made to estimate future costs for the years 2007 to 2013 and these were investigated using both the linear and higher order polynomial least squares regression analyses [11]. Using proportion of variance explained as a measure of goodness of fit of the models, the linear least squares analyses produced the best fit and was therefore presented in this paper. The projections were based on the trends observed over 1997–2006 and three scenarios were investigated: the *first* scenario extrapolated total annual population costs 1997–2006 to 2007–2013. The *second* scenario extrapolated the total number of PLHIV who used HIV services between 1997 and 2006 to 2007 and 2013. The average annual cost of treating a PLHIV across all stages of HIV infection in 2006 was calculated and this was multiplied by the projected numbers of PLHIV using NHS services for the years 2007–2013. The *third* scenario extrapolated PLHIV for each of the three stages of HIV infection from 1997–2006 to 2007–2013. Average 2006 annual cost of treatment and care for stage of HIV infection was used to extrapolate cost 2007–2013 by stage of HIV infection. Total projected annual treatment costs were obtained by adding annual population costs of each of the three stages of HIV infection across all three stages.

Results

26,033 PLHIV were managed in 14 UK HIV centres between 1997 and 2006. Seventy six percent of the study sample were men and 51% of all PLHIV were Caucasian. Of those whose sexual orientation was known, 62% were men who have sex with men (MSM), while 4.5% were known to be or have been injecting drug users (IDUs). Seventy nine percent of the HIV subjects had attended HIV centres in London for HIV care, while 15% were known to have attended more than one HIV centre within the UK during the study period.

Use of Hospital Services, 1997–2010

Annual Mean Number of Inpatient Days. Average mean number of IP days during the study period was 2.1 PPY for asymptomatic patients, which did not change substantially over time. Average mean number of IP days for symptomatic non-AIDS patients increased from 1.8 in 1997 to 2.7 PPY in 2006, while the average number of IP days for AIDS patients decreased from 7.7 in 1997 to 6.7 PPY in 2002 but increased to 10.9 in 2006 (Figure 1).

Annual Mean Number of Outpatient Visits. Average mean number of OP visits for asymptomatic patients was 6.5 PPY which did not change substantially over time, nor did the average mean number of OP visits for symptomatic non-AIDS patients at around 8.3 PPY. For AIDS patients, the mean number of OP visits decreased from 11.8 in 1997 to 7.0 PPY in 2006 (Figure 2).

Annual Mean Number of Dayward Visits. The average mean number of DW visits for asymptomatic patients increased from 0.3 in 1997 to 1.3 PPY in 2006. The average mean number of DW visits for symptomatic non-AIDS patients remained constant at 0.7 PPY, while for AIDS patients the average mean DW visits increased from 1.5 in 1997 to 2.0 PPY in 2006, having first decreased to 0.6 in 2000 (Figure 3).

Annual Cost of Treatment and Care Services by Type of ART

Treatment and care costs for PLHIV at different stage of HIV infection and different treatment regimens increased over time (Table 1).

Mono-therapy. For asymptomatic individuals in 1997 the annual cost of care was £8,308, which increased to £10,020 in 2006. For those with symptomatic non-AIDS, the 1997 cost of £12,076 decreased to £11,487, while for AIDS patients on mono-therapy, the annual costs increased from £30,717 in 1997 to £32,760 by 2006.

Dual-therapy. For asymptomatic PLHIV on dual therapy, the 1997 cost of £11,376 increased to £13,351. For patients with symptomatic non-AIDS, the annual cost increased from £14,685 in 1997 to £15,692 in 2006, while for AIDS patients on dual therapy, this increased from £33,726 in 1997 to £36,580 per patient-years in 2006.

Triple-Therapy. For asymptomatic PLHIV on triple therapy, annual costs increased from £16,347 to £18,280 in 2006. For patients with symptomatic non-AIDS annual costs increased from £19,806 to £21,597 in 2006, while for AIDS patients annual costs varied from £38,887 in 1997 to £41,747 in 2006.

Quadruple-or-more-Therapy. Annual cost for those asymptomatic PLHIV on quadruple-or-more therapy ranged from

£18,839 in 1997 to £23,775 in 2006. Similarly annual costs increased from £22,724 to £25,135 for PLHIV with symptomatic non-AIDS, while for AIDS patients annual costs increased from £41,383 to £48,055 in 2006.

It was of interest to note that the proportion spent on ART did not change significantly over time for any of three stages of HIV infection nor for the four ART treatment categories (Table 1).

Population Cost Treatment and Care 1997–2006 and 2007–2013

People Living With HIV Using NHS Services. The total number of PLHIV who used NHS services for treatment and care increased from 16,075 patients in 1997 to 52,083 by 2006, an increase that was seen across all stages of HIV infections. However, the proportion of asymptomatic PLHIV increased from 38% to 49% between 1997 and 2006, with the proportion of symptomatic non-AIDS patients and AIDS patients both decreasing, from 34% to 28% and from 28% to 23% respectively between 1997 and 2006 (Table 2).

Annual Population Costs 1997–2006. The population costs increased from £104 million in 1997 to £483 million in 2006 (Figure 4). If an estimate for community care costs was included, population costs rose from £164 million in 1997 to £683 million in 2006 (Figure 5).

In 1997 the total population cost for treating asymptomatic PLHIV was estimated at £22 million which increased to £162 million in 2006, while proportionally their annual cost increased from 21% in 1997 to 33% in 2006. Annual treatment costs for patients with symptomatic non-AIDS also increased, from £39 million to £146 million, but less dramatically compared with asymptomatic PLHIV; proportionally this group generated 37% of population costs in 1997, which decreased to 30% in 2006. For AIDS patients, annual population costs increased from £43 million to £176 million in 2006, but proportionally costs generated by this group decreased from 42% in 1997 to 36% by 2006.

Projected Annual Population Costs 2007–2013. The *first* scenario, which projected the annual population costs from 1997–2006 estimated that by 2013 the annual direct population cost would increase to £758 million or £1,065 million if community care costs were included (Figures 4 and 5).

The *second* scenario was based on the projected increase in total number of PLHIV by 2013. Multiplying the estimated number of PLHIV using NHS services by 2013 by the average 2006 per

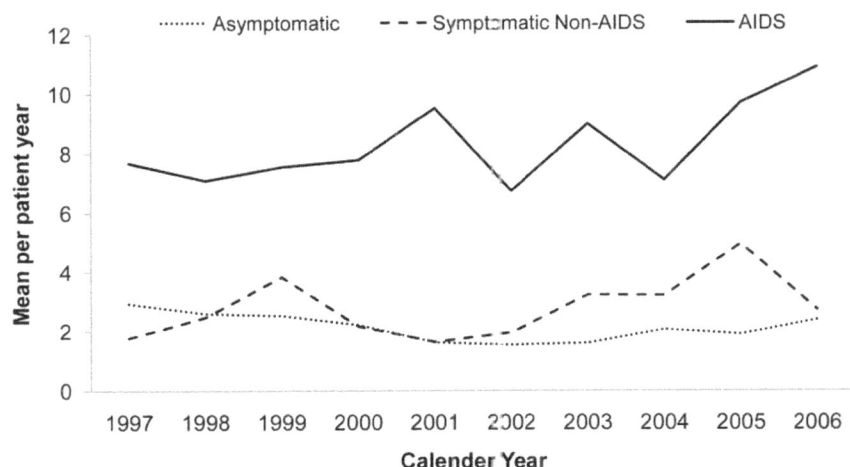

Figure 1. Mean Inpatient Days per Patient-year by Stage of HIV Infection and Year.

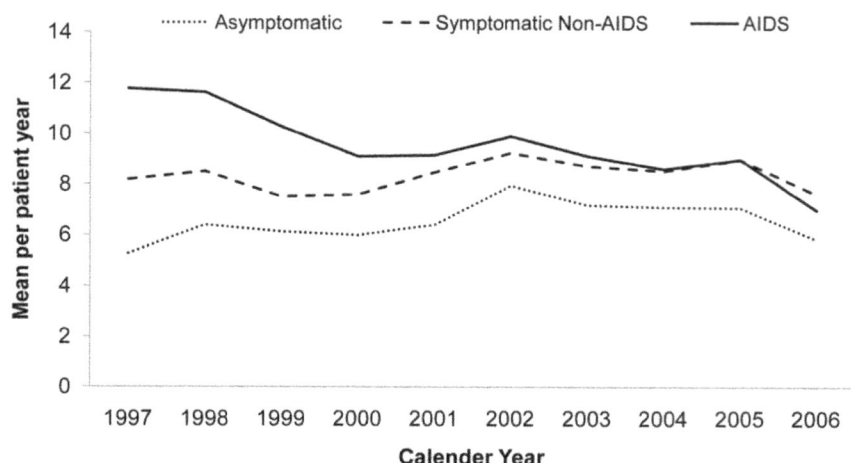

Figure 2. Mean Outpatient Visits Per Patient-year by Stage of HIV Infection and Year.

patient-year costs, the annual population cost was estimated to increase to £727 million by 2013, or £1,027 million when including community care costs (Figures 4 and 5).

For the *third* scenario, the number of PLHIV by stage of HIV infection were projected and multiplied by the average annual 2006 cost for each stage and a total annual population cost of £721 million was estimated by 2013, or £1,019 million including community care (Figures 4 and 5).

Discussion

This study estimated that the direct population cost for treatment and care of PLHIV in the UK has risen 4.6 fold between 1997 and 2006, from £104 million to £483 million respectively. The number of PLHIV using NHS services during this period tripled from 16,075 to 52,083 PLHIV: the greatest increase was seen among asymptomatic PLHIV and less so among PLHIV with symptomatic non-AIDS or AIDS.

There has been an increase in mean annual IP days and DW visits among AIDS patients, while number of OP visits declined. Increased use of IP services was also observed among PLHIV with symptomatic non-AIDS while asymptomatic PLHIV used more

DW services over time. These increases in annual cost of treatment and care over time were most pronounced for AIDS patients on quadruple-or-more ART. This may be due to these ART-experienced patients having to use more IP and DW services, as well as their increased use of new and more expensive ARVs in the second half of the study period.

The majority of patients were seen in London clinics and this may have skewed our findings, though overall costs did not seem to differ substantially between London and out-of-London sites during the study period [9]. This analysis is furthermore contingent on the fact that most if not all PLHIV using NHS services during the study, were diagnosed and reported to the HPA. Examples were described in the methods section of how some of the HPA data had to be adjusted because of missing data.

When the annual population costs were projected using three different methods, the estimated population costs increased to between £721 million and £758 million by 2013, a 1.5 fold increase from the 2006 baseline. The three scenarios produced similar estimates, with only a 5% difference between the lowest and highest estimates. The accuracy of these estimated projected figures of PLHIV using NHS services were compared with more recently figures published by HPA [12]. The recent HPA figures

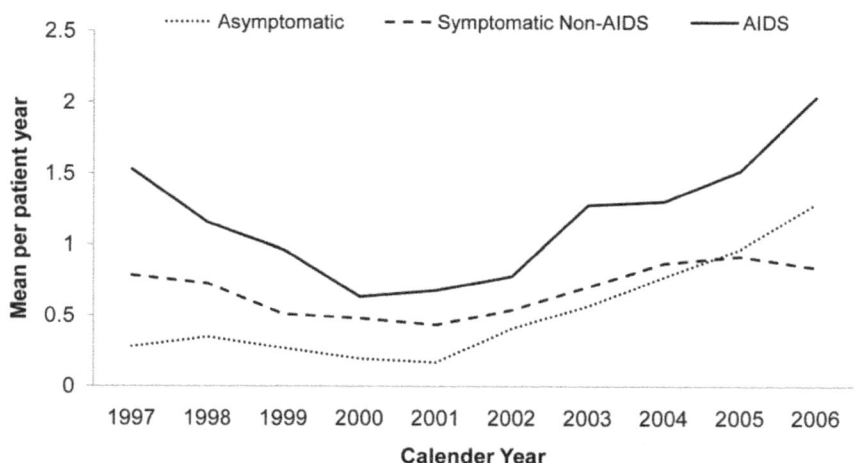

Figure 3. Mean Dayward Visits Per Patient-year by Stage of HIV Infection and Year.

Table 1. Annual cost of treatment and care by Stage of HIV Infection and different types of Anti-Retroviral Therapy in UK pound, 2006 UK prices and proportion of cost due to Antiretroviral Therapy (%).

Year	Monotherapy			Dual therapy			Triple therapy			Quadruple or more therapy		
	Asymp-tomatic	Symptomatic Non AIDS	AIDS	Asymp-tomatic	Symptomatic Non AIDS	AIDS	Asymp-tomatic	Symptomatic Non AIDS	AIDS	Asymp-tomatic	Symptomatic Non AIDS	AIDS
1997	£8,308	£12,076	£30,717	£11,376	£14,685	£33,726	£16,347	£19,806	£38,887	£18,839	£22,724	£41,383
	(46%)	(36%)	(13%)	(61%)	(47%)	(21%)	(73%)	(61%)	(31%)	(76%)	(66%)	(35%)
1998	£8,642	£13,008	£29,609	£11,660	£15,907	£32,467	£16,542	£21,006	£37,626	£19,528	£23,970	£40,621
	(48%)	(34%)	(15%)	(62%)	(46%)	(22%)	(73%)	(59%)	(33%)	(77%)	(54%)	(38%)
1999	£8,552	£13,481	£30,431	£11,619	£16,553	£33,542	£16,506	£21,980	£38,483	£19,894	£25,140	£42,005
	(50%)	(29%)	(14%)	(63%)	(43%)	(22%)	(74%)	(57%)	(32%)	(78%)	(52%)	(38%)
2000	£8,083	£11,299	£29,274	£10,981	£14,352	£32,423	£15,941	£19,683	£37,242	£18,734	£22,476	£40,380
	(51%)	(33%)	(14%)	(64%)	(47%)	(22%)	(75%)	(62%)	(32%)	(79%)	(56%)	(38%)
2001	£7,859	£11,489	£32,229	£10,906	£14,310	£35,493	£15,827	£19,521	£39,981	£20,613	£23,709	£44,911
	(52%)	(35%)	(13%)	(65%)	(47%)	(21%)	(76%)	(62%)	(30%)	(82%)	(58%)	(37%)
2002	£8,145	£11,901	£29,059	£11,358	£14,314	£32,164	£16,257	£19,954	£36,978	£21,449	£26,414	£42,235
	(49%)	(35%)	(14%)	(64%)	(46%)	(22%)	(75%)	(61%)	(32%)	(81%)	(71%)	(41%)
2003	£8,176	£13,435	£32,227	£11,319	£15,611	£35,454	£16,422	£21,474	£40,221	£21,747	£26,089	£45,831
	(49%)	(34%)	(13%)	(64%)	(43%)	(21%)	(75%)	(59%)	(30%)	(81%)	(56%)	(39%)
2004	£8,774	£12,272	£28,988	£11,777	£15,483	£32,206	£17,254	£21,621	£37,311	£22,827	£26,659	£43,436
	(48%)	(28%)	(15%)	(61%)	(43%)	(23%)	(74%)	(59%)	(34%)	(80%)	(57%)	(43%)
2005	£8,685	£12,192	£30,566	£11,864	£17,048	£33,864	£16,930	£22,713	£39,045	£22,979	£28,603	£45,661
	(50%)	(17%)	(14%)	(64%)	(41%)	(22%)	(74%)	(56%)	(32%)	(81%)	(55%)	(42%)
2006	£10,020	£11,482	£32,760	£13,351	£15,692	£36,580	£18,280	£21,597	£41,747	£23,775	£25,135	£48,055
	(43%)	(23%)	(11%)	(58%)	(43%)	(20%)	(69%)	(59%)	(30%)	(76%)	(72%)	(39%)

Table 2. Number of People Living with HIV Using NHS Services by Stage of HIV 1997–2006 [4] and Projected Figures for 2007–2013 (in italics).

Year	HIV Population (%)			
	Asymptomatic	Symptomatic non-AIDS	AIDS	Total
1997	6,124 (38%)	5,384 (34%)	4,567 (28%)	16,075
1998	5,835 (32%)	6,975 (38%)	5,525 (30%)	18,335
1999	6,833 (33%)	7,994 (37%)	6,288 (30%)	21,114
2000	8,055 (35%)	8,347 (37%)	6,338 (28%)	22,740
2001	10,015 (38%)	9,088 (34%)	7,253 (28%)	26,356
2002	12,787 (40%)	10,635 (34%)	8,115 (26%)	31,537
2003	15,932 (43%)	11,544 (32%)	9,203 (25%)	36,679
2004	18,794 (45%)	12,834 (31%)	10,009 (24%)	41,637
2005	21,656 (46%)	14,590 (31%)	10,779 (23%)	47,025
2006	25,385 (49%)	14,750 (28%)	11,947 (23%)	52,083
2007	25,485 (47%)	15,979 (30%)	12,378 (23%)	53,842
2008	27,729 (48%)	17,027 (29%)	13,173 (23%)	57,930
2009	29,974 (48%)	18,075 (29%)	13,969 (23%)	62,018
2010	32,218 (49%)	19,123 (29%)	14,764 (22%)	66,106
2011	34,462 (49%)	20,171 (29%)	15,560 (22%)	70,194
2012	36,707 (49%)	21,219 (29%)	16,355 (22%)	74,282
2013	38,951 (50%)	22,267 (28%)	17,151 (22%)	78,370

were 56,377, 57,930 and 62,018 for 2007, 2008 and 2009 respectively; the estimated figures were 53,842, 57,930 and 62,018 for respective years, an underestimate of 5% for each year.

Another potential source of error for estimating the population cost was the extent that HIV- services also used generic, non-HIV services to operate. While the unit costs include facility-level overheads, other general costs covered by the NHS, such as its drug procurement system, general staff training and other more general non-HIV indirect support, may not have been included in these estimates. However, these points suggest that the estimates produced in this study are likely to underestimate the true population cost of delivering HIV services in the NHS.

At the end of 2008 the number of people living with HIV in the UK was estimated to be 83,000, of whom an estimated 27% were unaware of being infected [3]; 7,298 people were newly diagnosed with HIV in 2008, or 9% of the estimated 83,000 PLHIV in the UK and 12% of the 61,213 PLHIV reportedly using NHS services during 2008. A recent study in the UK, confirmed the benefit for starting ART early with CD4 count <350 cells/mm^3 [13]. The annual cost of treatment and care, for those who started ART with a CD4 count >200 cells/mm^3, is 30–35% less than for those who start ART with a CD4 count ≤ 200 cells/mm^3. However, between 1996 and 2006, of 5,541 PLHIV who started first-line therapy, 55% were diagnosed with a CD4 count ≤ 200 cells/mm^3, many of whom were Black Africans [13]. It is likely that many of the PLHIV, who are currently unaware of being infected, may well present late in their disease course with a CD4 count ≤ 200 mm^3. Starting more PLHIVs with a CD4 count <350 cells/mm^3 will increase the number of people receiving HAART, which will initially add to

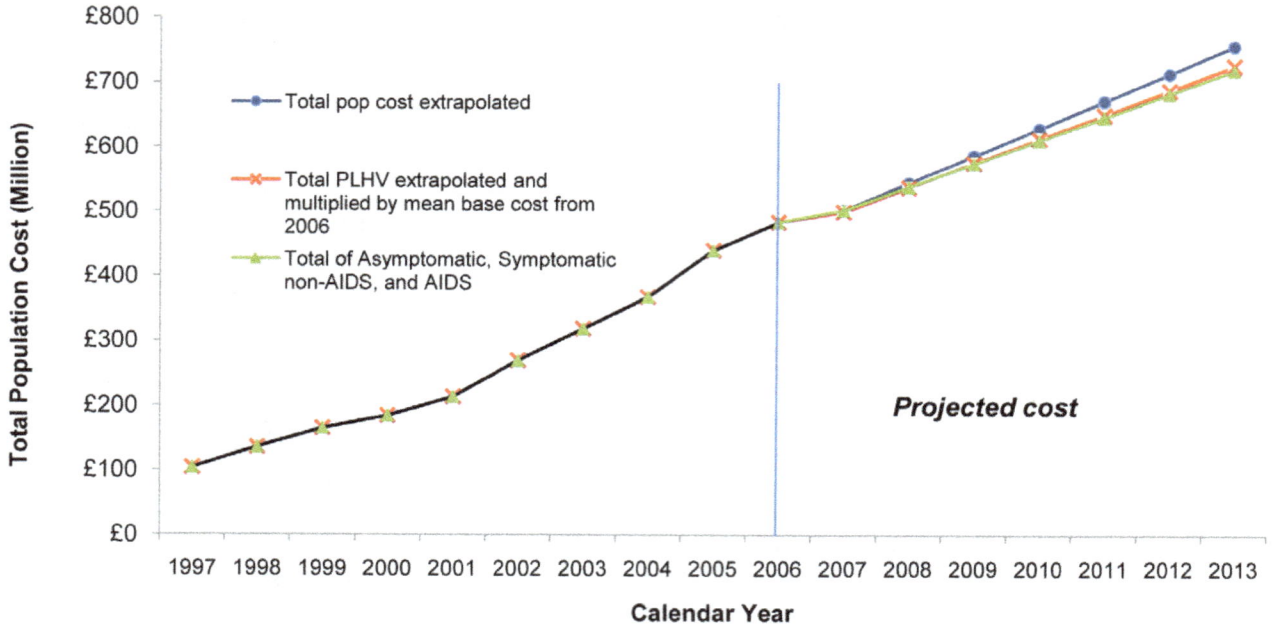

Figure 4. Annual Average UK Direct Population Cost 1997–2006 and Projections 2007–2013 based on three Scenarios (UK 2006 prices).

the financial burden of the NHS. However, starting PLHIV on cost-effective regimens earlier, will maintain them in better health, resulting in the use of fewer health or social services and thereby generating fewer treatment and care costs, while enabling them to remain socially and economically active members of society.

Increasing population costs for HIV treatment and care are raising serious concerns in high-income countries, especially as

many are going through periods of cutting public expenditure [14] as a consequence of the global economic downturn. This issue is even more pertinent for middle- and lower-income countries. As part of universal access, many of these countries have been increasing treatment and care services and the number of PLHIV currently on ART has reached 5 million PLHIV [15]. While this constitutes a great success, if countries want to continue to increase their ART coverage the issue of providing sustainable quality

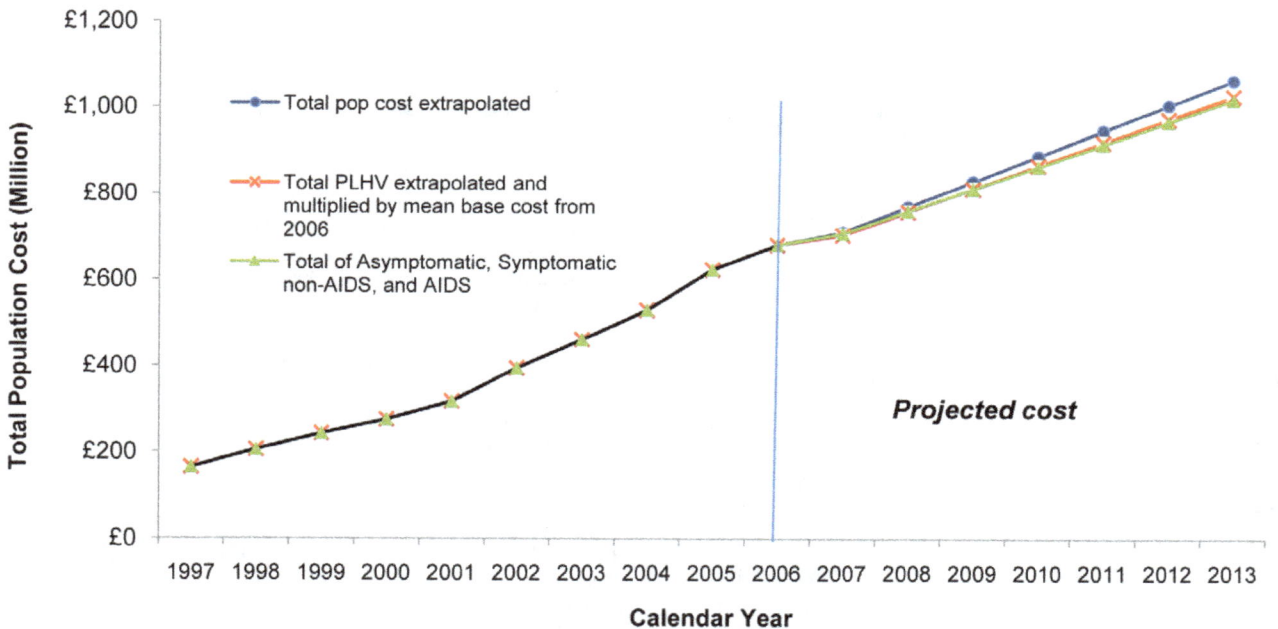

Figure 5. Annual Average UK Population Cost 1997–2006 and Projections 2007–2013 based on three Scenarios all including Community Care Costs (UK 2006 prices).

services in the context of limited country resources raises serious questions. Lessons from high-income countries teach us that increased coverage is going to result in increased population costs. Will these countries be able to provide ART free-at-point of delivery on a life-long basis, as is the underlying assumption in high-income countries [16]? The recent change in WHO criteria to start ART when CD4 count <350 cells/mm^3 [17] increases the number of PLHIV in need of starting on ART, and also raises the ethical issue whether PLHIV with more severe HIV disease should receive ART first, or should PLHIV with higher CD4 counts have preference because their treatment and care costs are less than those with higher CD4 counts? Starting ART early is effective [18] and cost-effective [8,19] in resource limited settings and if ART is focused on these PLHIV, one could argue that there will be more resources available that will enable more PLHIV to be receiving ART, while allowing them to remain socially and economically active. These are some of the issues, which countries and resource-limited ones in particular, will have to face. Furthermore, many low-income countries will need to make these choices with the knowledge that many of them, at least for the foreseeable future, will continue to be reliant on donor agencies or countries to sustain their treatment and care services [20].

Trying to curtail the costs of service provision is one measure by which one could try and curtail the population cost. Measures which are being used range from sending laboratory test results by email, home delivery of the drugs to the patient, which is exempted from VAT in the UK, to using the most cost-effective regimens [13]. Even if the costs could be brought down, without reducing the quality of services provided, the fact that the number of new people being infected with HIV continue to outpace those being put on ART, will continue to drive up population cost for HIV services.

Only greater prevention efforts will reduce the number of people becoming infected with HIV. A recent study from the US suggests that even if incidence is reduced drastically, the number of people newly infected with HIV will continue to increase [21]. While putting PLHIV on ART will reduce their infectivity and contribute to reducing the incidence of people newly infected with HIV [22], this in itself will not be sufficient to reduce incidence in a large number of settings. Only comprehensive prevention strategies, responding directly to the epidemic dynamics operating in each country, will be able to reduce HIV incidence [23]. It is now recognized that in most instances a combination of prevention interventions are going to be required to achieve significant reductions in HIV-incidence [24]. While recent biomedical interventions - like male-circumcision [25], the development of a vaccine [26], microbicides [27] and pre-exposure chemoprophylaxis [28] – constitute important advances, they are going to be most successful when juxtaposed with relevant behavioral and structural changes [24]. One of the findings of the Second Independent Evaluation of the UN Joint Programme on HIV/AIDS highlighted the relative lack of success of global prevention programmes, including in high-income countries, and recommended a greater emphasis on making prevention more effective and efficient [29]. Policy makers and other relevant stakeholders need to use evidence-informed HIV prevention, treatment and care strategies to ensure that PLHIV have full access to the treatments that they need based on their clinical condition, which will prolong life, reduce morbidity, reduce transmission and ultimately deliver the best for both the individual and public health agendas.

Author Contributions

Conceived and designed the experiments: EJB SM MY BG. Performed the experiments: TC PS JA GB RB MF GK MJ BM AP AT JW DW IW. Analyzed the data: SM RM GL EJB. Contributed reagents/materials/analysis tools: SM EJB RM GL. Wrote the paper: EJB SM RM MY BG.

References

1. European Centre for Disease Prevention and Control/WHO Regional Office for Europe (2009) HIV/AIDS surveillance in Europe 2008. Stockholm: European Centre for Disease Prevention and Control. 24–25. Available:http://www.euro.who.int/document/e93034.pdf Accessed November 2010.

2. Beck EJ, Mandalia S, Youle M, Brettle R, Fisher M, et al. 2008) Treatment Outcome and Cost-effectiveness of different HAART Regimens in the UK 1996–2002. International Journal of STD & AIDS 19: 297–304.

3. Health Protection Agency (2009) HIV in the United Kingdom: 2009 Report, London UK. Available: http://www.hpa.org.uk/web/HPAweb&HPAweb Standard/HPAweb_C/1259151891866. Accessed November 2010.

4. Health Protection Agency: Survey of Prevalent HIV Infections Diagnosed (SOPHID): Data tables 2008, London UK, 2009.

5. Beck EJ, Mandalia S (2003) The Cost of HIV Treatment and Care in England since HAART: Part 1. British Journal of Sexual Medicine 27(1): 19–21.

6. Beck EJ, Mandalia S (2003) The Cost of HIV Treatment and Care in England since HAART: Part 2. British Journal of Sexual Medicine 27(2): 21–23.

7. Beck EJ, Mandalia S, Gaudreault M, Brewer C, Zowall H, et al. (2004) The Cost-effectiveness of HAART, Canada 1991-2001. AIDS 18 2411–9.

8. Badri M, Maartens G, Mandalia S, Bekker L-G Penrod JR, et al. (2006) Cost-effectiveness of Highly Active Antiretroviral Therapy in South Africa. Plos Medicine 3: e4.

9. Beck EJ, Mandalia S, Lo G, Youle M and Gazzard B for the NPMS-HHC Steering Group (2008) Use and Cost of HIV Service Provision in UK NPMS-HHC Sites: aggregate analyses January 1996–2006. NPMS-HHC Coordinating and Analytic Centre, St. Stephen's Centre, Chelsea and Westminster Hospital Trust, London, UK.

10. Beck EJ, Miners AH (2001) Effectiveness and Efficiency in the Delivery of HIV Services: economic and related considerations in The Effective Management of HIV Disease, Gazzard B, Johnson M, Miles A, eds. London: Aesculapius Medical Press. pp 113–38.

11. Aldrich, John (2005) Fisher and Regression. Statistical Science 20(4): 401–417.

12. Health Protection Agency (2010) Survey of Prevalent HIV Infections Diagnosed (SOPHID): Data tables 2009, London UK. Available: http://www.hpa.org.uk/web/HPAwebFile/HPAweb_C/1221482342808. Accessed November 2010.

13. Beck EJ, Mandalia S, Lo Gary, Sharott P, Youle M, et al. (2010) PI$_{boosted}$ or NNRTI as first-line HAART regimens? Lessons from the UK. XVIII International AIDS Conference, Vienna, Austria: Abstract THPE0084.

14. Feature (2010) White paper: More brickbats than bouquets? BMJ;341:c3977. Available: http://www.bmj.com/cgi/content/full/341/jul28_2/c3977 Accessed November 2010.

15. WHO (2010) More than five million people receiving HIV treatment. Geneva, Available: http://www.who.int/mediacentre/news/releases/2010/hiv_treat ment_20100719/en/index.html Accessed November 2010.

16. Beck EJ, Walensky RP (2008) The Outcome and Impact of Ten Years of HAART, in: Zuniga JM, Whiteside A, Ghaziani A, Bartlett JG, eds. Oxford, UK: A Decade of HAART Oxford University Press. pp 45–62.

17. WHO (2010) Antiretroviral therapy for HIV infection in adults and adolescents, Recommendations for a public health approach, 2010 revision. Geneva, Available: http://whqlibdoc.who.int/publications/2010/9789241599764_eng.pdf. Accessed November 2010.

18. Severe P, Juste MAJ, Ambroise A, Eliacin L, Marchand C, et al. (2010) Early versus Standard Antiretroviral Therapy for HIV-Infected Adults in Haiti, New England Journal of Medicine 363: 257–65.

19. Loubiere S, Meiners C, Sloan C, Freedberg KA, Yazdanpanah Y (2010) Economic evaluation of ART in resource-limited countries. Curr Opin HIV AIDS 5: 225–31.

20. Hecht R, Bollinger L, John Stover J, William McGreevey W, Muhib F, et al. (2009) Critical Choices In Financing The Response To The Global HIV/AIDS Pandemic. Health Affairs 28: 1591–1605.

21. Hall HI, Green TA, Wolitski RJ, Holtgrave DR, Rhodes P, et al. (2010) Estimated Future HIV Prevalence, Incidence, and Potential Infections Averted in the United States: A Multiple Scenario Analysis. J Acquir Immune Defic Syndr 55: 271–6.

22. Montaner JSG, Lima VD, Barrios R, Yip B, Wood E, et al. (2010) Association of highly active antiretroviral therapy coverage, population viral load, and yearly new HIV diagnoses in British Columbia, Canada: a population-based study, Lancet. Available: http://press.thelancet.com/hivbc.pdf. Accessed November 2010.

23. Report of the Secretary-General (2010) Progress made in the implementation of the Declaration of Commitment on HIV/AIDS and the Political Declaration on

HIV/AIDS. Sixty-fourth session of the General assembly, Agenda item 44, Implementation of the Declaration of Commitment on HIV/AIDS and the Political Declaration on HIV/AIDS, United Nations, New York, US.

24. Hankins CA, de Zalduondo BO (2010) Combination prevention: a deeper understanding of effective HIV prevention, AIDS, 24(suppl 4): S70–S80.

25. Kahn JG, Marseille E, Auvert B (2006) Cost-effectiveness of male circumcision for HIV prevention in a South African setting. PLoS Med 3(12): e517.

26. Rerks-Ngarm S, Pitisuttithum P, Nitayaphan S, Kaewkungwal J, Chiu J, et al. (2009) for the MOPH–TAVEG Investigators. Vaccination with ALVAC and AIDSVAX to Prevent HIV-1 Infection in Thailand N Engl J Med 361: 1–12.

27. Baleta A (2010) Antiretroviral vaginal gel shows promise against HIV, Lancet. Available: http://download.thelancet.com/flatcontentassets/pdfs/S0140673610611233.pdf. Accessed November 2010.

28. Grant RM, Lama JR, Anderson PL, McMahan V, Liu AY, et al. (2010) Preexposure Chemoprophylaxis for HIV Prevention in Men Who Have Sex with Men NEJM. Available: http://www.nejm.org/doi/pdf/10.1056/NEJMoa1011205 Accessed November 2010 363: 1–13.

29. Poate D, Paul Balogun P, Attawell K (2009) UNAIDS Second Independent Evaluation 2002–2008, Final Report, ITAD and HLPS, UK. Available: http://data.unaids.org/pub/BaseDocument/2009/20091002_sie_final_report_en.pdf. Accessed November 2010.

15

Frailty, HIV Infection, and Mortality in an Aging Cohort of Injection Drug Users

Damani A. Piggott[1,2]*, Abimereki D. Muzaale[1,2], Shruti H. Mehta[2], Todd T. Brown[1,2], Kushang V. Patel[3], Sean X. Leng[1], Gregory D. Kirk[1,2]

1 Johns Hopkins University School of Medicine, Baltimore, Maryland, United States of America, **2** Johns Hopkins Bloomberg School of Public Health, Baltimore, Maryland, United States of America, **3** University of Washington School of Medicine, Seattle, Washington, United States of America

Abstract

Background: Frailty is associated with morbidity and premature mortality among elderly HIV-uninfected adults, but the determinants and consequences of frailty in HIV-infected populations remain unclear. We evaluated the correlates of frailty, and the impact of frailty on mortality in a cohort of aging injection drug users (IDUs).

Methods: Frailty was assessed using standard criteria among HIV-infected and uninfected IDUs in 6-month intervals from 2005 to 2008. Generalized linear mixed-model analyses assessed correlates of frailty. Cox proportional hazards models estimated risk for all-cause mortality.

Results: Of 1230 participants at baseline, the median age was 48 years and 29% were HIV-infected; the frailty prevalence was 12.3%. In multivariable analysis of 3,365 frailty measures, HIV-infected IDUs had an increased likelihood of frailty (OR, 1.66; 95% CI, 1.24–2.21) compared to HIV-uninfected IDUs; the association was strongest (OR, 2.37; 95% CI, 1.62–3.48) among HIV-infected IDUs with advanced HIV disease (CD4<350 cells/mm3 and detectable HIV RNA). No significant association was seen with less advanced disease. Sociodemographic factors, comorbidity, depressive symptoms, and prescription drug abuse were also independently associated with frailty. Mortality risk was increased with frailty alone (HR 2.63, 95% CI, 1.23–5.66), HIV infection alone (HR 3.29, 95% CI, 1.85–5.88), and being both HIV-infected and frail (HR, 7.06; 95%CI 3.49–14.3).

Conclusion: Frailty was strongly associated with advanced HIV disease, but IDUs with well-controlled HIV had a similar prevalence to HIV-uninfected IDUs. Frailty was independently associated with mortality, with a marked increase in mortality risk for IDUs with both frailty and HIV infection.

Editor: Alan Landay, Rush University, United States of America

Funding: This work was supported by the National Institutes of Health (grants RC1-AI-086053, R01-DA-04334, and R01-DA-12568). The funders had no role in study design, data collection and analysis, decision to publish, or preparation of the manuscript.

Competing Interests: The authors have declared that no competing interests exist.

* E-mail: dpiggott@jhsph.edu

Introduction

Frailty is a clinical syndrome which increases in prevalence with age and identifies older persons at higher risk for falls, disability, institutionalization, and death [1,2]. Conceptualized as a state of diminished reserves due to deficits across multiple physiologic systems, frailty leads to an increased vulnerability and limited adaptability to internal and external stressors [1,2]. A frailty phenotype, operationalized by Fried and colleagues, predicts adverse clinical outcomes in geriatric populations [3,4].

Since the advent of highly active antiretroviral therapy (HAART), improved survival of HIV-infected individuals has led to an increasing prevalence of older persons living with HIV [5,6]. However, several studies suggest that even with guideline concordant care, HIV-infected persons have reduced life expectancy relative to the general population and to HIV-uninfected controls with similar behavioral risk [7,8].

An estimated 3.4 million persons in the U.S. report injecting drugs at some time in their lifetime and this population of injection drug users (IDUs) has also been aging [9]. IDUs have decreased survival attributable to HIV and to other behaviorally-associated comorbid disease [10,11,12].

Limited data exist regarding the determinants of frailty among HIV-infected and drug using populations. A higher prevalence of a modified frailty-related phenotype was observed for HIV-infected men who have sex with men (MSM) compared to HIV-uninfected MSM [13]. An increased prevalence of frailty was also seen among HIV-infected women with limited immunological recovery [14], while in an urban HIV clinic setting, frailty was associated with prior opportunistic infections [15]. To date, no studies have examined frailty in an IDU population. Moreover, while frailty increases mortality risk in older HIV-uninfected persons, the effect of frailty on mortality among HIV-infected and at risk IDUs is unknown.

Ensuring the healthy aging of HIV-infected and at-risk persons may be facilitated by earlier interventions among persons at greatest risk for adverse age-associated clinical outcomes. In the current study, we postulated that frailty may be an appropriate phenotype to identify this high-risk subset. Incorporating the objective criteria originally proposed by Fried, we sought to characterize the demographic, behavioral, and clinical correlates of frailty in an aging cohort of HIV-infected and HIV-uninfected IDUs, and to assess the impact of frailty on mortality in this population.

Methods

Study Participants

The AIDS Linked to the IntraVenous Experience (ALIVE) cohort has prospectively followed persons with a history of injecting drugs in a community-recruited cohort since 1988. IDUs aged 18 years or older were recruited through street-based efforts from 1988 through 2008 as previously detailed [16,17]. The ALIVE study has been continually approved by the Johns Hopkins Institutional Review Board, and all participants provided written informed consent.

Data Collection

At semi-annual visits, ALIVE participants completed standardized questionnaires and underwent clinical examination. Detailed information obtained at each follow-up visit included socioeconomic, behavioral, and clinical parameters for the prior 6 month period. Substance use including alcohol, tobacco and illicit injection and non-injection drug use were assessed by participant self report of behaviors in the prior 6 month period. Comorbid conditions ascertained included obesity (defined as a body mass index [BMI] ≥ 30) and participant self-report of any provider diagnosis of diabetes, hypertension, or cerebrovascular, cardiovascular, renal, chronic lung, malignant, or liver disease. Hazardous alcohol use was assessed using the Alcohol Use Disorders Identification Test (AUDIT) [18]. Depressive symptoms were assessed using the Center for Epidemiological Studies Depression Scale (CES-D) [19]. Prescription drug abuse was by participant self report of abuse of drugs prescribed to them by a physician in the last year [20]. HAART was defined as use of at least 3 antiretroviral drugs, 1 of which was a nonnucleoside reverse-transcriptase inhibitor, tenofovir, abacavir, or a protease inhibitor and was reflective of use in the prior 6 months [21].

At each visit, HIV-uninfected persons had antibodies to HIV-1 assayed by enzyme-linked immunosorbent assay, with Western blot confirmation. CD4 cell counts were measured on HIV-infected persons at each visit using flow cytometry, and plasma HIV-1 RNA levels determined using reverse-transcriptase PCR methods. Mortality was assessed through linkage to the National Death Index (NDI) with review of death certificates to confirm correct matches.

Frailty Assessment

Frailty was assessed using the 5 original Fried criteria: slow gait, decreased grip strength (weakness), poor endurance (exhaustion), low physical activity, and physical shrinking (weight loss) (Table S1) [3]. Frailty assessment was routinely performed in ALIVE at six month intervals from July 2005 through the study period (91% of person-visits assessed), except that in March 2007 the assessment interval was altered to an annual basis until funding was secured to allow semi-annual assessment again in January 2008. For the physical activity domain, in lieu of the Minnesota Activity assessment of kilocalorie expenditure utilized by Fried, we incorporated the self-reported response to a standardized question on physical limitations as previously characterized in the Multicenter AIDS Cohort Study (MACS) [13,22]. Physical

shrinking at each visit was defined as measured weight loss of $\geq 5\%$ body weight from the prior study visit. For analysis, we included weight assessments that were 5 to 12 months from the last measurement (95% of all measurements). Each frailty parameter was considered as a binary variable (0, 1) and summed to obtain a frailty score; ≥ 3 was considered frail, 1 or 2 considered prefrail, and scores of 0 considered robust.

Statistical Analysis

We compared participant characteristics by HIV status and by frailty status at baseline and by person-visits. For each person-visit, frailty was treated as a 3 category outcome (robust, prefrail, frail). Using all person-visits, generalized linear mixed models estimated associations of sociodemographic, behavioral, and clinical factors with the frailty phenotype, comparing frail to robust and prefrail to robust. To account for the intra-person correlation within the repeated frailty measures, participants were incorporated as random effects, with other covariates considered fixed effects [23]. Age was included as a continuous variable. Given the predominance of African Americans in the cohort, self-reported race was dichotomized as African American versus other. Depressive symptomatology was assessed using a modified version of the CES-D scale, removing the 2 items included in the frailty assessment and adjusting the score to consider ≥ 21 as indicative of depressive symptoms. In sensitivity analyses using variable CES-D cutpoints or including the frailty-associated items, findings were not significantly changed. An AUDIT score of ≥ 8 was considered to be indicative of hazardous alcohol use [18]. In sensitivity analyses excluding the period of annual frailty assessment, no substantive changes to the covariate associations with prefrailty and frailty were observed.

To evaluate the relationship between prefrailty and frailty with all-cause mortality, Kaplan-Meier survival analyses and Cox proportional hazards regression models were performed. The index (baseline) visit, defined as the first visit for which frailty was measured, was the time origin with observation until date of death or for those remaining alive, December 31, 2008. Frailty status, CD4 count, and HIV viral load were considered as time-varying covariates. To evaluate the independent and joint effects of HIV and frailty on mortality, we constructed a 4-category variable combining HIV status (positive/negative) with frailty status (frail if score ≥ 3; nonfrail if score 0–2). Given the lack of association of prefrailty (frailty score 1–2) with increased risk of mortality relative to the robust group, we combined the robust group with the prefrail group to create the "nonfrail" group for this 4-category variable. Unadjusted hazard ratios were estimated, with multivariable models constructed based on inclusion of variables found to be associated with the outcome and of variables considered a priori to be important predictors of mortality. The proportional hazards assumption was found to be reasonable by graphical assessment. Analyses were performed using STATA (version 11; Stata Corp., College Station, TX).

Results

A total of 1230 ALIVE participants contributed 3365 person-visits (median of 3 frailty measurements; IQR, 2–4). At initial frailty assessment, the median age of participants was 48 years (IQR, 42.9, 52.5), 89% were African American, 66% were male and 29% were HIV-infected. Of the 3365 person-visits (Table 1), 31% were among HIV-infected persons, with a median CD4 cell count of 296 (IQR, 168, 475) cells/uL, and a median viral load of 2.7 (IQR, 1.6, 4.4) $\log_{10}$ copies/ml. Recent HAART use was reported at 54% of visits.

Table 1. Characteristics of 1230 ALIVE Participants at 3365 Study Visits, by HIV Status[a].

	HIV-uninfected N = 2306 visits	HIV-infected N = 1059 visits
	No. (%)	No. (%)
Age, median (IQR), y	49.3 (44.2, 54.0)	48.7 (44.6, 52.8)
Female	751 (32.6)	388 (36.6)
African American	2074 (89.9)	1017 (96.0)
Less than high school education	1318 (57.2)	682 (64.9)
Not married/common law	2109 (91.5)	1004 (95.4)
Homeless[b]	280 (12.2)	112 (10.6)
Hazardous alcohol use[b]	530 (23.0)	196 (18.5)
Recent injection drug use[b]	925 (40.1)	331 (31.3)
Any non-injection drug use[b]	1055 (45.8)	345 (32.6)
Recent tobacco use[b]	1894 (82.2)	851 (80.7)
Prescription drug abuse[c]	244 (10.6)	58 (5.5)
Depressive symptoms[b]	491 (21.3)	212 (20.0)
# Comorbid Conditions[d]		
0–1	1636 (72.2)	770 (73.8)
2	373 (16.5)	173 (16.6)
≥3	257 (11.3)	101 (9.7)
CD4+ cell count, median (IQR)		296 (168, 475)
HIV RNA, median (IQR), log_{10} copies/ml		2.66 (1.60, 4.43)
Median CD4+ nadir (IQR)		135 (53, 230)
Recent HAART[b]		572 (54.2)

Abbreviations: HAART, highly active antiretroviral therapy; IQR, interquartile range; y, years; Hazardous alcohol use, score of ≥8 on the AUDIT; Depressive symptoms, score of ≥21 on the CES-D.
[a]Data are no. (%) of participants, unless otherwise indicated.
[b]Reflect characteristics within the previous 6 months.
[c]Reflect characteristics within the prior year.
[d]Diabetes, Hypertension, Cerebrovascular accident, Cardiovascular disease, Renal disease, Chronic obstructive pulmonary disease, Cancer, Obesity, Liver disease.

At the index visit, 12.3% of participants were classified as frail and 62.1% as prefrail. Among all 3365 person-visits, 12.4% (417 person-visits) met criteria for frailty and 60% (2020 person-visits) criteria for prefrailty. Univariate and multivariate associations with frailty and prefrailty are shown in Table 2. In multivariable analysis, frailty was significantly associated with older age, female gender, lower educational attainment, absence of a cohabitating partner, depressive symptoms, and increased number of comorbid conditions (Table 2). In univariate analysis, frailty was associated with hazardous alcohol use, being homeless, and non-injection use of illicit drugs. However, these associations did not retain significance in multivariable analyses. HIV infection was associated with a 66% greater likelihood of frailty (OR, 1.66; 95% CI, 1.24–2.21) (Table 2, Model A). In further analysis of HIV disease status (Table 2, Model B), having both immunosuppression (CD4 count <350 cells) and a detectable viral load was significantly associated with frailty (OR, 2.37; 95% CI, 1.62–3.48). There was no significant difference in frailty between HIV-uninfected person-visits and those of HIV-infected persons with a CD4 count ≥350 cells and an undetectable viral load while modest, but non-significant associations were seen for HIV-infected IDUs with

either lower CD4 counts only or detectable viral load only. In joint analysis of current and nadir CD4 count, current CD4 count but not CD4 nadir was found to be significantly associated with frailty (data not shown). In separate adjusted models, HIV-infected IDUs not receiving HAART had a substantially greater likelihood of frailty (OR, 1.91; 95% CI, 1.32–2.75) compared to HIV-uninfected IDUs, although this association was substantially attenuated but remained significant with recent HAART usage (OR, 1.45; 95% CI, 1.01–2.07) (Table 2, Model C). In models stratifying by severity of HIV disease, frailty was consistently associated with advanced (but not less advanced) HIV disease irrespective of HAART use.

In adjusted analysis of prefrailty, factors significantly associated with frailty generally remained similarly associated, but the associations were more modest in magnitude (Table 2), with the exception that comorbidity was not associated with prefrailty. HIV-infected IDUs had a 38% greater likelihood of prefrailty compared to HIV-uninfected IDUs (OR, 1.38; 95% CI, 1.11–1.70), and having a CD4 count<350 and detectable HIV viral load was significantly associated with prefrailty (OR, 1.79; 95% CI, 1.33–2.39).

During prospective evaluation of the relationship of frailty and prefrailty with mortality, we observed 73 deaths over 2644 person-years for a mortality rate of 2.8 per 100 person-years. Overall, frail persons had substantially higher mortality compared to persons that were either prefrail or robust (Figure 1). Adjusting for sociodemographic factors in Cox proportional hazards models, frailty (HR, 2.77; 95% CI, 1.32–5.81), having 3 or more comorbid conditions (HR, 2.97; 95%CI, 1.65–5.35) and HIV infection (HR, 3.05; 95%CI, 1.89–4.93) were independently associated with mortality (Table 3, Model A). Controlling for frailty status and comorbidity, HIV-infected IDUs with advanced disease had notably increased mortality risk (HR, 5.83; 95% CI, 3.48–9.74), with no significantly increased risk of death for those with less advanced HIV disease compared to HIV negatives (Table 3, Model B). The prefrail state was not a significant predictor of death in these models. In models with HIV-uninfected, nonfrail persons as the referent group (Figure 2; Table 3, Model C) being HIV-infected or being frail conferred an increased mortality risk with an approximately 3-fold magnitude for each. Persons that were both HIV-infected and frail had an over 7-fold increased risk of death (HR, 7.06; 95% CI, 3.49–14.3)

Discussion

In this study, we incorporated standardized assessment of frailty into a community cohort of HIV-infected and epidemiologically-comparable HIV-uninfected IDUs. We identified a frailty prevalence of 12.3% and found that HIV infection, particularly advanced disease stage with lower CD4 cell counts and the absence of ART or virological suppression, was strongly associated with frailty. Despite our cohort being relatively young compared to geriatric populations where frailty has been shown to presage adverse clinical outcomes, frailty was independently associated with increased mortality risk in prospective analysis even after accounting for sociodemographic variables, comorbidity, and HIV infection. Moreover, the combined effect of frailty and HIV on mortality appeared to exceed what one would expect from the additive effect of the individual exposures. In summary, these findings suggest that frailty is a useful phenotype for investigating aging among HIV-infected IDUs and could potentially identify individuals at high-risk for adverse outcomes among these highly vulnerable groups. Our data also raise the possibility that optimal

Table 2. Factors Associated with Frailty and Prefrailty among 3365 ALIVE Study Person-Visits[a].

Model A. Odds of Frailty and Prefrailty by Sociodemographic, Behavioral, and Clinical Risk Factors[b]

	Prefrail	Prefrail	Frail	Frail
	Unadjusted	Adjusted	Unadjusted	Adjusted
	OR (95% CI)	OR (95% CI)	OR (95% CI)	OR (95% CI)
Age (per year)	1.00 (0.99, 1.01)	1.02 (1.00, 1.03)	1.03 (1.01, 1.05)	1.05 (1.03, 1.07)
Female	1.24 (1.02, 1.51)	1.17 (0.95, 1.45)	1.62 (1.23, 2.13)	1.44 (1.07, 1.94)
African American	0.72 (0.52, 1.00)	0.72 (0.50, 1.04)	0.76 (0.47, 1.23)	0.67 (0.40, 1.13)
Less than high school education	1.27 (1.05, 1.54)	1.25 (1.03, 1.52)	1.43 (1.09, 1.87)	1.48 (1.12, 1.95)
Not married/common law	1.56 (1.08, 2.23)	1.57 (1.08, 2.29)	1.77 (1.02, 3.06)	2.05 (1.16, 3.60)
Homeless[d]	1.23 (0.93, 1.61)	–	1.49 (1.06, 2.11)	–
Hazardous alcohol use[d]	1.20 (0.98, 1.48)	–	1.47 (1.12, 1.92)	–
Recent injection drug use[d]	1.04 (0.87, 1.23)	–	1.00 (0.79, 1.27)	–
Any non-injection drug use[d]	1.21 (1.01, 1.44)	–	1.38 (1.09, 1.75)	–
Recent tobacco use[d]	1.11 (0.88, 1.41)	–	1.32 (0.94, 1.85)	–
Prescription drug abuse[e]	1.66 (1.20, 2.29)	1.50 (1.05, 2.14)	2.14 (1.45, 3.14)	1.70 (1.11, 2.59)
Depressive symptoms[d]	2.23 (1.77, 2.81)	2.11 (1.66, 2.69)	4.70 (3.58, 6.16)	4.40 (3.31, 5.84)
# Comorbid conditions[f]				
0–1	Ref	Ref	Ref	Ref
2	1.08 (0.85, 1.38)	1.05 (0.82, 1.35)	1.87 (1.40, 2.49)	1.70 (1.26, 2.30)
≥3	1.18 (0.87, 1.60)	1.10 (0.80, 1.51)	2.67 (1.84, 3.87)	2.06 (1.39, 3.05)
HIV negative	Ref	Ref	Ref	Ref
HIV positive	1.34 (1.09, 1.64)	1.38 (1.11, 1.70)	1.53 (1.15, 2.02)	1.66 (1.24, 2.21)

Model B. Odds of Frailty and Prefrailty by CD4 and VL Strata[c]

	Prefrail	Prefrail	Frail	Frail
	Unadjusted	Adjusted	Unadjusted	Adjusted
	OR (95% CI)	OR (95% CI)	OR (95% CI)	OR (95% CI)
HIV negative	Ref	Ref	Ref	Ref
CD4≥350, VL UD	1.10 (0.79, 1.55)	1.18 (0.82, 1.69)	1.03 (0.64, 1.65)	1.09 (0.67, 1.77)
CD4<350, VL UD	1.23 (0.82, 1.84)	1.33 (0.89, 2.00)	1.35 (0.81, 2.25)	1.47 (0.86, 2.51)
CD4≥350, VL+	1.06 (0.71, 1.58)	1.04 (0.69, 1.56)	1.33 (0.80, 2.22)	1.37 (0.80, 2.36)
CD4<350, VL+	1.76 (1.33, 2.33)	1.79 (1.33, 2.39)	2.12 (1.46, 3.07)	2.37 (1.62, 3.48)

Model C. Odds of Frailty and Prefrailty by HAART status[c]

	Prefrail	Prefrail	Frail	Frail
	Unadjusted	Adjusted	Unadjusted	Adjusted
	OR (95% CI)	OR (95% CI)	OR (95% CI)	OR (95% CI)
HIV negative	Ref	Ref	Ref	Ref
HAART+	1.30 (1.01, 1.67)	1.40 (1.08, 1.81)	1.27 (0.90, 1.80)	1.45 (1.01, 2.07)
No HAART[d]	1.38 (1.07, 1.80)	1.35 (1.03, 1.77)	1.87 (1.31, 2.65)	1.91 (1.32, 2.75)

Abbreviations : HAART, highly active antiretroviral therapy; VL, HIV viral load; UD, undetectable, <50 HIV RNA copies/ml; Hazardous alcohol use, score of ≥8 on the AUDIT; Depressive symptoms, score of ≥21 on the CES-D.
– Not included in final model/not significant in adjusted analyses.
[a]Data are given as unadjusted and adjusted odds ratios (95% confidence interval).
[b]Adjusted for age, gender, race, education, marital status, prescription drug abuse, depressive symptoms, # comorbid conditions and HIV status.
[c]Adjusted for age, gender, race, education, marital status, prescription drug abuse, depressive symptoms, and # comorbid conditions.
[d]Reflect characteristics within the previous 6 months.
[e]Reflect characteristics within the prior year.
[f]Diabetes, Hypertension, Cerebrovascular accident, Cardiovascular disease, Renal disease, Chronic obstructive pulmonary disease, Cancer, Obesity, Liver disease.

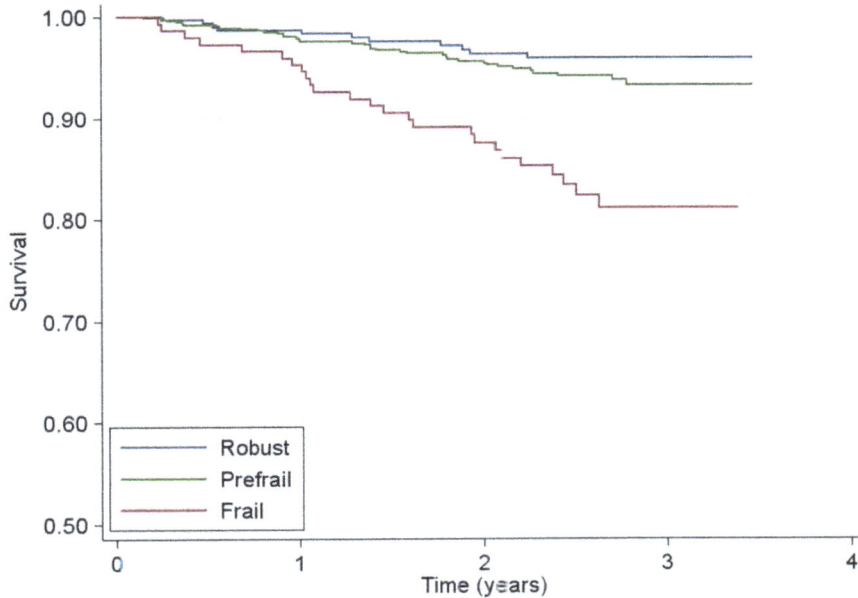

Figure 1. Survival by Frailty Status in the ALIVE cohort. Kaplan Meier Survival Curve Estimates for 1230 ALIVE Participants from July 2005 to December 2008. Robust participants had a frailty score of 0; prefrail participants had a frailty score of 1–2; frail participants had a frailty score of 3–5.

HIV care with virological suppression could attenuate the development of frailty.

Aberrant inflammation and immune dysregulation have been hypothesized to characterize the natural process of aging as well as underlie the pathogenesis of chronic HIV disease [24]. Based on emerging epidemiologic, clinical, and mechanistic evidence, inflammation and immune dysfunction are postulated to play a central role in frailty pathophysiology among older HIV-uninfect-ed adults [25,26,27]. We find that HIV-infected IDUs with well-controlled HIV disease are no more likely to be frail than similar individuals without HIV infection. In contrast, the likelihood of frailty was significantly higher with advanced HIV disease with inadequate virologic control. These results suggest that HIV infection without effective treatment may represent a significant, modifiable risk factor for frailty. Thus, together with data from other HIV cohorts [13,14], these findings suggest a putative role

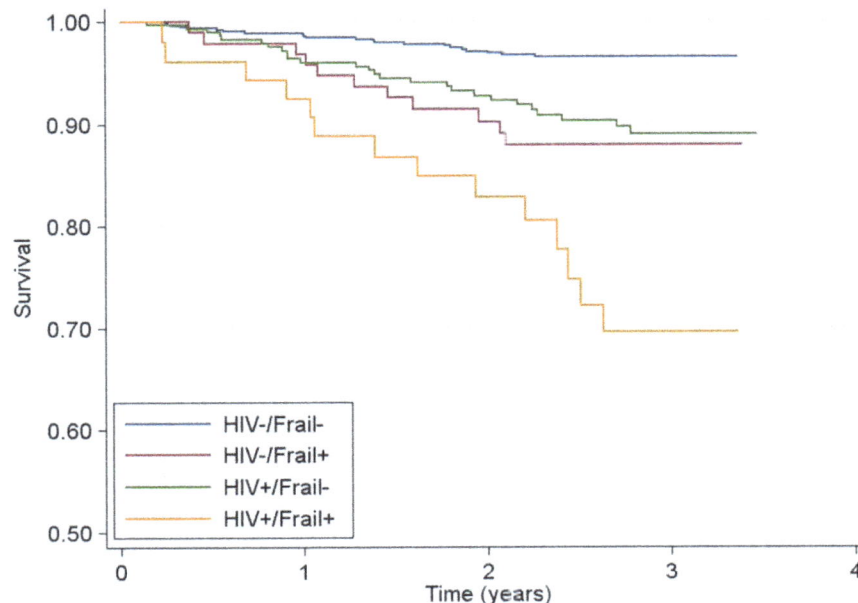

Figure 2. Survival by Frailty and HIV Status in the ALIVE cohort. Kaplan Meier Survival Curve Estimates for 1230 ALIVE Participants from July 2005 to December 2008. Frail- participants had a frailty score of 0–2; Frail+ participants had a frailty score of 3–5.

Table 3. Mortality Risk associated with Frailty and HIV among ALIVE Participants[a].

	Unadjusted	Adjusted
	HR (95% CI)	HR (95% CI)
Model A[b]		
Age (per year)	1.05 (1.01, 1.08)	1.04 (1.00, 1.08)
Female	1.55 (0.98, 2.46)	1.23 (0.74, 2.02)
African American	1.03 (0.45, 2.38)	0.76 (0.33, 1.77)
Less than high school education	0.86 (0.54, 1.37)	0.79 (0.49, 1.27)
# Comorbid conditions		
0–1	Ref	Ref
2	1.77 (0.95, 3.28)	1.39 (0.73, 2.63)
≥3	4.10 (2.39, 7.03)	2.97 (1.65, 5.35)
HIV positive	2.83 (1.78, 4.49)	3.05 (1.89, 4.93)
Frailty status[d]		
Robust	Ref	Ref
Prefrail	1.46 (0.74, 2.86)	1.24 (0.63, 2.45)
Frail	4.38 (2.16, 8.90)	2.77 (1.32, 5.81)
Model B[c]		
HIV status		
HIV negative	Ref	Ref
CD4≥350, VL UD	0.68 (0.16, 2.83)	0.60 (0.14, 2.55)
CD4<350, VL UD	1.05 (0.25, 4.39)	1.18 (0.28, 4.95)
CD4≥350, VL+	1.12 (0.34, 3.65)	1.38 (0.42, 4.54)
CD4<350, VL+	4.89 (3.01, 7.97)	5.83 (3.48, 9.74)
Frailty status[d]		
Robust	Ref	Ref
Prefrail	1.46 (0.74, 2.86)	1.13 (0.57, 2.22)
Frail	4.38 (2.16, 8.90)	2.20 (1.03, 4.68)
Model C[c]		
HIV/Frailty status[d]		
HIV negative/nonfrail	Ref	Ref
HIV negative/frail	3.45 (1.67, 7.12)	2.63 (1.23, 5.66)
HIV positive/nonfrail	2.85 (1.62, 5.04)	3.29 (1.85, 5.88)
HIV positive/frail	8.31 (4.25, 16.3)	7.06 (3.49, 14.3)

[a]Data are given as unadjusted and adjusted hazard ratios (95% confidence interval).
[b]Adjusted for age, gender, race, education, # comorbid conditions, HIV status and frailty status.
[c]Adjusted for age, gender, race, education and # comorbid conditions.
[d]Robust participants had a frailty score of 0; prefrail participants had a frailty score of 1–2; frail participants had a frailty score of 3–5; nonfrail participants had a frailty score of 0–2.

for HAART in arresting the progression to frailty. HAART has been shown to have a significant impact on morbidity and mortality for HIV-infected populations in general and HIV-infected IDUs specifically [28,29,30,31,32]. The negative impact of late initiation of care and premature interruption of HAART on survival has also been well defined [7,33,34]. Engagement in care and adherence to antiretroviral regimens continue to be a daunting challenge for the HIV-infected population [35]. These effects are exacerbated among IDUs, who tend to have later diagnosis, poorer access to care, lower HAART uptake, more limited adherence, and frequent treatment interruptions with

significant consequences for HIV-related morbidity and mortality [17,36,37,38,39,40,41]. With less successful navigation of the HIV care continuum, HIV-infected IDUs remain at higher risk for HIV/AIDS progression, and by extension may suffer increased progression to frailty with its consequent adverse outcomes. Future investigations will need to elucidate the underlying mechanisms of frailty development in the setting of HIV and determine whether earlier ART may be effective for frailty prevention.

We found that frailty was independently associated with an increased risk of death among HIV-infected and at risk IDUs. These findings are particularly notable given that the median age of this cohort was 48 years. Frailty has been primarily linked to mortality and other adverse outcomes in significantly older cohorts (predominantly 65 years of age and older) [3,4]. Consistent with our data, a frailty related construct has demonstrated increased mortality risk in younger populations in 2 recent studies [22,42]. As comprehensive treatment for HIV infection evolves beyond a focus primarily on viral suppression and broadens to consider management of multiple chronic conditions to achieve healthy aging, assessment tools beyond HIV RNA and CD4 counts will be increasingly needed. Frailty may improve risk stratification and inform appropriate clinical management for aging, complex care patients living with HIV. Further, the joint impact of frailty and HIV infection on mortality suggests that efforts to reduce mortality risk through both frailty and HIV targeted interventions may translate into significant survival benefit.

Besides HIV disease markers, we found that depressive symptoms and prescription drug abuse were associated with both frailty and prefrailty. Previously, we have documented self-medication with 'street' drugs for symptoms in this population [43]. Although directionality of these associations cannot be determined in the current analysis, it will be important to examine whether frailty interventions alleviate associated pain or other symptoms and lead to improved health-related quality of life.

Consistent with studies of frailty in HIV-uninfected older adults [3,44], we observed that advancing age, female gender, lower educational attainment, and increased number of comorbid conditions were associated with frailty within this IDU population. The absence of a cohabiting life partner may be a putative measure of social isolation with which frailty has also been previously associated [3]. As with HIV, dysregulated inflammation has been associated with age and socioeconomic status [24,45,46,47]. Further, hormonal influences have been postulated to play an important role in age-associated changes in inflammation among women [48,49]. Whether hormonally mediated changes in inflammation account for sex-specific differences in frailty prevalence remains to be determined. However, inflammation may be a predominant pathway by which these factors could contribute to progression to a frail state.

Prefrailty is considered to be an intermediate state that presages progression to frailty in geriatric populations [3]. Therefore, the prefrail state may provide a window of opportunity when interventions could mitigate adverse clinical outcomes. We observed consistent, although attenuated, associations of prefrailty with HIV disease and other frailty risk factors; however, prefrailty was not predictive of mortality. A larger study size or longer duration may allow identification of incremental mortality risk with prefrailty. Further follow-up also is needed to define the likelihood of transition from prefrailty to frailty among HIV-infected persons. These data will be vital to inform development of interventions to reverse or slow progression to frailty. The high prevalence of almost two-thirds of our participants with prefrailty is consistent with other studies and provides a large target population for intervention [3,4].

Our study had several limitations. Debate persists on the optimal criteria for defining frailty [50]. The frailty phenotype employed in this study closely approximated the original Fried criteria, with objective measurement of weight loss, gait speed, and grip strength. Consistent with prior studies, we substituted a self-reported measure of low physical activity [13,22]. Our weight loss parameter did not discern intentionality; however, similarly constructed frailty constructs had predictive validity roughly equivalent to the original Fried phenotype in elderly HIV-uninfected persons [4,51]. As we used weight loss of ≥5% since last study visit (median of 6 months), our threshold for meeting this criteria required greater weight loss than the original criteria. Given the observational nature of the study and lack of temporality for HIV-frailty associations, caution is needed regarding inferences of causality. Our cohort is a predominantly African American, urban IDU cohort and as such, our findings may not be fully generalizable to other HIV-infected populations. However, significant relationships between frailty (and a frailty-related phenotype) and advanced HIV disease have been noted in several non-IDU cohorts [13,14,15]. Further, we have observed a similar relationship between frailty and non-HIV-related factors in our population as reported from older HIV-uninfected populations [3,44]. Whether similar biological mechanisms underlie the development of frailty for these different groups needs to be further investigated. Nevertheless, this population does represent those individuals particularly vulnerable to disparities in access to care and key adverse health care outcomes for whom appropriately targeted frailty interventions could have substantial clinical impact.

Improved understanding of frailty in high-risk populations may translate into clinical utility as well as strengthen our scientific understanding of the aging process. Despite improving survival and recent aging trends, HIV-infected and at risk IDUs continue to experience marked socioeconomic challenges with persistent disparities in treatment access, morbidity and mortality outcomes [10,11,17,21,52]. Frailty assessment may prove useful in identifying those persons at greatest risk for premature death and allow appropriate intervention. Whether HIV infection and frailty share a single common pathway to premature death remains to be determined. However, elucidation of the mechanisms underlying frailty development may provide substantial opportunities for realizing the healthy aging of HIV-infected and drug using populations, with potential additional benefit to the general aging population.

Supporting Information

Table S1   Characterization of the Frailty Phenotype in the AIDS Linked to the IntraVenous Experience (ALIVE) Cohort.

Author Contributions

Edited and critically revised the manuscript: DP AM SM TB KP SL GK. Conceived and designed the experiments: DP AM SM TB KP SL GK. Performed the experiments: DP SM KP GK. Analyzed the data: DP AM GK. Contributed reagents/materials/analysis tools: SM GK. Wrote the paper: DP GK.

References

1. Fried LP, Ferrucci L, Darer J, Williamson JD, Anderson G (2004) Untangling the concepts of disability, frailty, and comorbidity: implications for improved targeting and care. J Gerontol A Biol Sci Med Sci 59: 255–263.
2. Xue QL (2011) The frailty syndrome: definition and natural history. Clin Geriatr Med 27: 1–15.
3. Fried LP, Tangen CM, Walston J, Newman AB, Hirsch C, et al. (2001) Frailty in older adults: evidence for a phenotype. J Gerontol A Biol Sci Med Sci 56: M146–156.
4. Bandeen-Roche K, Xue QL, Ferrucci L, Walston J, Guralnik JM, et al. (2006) Phenotype of frailty: characterization in the women's health and aging studies. J Gerontol A Biol Sci Med Sci 61: 262–266.
5. High KP, Brennan-Ing M, Clifford DB, Cohen MH, Currier J, et al. (2012) HIV and aging: state of knowledge and areas of critical need for research. A report to the NIH Office of AIDS Research by the HIV and Aging Working Group. J Acquir Immune Defic Syndr 60 Suppl 1: S1–18.
6. Mills EJ, Barnighausen T, Negin J (2012) HIV and aging—preparing for the challenges ahead. N Engl J Med 366: 1270–1273.
7. Losina E, Schackman BR, Sadownik SN, Gebo KA, Walensky RP, et al. (2009) Racial and sex disparities in life expectancy losses among HIV-infected persons in the united states: impact of risk behavior, late initiation, and early discontinuation of antiretroviral therapy. Clin Infect Dis 49: 1570–1578.
8. Lohse N, Hansen AB, Pedersen G, Kronborg G, Gerstoft J, et al. (2007) Survival of persons with and without HIV infection in Denmark, 1995–2005. Ann Intern Med 146: 87–95.
9. Armstrong GL (2007) Injection drug users in the United States, 1979–2002: an aging population. Arch Intern Med 167: 166–173.
10. Wolfe D, Carrieri MP, Shepard D (2010) Treatment and care for injecting drug users with HIV infection: a review of barriers and ways forward. Lancet 376: 355–366.
11. Degenhardt L, Hall W, Warner-Smith M (2006) Using cohort studies to estimate mortality among injecting drug users that is not attributable to AIDS. Sex Transm Infect 82 Suppl 3: iii56–63.
12. Kohli R, Lo Y, Howard AA, Buono D, Floris-Moore M, et al. (2005) Mortality in an urban cohort of HIV-infected and at-risk drug users in the era of highly active antiretroviral therapy. Clin Infect Dis 41: 864–872.
13. Desquilbet L, Jacobson LP, Fried LP, Phair JP, Jamieson BD, et al. (2007) HIV-1 infection is associated with an earlier occurrence of a phenotype related to frailty. J Gerontol A Biol Sci Med Sci 62: 1279–1286.
14. Terzian AS, Holman S, Nathwani N, Robison E, Weber K, et al. (2009) Factors associated with preclinical disability and frailty among HIV-infected and HIV-uninfected women in the era of cART. J Womens Health (Larchmt) 18: 1965–1974.
15. Onen NF, Agbebi A, Shacham E, Stamm KE, Onen AR, et al. (2009) Frailty among HIV-infected persons in an urban outpatient care setting. J Infect 59: 346–352.
16. Vlahov D, Anthony JC, Munoz A, Margolick J, Nelson KE, et al. (1991) The ALIVE study, a longitudinal study of HIV-1 infection in intravenous drug users: description of methods and characteristics of participants. NIDA Res Monogr 109: 75–100.
17. Salter ML, Lau B, Go VF, Mehta SH, Kirk GD (2011) HIV infection, immune suppression, and uncontrolled viremia are associated with increased multimorbidity among aging injection drug users. Clin Infect Dis 53: 1256–1264.
18. Saunders JB, Aasland OG, Babor TF, de la Fuente JR, Grant M (1993) Development of the Alcohol Use Disorders Identification Test (AUDIT): WHO Collaborative Project on Early Detection of Persons with Harmful Alcohol Consumption-II. Addiction 88: 791–804.
19. Weissman MM, Sholomskas D, Pottenger M, Prusoff BA, Locke BZ (1977) Assessing depressive symptoms in five psychiatric populations: a validation study. Am J Epidemiol 106: 203–214.
20. Skinner HA (1982) The drug abuse screening test. Addict Behav 7: 363–371.
21. Mehta SH, Kirk GD, Astemborski J, Galai N, Celentano DD (2010) Temporal trends in highly active antiretroviral therapy initiation among injection drug users in Baltimore, Maryland, 1996–2008. Clin Infect Dis 50: 1664–1671.
22. Desquilbet L, Jacobson LP, Fried LP, Phair JP, Jamieson BD, et al. (2011) A Frailty-Related Phenotype Before HAART Initiation as an Independent Risk Factor for AIDS or Death After HAART Among HIV-Infected Men. J Gerontol A Biol Sci Med Sci.
23. Rabe-Hesketh S, Skrondal A (2008) Multilevel and Longitudinal Modeling Using Stata. College Station, TX: Stata Press.
24. Deeks SG (2011) HIV infection, inflammation, immunosenescence, and aging. Annu Rev Med 62: 141–155.
25. Yao X, Li H, Leng SX (2011) Inflammation and immune system alterations in frailty. Clin Geriatr Med 27: 79–87.
26. Leng SX, Xue QL, Tian J, Walston JD, Fried LP (2007) Inflammation and frailty in older women. J Am Geriatr Soc 55: 864–871.
27. Walston J, McBurnie MA, Newman A, Tracy RP, Kop WJ, et al. (2002) Frailty and activation of the inflammation and coagulation systems with and without clinical comorbidities: results from the Cardiovascular Health Study. Arch Intern Med 162: 2333–2341.
28. Detels R, Munoz A, McFarlane G, Kingsley LA, Margolick JB, et al. (1998) Effectiveness of potent antiretroviral therapy on time to AIDS and death in men with known HIV infection duration. Multicenter AIDS Cohort Study Investigators. JAMA 280: 1497–1503.
29. Hammer SM, Squires KE, Hughes MD, Grimes JM, Demeter LM, et al. (1997) A controlled trial of two nucleoside analogues plus indinavir in persons with

human immunodeficiency virus infection and CD4 cell counts of 200 per cubic millimeter or less. AIDS Clinical Trials Group 320 Study Team. N Engl J Med 337: 725–733.

30. Murphy EL, Collier AC, Kalish LA, Assmann SF, Para MF, et al. (2001) Highly active antiretroviral therapy decreases mortality and morbidity in patients with advanced HIV disease. Ann Intern Med 135: 17–26.

31. Vlahov D, Galai N, Safaeian M, Galea S, Kirk GD, et al. (2005) Effectiveness of highly active antiretroviral therapy among injection drug users with late-stage human immunodeficiency virus infection. Am J Epidemiol 161: 999–1012.

32. Wood E, Hogg RS, Lima VD, Kerr T, Yip B, et al. (2008) Highly active antiretroviral therapy and survival in HIV-infected injection drug users. JAMA 300: 550–554.

33. Kitahata MM, Gange SJ, Abraham AG, Merriman B, Saag MS, et al. (2009) Effect of early versus deferred antiretroviral therapy for HIV on survival. N Engl J Med 360: 1815–1826.

34. Giordano TP, Gifford AL, White AC Jr, Suarez-Almazor ME, Rabeneck L, et al. (2007) Retention in care: a challenge to survival with HIV infection. Clin Infect Dis 44: 1493–1499.

35. Gardner EM, McLees MP, Steiner JF, Del Rio C, Burman WJ (2011) The spectrum of engagement in HIV care and its relevance to test-and-treat strategies for prevention of HIV infection. Clin Infect Dis 52: 793–800.

36. Wood E, Hogg RS, Harrigan PR, Montaner JS (2005) When to initiate antiretroviral therapy in HIV-1-infected adults: a review for clinicians and patients. Lancet Infect Dis 5: 407–414.

37. Nijhawan A, Kim S, Rich JD (2008) Management of HIV infection in patients with substance use problems. Curr Infect Dis Rep 10: 432–438.

38. Arnsten JH, Demas PA, Grant RW, Gourevitch MN, Farzadegan H, et al. (2002) Impact of active drug use on antiretroviral therapy adherence and viral suppression in HIV-infected drug users. J Gen Intern Med 17: 377–381.

39. Celentano DD, Vlahov D, Cohn S, Shadle VM, Obasanjo O, et al. (1998) Self-reported antiretroviral therapy in injection drug users. JAMA 280: 544–546.

40. Kavasery R, Galai N, Astemborski J, Lucas GM, Celentano DD, et al. (2009) Nonstructured treatment interruptions among injection drug users in Baltimore, MD. J Acquir Immune Defic Syndr 50: 360–366.

41. Mathers BM, Degenhardt L, Ali H, Wiessing L, Hickman M, et al. (2010) HIV prevention, treatment, and care services for people who inject drugs: a systematic review of global, regional, and national coverage. Lancet 375: 1014–1028.

42. Rockwood K, Song X, Mitnitski A (2011) Changes in relative fitness and frailty across the adult lifespan: evidence from the Canadian National Population Health Survey. CMAJ 183: E487–494.

43. Khosla N, Juon HS, Kirk GD, Astemborski J, Mehta SH (2011) Correlates of non-medical prescription drug use among a cohort of injection drug users in Baltimore City. Addict Behav 36: 1282–1287.

44. Szanton SL, Seplaki CL, Thorpe RJ Jr, Allen JK, Fried LP (2010) Socioeconomic status is associated with frailty: the Women's Health and Aging Studies. J Epidemiol Community Health 64: 63–67.

45. Carroll JE, Cohen S, Marsland AL (2011) Early childhood socioeconomic status is associated with circulating interleukin-6 among mid-life adults. Brain Behav Immun.

46. Nazmi A, Victora CG (2007) Socioeconomic and racial/ethnic differentials of C-reactive protein levels: a systematic review of population-based studies. BMC Public Health 7: 212.

47. Koster A, Bosma H, Penninx BW, Newman AB, Harris TB, et al. (2006) Association of inflammatory markers with socioeconomic status. J Gerontol A Biol Sci Med Sci 61: 284–290.

48. Joseph C, Kenny AM, Taxel P, Lorenzo JA, Duque G, et al. (2005) Role of endocrine-immune dysregulation in osteoporosis, sarcopenia, frailty and fracture risk. Mol Aspects Med 26: 181–201.

49. Singh T, Newman AB (2011) Inflammatory markers in population studies of aging. Ageing Res Rev 10: 319–329.

50. Rodriguez-Manas L, Feart C, Mann G, Vina J, Chatterji S, et al. (2012) Searching for an Operational Definition of Frailty: A Delphi Method Based Consensus Statement. The Frailty Operative Definition-Consensus Conference Project. J Gerontol A Biol Sci Med Sci.

51. Ensrud KE, Ewing SK, Taylor BC, Fink HA, Cawthon PM, et al. (2008) Comparison of 2 frailty indexes for prediction of falls, disability, fractures, and death in older women. Arch Intern Med 168: 382–389.

52. Crystal S, Akincigil A, Sambamoorthi U, Wenger N, Fleishman JA, et al. (2003) The diverse older HIV-positive population: a national profile of economic circumstances, social support, and quality of life. J Acquir Immune Defic Syndr 33 Suppl 2: S76–83.

16

Investigation Outcomes of Tuberculosis Suspects in the Health Centers of Addis Ababa, Ethiopia

Amare Deribew[1]*, Nebiyu Negussu[2], Zenebe Melaku[3], Kebede Deribe[4]

1 Department of Epidemiology, Jimma University, Jimma, Ethiopia, 2 Somali Regional Health Bureau, Jijiga, Ethiopia, 3 International Center for AIDS Care and Treatment Program (ICAP), Addis Ababa, Ethiopia, 4 Department of General Public Health, Jimma University, Jimma, Ethiopia

Abstract

Background: Little is known about the prevalence of tuberculosis (TB) and HIV among TB suspects in primary health care units in Ethiopia.

Methods: In the period of February to March, 2009, a cross sectional survey was done in 27 health centers of Addis Ababa to assess the prevalence of TB and HIV among TB suspects who have $> = 2$ weeks symptoms of TB such as cough, fever and weight loss. Diagnosis of TB and HIV was based on the national guidelines. Information concerning socio-demographic variables and knowledge of the respondents about TB was collected using pretested questionnaire.

Results: Of the 545 TB suspects, 506 (92.7%) of them participated in the study. The prevalence of both pulmonary and extra pulmonary TB was 46.0% (233/506). The smear positivity rate among pulmonary TB suspect was 21.3%. Of the TB suspects, 298 (58.9%) of them were tested for HIV and 27.2% (81/298) were HIV seropositive. Fifty percent of the HIV positive TB suspects had TB. TB suspects who had a contact history with a TB patient in the family were 9 times more likely to have TB than those who did not have a contact history, [OR = 9.1, (95%CI:4.0, 20.5)]. Individuals who had poor [OR = 5.2, (95%C : 2.3, 11.2)] and fair knowledge [OR = 3.7, (95%CI: 1.3, 10.4)] about TB were more likely to have TB than individuals who had good knowledge.

Conclusion: In conclusion, the prevalence of TB among TB suspects with duration of 2 or more weeks is high. Fifty percent of the HIV positive TB suspects had TB. Case finding among TB suspects with duration of 2 or more weeks should be intensified particularly among those who have a contact history with a TB patient.

Editor: Cesar V. Munayco, Dirección General de Epidemiología, Peru

Funding: The study was funded by Jimma University. The funder had no role in the study design, data collection, and analysis, decision to publish or preparation of the manuscript.

Competing Interests: The authors have declared that no competing interests exist.

* E-mail: amare_deribew@yahoo.com

Introduction

One third of the global population is infected by *mycobacterium tuberculosis*. Eighty percent of the total new tuberculosis (TB) in the world are found in 22 high burden countries[1]. Since the last 50 years, TB has been recognized as a major public health problem of Ethiopia[2]. The World Health Organization (WHO) estimated that Ethiopia is the seventh high burden country in terms of incidence cases of TB[1].

Low case detection rate (34%) of smear positive TB[2], high burden of TB/HIV co-infection, ranging from 25% to 57% [3,4,5,6,7] and the emergence of multi-drug resistance TB pose serious challenges for the TB control program in Ethiopia[1,2]. The country has been implementing the TB/HIV collaborative activities such as screening of TB patients for HIV, intensified TB case finding among HIV patients and joint coordination of the two diseases since 2007[8].

Screening of TB suspects using symptom based questionnaires provides a quick, cheap and convenient way to identify individuals at a high risk of tuberculosis (TB). Individuals identified as TB suspects by the simple clinical algorithm need to be investigated further using definitive tests such as sputum microscopy, chest radiography and, TB culture if it is available. More recently, provider-initiated TB screening (i.e. active case-finding) has become an important part of HIV care in resource-poor settings including Ethiopia [9–14]. Ruling out active TB is necessary both for individual patient management and for TB infection control. In patients starting antiretroviral therapy, undiagnosed TB is common and carries a substantially increased risk of death or hospitalization in the first few months of treatment [14,15].

In Ethiopia, little is known about the prevalence of TB, HIV and TB/HIV co-infection among TB suspects with duration of cough of two or more weeks in the primary health care units (health centers). The objective of this study was to evaluate the prevalence of TB and HIV among TB suspects in Addis Ababa using simple symptom based questionnaire. Participants who were identified as TB suspects were further investigated for TB and HIV using sputum analysis and rapid HIV testing.

Methods

Setting and period

The study was conducted from February to March, 2009 in twenty-seven public health centers (primary health care units) in Addis Ababa, the capital city of the Federal democratic Republic of Ethiopia. These health centers provide curative and preventive health services for the community of Addis Ababa which has an estimated total population of 2,917,295[16].

Study design

A facility based cross-sectional study was conducted in 27 health centers in Addis Ababa.

Study population and sampling

Study participants were 545 adult pulmonary TB or extrapulmonary TB (TB lymphadenitis) suspects (> = 15 years) identified in the study health centers. Other forms of extrapulmonary TB suspects were excluded from the study. Considering resources, the sample size was estimated using a single proportion sample size formulae by considering the following parameters: prevalence of TB among adult pulmonary TB suspects of 29% [6], 95% CI, and 4% of margin of error and 10% for the non-response rate.

Measurement

TB suspects were identified using a pre-tested questionnaire. TB suspects were defined as individuals who had cough of ≥2 weeks OR two or more of the following symptoms: *weight loss, fever, excessive night sweats and painless swelling of cervical or axillary lymph nodes* of more than 2 weeks. Diagnosis of TB among TB suspects was based on the national TB guideline[2]. Three consecutive sputum samples (spot-morning-spot) were collected and examined for the presence of Acid Fast Bacilli (AFB) using the standard Ziehl-Neelsen method[17]. As a quality control method, the entire positive and 10% of the negative slides were re-read by experienced laboratory technicians. Pulmonary TB suspects who had two smear positive results were categorized as smear positive. TB suspects who had three negative smears and suggestive X-ray findings or failure to respond to an antibiotic trials were categorized as smear negative pulmonary TB. TB lymphadenitis was diagnosed based on clinical parameters and cytological examination obtained by fine needle aspiration. Diagnosis of HIV was based on national guideline and the detail procedure is published elsewhere[18].

Information concerning the socio-demographic and knowledge of patients on TB was collected by trained general practitioners or nurses using a pretested and previously used questionnaire [19]. The questionnaire was originally developed in English and translated to Amharic (local language). To ensure consistency, the questionnaire was retranslated to English by another person who was blind to the original questionnaire. There were 24 knowledge questions about TB. The questions focused on sign and symptoms, preventive methods, treatment of TB. For each question 0 is given for incorrect answers and 1 for correct answers. A person was considered to have good, fair or poor knowledge if he/she answered respectively more than 75%, 50–75%, or less than 50% of the questions correctly.

Data analysis

Data were entered into SPSS Version 16.0 statistical software. Univariate analysis was done to describe the socio-demographic characteristics of the study participants and prevalence of TB. A bivariate analysis using binary logistic regression was done to determine the presence of a statistically significant association between explanatory variables and the outcome variables (presence of TB or HIV). To identify independently associated factors, multiple logistic regression model was produced by taking presence of TB as outcome variable. All explanatory variables that were associated with the outcome variable in the bivariate analysis

(P = ≤0.2) and variables consistently found to be associated with occurrence of TB in other studies were included in the logistic regression model. Odds Ratio (OR) and their 95% Confidence Intervals (CI) were calculated.

Ethical consideration

Ethical clearance was obtained from the ethical committee of Jimma University and the Addis Ababa health bureau. Written consent was obtained from each participants and confidentiality was assured for all the information provided. Identification of a participant was only through numerical codes.

Results

Prevalence of TB among TB suspects

Of the total TB suspects during the study period (n = 545), 506(92.7%) of them participated in the study. The prevalence of both pulmonary and extra pulmonary TB was 46.0% (233/506). Of the TB patients, 100(42.9%), 96(41.2%) and 37(15.9) had smear positive, smear negative and extra pulmonary TB. The smear positivity rate among pulmonary TB suspect was 21.3% (100/469).

There was no difference in sex, age, literacy status, occupation and marital status between patients with and without evidence of TB (**Table-1**).

HIV prevalence among TB suspects

Of the TB suspects, 298(58.9%) of them were tested for HIV. The prevalence of HIV was 27.2% (81/298). The HIV positive and negative individuals had no significant differences concerning sex, educational status, and marital status. Larger proportion of housewives and merchants were HIV positive (P = 0.025). The prevalence of HIV was higher in the age group of 25–34 and > = 50 years (P = 0.014). Fifty percent of the HIV positive (41/81) and 48.4%(105/217) of the HIV negative TB suspects had TB (P = 0.32) (**Table-2**).

The association between symptoms and occurrence of pulmonary TB

There was no statistically significant association between chronic cough, night sweating, loss of appetite, weight loss, and fever with the occurrence of pulmonary TB. Those who had chest pain were 1.5 times more likely to have pulmonary TB than those who did not have chest pain, [OR = 1.5, (95%CI: 1.0, 2.28)] (**Table-3**).

Factors associated with pulmonary TB

TB suspects who had a contact history with a TB patient in the family were 9 times more likely to have TB than those who did not have a contact history, [OR = 9.1,(4.0, 20.5)]. Individuals who had poor [OR = 5.2, (95%CI: 2.3, 11.2)] and fair knowledge [OR = 3.7, (95%CI: 1.3, 10.4)] about TB were more likely to have TB than individuals who had good knowledge. Number of people per room in a household, and smoking did not have association with the occurrence of TB (**Table-3**).

Discussion

In this study several important findings were observed. The prevalence of both pulmonary and extra pulmonary TB among suspects was 46.0%. The smear positivity rate among pulmonary TB suspect was 21.3%. Of the TB suspects, 27.2% were found to be HIV positive. Half of the HIV positive TB suspects had TB. Low knowledge of TB and contact history were predictors of

Table 1. Association of socio-demographic characteristics and TB Addis Ababa, March 2009.

Socio-demographic variables	Presence of TB Disease		P-value
	Yes, no (%)	No, n (%)	
Sex			0.89
Males	113(48.5)	134(49.1)	
Females	120(51.5)	139(50.9)	
Age in years			0.59
15–24	64(27.5)	63(23.1)	
25–34	67(28.8)	78(28.6)	
35–49	68(29.2)	83(30.4)	
>=50	34(14.6)	49(17.9)	
Educational status			0.57
Illiterate	67(28.8)	96(35.2)	
Can read and write	95(40.8)	99(36.3)	
Elementary	22(9.4)	21(7.7)	
High school	38(16.3)	46(16.8)	
Above high school	11(4.7)	11(4.0)	
Occupation			0.89
House wives	56(24.0)	65(23.8)	
Merchant	32(13.7)	44(16.1)	
Government employee	30(12.9)	32(11.7)	
Day laborers	97(41.6)	107(39.2)	
Jobless	18(7.7)	25(9.2)	
Marital status			0.22
Single	104(44.6)	102(37.4)	
Married	97(41.6)	124(45.4)	
Divorced	32(13.7)	47(17.2)	

(n = 506).

Table 2. Association of socio-demograph c characteristics and HIV serostatus Addis Ababa, March 2009.

Socio-demographic variables	HIV serostatus		P-value
	Positive, no (%)	Negative, no (%)	
Sex			0.71
Males	40(49.4)	102(47.0)	
Females	41(50.6)	115(53.0)	
Age in years			0.014
15–24	10(12.3)	61(28.1	
25–34	32(39.5)	62(28.6	
35–49	23(28.4)	67(30.9	
>=50	16(19.8)	27(12.4	
Educational status			0.84
Illiterate	26(32.1)	61(28.1	
Can read and write	34(42.0)	87(40.1	
Elementary	6(7.4)	23(10.6	
High school	12(14.8)	34(15.7	
Above high school	3(3.7)	12(5.5)	
Occupation			0.025
House wives	21(25.9)	49(22.6	
Merchant	15(18.5)	38(17.5	
Government employee	12(14.8)	32(14.7	
Day laborers	22(27.2)	89(41.0	
Jobless	11(13.6)	9(4.1)	
Marital status			0.35
Single	29(35.8)	93(42.9	
Married	36(44.4)	94(43.3	
Divorced	16(19.8)	30(13.8	
Infection with TB			0.32
No TB	40(49.4)	112(51.6	
Pulmonary TB	31(38.3)	90(41.5)	
Extra pulmonary TB	10(12.3)	15(6.9)	
Both PTB and ETB	40(49.4)	102(47.0	

(n = 298).

active TB among suspects. None of the single TB symptoms were associated with occurrence of pulmonary TB.

The smear positivity rate in our study (21.3%) was higher than previous reports in Mali (10%)[20], Ethiopia (15 6%)[21] and Mexico (7.5%) [22], however a high (47.8%) prevalence was observed among patients with cough of more than 3 weeks in Latin America [23]. The prevalence of pulmonary TB in this study is also higher than the finding of Bruchfeld et al who identified a prevalence of 19% using microscopy among TB suspects who had cough of more than 3 weeks in Ethiopia[6]. The prevalence of TB among suspects in the health institution is also higher than the prevalence in the general population of urban[24,25] and rural[26] Ethiopia. The prevalence of HIV among TB suspects (27%) was comparable with the finding of Yassin et al in south Ethiopia[7], but lower than the reports of Odhiambo et al in Kenya (61%)[27], and Srikantiah et al in Uganda (42%)[28]. The difference could be due to the difference in the general HIV prevalence in the countries. The proportion of extra pulmonary TB(15.9%) in this study is lower compared to the national estimate (34%)[2]. The difference could be due to over diagnosis of extrapulmonary TB in rural health centers in Ethiopia where there is no laboratory facilities.

In this study, there was no statistically significant association between HIV and TB disease. Results on the association between HIV and TB among TB suspects are conflicting. A study in Kenya revealed no association between HIV and TB[27]. On the other hand, a study in Uganda[28] showed that HIV prevalence was higher among non-TB patients than TB patients, Brushfeld et al in Ethiopia showed that HIV patients were more likely to have TB than HIV negative individuals[6]. The peak HIV prevalence is in the age group of 35–45 which is consistent with previous report[6]. HIV prevalence is higher among housewives compared to the others. Previous assessment showed that housewives are among the most at high risk groups for HIV infection as a result of the extramarital unprotected sexual affairs of their partners[29,30].

Cough, fever, weight loss and night sweating do not predict the presence of active TB among TB suspects in this study. Recent reports showed that single symptoms of TB such as cough or fever are not sensitive and specific enough to predict the presence of TB. A combination of symptoms should be evaluated for the presence of TB[31,32].

Table 3. Association of symptoms with the occurrence of pulmonary TB, Addis Ababa, March 2009.

Variables	Presence of TB disease		Crude OR (95%CI)	Adjusted OR (95% CI)
	Yes, no (%)	No, no (%)		
Cough				
Yes	181(92.3)	245(89.7)	1.37(0.72,2.65)	-
No	15(7.7)	28(10.3)	1	
Night sweating				
Yes	84(42.9)	130(47.6)	0.82 (0.57.1.19)	-
No	112(57.1)	143(52.4)	1	
Loss of appetite				
Yes	40(20.4)	70(25.6)	0.74(0.47,1.15)	-
No	156(79.6)	203(74.4)	1	
Weight loss				
Yes	37(18.9)	63(23.1)	0.77(0.49,1.22)	-
No	159(81.1)	21(7.7)	1	
Fever				
Yes	33(16.8)	41(15.0)	1.20(0.69,1.88)	-
No	163(83.2)	232(85.0)	1	
Shortness of breath				
Yes	10(5.1)	7(2.6)	2.0(0.76,5.46)	-
No	186(94.9)	266(97.4)	1	
Chest pain				
Yes	63(32.1)	65(23.8)	1.50(1.0,2.28)	-
No	133(67.9)	208(76.2)	1	
Contact with TB patient				
No	138(70.4)	256(93.8)	1	1
Yes	58(29.6)	17(6.2)	5.2(2.9,9.2)	9.1(4.0,20.5)
Knowledge about TB				
Good	16(8.2)	84(30.8)	1	1
Fair	23(11.7)	30(11.0)	4.0(1.8,8.6)	3.7(1.3,10.4)
Poor	157(80.1)	159(58.2)	6.4 (3.6,11.4)	5.2(2.3,11.2)
HIV status				
Negative	90(74.4)	112(73.7)	1	1
Positive	31(25.6)	40(26.3)	1.1(0.6,1.8)	0.8(0.4,1.5)
Number of people per room in a house(average = 2.3 persons/room)				
Below average	110(61.7)	168(61.5)	1	1
Above average	86(56.1)	105(38.5)	1.1(0.8,1.6)	1.3(0.7,2.2)
Smoking				
No	171(87.2)	241(88.3)	1	1
Yes	25(12.8)	32(11.7)	1.1(0.6,1.8)	1.2(0.5,2.7)

(n = 469).

Knowledge of the TB suspects and a contact history were the two major risk factors for active TB in this study population. Individuals who had good knowledge about the transmission methods of TB might protect themselves from the diseases. Several previous reports have shown that contact history is a strong risk factors for the development of active TB[33,34,35]. Number of persons per room which is a proxy indicator of crowding does not predict active TB which is similar to a study conducted in southwest Ethiopia (unpublished data). Frequency and intimacy of contact may be important predictors than the crowding index. History of smoking does not have an association with active pulmonary TB which is in contrast to many literatures[36,37] but in agreement with a study done in Ethiopia.

This study clearly indicated the importance of collaboration of the two diseases. In Africa where the prevalence of both diseases is high, it is quite important to consider both diseases in programming interventions and disease management. Separate planning of individual diseases will result a clear missed opportunities. In our study contact history is a predictor of active TB. This signifies the importance of contact tracing, to identify the contacts of index cases and possible treatment of latent TB cases.

Inclusion of all the health centers in Addis Ababa, use of primary data, and adequate sample size are some of the strength of this study. However, this study has some limitations. First, culture was not done which may introduce misclassification bias. Second, we couldn't follow the outcome of the non-TB patients. Third, we did not measure previous history of TB which might have implication for the finding.

In conclusion, the prevalence of TB among TB suspects is high. Fifty percent of the HIV positive TB suspects had TB. Knowledge and contact history with a TB patient in the family were strong

predictors of TB. Case finding among TB suspects should be intensified particularly among those who have contact history with a TB patient in the family.

Acknowledgments

The authors acknowledge the study participants and health institutions for their unreserved support to give the necessary information.

Author Contributions

Conceived and designed the experiments: AD. Performed the experiments: NN AD. Analyzed the data: AD NN KD. Contributed reagents/materials/analysis tools: AD NN ZM. Wrote the paper: AD NN ZM KD.

References

1. World Health Organization (2009) Global tuberculosis control: epidemiology, strategy, financing, WHO report 2009. Geneva, World Health Organization WHO/HTM/TB/2009.411.
2. Federal Ministry of Health Ethiopia (2007) TB, eprosy and T3/HIV prevention and control program manual, fourth edition. Addis Ababa, Ethiopia.
3. Kassu A, Mengistu G, Ayele B, Diro E, Mekonnen F, et al. (2007) Coinfection and clinical manifestations of tuberculosis in human immunodeficiency virus-infected and -uninfected adults at a teaching hospital, northwest Ethiopia. J Microbiol Immunol Infect 40: 116–122.
4. Ayenew A, Leykun A, Colebunders R, Deribew A (2010) Predictors of HIV testing among patients with tuberculosis in North West Ethiopia: a case-control study. PLoS One 5: e9702.
5. Datiko DG, Lindtjorn B (2009) Health extension workers improve tuberculosis case detection and treatment success in southern Ethiopia: a community randomized trial. PLoS One 4: e5443.
6. Bruchfeld J, Aderaye G, Palme IB, Bjorvatn B, Britton S, et al. (2002) Evaluation of outpatients with suspected pulmonary tuberculosis in a high HIV prevalence setting in Ethiopia: clinical, diagnostic and epidemiological characteristics. Scand J Infect Dis 34: 331–337.
7. Yassin MA, Takele L, Gebresenbet S, Girma E, Lera M, et al. (2004) HIV and tuberculosis coinfection in the southern region of Ethiopia: a prospective epidemiological study. Scand J Infect Dis 36: 670–673.
8. World Health Organization (2004) Interim policy on collaborative TB/HIV activities. World Health Organization, WHO/HTM/TB/2004.330.
9. World Health Organization (2006) Improving the diagnosis and treatment of smear-negative pulmonary and extrapulmonary tuberculosis among adults and adolescents. Recommendations for HIV-prevalent and resource-constrained settings. Geneva, http//:www.who.int/gtb.
10. World Health Organization (2004) Interim policy on collaborative TB/HIV activities Geneva: World Health Organization (WHO/HTM/TB/2004.33).
11. Mohammed A, Ehrlich R, Wood R, Cilliers F, Maartens G (2004) Screening for tuberculosis in adults with advanced HIV infection prior to preventive therapy. Int J Tuberc Lung Dis 8: 792–5.
12. Day JH, Charalambous S, Fielding KL, Hayes RJ, Churchyard GJ, et al. (2006) Screening for tuberculosis prior to isoniazid preventive therapy among HIV-infected gold miners in South Africa. Int J Tuberc Lung Dis 10: 523–9.
13. Lawn SD, Myer L, Bekker LG, Wood R (2006) Burden of tuberculosis in an antiretroviral treatment programme in sub-Saharan Africa: impact on treatment outcomes and implications for tuberculosis control. AIDS 20: 1605–12. doi: 10.1097/01.aids.0000238406.93249.cd.
14. Bonnet MM, Pinoges LL, Varaine FF, Oberhauser BB, O'Brien DD, et al. (2006) Tuberculosis after HAART initiation in HIV-positive patients from five countries with a high tuberculosis burden. AIDS 20: 1275–9. doi: 10.1097/01.aids.0000232235.26630.ee.
15. Lawn SD, Myer L, Bekker LG, Wood R (2007) Tuberculosis-associated immune reconstitution disease: incidence, risk factors and impact in an antiretroviral treatment service in South Africa. AIDS 21 335–41. doi: 10.1097/QAD.0-b013e328011efac.
16. Central Statistical Authority, Ethiopia (2008) Summary and Statistical Report of the 2007 Population and Housing Census Results.
17. Authority, Ethiopia (2000) Sputum examination for tuberculosis by direct microscopy in low income countries: 5th ed. Paris, France IUATLD.
18. Deribew A, Negussu N, Kassahun W, Apers L Colebunders R (2010) Uptake of provider initiated counseling and testing among suspects of tuberculosis, Ethiopia. Int J Tuberc Lung Dis 14(10): 1–5.
19. Wondimu T, W/Michael K, Kassahun W, Getachew S (2007) Delay in initiating tuberculosis treatment and factors associated among pulmonary

20. tuberculosis patients in East Wollega, Western Ethiopia. Ethiop J Health Dev 21(2): 148–156.
20. Banda HT, Harries AD, Welby S, Boeree MJ, Wirima JJ, et al. (1998) Prevalence of tuberculosis in TB suspects with short duration of cough. Trans R Soc Trop Med Hyg 92: 161–163.
21. Wesen A, Mitike G (2009) Screening and case detection for tuberculosis among people living with HIV in Addis Ababa, Ethiopia. Ethiop Med J 47: 109–115.
22. Sánchez-Pérez H, Flores-Hernández J, Jansá J, Caylá, Martín-Mateo M (2001) Pulmonary tuberculosis and associated factors in areas of high levels of poverty in Chiapas, Mexico. Int J Epidemiol 30(2): 386–93.
23. Romero-Sandoval NC, Flores-Carrera OF, Sánchez-Férez HJ, Sánchez-Pérez I, Mateo MM (2007) Pulmonary tuberculosis in an indigenous community in the mountains of Ecuador. Int J Tuberc Lung Dis 11(5): 550–5.
24. Shargie EB, Morkve O, Lindtjorn B (2006) Tuberculosis case-finding through a village outreach programme in a rural setting in southern Ethiopia: community randomized trial. Bull World Health Organ 84: 112–119.
25. Yimer S, Holm-Hansen C, Yimaldu T, Bjune G (2009) Evaluating an active case-finding strategy to identify smear-positive tuberculosis in rural Ethiopia. Int J Tuberc Lung Dis 13: 1399–1404.
26. Demissie M, Zenebere B, Berhane Y, Lindtjorn B (2002) A rapid survey to determine the prevalence of smear-positive tuberculosis in Addis Ababa. Int J Tuberc Lung Dis 6: 580–584.
27. Odhiambo J, Kizito W, Njoroge A, Wambua N, Nganga L, et al. (2008) Provider-initiated HIV testing and counselling for TB patients and suspects in Nairobi, Kenya. Int J Tuberc Lung Dis 12: 63–68.
28. Srikantiah P, Lin R, Walusimbi M, Okwera A, Luzze H, et al. (2007) Elevated HIV seroprevalence and risk behavior among Ugandan TB suspects: implications for HIV testing and prevention. Int J Tuberc Lung Dis 11: 168–174.
29. Federal Ministry of Health, Ethiopia (2005) Behavioral Surveillance Survey 2005. Addis Ababa, Ethiopia.
30. Shabbir I, Larson CP (1995) Urban to rural routes of HIV infection spread in Ethiopia. J Trop Med Hyg 98: 338–342.
31. Cain KP, McCarthy KD, Heilig CM, Monkongdee P, Tasaneeyapan T, et al. (2010) An algorithm for tuberculosis screening and diagnosis in people with HIV. N Engl J Med 362: 707–716.
32. Shah NS, Anh MH, Thuy TT, Duong Thom BS, Linh T, et al. (2008) Population-based chest X-ray screening for pulmonary tuberculosis in people living with HIV/AIDS, An Giang, Vietnam. Int J Tuberc Lung Dis 12: 404–410.
33. Lienhardt C, Fielding K, Sillah J, Tunkara A, Donkor S, et al. (2003) Risk factors for tuberculosis infection in sub-Saharan Africa: a contact study in The Gambia. Am J Respir Crit Care Med 168: 448–455.
34. Lienhardt C, Fielding K, Sillah JS, Bah B, Gustafson P, et al. (2005) Investigation of the risk factors for tuberculosis: a case-control study in three countries in West Africa. Int J Epidemiol 34: 914–923.
35. Hill PC, Jackson-Sillah D, Donkor SA, Otu J, Adegbola RA, et al. (2006) Risk factors for pulmonary tuberculosis: a clinic-based case control study in The Gambia. BMC Public Health 6: 156.
36. Ariyothai N, Podhipak A, Akarasewi P, Tornee S, Smithtikarn S, et al. (2004) Cigarette smoking and its relation to pulmonary tuberculosis in adults. Southeast Asian J Trop Med Public Health 35: 219–227.
37. Lin HH, Ezzati M, Chang HY, Murray M (2009) Association between tobacco smoking and active tuberculosis in Taiwan: prospective cohort study. Am J Respir Crit Care Med 180: 475–480.

17

A Cross-Sectional Study of Disclosure of HIV Status to Children and Adolescents in Western Kenya

Rachel C. Vreeman[1,2]*, **Michael L. Scanlon[1,2]**, **Ann Mwangi[2,3]**, **Matthew Turissini[1,2]**, **Samuel O. Ayaya[2,4]**, **Constance Tenge[2,4]**, **Winstone M. Nyandiko[2,4]**

1 Children's Health Services Research, Department of Pediatrics, Indiana University School of Medicine, Indianapolis, Indiana, United States of America, 2 USAID-Academic Model Providing Access to Healthcare (AMPATH), Eldoret, Kenya, 3 Department of Behavioral Science, School of Medicine, College of Health Sciences, Moi University, Eldoret, Kenya, 4 Department of Child Health and Paediatrics, School of Medicine, College of Health Sciences, Moi University, Eldoret, Kenya

Abstract

Introduction: Disclosure of HIV status to children is essential for disease management but is not well characterized in resource-limited settings. This study aimed to describe the prevalence of disclosure and associated factors among a cohort of HIV-infected children and adolescents in Kenya.

Methods: We conducted a cross-sectional study, randomly sampling HIV-infected children ages 6–14 years attending 4 HIV clinics in western Kenya. Data were collected from questionnaires administered by clinicians to children and their caregivers, supplemented with chart review. Descriptive statistics and disclosure prevalence were calculated. Univariate analyses and multivariate logistic regression were performed to assess the association between disclosure and key child-level demographic, clinical and psychosocial characteristics.

Results: Among 792 caregiver-child dyads, mean age of the children was 9.7 years (SD = 2.6) and 51% were female. Prevalence of disclosure was 26% and varied significantly by age; while 62% of 14-year-olds knew their status, only 42% of 11-year-olds and 21% of 8-year-olds knew. In multivariate regression, older age (OR 1.49, 95%CI 1.35–1.63), taking antiretroviral drugs (OR 2.27, 95%CI 1.29–3.97), and caregiver-reported depression symptoms (OR 2.63, 95%CI 1.12–6.20) were significantly associated with knowing one's status. Treatment site was associated with disclosure for children attending one of the rural clinics compared to the urban clinic (OR 3.44, 95%CI 1.75–6.76).

Conclusions: Few HIV-infected children in Kenya know their HIV status. The likelihood of disclosure is associated with clinical and psychosocial factors. More data are needed on the process of disclosure and its impact on children.

Editor: Julian W. Tang, Alberta Provincial Laboratory for Public Health/University of Alberta, Canada

Funding: This research was supported in part by a grant (K23MH087225) to Dr. Rachel Vreeman from the NIMH and by the USAID-AMPATH Partnership from the United States Agency for International Development as part of the President's Emergency Plan for AIDS Relief (PEPFAR). The funders had no role in study design, data collection and analysis, decision to publish, or preparation of the manuscript.

Competing Interests: The authors have declared that no competing interests exist.

* E-mail: rvreeman@iupui.edu

Introduction

In 2011, the World Health Organization (WHO) estimated there were 3.4 million children under 15 years of age living with the Human Immunodeficiency Virus (HIV), while an estimated 330,000 children were newly infected in 2011 alone. [1] The advent of antiretroviral therapy (ART) and expanded access to treatment have resulted in more HIV-infected children reaching adolescence and adulthood, [2] especially in resource-limited settings like sub-Saharan Africa, which is home to over 90% of the pediatric HIV-infected population. [1] As HIV-infected children live longer, emerging challenges to comprehensive pediatric HIV care include supporting high rates of adherence to treatment, preventing secondary transmission and promoting overall physical and mental health. [3] For these children, learning about their HIV diagnosis - often referred to as disclosure - is an important step towards long-term disease management and necessary for the transition from pediatric care into adolescent and adult care settings. [4].

In the United States, recommendations for disclosure of HIV status to children endorse a gradual process of giving age-appropriate information as the child develops the cognitive and emotional maturity to process this information. [5] Globally, institutions such as the WHO have issued similar guidelines, [6] but there are few published data on standardized, culturally appropriate disclosure protocols in resource-limited settings. A recent review on disclosure of HIV status to children found that lower proportions of children in low- and middle-income countries (LMIC) knew their status compared to those in high-income countries and among those that did know, children in LMIC reported learning it at older ages. [7] Of the 21 studies included for review by Pinzon-Iregui et al. that reported prevalence of disclosure, median prevalence of disclosure among similarly aged children was 20% in studies conducted in LMIC and 43% in high-income countries, while median age of disclosure was 9.6 years in

Caregiver Questionnaire Items

1. Does the child know that he/she comes to the AMPATH clinic for HIV care?
2. Does the child know that he/she has HIV?
3. Does the child know that the name of his/her illness is HIV?
4. Does the child know that he/she is taking medicines for HIV?
5. If the child does not know that he/she has HIV, what explanation do you give for coming to the clinic or for taking medicines?
6. Does the child ever ask questions about why he/she has to take medicines?
7. Does the child ever refuse to take the medicines he/she is supposed to take?
8. Do you ever not give the medicines because you do not want to give them in front of other people?
9. Do you ever have problems with giving the medicines because the child does not know why he/she is taking them?
10. Does the child ever have problems taking the medicines on time or taking them every day?
11. Do other children avoid playing with the child because of his/her HIV status?
12. Do other children tease or call the child hurtful names because of his/her HIV status?
13. Has your child been rejected by friends or family because of his/her illness?
14. Does your child seem to have little interest or pleasure in doing things lately?
15. Has your child been feeling down, depressed, or hopeless?

Child Questionnaire Items

Items 1-8 were administered to ALL children.
1. Why do you come for visits at the AMPATH clinic?
2. Do you know what your illness is called?
3. Why do you have to take medicines?
4. Do you ever miss taking the medicines that you are supposed to take?
5. Do you ever refuse to take the medicines that you are supposed to take?
6. Do you ever not take the medicines because you do not want to take them in front of other people?
7. Do you ever have problems taking the medicines because you do not know why you are taking them?
8. Do you ever have problems taking the medicines on time or taking them every day?

Items 9-17 were administered to ONLY disclosed children (answered 'HIV' to Item 1-3)
9. Have you been told that your illness is HIV?
10. Before you knew that you had HIV, did you ask questions about why you had to take the medicines?
11. Do you still have questions about why you have to take medicines?
12. Do other children avoid playing with you because of your HIV status?
13. Do other children tease or call you hurtful names because of your HIV status?
14. Have you ever been rejected by friends or family because of your illness?
15. Do you seem to have little interest or pleasure in doing things lately?
16. Have you been feeling down, depressed, or hopeless?
17. Who informed you of your HIV status?

Figure 1. Disclosure questionnaire items.

LMIC and 8.3 years in high-income countries. Caregivers in both resource-poor and resource-rich settings report weighing the potential risks and benefits of disclosure. While the child's increasing age, independence and concerns about medication adherence may motivate caregivers to disclose, caregivers often have fears about the negative emotional effects of disclosure and HIV-related stigma and discrimination. Few studies have measured the actual impact of disclosure on children's clinical, emotional and psychosocial outcomes. [8] Anecdotal evidence from qualitative and quantitative studies suggests both positive and negative effects of disclosure on disease progression, adherence to ART, caregiver-child relationships, access to social support and psychological health outcomes.

As children in HIV care systems mature through adolescence, more data on disclosure of their HIV status in resource-limited settings are needed. These data will help inform the design and adoption of culturally-relevant guidelines which providers and other health professionals can use to support caregivers and children through this difficult process. Previously, we reported the results of a pilot study on the prevalence of disclosure among 270 HIV-infected children at a single urban clinic in western Kenya [9] under the umbrella of the Academic Model Providing Access to Healthcare (AMPATH), one of the largest HIV care systems in sub-Saharan Africa. This article describes the results of the parent study that assessed the prevalence of disclosure and factors associated with disclosure among a larger sample drawn from 4 urban and rural AMPATH clinics across western Kenya.

Methods

Study Design

We conducted a cross-sectional study using assessments of a random sample of caregivers and their HIV-infected children ages 6–14 years receiving care at four AMPATH clinics in western Kenya. Clinicians independently administered a 17-item questionnaire to HIV-infected children and a 15-item questionnaire to their caregivers at routine clinic visits to assess disclosure status, ART adherence, stigma and depression (see Figure 1 for full set of caregiver and child questionnaire items on the Disclosure Questionnaire). Children were asked to leave the examination room when clinicians were administering the questionnaire to caregivers to avoid accidental disclosure. All children were asked general questions about reasons for receiving care and disclosure status, but only children who self-reported knowing their HIV status were asked questions about HIV-related stigma and depression. Caregivers were asked to respond to HIV-related stigma and depression as experienced by their children. Depression symptoms were evaluated using the PHQ-2 questions, [10] but other questionnaire items were developed in this setting. Demographic and clinical characteristics of child participants were extracted from chart review. Age, weight, orphan status, medications, and duration of enrollment in AMPATH were calculated at study visit. The most recent CD4 count and CD4 percentage (CD4%) in a child's medical chart was used. No demographic or other data were collected for caregivers. The study was approved by the Institutional Review Board at Indiana University School of Medicine in Indianapolis, Indiana, USA and by the Institutional Research and Ethics Committee at Moi University School of Medicine in Eldoret, Kenya. Consent and assent were waived for this study as the questionnaires were administered during routine visits with clinicians and the assessments were in line with AMPATH's protocol to begin routine collection of disclosure data. Both the Institutional Review Board at Indiana University School of Medicine and the

Institutional Research and Ethics Committee at Moi University School of Medicine approved the waiving of consent and assent for this study. Data were collected from July 2011 to June 2012.

Setting

AMPATH is a partnership between Moi University School of Medicine, Moi Teaching and Referral Hospital (MTRH) and a consortium of North American academic medical centers led by Indiana University. [11] As of January 2013, AMPATH provides comprehensive HIV care, including free ART and psychosocial and nutritional support, to over 55,000 HIV-infected adults and 15,000 pediatric patients in 56 clinics and satellite sites across western Kenya. AMPATH's protocol on disclosure of HIV status to children recommends initiating disclosure for all children who are 10 years and above but the decision to disclose is ultimately left to the child's caregiver. Caregivers are invited to private and group disclosure counseling sessions and offered support at the clinic that includes information about HIV, discussing worries, fears and potential advantages of disclosure and making a disclosure plan. Children over 14 years of age, those without caregivers and those at risk of endangering themselves through poor adherence or others through sexual activity are often identified for enhanced disclosure counseling.

Study Participants

The study population was caregivers and their HIV-infected children ages 6 to 14 years who were enrolled in care at 4 AMPATH clinics: MTRH, Kitale, Turbo, and, Webuye. These clinics were selected because they are among AMPATH's largest pediatric sites and treat geographically and ethnically diverse patient populations. A "caregiver" was defined as someone responsible for the well-being of the child, who brought the child to clinic, and who was knowledgeable about the child's HIV care behaviors (e.g., adherence to ART). HIV infection was defined as having one positive HIV DNA PCR test or one positive HIV ELISA antibody test. A patient randomization module within the electronic health record system was used to select a random sample of HIV-infected patients ages 6 to 14 years enrolled in care at the 4 study clinics. Disclosure status was not recorded in the electronic data and was not considered in the inclusion criteria. The minimum age limit was based on a previous pilot study that included a subset of this population [9] while the maximum age limit was selected because children aged 15 years and above are often treated in adult care settings where HIV disclosure is assumed. No incentives were provided to study participants for participation.

Outcomes

The outcome variable was children's disclosure status, defined as a binomial variable of "disclosed" versus "not disclosed." Children were considered disclosed if the caregiver answered "yes" to any of the questions about the child knowing about their HIV status (see Figure 1, Caregiver Items 1–4) or if the child reported HIV as the reason he/she comes to clinic or takes medications, the name of his/her illness or if he/she reported being told their illness is HIV (see Figure 1, Child Items 1–3, 9).

Data Analysis

Descriptive statistics were calculated and the prevalence of disclosure was described for child participants and within subcategories by age. Univariate analyses with Pearson's chi-squared (χ^2) tests were used to investigate associations between a child's disclosure status and child-level demographic, clinical and psychosocial characteristics. Multivariate analyses were then conducted using logistic regression with odds ratios (OR) and 95% confidence intervals (95%CI). As this was a largely exploratory analysis, we included the entire set of variables in the multivariate model whether they were significant in univariate analyses or not. Binomial variables were calculated to describe child-level adherence, stigma and depression based on child and caregiver responses.

"Non-adherence" was defined as any missed doses in the past 30 days by caregiver-report or child-report on the standard AMPATH clinical encounter form or any indication of adherence difficulties reported by caregivers (see Figure 1, Caregiver Items 7–10) or children (see Figure 1, Child Items 4–8) on the Disclosure Questionnaire. "Stigma" was defined as any indication of child-experienced stigma from the caregiver (see Figure 1, Caregiver Items 11–13) or the child (see Figure 1, Child Items 12–14) and "depression" was defined by any indication of child depression symptoms as reported by the caregiver (see Figure 1, Caregiver Items 14, 15) or the child (see Figure 1, Child Items 15, 16) using the PHQ-2. All statistical analyses were performed using STATA version 10.0 (StataCorp LP, College Station, Texas, USA).

Results

Characteristics of Child Participants

Among 792 children, mean age was 9.8 years (SD = 2.6) and 51% were female (Table 1). Children had a mean weight-for-age Z-score (WAZ) of −1.3 (SD = 1.2). Almost half of the children were orphans (48%) with orphan defined as having a deceased biological mother, having a deceased biological father or having both. The biological mother was the caregiver for a little over half of the children (60%). Most children were on ART (79%), while only 16 children (2%) were also taking anti-tuberculosis medication. Children had a mean duration of enrollment in an AMPATH clinic of 48 months (SD = 25.3) and mean CD4% of 28% (SD = 0.16). Only 8% of children had indications of non-adherence to ART on the standard clinical encounter form.

Prevalence of Disclosure

The overall prevalence of disclosure was 26%. The proportion of children who knew their status was greater among older children compared to young children. Disclosure by age is shown in Table 1. While only 9% of 6- to 7-year olds knew their status, 33% of 10- to 11-year olds and 56% of 13- to 14-year olds reported knowing their status (Figure 2). The prevalence of disclosure also differed by clinic: disclosure prevalence was highest at Webuye (40%) and lowest at MTRH (17%).

Association between Disclosure and Child Characteristics

In univariate analyses, older age (p<.01), being an orphan (p = .04), having a lower CD4 count (p = .03), being on ART (p = .01), ethnic group (p<.01) and treatment site (p<.01) were all significantly associated with knowing one's status (Table 1). While disclosure status was not associated with adherence either reported on the clinical encounter form or by caregivers, disclosure was associated with child-reported adherence (p = .03) with disclosed children reporting more non-adherence than non-disclosed children (Table 2). Caregiver-reported child-experienced stigma and child depression symptoms were both significantly associated with disclosure; while only 2% caregivers of non-disclosed children reported stigma and 4% reported depression symptoms, 10% of caregivers of disclosed children reported stigma (p<.01) and 12% reported depression symptoms (p<.01).

In multivariate analyses, variables significantly associated with disclosure were a child's older age (OR 1.5, 95%CI 1.3–1.6), being on ART (OR 2.3, 95%CI 1.3–4.0), and caregiver-reported child depression symptoms (OR 2.6, 95%CI 1.1–6.2) (Table 3). Treatment site was also associated with disclosure at two clinics; being treated at Webuye compared to MTRH was significantly associated with disclosure (OR 3.4, 95%CI 1.7–6.8). Children with a deceased father tended to be more likely to know their status than non-orphans (OR 1.6, 95%CI 0.9–2.8), as did children with caregivers who reported experiences of HIV stigma (OR 2.4, 95%CI 0.9–6.2), but neither test reached statistical significance. Gender, primary caregiver, CD4%, duration enrolled in AMPATH, malnutrition and adherence were not associated with disclosure in multivariate regression.

Child versus Caregiver-reported Variables

Child-reported versus caregiver-reported variables related to disclosure status, adherence to ART, and experiences of stigma and depression were analyzed to identify discrepancies. Caregivers were more likely to report that the child knew their HIV status (p<.01), had poor adherence (p<.01), and had experiences with HIV-related stigma (p<.01) and depression symptoms (p<.01) compared to children's self-reports.

Discussion

As children with HIV survive into adolescence and adulthood at unprecedented rates, disclosure of HIV status is an essential component of pediatric HIV care and long-term disease management. This study investigated the prevalence and correlates of disclosure of HIV status to children in 4 clinics in western Kenya. We found a minority of children aged 6–14 years knew their status, consistent with findings from studies in Ghana, [12] Uganda, [13] and a previous study in Nairobi, Kenya, which found prevalence of disclosure to be 19% among 271 children with a median age of 9 years. [14] We did, however, find higher rates of disclosure in this expanded sample compared to rates of disclosure in a pilot study that revealed only 11% of children (median age 9.3 years) knew their HIV status. The results of this study prompted a program-wide reevaluation of AMPATH disclosure protocols and retraining of clinic-level staff. We are also now in the process of evaluating a 2–year disclosure intervention that includes further training of disclosure staff, employment of dedicated disclosure counselors and tailored disclosure curricula and materials.

Our study revealed a number of associations between disclosure status and demographic and clinical characteristics. Older children knew their status more frequently than younger children, likely as a result of increasing maturity, independence and responsibility for self-care that required knowledge of their status. For example, our finding that those on ART were significantly more likely to know their status may reflect disclosure following increased disease management activities like taking ART. We did not find any associations between disclosure status and clinical indicators like CD4 count and WHO disease stage. A study among Thai adolescents found that while disclosure was associated with CD4% below 30% in multivariate analysis, disclosure status was not associated with virologic outcomes. [15] In contrast, a study in Romania found that children who did not know their HIV status were at higher risk for disease progression, measured by CD4 count decline and death compared to disclosed children. [16] Other clinic-level factors like retention in care may also be associated with disclosure status and are important to understand, however, we did not evaluate retention in care in this study.

Table 1. Demographic and Clinical Characteristics of Child Participants by Disclosure Status.

Variable	Disclosed No (N = 588)		Disclosed Yes (N = 204)		P-Value†
	N	%	N	%	
Gender					
Female	298	51%	107	52%	0.663
Male	290	49%	97	48%	
On ART					
Yes	450	24%	174	86%	0.006*
No	138	76%	29	14%	
On Anti-TB					
Yes	14	2%	2	1%	0.221
No	572	98%	201	99%	0.221
WHO Stage					
1	135	23%	64	32%	0.079
2	142	24%	41	20%	
3	271	46%	89	44%	
4	39	7%	9	4%	
Orphan Status					
Both parents living	325	55%	91	45%	0.043*
Both parents dead	70	12%	35	17%	
Mother dead	57	10%	23	11%	
Father dead	79	13%	28	19%	
Do not know	57	10%	17	8%	
Caregiver					
Mother	347	59%	104	51%	0.382
Father	56	9%	19	9%	
Aunt/Uncle	69	125	28	14%	
Grandparent	52	9%	19	9%	
Sibling	18	3%	9	5%	
Children's Home	15	3%	8	4%	
Other	31	5%	17	8%	
Ethnic Group					
Kalenjin	168	29%	36	17%	0.001*
Kikuyu	69	12%	18	9%	
Luhya	265	45%	126	62%	
Luo	47	8%	12	6%	
Other	39	6%	12	6%	
Clinic					
MTRH	223	38%	47	23%	<0.001*
Kitale	123	21%	44	22%	
Turbo	132	22%	40	19%	
Webuye	110	19%	73	36%	
Adherence on Clinic Encounter (30-day recall)					
Adherent	542	92%	185	91%	0.504
Non-adherent	46	8%	19	9%	
	Mean	SD	Mean	SD	
Age (years)	9.4	2.2	11.4	2.3	<0.001*

Table 1. Cont.

Variable	Disclosed No (N = 588)		Disclosed Yes (N = 204)		P-Value†
	N	%	N	%	
Time enrolled at AMPATH clinic (months)	47.9	24.9	47.6	24.9	0.967
CD4 Count	753.5	453.4	712.3	386.3	0.035*
CD4%	0.29	0.18	0.27	0.10	0.582

†Univariate analyses using Pearson's chi-squared tests.
*Significant at the p<0.05 level.

The relationship between adherence to ART and disclosure is not well described and studies report mixed results.[17–19] There are several reasons disclosure might be associated with non-adherence. Disclosure is a traumatic event for many children and can be accompanied by feelings of anger, hopelessness and rebellion, which may lead to temporary or longer-term adherence problems. The negative effects of HIV-related stigma, including efforts to keep the diagnosis secret by hiding or not taking medicines, may also impact adherence to therapy for disclosed children more than non-disclosed children. Adherence issues may be compounded by other adolescent-specific factors such as increased incidence of depression [20] and generally poorer medication adherence among this age group. [21] On the other hand, there are also reasons to believe disclosure may lead to improved adherence, including increased responsibility over medication-taking and better access to social support. Pediatric HIV providers often recommend disclosure of HIV status to children as necessary to building trusting provider-patient and family relationships and developing disease management skills that facilitate adherence. [22] In the only longitudinal study to assess adherence pre- and post-disclosure, Blasini et al reported that approximately 58% of children and their caregivers reported that adherence improved post-disclosure; however, adherence was assessed by self- and proxy-report among a small sample of only 40 children and clinicians felt that adherence improved in only 25% of cases. [23] Furthermore, since the study assessed disclosure after an intensive, supportive disclosure intervention, its results may not be representative of the majority of disclosure experiences.

Our finding that reports of adherence differed significantly depending on whether adherence was caregiver-reported or child-reported is indicative of the ongoing difficulties of clinic-level staff in resource-limited settings to accurately assess adherence to ART. A systematic review on adherence to ART found that adherence assessment items are rarely validated, that proxy-reports (i.e., caregiver-reports) often overestimate adherence and that children report more non-adherence than their caregivers do. [24] In our study, children reported less non-adherence than their caregivers, but these findings may be shaped by several cultural-specific biases. In particular, children in this setting with strong cultural traditions requiring children to obey authority figures (i.e., caregivers and clinicians) may be more vulnerable to social desirability pressure to report higher adherence. [25] In addition, despite clinical protocols recommending private interviewing of children about adherence, children are seldom questioned in private as was required for completion of the evaluations within this study. Finally, many of the children involved in this study were in the care of their grandparents and other extended family members rather than their biological parents. These non-parent caregivers may feel less pressure to report adherence.

Few studies investigate the psychosocial impact of disclosure in resource-limited settings. While this study was not designed to assess the impact by pre- and post-disclosure characteristics, we found higher rates of experiences of HIV-related stigma and depression symptoms among disclosed children, although only depression symptoms were significantly associated with disclosure in multivariate regression. This finding contradicts the findings of studies from the US and Zambia that suggest non-disclosed

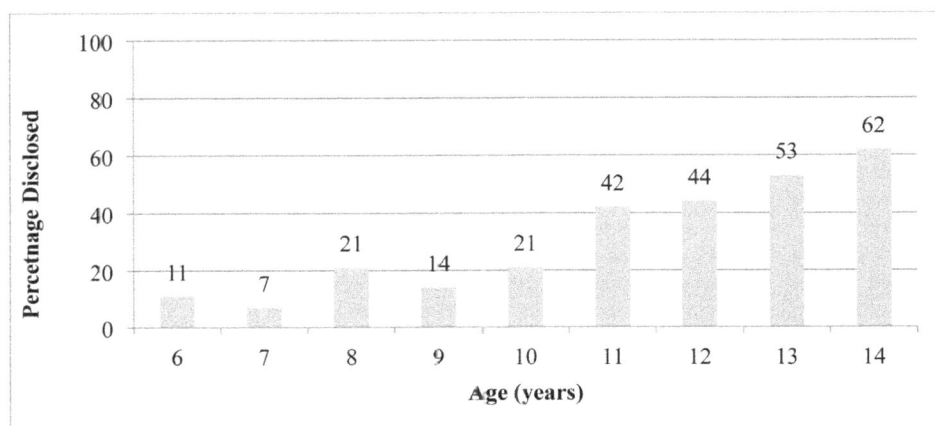

Figure 2. Prevalence of disclosure by age.

Table 2. Indicators of Adherence, Stigma and Depression by Caregiver- and Child-Report.

Variable	Disclosed No (N = 588)		Disclosed Yes (N = 204)		P-Value†
	N	%	N	%	
Caregiver-Reported Variables:					
Combined Adherence					
Adherent	280	48%	92	45%	0.534
Non-adherent	308	52%	112	55%	
Combined Stigma					
No reported stigma	575	98%	184	90%	<0.001*
Reported stigma	13	2%	20	10%	
Combined Depression					
No reported depression	566	96%	180	88%	<0.001*
Reported depression	22	4%	24	12%	
Child-Reported Variables:					
Combined Adherence					
Adherent	488	83%	155	76%	0.027*
Non-adherent	100	17%	49	24%	
Combined Stigma**					
No reported stigma	–	–	189	93%	–
Reported stigma	–	–	15	7%	–
Combined Depression**	–	–			–
No reported depression	–	–	195	96%	–
Reported depression	–	–	9	4%	–

†Univariate analyses using Pearson's chi-squared tests.
*Significant at the p<0.05 level.
**Only disclosed children were asked questions about stigma and depression.

children have increased levels of psychological distress, including anxiety and depression, internalizing behavioral problems and poorer psychological adjustment compared to children that know their status.[26–28] In one of the few longitudinal studies measuring the psychosocial impact of disclosure, Butler et al found no significant association between caregiver-reported quality of life indicators pre- and post-disclosure among 395 perinatally HIV-infected children in the US Pediatric AIDS Clinical Trials Group 219C. [29] Our findings highlight the need to investigate the impact of disclosure on emotional and mental health outcomes in settings like Kenya so that appropriate support services can be provided.

Significant variations in the prevalence of disclosure among the clinics included in this study deserve further attention. Our analyses may not capture significant clinic-level factors, such as clinic staff motivated or experienced in disclosure; cultural factors such as varying populations of ethnic groups with differing perspectives on disclosure; or other structural factors like urban versus rural characteristics and transportation time and cost to clinic. In our sample, the prevalence of disclosure was highest at Webuye (39.9%), one of the rural satellite clinics, and was significantly lower at MTRH (17.4%), the second largest referral hospital in the country located in an urban center. Interestingly, caregivers of children attending Webuye clinic also reported significantly higher medication adherence (63.4%) than caregivers of children at MTRH (28.8%). We are aware of at least one nurse counselor at the Webuye clinic who expressed high interest in disclosure and its impact on care, which may contribute to the clinic's higher rates of disclosure. While AMPATH clinics routinely offer counseling (including disclosure counseling) and support group services to children and their caregivers, we did not investigate differences in clinic-level services or their utilization by study group participants. Identifying clinic-level factors that promote or impede disclosure may help shape best practices for pediatric HIV care.

Many factors influence how and when caregivers decide to disclose to a child. This study did not assess caregiver perspectives on disclosure; however, previous qualitative work in this setting found that caregivers of HIV-infected children weighed potential risks and benefits as they made their decisions about when to disclose. [30] Perceived risks in this setting included the child being too young to understand, negative emotional consequences for the child and the subsequent disclosure of the child's status to others, resulting in stigma and discrimination. At least one study found that children who disclosed their status to friends over the study period showed greater improvements in CD4 cell counts than children who had not disclosed, which may suggest better health outcomes after engaging social support. [31] On the other hand, caregivers believed that disclosure might lead to positive changes, including the child asking fewer questions, improved adherence to medications, and better access to social support. These findings are consistent with perspectives of caregivers in other resource-rich and resource-limited settings, who identify similar risks and benefits of disclosure. [7] While not significant, we found some indication that disclosure status varies by ethnic group in our setting in western Kenya. More qualitative data are needed to further explore how cultural beliefs may impact decisions about how and when to disclose HIV status to children in this setting.

Table 3. Factors Associated with Disclosure Status in Multivariate Regression Model.

Variable	Odds Ratio	95% Confidence Interval
Female vs. Male	0.81	0.55–1.20
Age	1.49	1.35–1.63*
On ART (Yes vs. No)	2.26	1.29–3.97*
On Anti-TBs (Yes vs. No)	0.15	0.01–2.50
Time enrolled at AMPATH clinic	1.00	0.99–1.01
CD4%	0.54	0.14–2.05
Orphan Status		
Total orphan vs. Non-orphan	1.19	0.49–2.90
Mother dead vs. Non-orphan	0.87	0.39–1.97
Father dead vs. Non-orphan	1.62	0.92–2.85
Parent status unknown vs. Non-orphan	1.35	0.53–3.48
Malnutrition		
Mild malnutrition vs. Normal	1.06	0.66–1.71
Moderate malnutrition vs. Normal	1.07	0.61–1.89
Severe malnutrition vs. Normal	0.75	0.26–2.16
Disease Stage		
WHO Stage II vs. WHO Stage I	0.62	0.35–1.09
WHO Stage III vs. WHO Stage I	0.72	0.43–1.21
WHO Stage IV vs. WHO Stage I	0.41	0.15–1.08
Ethnic Group		
Kikuyu vs. Kalenjin	1.42	0.66–3.12
Luhya vs. Kalenjin	1.66	0.95–2.90
Luo vs. Kalenjin	1.74	0.72–4.20
Clinic		
Webuye vs. MTRH	3.44	1.75–6.76*
Kitale vs. MTRH	1.94	0.96–3.92
Turbo vs. MTRH	1.50	0.76–2.95
Caregiver-reported variables		
Non-adherent vs. Adherent	1.31	0.86–1.98
Reported stigma vs. No reported stigma	2.39	0.93–6.18
Reported depression vs. No reported depression	2.63	1.12–6.20*

*Significant in multivariate regression (95%CI does not include 1.00).

This study had a number of limitations for consideration. One limitation was that we did not assess the prevalence of partial disclosure, where a child has incomplete information about HIV, which may be part of an age-appropriate disclosure process. [32] We counted any knowledge of HIV as a reason for treatment as disclosure. In other cases, caregivers or healthcare providers may give inaccurate information regarding the child's diagnosis, such as attributing the illness, medication or clinic responsibilities to a different, often less-stigmatized condition like tuberculosis. Investigating how partial disclosure and misinformation are used by caregivers and healthcare providers and the impact on full disclosure, clinical outcomes, and psychosocial outcomes are important to understand. We also did not consider whether time since diagnosis or duration on ART were associated with disclosure of HIV status. In this setting, the vast majority of children are perinatally infected and thus diagnosed at birth or shortly thereafter but age at ART initiation varies from child to child. Time since diagnosis and duration on ART may be important factors associated with

disclosure [33] and should be investigated in this setting. Another potential limitation of this study was the validity of the proxy- and self-reports for obtaining information on disclosure status, adherence, and experiences of stigma and depression. Validated measures for assessing disclosure status do not exist, so we attempted to use a variety of questionnaire items, evaluating potential aspects of disclosure such as whether the child knew their disease, the name of their disease, why they took medicines, or why they attended clinic. We used the PHQ-2 depression screening questions because they have reasonable validity and reliability among HIV-infected adults in western Kenya [34] and adolescents in the US [35] but there are no such studies on depression screening among children and adolescents in this setting. No validated measures for HIV-related stigma currently exist for this population. [36] Data related to disclosure were collected in the context of a routine HIV clinic visit, which limits the data points available. It is also possible that the caregivers or children may have been hesitant to discuss disclosure status, adherence, stigma, or depression symptoms with their regular clinician. Nonetheless, our intent was to make these discussions a routine part of the clinical encounter between clinician and family or patient, and asking these questions as part of the clinical visit modeled that patient-physician interaction. Finally, the cross-sectional design of this study did not allow us to measure disclosure rates of HIV status to children, causal pathways of disclosure or the potential impact of disclosure on clinical and psychosocial outcomes. Longitudinal cohort studies on disclosure of HIV status in this setting are urgently needed to answer these important questions as more HIV-infected children and adolescents make the difficult transition to adulthood.

Conclusions

This sample from a large, pediatric HIV care program in sub-Saharan Africa suggests a low prevalence of disclosure of HIV status to children, while highlighting how disclosure may be related to key outcomes such as medication adherence, experi-ences of stigma, and symptoms of depression. More data are needed to better understand the impact of disclosure and to inform disclosure support interventions as children and their families go through this challenging process.

Acknowledgments

The views expressed in this article are those of the authors and do not necessarily represent the view of the Indiana University School of Medicine or the Moi University School of Medicine. The authors have no conflicts of interest to disclose. We acknowledge the significant work of key clinicians in promoting and evaluating disclosure to Kenyan children, including Irene Marete, Edith Apondi, Peter Gisore, Lucy Warui, Mary Rugut, Victor Cheboi, and Christine Mukhwana.

Author Contributions

Conceived and designed the experiments: RV MT SA CT WN. Analyzed the data: RV MS AM. Contributed reagents/materials/analysis tools: RV MT AM CT WN. Wrote the paper: RV MS WN AM SA MT CT.

References

1. World Health Organization (2011) Progress Report 2011: Global HIV/AIDS Response. Geneva, Switzerland WHO, UNICEF, UNAIDS.
2. Brady MT, Oleske JM, Williams PL, Elgie C, Mofenson LM, et al. (2010) Declines in mortality rates and changes in causes of death in HIV-1-infected children during the HAART era. J Acquir Immune Defic Syndr 53(1): 86–94. doi: 10.1097/QAI.0b013e3181b9869f.
3. Havens J, Mellins C, Hunter J (2002) Psychiatric Aspects of HIV/AIDS in childhood and adolescence. In: Rutter M, Taylor F, editors. Child and Adolescent Psychiatry: Modern Approaches Oxford: Blackwell. 828–841.
4. Wiener L, Mellins CA, Marhefka S, Battles HB (2007) Disclosure of an HIV diagnosis to children: history, current research, and future directions. J Dev Behav Pediatr 28(2): 155–166. doi: 10.1097/01. DBP.0000267570.87564.cd.
5. American Academy of Pediatrics Committee on Pediatrics AIDS (1999) Disclosure of illness status to children and adolescents with HIV infection. Pediatrics 103(1): 164–166. PMID: 9917458.
6. World Health Organization (2011) Guideline on HIV Disclosure Counselling for Children up to 12 Years of Age. Geneva, Switzerland: World Health Organization.
7. Pinzon-Iregui MC, Beck-Sague CM, Malow RM (2013) Disclosure of Their HIV Status to Infected Children: A Review of the Literature. J Trop Pediatr 59(2): 84–89. doi: 10.1093/tropej/fms052.
8. Vreeman RC, Gramelspacher AM, Gisore PO, Scanlon ML, Nyandiko WM (2013) Disclosure of HIV status to children in resource-limited settings: a systematic review. J Int AIDS Soc 1618466. doi: 10.7448/IAS.16.1.18466.
9. Turissini ML, Nyandiko WM, Ayaya SO, Marete I, Mwangi A, et al. (2013) The prevalence of disclosure of HIV status to HIV-infected children in western Kenya. J Ped Infect Dis 2(2): 136–143. doi: 10.1093/jpids/pit024.
10. Kroenke K, Spitzer RL, Williams JB (2003) The Patient Health Questionnaire-2: validity of a two-item depression screener. Med Care 41(11): 1284–1292. doi: 10.1097/01. MLR.0000093487.78664.3C.
11. Einterz RM, Kimaiyo S, Mengech HN, Khwa-Otsyula BO, Esamai F, et al. (2007) Responding to the HIV pandemic: the power of an academic medical partnership. Acad Med 82(8): 812–818. doi: 10.1097/ACM.0b013e3180cc29f1.
12. Kallem S, Renner L, Ghebremichael M, Paintsil E (2011) Prevalence and pattern of disclosure of HIV status in HIV-infected children in Ghana. AIDS Behav 15(6): 1121–1127. doi: 10.1007/s10461-010-9741-9.
13. Bikaako-Kajura W, Luyirika E, Purcell DW, Downing J, Kaharuza F, et al. (2006) Disclosure of HIV status and adherence to daily drug regimens among HIV-infected children in Uganda. AIDS Behav 10(4 Suppl): S85–93. doi: 10.1007/s10461-006-9141-3.
14. John-Stewart GC, Wariua G, Beima-Sofie KM, Richardson BA, Farquhar C, et al. (2013) Prevalence, perceptions, and correlates of pediatric HIV disclosure in an HIV treatment program in Kenya. AIDS Care 25(9): 1067–1076. doi: 10.1080/09540121.2012.749333.
15. Sirikum C, Sophonphan J, Chuanjaroen T, Lakonphon S, Srimuan A, et al. (2013) HIV disclosure and its effects on treatment outcomes in HIV-infected Thai children and adolescents. 5th International Workshop on HIV Pediatrics 28–29 June 2013; Kuala Lumpur, Malaysia.
16. Ferris M, Burau K, Schweitzer AM, Mihale S, Murray N, et al. (2007) The influence of disclosure of HIV diagnosis on time to disease progression in a cohort of Romanian children and teens. AIDS Care 19(9): 1088–1094. doi: 10.1080/09540120701367124.
17. Hammami N, Nostlinger C, Hoeree T, Lefevre P, Jonckheer T, et al. (2004) Integrating adherence to highly active antiretroviral therapy into children's daily lives: a qualitative study. Pediatrics 114(5): e591–597. doi: 10.1542/peds.2004-0085.

18. Marhefka SL, Tepper VJ, Brown JL, Farley JJ (2006) Caregiver psychosocial characteristics and children's adherence to antiretroviral therapy. AIDS Patient Care STDS 20(6): 429–437. doi: 10.1089/apc.2006.20.429.
19. Mellins CA, Brackis-Cott E, Dolezal C, Abrams EJ (2004) The role of psychosocial and family factors in adherence to antiretroviral treatment in human immunodeficiency virus-infected children. Pediatr Infect Dis J 23(11): 1035–1041. doi: 10.1097/01.inf.0000143646.15240.ac.
20. Haberer J, Mellins C (2009) Pediatric adherence to HIV antiretroviral therapy. Curr HIV/AIDS Rep 6(4): 194–200. doi: 10.1007/s11904-009-0026-8.
21. Murphy DA, Wilson CM, Durako SJ, Muenz LR, Belzer M, et al. (2001) Antiretroviral medication adherence among the REACH HIV-infected adolescent cohort in the USA. AIDS Care 13(1): 27–40. doi: 10.1080/09540120020018161.
22. Brackis-Cott E, Mellins CA, Abrams E, Reval T, Dolezal C (2003) Pediatric HIV medication adherence: the views of medical providers from two primary care programs. J Pediatr Health Care 17(5): 252–260. doi: 10.1016/S0891-5245(02)8813-4.
23. Blasini I, Chantry C, Cruz C, Ortiz L, Salabarria I, et al. (2004) Disclosure model for pediatric patients living with HIV in Puerto Rico: design, implementation, and evaluation. J Dev Behav Pediatr 25(3): 181–189. PMID: 15194903.
24. Vreeman RC, Wiehe SE, Pearce EC, Nyandiko WM (2008) A systematic review of pediatric adherence to antiretroviral therapy in low- and middle-income countries. Pediatr Infect Dis J 27(8): 686–691. doi: 10.1097/IN-F.0b013e31816dd325.
25. Wagner G, Miller LG (2004) Is the influence of social desirability on patients' self-reported adherence overrated? J Acquir Immune Defic Syndr 35(2): 203–204. PMID: 14722455.
26. Bachanas PJ, Kullgren KA, Schwartz KS, Lanier B, McDaniel JS, et al. (2001) Predictors of psychological adjustment in school-age children infected with HIV. J Pediatr Psychol 26(6): 343–352. doi: 10.1093/jpepsy/26.6.343.
27. Riekert KA, Wiener L, Battles HB (1999) Prediction of Psychological Distress in School-Age Children with HIV. Children's Health Care 28(3): 201–220. doi: 10.1207/s15326888chc2803_1.
28. Menon A, Glazebrook C, Campain N, Ngoma M (2007) Mental health and disclosure of HIV status in Zambian adolescents with HIV infection: implications for peer-support programs. J Acquir Immune Defic Syndr 46(3): 349–354. doi: 10.1097/QAI.0b013e3181565df0.
29. Butler AM, Williams PL, Howland LC, Storm D, Hutton N, et al. (2009) Impact of disclosure of HIV infection on health-related quality of life among children and adolescents with HIV infection. Pediatrics 123(3): 935–943. doi: 10.1542/peds.2008-1290.
30. Vreeman RC, Nyandiko WM, Ayaya SO, Walumbe EG, Marrero DG, et al. (2010) The Perceived Impact of Disclosure of Pediatric HIV Status on Pediatric Antiretroviral Therapy Adherence, Child Well-Being, and Social Relationships in a Resource-Limited Setting. AIDS Patient Care STDS 24(10): 639–649. doi: 10.1089/apc.2010.0079.
31. Funck-Brentano I, Costagliola D, Seibel N, Straub E, Tardieu M, et al. (1997) Patterns of disclosure and perceptions of the human immunodeficiency virus in infected elementary school-age children. Arch Pediatr Adolesc Med 151(10): 978–985. doi: 10.1001/archpedi.1997.02170470012002.
32. Funck-Brentano I (1995) Informing a child about his illness in HIV infection: words and meaning. La Psychiatrie de l'enfant 38(1): 109–139. PMID: 8559848.
33. Madiba S (2012) Patterns of HIV diagnosis disclosure to infected children and family members: Data from a paediatric antiretroviral program in South Africa. World Journal of AIDS 2(3): 212–221. doi: 10.4236/wja.2012.23027.

34. Monahan PO, Shacham E, Reece M, Kroenke K, Ong'or WO, et al. (2009) Validity/reliability of PHQ-9 and PHQ-2 depression scales among adults living with HIV/AIDS in western Kenya. J Gen Intern Med 24(2): 189–197. doi: 10.1007/s11606-008-0846-z.

35. Richardson LP, Rockhill C, Russo JE, Grossman DC, Richards J, et al. (2010) Evaluation of the PHQ-2 as a brief screen for detecting major depression among adolescents. Pediatrics 125(5): e1097–1103. doi: 10.1542/peds.2009–2712.

36. Mahajan AP, Sayles JN, Patel VA, Remien RH, Sawires SR, et al. (2008) Stigma in the HIV/AIDS epidemic: a review of the literature and recommendations for the way forward. AIDS (Suppl 2): S67–79. doi: 10.1097/01.aids. 0000327438.13291.62.

18

High Uptake of Systematic HIV Counseling and Testing and TB Symptom Screening at a Primary Care Clinic in South Africa

Annelies Van Rie[1]*, Kate Clouse[1], Colleen Hanrahan[1], Katerina Selibas[2], Ian Sanne[2], Sharon Williams[3], Peter Kim[3], Jean Bassett[4]

1 Department of Epidemiology, University of North Carolina at Chapel Hill, Chapel Hill, North Carolina, United States of America, **2** Clinical HIV Research Unit, University of the Witwatersrand, Johannesburg, South Africa, **3** National Institute of Allergy and Infectious Diseases, National Institutes of Health, Bethesda, Maryland, United States of America, **4** Witkoppen Health and Welfare Center, Johannesburg, South Africa

Abstract

Background: Timely diagnosis and treatment of tuberculosis (TB) and HIV is important to reduce morbidity and mortality, and break the cycle of ongoing transmission.

Methods: We performed an implementation research study to develop a model for systematic TB symptom screening and HIV counseling and testing (HCT) for all adult clients at a primary care clinic and prospectively evaluate the 6-month coverage and yield, and 18-month sustainability at a primary care clinic in Johannesburg, South Africa.

Results: During the first 6 months, 26,515 visits occurred among 12,078 adults. The proportion of adults aware of their HIV status was 43.7% at the start of the first visit, increased to 84.6% at the end of the first visit, and to 90% at end of any visit during the first 6 months. During these 6 months, 1042 clients were newly diagnosed with HIV. HIV prevalence was 22.9% among those newly tested, and 58.9% among all adult clinic clients. High coverage of systematic HCT was sustained across all 18 months. Coverage of systematic HIV-stratified TB symptom screening during first 6-months was also high (89.6%) but only 35.0% of those symptomatic were screened by sputum. During these 6-months, 90 clients had a positive Xpert MTB/RIF assay, corresponding to a TB prevalence of 0.4% among all 23,534 clients TB symptom-screened and 2.8% among the 3,284 clients with a positive TB symptom screen. The initial high coverage of TB symptom screening was not sustained, with coverage of TB symptom screening dropping after the first six months to 70% and assessment by sputum dropping to 15%.

Conclusion: Routine, systematic HCT and HIV-stratified TB symptom screening is feasible at primary care level. Systematic HCT doubled the proportion of clients with known HIV status. While HCT was sustainable, coverage of systematic TB screening dropped significantly after the first 6 months of implementation.

Editor: Nitika Pant Pai, McGill University Health Centre, McGill University, Canada

Funding: This work was supported by PEPFAR and the National Institutes of Health grant UM1 AI069463, and by the United States Agency for International Development grants to Right to Care: 674-A-00-08-00007 and 674-A-12-00020, and to Witkoppen Health and Welfare Center: 674-A-12-00033. The funders had no role in data collection, analysis, or decision to publish.

Competing Interests: The authors have declared that no competing interest exists.

* Email: Vanrie@email.unc.edu

Introduction

The global burden of tuberculosis (TB) and human immunodeficiency virus (HIV) remains enormous. In 2012, there were an estimated 35.3 million people living with HIV (PLWH), 2.3 million new HIV infections, 1.3 million AIDS deaths, 8.6 million new cases of TB, and 1.3 million TB deaths, including 320,000 among PLWH [1,2]. In sub-Saharan Africa, there is a high prevalence of undiagnosed TB in the community [3–5], many people are unaware of their HIV status [6], and people often enter care at advanced stages of disease [7], suggesting that the current public health approach to diagnosis of TB and HIV is insufficient.

HIV counseling and testing (HCT) is predominantly delivered through voluntary counseling and testing or provider-initiated counseling and testing (PICT). Even though the World Health

Organization (WHO) recommends PICT for all people visiting a health facility [8], PICT in health care facilities in high burden countries is mainly targeted at individuals presenting for antenatal, TB or STI care [9]. Alternative approaches such as testing contacts of index cases, mobile testing, door-to-door testing, and school-based testing can increase HIV case finding [10]. A similar situation holds for TB, with suboptimal case finding using the conventional approach of passive case finding among people presenting to health facilities with symptoms suggestive of TB [1,11]. In pursuit of a more active approach to TB case detection, the WHO recommends intensified case finding among PLWH and close contacts of individuals with infectious TB [12,13]. Mobile TB screening, door-to-door screening, school-based programs, and community sputum collection point programs have been evaluated but are not routinely implemented [4,14,15].

Despite high rates of missed TB and HIV case finding at health facilities [16–19], few studies have evaluated the impact of systematic TB symptom screening and HCT for all clients, independent of the presence of risk factors. We aimed to develop a primary care model for systematic TB and HIV screening for all adults presenting to a primary care clinic. We evaluated the model's impact on knowledge of HIV status of clinic clients, HIV and TB case finding, and assessed feasibility and sustainability at a primary care clinic in Johannesburg, South Africa.

Methods

Ethics statement

The study was approved by the Institutional Review Board of the University of North Carolina at Chapel Hill, USA, and the Human Research Ethics Committee of the University of the Witwatersrand, Johannesburg, South Africa. Clinic clients provided written consent for use of routine clinic data for research purposes.

Study setting

The prospective implementation research study took place at the Witkoppen Health and Welfare Centre (WHWC), a primary care clinic serving Diepsloot, a densely populated informal settlement community. Diepsloot, located in northern Johannesburg, is the 5th most deprived of the 420 geopolitical subdivisions of Gauteng Province, South Africa [20].

Prior to the intervention, clinic clients were referred for HIV counseling and testing either through self-request (voluntary HCT) or by their provider (PICT) who targeted clients of antenatal care, tuberculosis and sexually transmitted disease services. Symptom screening for the presence of prolonged cough and weight loss was initiated by the care provider at time of clinical evaluation, either systematically among PLWH or as part of targeted clinical assessment in others. Collection of sputum was performed if requested by the nurse or doctor.

Development of a primary care model for integrated routine screening for TB and HIV

Model development first involved meetings with the clinic leadership to discuss preliminary findings [18], map current patient flow, and identify possibilities for re-allocation of space and distribution of new tasks. Meetings were then held to receive input from clinic staff routinely involved in TB and HIV care and treatment. To establish the final model, an iterative process was implemented over a 12-month period using participatory quality improvement methods. Once the final model was developed, the TB symptom screening and HCT activities became routine clinic activities and were no longer supported or monitored by research staff.

Data collection

All data were collected as part of routine patient care. Data used in the analysis were retrieved from paper-based medical files and clinic registers, as well as electronic clinic records and laboratory data. Clinic files of all adults (age ≥18 years) visiting the clinic between 30 Jan 2012 and 27 July 2012 were reviewed and data were collected on age, gender, pregnancy status, nationality, employment, HIV status (known positive, negative test result in prior 3 month period, unknown), outcome of HCT (positive, negative, not done), CD4 count if newly diagnosed with HIV, outcome of HIV-stratified TB symptom screening (positive, negative, not done), collection of sputum (if positive symptom screen), and Xpert MTB/RIF result.

To determine long-term sustainability, an additional file review was performed for 162 clients randomly selected among those visiting the clinic between January 28 to February 1, 2013 and 142 clients visiting the clinic during July 29 to August 2, 2013.

Statistical analysis

Characteristics of clinic clients are described using proportions for categorical variables, and medians and interquartile ranges (IRQ) for continuous variables. Detailed analysis of uptake and results of HCT by prior HCT status was performed for all clinic clients at the time of their first visit to the clinic during the six-month period. To determine changes in weekly HIV and TB screening outcomes of all visits (including repeat visits by some clinic clients), linear regression modeling techniques were used, incorporating an autoregressive error model to correct for the time-series structure and autocorrelation. The model output consists of a slope estimate (β) corresponding to an increase or decrease per week during the 6-month period. For example, a β of 0.001 corresponds to an increase of 0.1% per week. Log-binomial regression modeling was used to identify factors associated with testing outcomes, with results presented as crude risk ratios (RR) and 95% confidence intervals (95%CI).

Results

Model development for integrated systematic screening for TB and HIV at primary care

During the iterative, 12-month participatory process, changes were made to leverage existing space and staff, simplify patient flow and reduce waiting times. Conditions agreed upon between investigators and clinic staff were to: (1) integrate activities into current clinic activities instead of creating separate screening officers [21] (2) make HIV counseling part of routine care and perform HIV testing in those with unknown HIV status unless the client refuses, (3) have HCT precede TB screening to allow HIV-stratified TB symptoms screening, and (4) perform HCT and TB symptom screening during the time people wait to see a nurse or clinician so that results are available at time of clinical evaluation. Two TB symptom checklist stamps were developed to guide health care workers in performing a rapid HIV-stratified TB screen. For PLWH, symptoms suggestive of TB were cough, fever, night sweats and loss of weight for any duration [12]. For HIV-negative individuals, prolonged (≥2 weeks) cough or fever, night sweats and substantial weight loss were considered suggestive of active TB.

The final model involved staff across the spectrum of clinic personnel. The administrative staff registering clinic clients at presentation reviewed the client's file to determine the individual's need for HCT. People who visited WHWC for the first time and returning clients without documented HIV-infected status or a documented HIV negative test performed more than three months prior were judged in need of HCT and referred for group HIV pretest counseling. Lay counselors performed HIV pretest counseling in small groups throughout the morning prior to a client's clinical evaluation. At the end of the group session, people were invited for one-on-one rapid HIV testing and post-test counseling in a private setting. Upon completion of post-test counseling, the counselor placed the appropriate TB symptom screen stamp in the patient's clinic file. It was then the task of the clinic staff performing the routine assessment of vitals (weight, temperature, blood pressure and pregnancy test) to complete the information in the TB symptom screen stamp and to follow the simple algorithm to determine which individuals had a positive TB symptom screen. The same staff decided whether collection of a sputum sample was indicated. Between July 1, 2011 and July 31,

2012, Xpert MTB/RIF assay was performed at point-of-care, with the goal to have the result ready by the time the patient was seen by the nurse or doctor. After August 1, 2012, sputum samples were transported to a centralized laboratory for analysis. If the first-line clinic staff did not request a sputum sample, the nurse of doctor could still request this upon completion of the history-taking and clinical exam.

Clinic population

A total of 26,515 visits by 12,078 adults occurred at the clinic during the 6-month period (30 Jan 2012 to 27 July 2012) after the model was finalized as described above. The majority (69.5%) of clinic clients were women, 16.8% of whom were pregnant (Table 1). Ages of clients spanned the entire adult range, with a median age of 35 years (IQR 28-43), and 13.7% being 50 years or older. Almost one in three (32.3%) were not of South African nationality, and half (51.7%) were unemployed.

Uptake of HIV counseling and testing

At time of arrival for the first clinic visit during the 6-month period, 41.2% (95%CI: 40.3–42.0%) of the 12,078 adults were known HIV positive, 2.5% (95%CI: 2.2–2.8%) had a documented HIV negative test within the past 3 months, and 54.7% (95%CI: 53.8–55.6%) had an unknown HIV status (Table 2). Of those with unknown HIV status, the vast majority (88.2%) had never been tested for HIV at WHWC. Of those with unknown status, 74.8% (95%CI: 73.6–75.9%) were tested during their first clinic visit. The proportion tested was higher for those never previously tested at WHWC (77.9%, 95% CI 76.8–79.0%) compared to those tested more than 3 months ago (51.7%, 95% CI 48.2–55.2%). All except one person with a prior negative HIV test had a repeat negative HIV test. Among the 4537 tested for the first time at the clinic,

1041 new cases of HIV were detected (22.9%, 95% CI 21.7–24.2%). The number needed to test to identify one new case of HIV was 4.7 among all 4940 clients tested and 6.3 among all 6603 clients who received pretest counseling. By the end of the first clinic visit during the 6-month period, 84.6% (95% CI 83.9–85.2%) of all adult clients were aware of their HIV status, of which 58.9% were HIV positive. Failure to receive a documented HIV status during the first clinic visit was not associated with gender (RR 0.97, 95%CI: 0.93–1.02) but was higher among younger clients (age<40 years, RR 1.25, 95% CI 1.19–1.30) and those with foreign nationality (RR 1.10, 95% CI 1.05–1.15).

To assess sustainability, we assessed changes over time in the proportion of clients knowledgeable of their HIV status by the end of *any* clinic visit (i.e. first and repeat visits) (Figure 1). During the 6-month period, 90.0% (95%CI: 89.7–90.4%) of clients were aware of their HIV status by the end of any visit. This proportion did not change during the 6-month period (β = 0.000) and remained similar 6 and 12 months later (92.6%, p = 0.27 and 86.0%, p = 0.12), suggesting long-term sustainability of routine HCT.

While the HIV prevalence among newly-tested clients at *any* visit decreased from an estimated 19.5% (95%CI: 10.5–28.3) to 16.4% (95%CI: 7.5–25.3) during the 6-month period (Figure 1), HIV prevalence among clients newly tested when visiting the clinic for the *first* time was 22.9% and increased from an estimated 19.5% (95%CI: 10.5–28.3) to 23.1% (95% CI: 11.4%–34.8%).

The median CD4 value at the time of a new HIV diagnosis was 260 cells/μl (IQR 136–412). Newly-diagnosed men had more advanced disease compared to women (221 CD4 cells/μl, IQR: 94–352 among men vs. 295 cells/μl, IQR: 169–427 among women, p<0.001).

Table 1. Characteristics of clients seeking care at a primary care clinic in Johannesburg, South Africa.

	Overall	Male	Female
Number of clinic visits	26515	7831	18684
Number of individual clinic clients, n (%)	12078	3687 (30.5)	8391 (69.5)
Number of visits per client, median (range)	2 (1–11)	2 (1–11)	2 (1–10)
Age at first visit			
Median (IQR)	35 (28–43)	36 (30–44)	34 (27–43)
18–29 years	3799 (31.5)	920 (24.2)	2879 (34.3)
30–39 years	4221 (35.0)	1375 (37.3)	2846 (33.9)
40–49 years	2407 (19.9)	876 (23.8)	1531 (18.3)
≥50 years	1651 (13.7)	516 (14.0)	1135 (13.5)
Pregnancy status at first visit, n (%)*			
Pregnant	—	—	1360 (16.8)
Not pregnant	—	—	6729 (83.2)
Nationality, n (%)#			
Born in South Africa	8172 (67.8)	2395 (65.1)	5777 (68.9)
Born outside of South Africa	3890 (32.3)	1285 (34.9)	2605 (31.1)
Employment status at first visit, n (%)**			
Employed	5827 (48.3)	1966 (53.4)	3861 (46.0)
Not employed	6246 (51.7)	1717 (46.6)	4529 (54.0)

IQR: interquartile range;
* pregnancy status missing in 302 (3.6%) of women;
#nationality missing in 16 (0.1%) individuals;
** employment status missing in 5 (0.0) individuals.

Table 2. Uptake and results of HIV counseling and testing among 12,078 individuals visiting a primary care clinic in Johannesburg, South Africa.

	Overall		Male		Female	
	N*	%*	N*	%*	N*	%*
HIV status at start of first visit						
Known positive	4972	41.2	1481	40.2	3491	41.6
Known negative (test ≤3 m)	304	2.5	51	1.4	253	3.0
Unknown	6603	54.7	2103	57.0	4500	53.6
Prior tested (>3 m)	779	11.8	134	6.4	645	14.3
Not tested previously	5824	88.2	1969	93.6	3855	85.7
Clinic file not found	199	1.7	52	1.4	147	1.8
Outcome of HCT (among those with unknown HIV status)						
Not tested	1663	25.2	592	28.2	1071	23.8
Tested	4940	74.8	1511	71.9	3429	76.2
All tested						
HIV positive	1042	21.1	354	23.4	688	20.1
HIV negative	3898	78.9	1157	76.6	2741	79.9
Prior test (>3 m) negative						
Tested	403	51.7	58	43.3	345	53.5
HIV positive	1	0.2	0	0.0	1	0.3
HIV negative	402	99.8	58	100.0	344	99.7
Not tested previously						
Tested	4537	77.9	1453	73.8	3084	80.0
HIV positive	1041	22.9	354	24.4	687	22.3
HIV negative	3496	77.1	1099	75.6	2397	77.7
Initial CD4 count if newly diagnosed with HIV						
Median (IQR) cells/μl	268	136–412	221	94–352	295	169–427
<50 cells/μl	87	8.3	46	13.0	41	6.0
50–199 cells/μl	262	25.1	109	30.8	153	22.2
200–350 cells/μl	283	27.2	92	26.0	191	27.8
>350 cells/μl	330	31.7	86	24.3	244	35.4
Missing	80	7.7	21	5.9	59	8.6
HIV status at end of clinic visit						
Known	10216	84.6	3043	82.5	7173	85.5
Known positive	6014	58.9	1835	60.3	4179	58.3
Known negative	4202	41.1	1208	39.7	2994	41.7
Unknown	1862	15.4	644	17.5	1218	14.5

* N and % unless indicated otherwise the estimated proportion.

Uptake of HIV-stratified TB symptom screening

Information on completion of a TB symptom screen was available for 26,279 clinic visits during the 6-month period (Table 3). A TB symptom screen was performed at 89.6% (95% CI 89.2–89.9%) of the visits (Figure 2). Of the 23,534 symptom screens performed, 14.0% (95% CI 13.5–14.4%) were positive. Among the 3284 visits with a positive TB symptom screen, a sputum specimen was collected in 1150 (35.0%, 95%CI: 33.4–36.7%), of which 90 (8.0%, 95% CI 6.5–9.7%) were positive for *Mycobacterium tuberculosis* on Xpert MTB/RIF. Overall, 90 cases of TB were detected, corresponding to a 7.8% case detection among the 1150 cases screened by sputum, 2.7% case detection rate among the 3284 clients with a positive symptom screen and 0.4% case detection among all 23534 clients screened for TB symptoms.

There was no difference in TB symptom screening by gender (RR 1.00. 95%CI: 0.99–1.01), but men were more likely to be investigated by sputum (RR 1.45, 95%CI: 1.31–1.62) and were twice as likely to test positive for *M. tuberculosis* (RR 2.24, 95%CI: 1.53–3.26). HIV-positive clients were more likely to be screened for TB symptoms (94.4%) compared to HIV-negative clients (84.3%); those with unknown HIV status were least likely to be screened (70.6%). Case detection rate was similar among the three groups (7.5%, 8.7% and 7.9% for HIV-positive, HIV-negative and HIV-unknown, respectively). The number of clients needed to symptom screen to identify one case of TB was 262 overall, 131 for male clients, 448 for female clients, 317 for HIV infected clients,

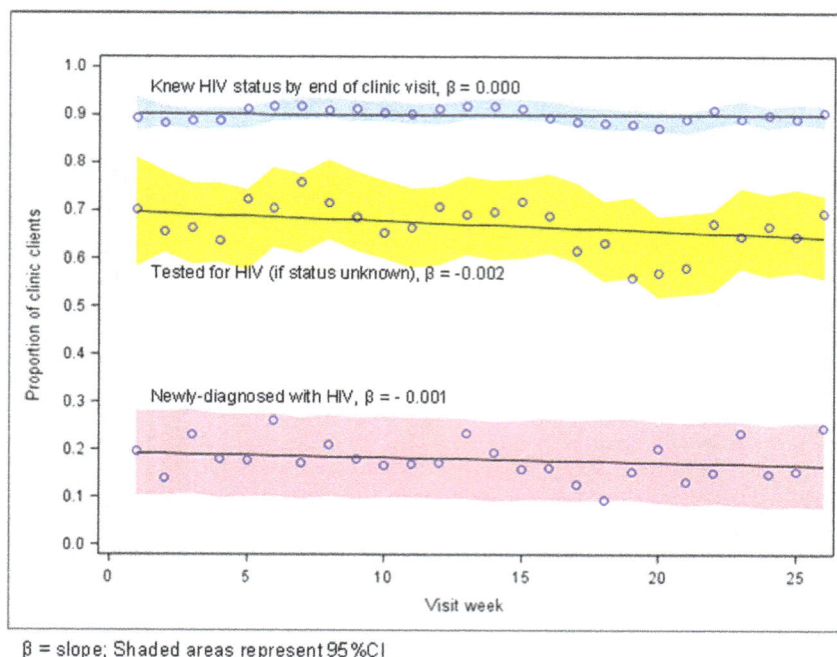

β = slope; Shaded areas represent 95%CI

Figure 1. Systematic HIV counseling and testing at primary care clinic in Johannesburg, South Africa: coverage, case detection and sustainability over a 26-week period.

239 for HIV uninfected clients and 116 for clients with unknown HIV status.

During the 6-month period, an increase over time was observed for the uptake of TB symptom screening (from an estimated 84.7 (95%CI: 79.1–90.3%) to 93.5% (95%CI: 88.2–98.7%), β = 0.004) and the proportion of TB suspects investigated by sputum (from an estimated 19.9% (95%CI: 9.5–38.9%) to 49.8% (95%CI: 34.1–65.4%), β = 0.012) (Figure 3). Associated with the increase in the proportion of clients assessed by sputum, the proportion Xpert MTB/RIF positive among those assessed by sputum decreased (β = −0.003) from an estimated 12.6% (95%CI: 4.3–24.7%) to 5.3% (95%CI: 0.0–17.5%).

TB screening coverage was not sustained long-term, with significantly lower proportion of clients screened for TB symptoms 6 and 12 months later (68.5% and 71.0%, respectively, p<0.001), and significantly lower proportion of TB suspects assessed by sputum 6 and 12 months later (15.3% and 13.6%, respectively, p = 0.090).

Discussion

In this study, the first to our knowledge to implement and evaluate a primary care model for integrated systematic HIV counseling and testing and TB symptom screening, we achieved high rates of TB symptom screening and HCT when implemented for all adult clients at a primary care clinic in South Africa, with 89.6% being screened for TB symptoms and 84.6% of people being aware of their HIV status by the end of their first clinic visit. Six months of systematic screening for HIV and TB resulted in the detection of 1042 cases of HIV, corresponding to a 22% HIV prevalence among those with unknown status, and 90 new cases of TB, corresponding to a 2.7% TB prevalence rate among those with a positive symptom screen.

Missed opportunities for HIV testing at health facilities are common, and only testing those perceived to be at high risk of

HIV can miss large numbers of PLWH [19]. Implementation of routine HCT doubled the proportion of individuals knowledgeable about their HIV status, from 43.7% at the start of the clients' first clinic visit to 84.6% by the end of the clinic visit. HCT uptake was higher than that reported for other facility-based HCT approaches, and similar to the 80–85% uptake achieved in community-based HCT programs [10].

HIV prevalence among those with unknown HIV status who accepted testing was 19.5%, slightly higher but not statistically different from the 16.1% estimated population HIV prevalence in Gauteng Province in 2011 [22]. This is in contrast with results of a meta-analysis, which found that the HIV positivity rate at facility-based HCT was, on average, double that of community-based HCT [10]. Despite high uptake, HCT did not result in high proportions of diagnoses at early stages of disease, with only 31.7% diagnosed at CD4 count >350 cells/μl, substantially lower than the 40.2% estimate in a meta-analysis of individuals diagnosed with CD4 count >350 through community-based HCT [10]. Taken together, these data suggest that systematic HIV testing at facility levels can reach similar case finding rates as community-based HCT but captures individuals at more advanced level of disease progression.

Reports of missed opportunities for TB case finding at primary care clinics suggest that TB case finding should not be limited to passive case finding or PLWH [17]. We achieved high (89.6%) coverage of HIV-stratified TB symptom screening of all clinic clients, suggesting operational feasibility under programmatic conditions. The proportion of individuals with positive symptom screen assessed by sputum (35%) was lower than expected, in part due to the frequent occurrence of unproductive cough. This is similar to findings at primary care clinics in Botswana, where only 35.3% of those with a positive symptom screen were referred for sputum smear microscopy or X-ray [23]. The TB case finding yield was relatively low, with 90 cases detected, representing 2.8% of the 3,284 clients with a positive TB symptom screen and 0.4%

Table 3. Uptake and results of TB symptom screening and sputum testing during 26,279 clinic visits at a primary care facility in Johannesburg, South Africa.

	All visits		Male		Female		HIV-positive		HIV negative		HIV-unknown	
	N	%	N	%	N	%	N	%	N	%	N	%
Screened for TB symptoms at visit*												
No	2745	10.5	803	10.3	1942	10.5	952	5.6	1023	15.7	770	29.4
Yes	23534	89.6	6962	89.7	16572	89.5	16181	94.4	5502	84.3	1851	70.6
Presence of TB symptoms among those screened												
No	20250	86.1	5778	83.0	14572	87.3	14145	87.4	4690	85.2	1415	76.5
Yes	3284	14.0	1184	17.0	2100	12.7	2036	12.6	812	14.8	436	23.5
Investigation by sputum among those with positive symptom screen												
No	2134	65.0	726	61.3	1408	67.0	1355	66.5	547	67.4	232	53.2
Yes	1150	35.0	458	38.7	692	33.0	681	33.5	265	32.6	204	46.0
Xpert result among those investigated by sputum**												
Negative	1030	89.8	393	86.0	637	92.3	609	89.7	238	89.8	183	90.2
Positive	90	7.9	53	11.6	37	5.4	51	7.5	23	8.7	16	7.9
Error or invalid	27	2.4	11	2.4	16	2.3	19	2.8	4	1.5	4	2.0

* Clinic file could not be located for 229 patients;
** Excludes 3 missing Xpert results.

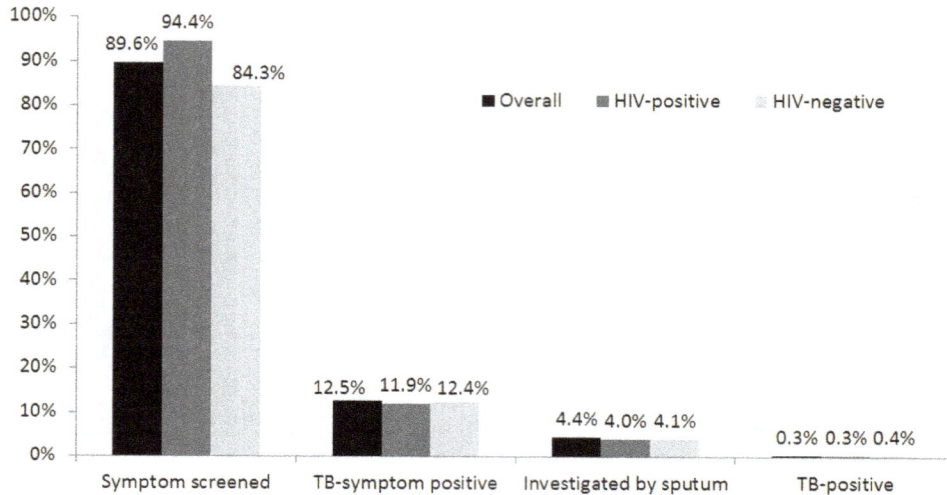

Figure 2. The TB screening cascade observed at 26,279 clinic visits at a primary care clinic in Johannesburg, South Africa. Black bars represent screenings in all clinic clients, dark grey bars represent screenings in HIV-positive clinic clients, and light grey bars represent screenings in HIV-negative clinic clients.

of the 23,534 clients screened. Operational feasibility but low yield of systematic TB symptom screening was also observed in other studies. In Botswana, 926 (8%) of 11,799 clinic clients had a positive symptom screen, 327 (35.3%) were referred for examinations (sputum smear microscopy or X-ray), and 19 (13.4% of those tested, 0.2% of those screened) were diagnosed with TB [23]. In outpatient departments of 32 hospitals in Swaziland [11], 14,998 (6%) of 251,867 clients screened positive and were tested using Xpert, 1499 (10% of those tested, 0.6% of those screened) were diagnosed with TB. In Afghanistan, 22,228 (2.5%) of 889,120 clinic attendees systematically screened for TB at 47 health

facilities were tested with smear microscopy of whom 1986 were diagnosed with TB (8.9% of those tested, 0.2% of those screened) [11].

In contrast to our findings of sustainability of systematic HCT, the high coverage of systematic TB screening was not sustained long term. The proportion of individuals symptom screened dropped from 89.6% to about 70% and the proportion with positive symptom screen assessed by sputum dropped from 35% to about 15%. Several factors may have contributed to this observation. First, whereas systematic HIV testing is part of a South Africa national testing campaign, systematic TB symptom

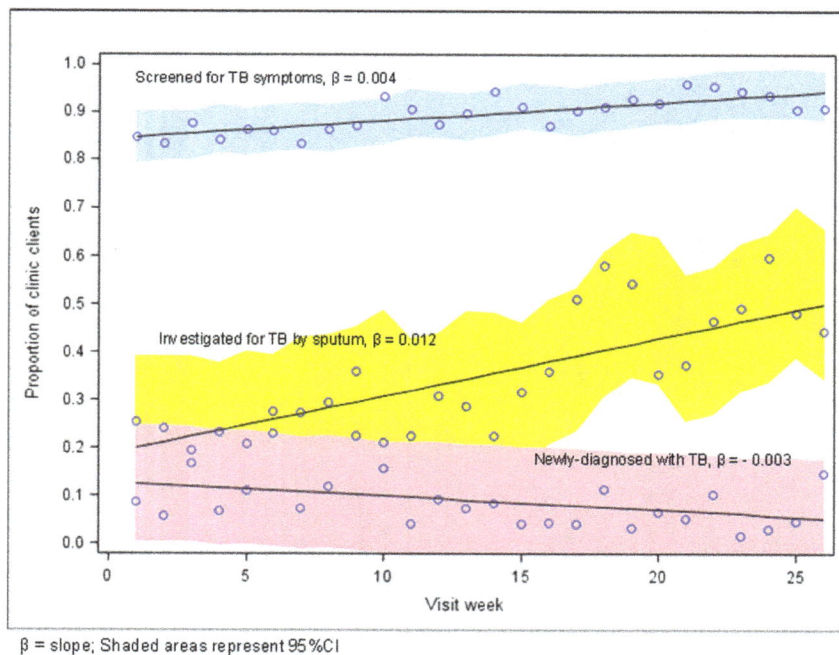

β = slope; Shaded areas represent 95%CI

Figure 3. Systematic TB symptom screening and assessment at primary care clinic in Johannesburg, South Africa: coverage, case detection, and sustainability over a 26-week period.

screening in all clinic clients is not recommended by the South African Department of Health. Second, the number needed to screen to detect one case is much higher for TB than HIV (262 versus 6), possibly resulting in a perception of higher effectiveness and thus stronger motivation for the health care workers to test for HIV compared to TB. Third, while Xpert MTB/RIF was performed at point-of-care during the study period samples were sent to a centralized laboratory after the first 6 months. Lack of immediate feedback on sputum results may further have decreased the motivation of the clinic staff to collect sputum for evaluation.

The large sample size, pragmatic approach and the evaluation under real-world conditions using non-research clinic staff to perform all activities are important strengths of our study. The interpretation of the findings however needs to take some limitations into account. The study was a single-site observational study without a control group. The impact of the intervention on HIV and TB diagnoses could therefore not be estimated as the proportion of new HIV and TB diagnoses that would have been made under standard of care was not known. We also do not know if missed diagnoses occurred among those who were not tested for HIV, those with a negative TB symptom screen, and clients with a positive symptom screen who were not assessed by sputum. Inclusion of a historical control using routine clinic statistics could provide some insights but would have inherent limitations due to differences in time periods assessed and use of different data collection standards. Finally, the available data did not allow us to estimate cost effectiveness of the program, or to assess the impact of the intervention on individual morbidity and mortality or transmission of TB and HIV at population level.

Conclusion

To date, efforts to curb the TB/HIV epidemic have focused on TB screening for PLWH and HCT for people diagnosed with active TB. While outreach screening activities have been shown to be effective, these programs require infrastructure development, complicate linkage to care, and sustainability under programmatic conditions of such programs can be hard to obtain. Improving TB and HIV case finding at health facilities may be a more affordable and sustainable first step to increase case finding in high burden settings. Key features likely contributing to our program's success were full integration of TB symptom screening and HCT into routine clinic activities, distribution of tasks across a range of clinic personnel, and timing of HCT and TB symptom screening during the time clinic clients waited to see a nurse or physician. Future research is needed to explore the epidemiological and contextual factors that improve the effectiveness of different tools and approaches to systematic TB screening at primary care.

Acknowledgments

We are deeply grateful to all patients and staff at Witkoppen Health and Welfare Center. We would also like to thank members of the research team: Veronica Modise, Bridgette Moatlhodi, and Violet Molepo. We thank Pierre Barker and Michèle Youngleson of the Institute for Healthcare Improvement for guidance and support regarding the use of quality improvement methods.

Author Contributions

Conceived and designed the experiments: AVR PK SW IS JB. Performed the experiments: JB KC CH KS. Analyzed the data: KC AVR CH. Wrote the paper: AVR KC CH JB PK. Collected data: KS CH.

References

1. WHO (2013) Global Tuberculosis Report Geneva, Switzerland.
2. UNAIDS (2012) Report on the Global AIDS Epidemic. UNAIDS.
3. Ayles H, Schaap A, Nota A, Sismanidis C, Tembwe R, et al. (2009) Prevalence of tuberculosis, HIV and respiratory symptoms in two Zambian communities: implications for tuberculosis control in the era of HIV. PLoS One 4: e5602.
4. Corbett EL, Bandason T, Duong T, Dauya E, Makamure B, et al. (2010) Comparison of two active case-finding strategies for community-based diagnosis of symptomatic smear-positive tuberculosis and control of infectious tuberculosis in Harare, Zimbabwe (DETECTB): a cluster-randomised trial. Lancet 376: 1244–1253.
5. Wood R, Middelkoop K, Myer L, Grant AD, Whitelaw A, et al. (2007) Undiagnosed tuberculosis in a community with high HIV prevalence: implications for tuberculosis control. Am J Respir Crit Care Med 175: 87–93.
6. WHO, UNAIDS, UNICEF (2011) Global HIV/AIDS repsonse. Epidemic update and health sector progress towards universal access. Progress report 2011.
7. Braitstein P, Brinkhof MW, Dabis F, Schechter M, Boulle A, et al. (2006) Mortality of HIV-1-infected patients in the first year of antiretroviral therapy: comparison between low-income and high-income countries. Lancet 367: 817–824.
8. WHO (2007) Guidance on provider-initiated HIV testing and counseling in health facilities Geneva.
9. Roura M, Watson-Jones D, Kahawita TM, Ferguson L, Ross DA (2013) Provider-initiated testing and counselling programmes in sub-Saharan Africa: a systematic review of their operational implementation. AIDS 27: 617–626.
10. Suthar AB, Ford N, Bachanas PJ, Wong VJ, Rajan JS, et al. (2013) Towards Universal Voluntary HIV Testing and Counselling: A Systematic Review and Meta-Analysis of Community-Based Approaches. PLoS Med 10: e1001496.
11. Uplekar M, Creswell J, Ottmani SE, Weil D, Sahu S, et al (2013) Programmatic approaches to screening for active tuberculosis. Int J Tuberc Lung Dis 17: 1248–1256.
12. WHO (2010) Guidelines for intensified tuberculosis case finding and isoniazid preventive therapy for people living with HIV in resource-contrained settings. Geneva, Switzerland: World Health Organization.

13. WHO (2012) Recommendations for investigating contacts of persons with infectious tuberculosis in low- and middle-income countries. World Health Organization. WHO/INT/TB/2012.9 WHO/INT/TB/2012.9.
14. Kranzer K, Lawn SD, Meyer-Rath G, Vassall A, Raditlhalo E, et al. (2012) Feasibility, yield, and cost of active tuberculosis case finding linked to a mobile HIV service in Cape Town, South Africa: a cross-sectional study. PLoS Med 9: e1001281.
15. Ayles H, Muyoyeta M, Du Toit E, Schaap A, Floyd S, et al. (2013) Effect of household and community interventions on the burden of tuberculosis in southern Africa: the ZAMSTAR community-randomised trial. Lancet.
16. Bassett IV, Wang B, Chetty S, Giddy J, Losina E, et al. (2010) Intensive tuberculosis screening for HIV-infected patients starting antiretroviral therapy in Durban, South Africa. Clin Infect Dis 51: 823–829.
17. Claassens MM, Jacobs E, Cyster E, Jennings K, James A, et al. (2013) Tuberculosis cases missed in primary health care facilities: should we redefine case finding? Int J Tuberc Lung Dis 17: 608–614.
18. Voss De Lima YP-S, Sanne I, Van Rie A (2010) Routine screening for TB and HIV by health care workers in primary care clinics. Lille, France. The International Unions Against Tuberculosis and Lung Diseases. pp. S111.
19. Fetene NW, Feleke AD (2010) Missed opportunities for earlier HIV testing and diagnosis at the health facilities of Dessie town, North East Ethiopia. BMC Public Health 10: 362.
20. De Wet T, Patel L, Korth M, Forrester C (2008) Johannesburg Poverty and Livelihoods Study. Johannesburg: Centre for Social Development in Africa, University of Johannesburg.
21. Khan AJ, Khowaja S, Khan FS, Qazi F, Lotia I, et al. (2012) Engaging the private sector to increase tuberculosis case detection: an impact evaluation study. Lancet Infect Dis 12: 608–616.
22. Health SANDo (2012) The National Antenatal Sentinel HIV and Syphilis Prevalence Survey, South Africa, 2011. Pretoria.
23. Bloss E, Makombe R, Kip E, Smit M, Chirenda J, et al. (2012) Lessons learned during tuberculosis screening in public medical clinics in Francistown, Botswana. Int J Tuberc Lung Dis 16: 1030–1032.

19

Linking Women Who Test HIV-Positive in Pregnancy-Related Services to HIV Care and Treatment Services in Kenya: A Mixed Methods Prospective Cohort Study

Laura Ferguson[1,2,3]*, Alison D. Grant[4], James Lewis[2], Karina Kielmann[5], Deborah Watson-Jones[4,6], Sophie Vusha[3], John O. Ong'ech[3,7], David A. Ross[2]

1 Institute for Global Health, University of Southern California, Los Angeles, California, United States of America, 2 MRC Tropical Epidemiology Group, Department of Infectious Disease Epidemiology, London School of Hygiene and Tropical Medicine, London, United Kingdom, 3 University of Nairobi Institute for Tropical and Infectious Diseases, Nairobi, Kenya, 4 Clinical Research Department, London School of Hygiene & Tropical Medicine, London, United Kingdom, 5 Institute for International Health & Development, Queen Margaret University, Edinburgh, United Kingdom, 6 Mwanza Intervention Trials Unit, National Institute for Medical Research, Mwanza, Tanzania, 7 Department of Obstetrics and Gynaecology, University of Nairobi, Nairobi, Kenya

Abstract

Introduction: There has been insufficient attention to long-term care and treatment for pregnant women diagnosed with HIV.

Objective and Methods: This prospective cohort study of 100 HIV-positive women recruited within pregnancy-related services in a district hospital in Kenya employed quantitative methods to assess attrition between women testing HIV-positive in pregnancy-related services and accessing long-term HIV care and treatment services. Qualitative methods were used to explore barriers and facilitators to navigating these services. Structured questionnaires were administered to cohort participants at enrolment and 90+ days later. Participants' medical records were monitored prospectively. Semi-structured qualitative interviews were carried out with a sub-set of 19 participants.

Findings: Only 53/100 (53%) women registered at an HIV clinic within 90 days of HIV diagnosis, of whom 27/53 (51%) had a CD4 count result in their file. 11/27 (41%) women were eligible for immediate antiretroviral therapy (ART); only 6/11 (55%) started ART during study follow-up. In multivariable logistic regression analysis, factors associated with registration at the HIV clinic within 90 days of HIV diagnosis were: having cared for someone with HIV (aOR:3.67(95%CI:1.22, 11.09)), not having to pay for transport to the hospital (aOR:2.73(95%CI:1.09, 6.84)), and having received enough information to decide to have an HIV test (aOR:3.61(95%CI:0.83, 15.71)). Qualitative data revealed multiple factors underlying high patient drop-out related to women's social support networks (e.g. partner's attitude to HIV status), interactions with health workers (e.g. being given unclear/incorrect HIV-related information) and health services characteristics (e.g. restricted opening hours, long waiting times).

Conclusion: HIV testing within pregnancy-related services is an important entry point to HIV care and treatment services, but few women successfully completed the steps needed for assessment of their treatment needs within three months of diagnosis. Programmatic recommendations include simplified pathways to care, better-tailored counselling, integration of ART into antenatal services, and facilitation of social support.

Editor: Stefan Baral, Johns Hopkins School of Public Health, United States of America

Funding: Funding to support this work came from the Economic and Social Research Council (UK)/Medical Research Council UK (www.esrc.ac.uk; www.mrc.ac.uk), the UK Department for International Development-supported Evidence for Action on HIV Treatment and Care Systems Research Programme (www.evidence4action.org), the Parkes Foundation (www.parkesfoundation.org.uk) and the University of London Central Research Fund (www.london.ac.uk). The funders had no role in study design, data collection and analysis, decision to publish, or preparation of the manuscript.

Competing Interests: The authors have declared that no competing interests exist.

* E-mail: laurafer@usc.edu

Introduction

Global attention to HIV testing in pregnancy has focused almost exclusively on prevention of mother-to-child transmission (PMTCT) of HIV. [1] Attention is now increasingly being paid to linking women who are diagnosed with HIV in antenatal or delivery services (collectively "pregnancy-related services") to long-term care and treatment for their own HIV infection. [2].

Based on the potential advantages to mother and infant of early initiation of maternal antiretroviral therapy (ART), [3] Kenya, along with many other countries, is considering the adoption of a policy of immediate lifelong ART for all women diagnosed with HIV during pregnancy (also known as "Option B+"). To maximize the potential benefits of Option B+, linkage into ART services following an HIV diagnosis in pregnancy-related services is required. However, a recent systematic literature review highlighted sub-optimal linkage into long-term HIV care and treatment services of women diagnosed with HIV during pregnancy. [4].

We carried out a retrospective cohort study in Naivasha Hospital, Kenya, between January 2008 and June 2010, finding high attrition along the pathway to HIV care and treatment: within six months of diagnosis with HIV in pregnancy-related services, only 153/892 (17%) women had registered at the on-site HIV clinic. Of 99 women with a recorded CD4 count, 53 were eligible for and only 21 (40%) initiated ART within six months of HIV diagnosis. [5] This review was based on manually-matched hospital records, potentially underestimating uptake of care in nearby health facilities.

We therefore recruited a cohort of HIV-positive women within pregnancy-related services in the same hospital and followed them prospectively, aiming to quantify uptake of long-term HIV care and treatment services while taking into account uptake of services at other nearby health facilities and to explore reasons underlying client attrition along the care continuum.

Methods

Ethics Statement

Ethical approval was provided by the University of Nairobi/ Kenyatta National Hospital Ethics Review Committee and the London School of Hygiene & Tropical Medicine Ethics Committee. Information sheets were read to all participants and written informed consent was obtained at enrolment and again for qualitative interviews. This included consent for researchers to access participants' medical records. Three women aged 16–17 participated, each of whom was deemed competent to provide informed consent; involvement of their parents was discussed and encouraged but refused by the participants. To preserve confidentiality, unique study numbers were assigned at enrolment and used in all active databases and documents. After the qualitative interviews, participants who were not engaged with HIV care were encouraged to attend clinic.

Setting

This study was carried out in Naivasha District Hospital, Rift Valley Province, Kenya. Among women in Rift Valley Province, HIV prevalence is 6.3%, [6] while in the study hospital the estimated HIV prevalence of HIV among antenatal attendees is 4% (based on routine hospital data, 2009–10).

According to Kenyan national guidelines at the time of the study, pregnant women with unknown HIV status should have been offered provider-initiated rapid HIV testing and counselling. [7] Women who tested HIV-positive should have been given nevirapine (an intra-partum dose for themselves and a post-natal course for their infant). Lifelong ART, provided free, was recommended for pregnant women with a CD4 count ≤ 350 cells/mm^3 and could be initiated within two days of diagnosis. [7,8].

Naivasha Hospital policy at the time stated that, immediately following diagnosis with HIV in antenatal care (ANC), women should have been accompanied by the ANC nurse to the on-site HIV clinic for clinical staging, a two-week prescription of antenatal zidovudine (AZT) and cotrimoxazole, and referral to the on-site laboratory for CD4 count testing and then on to the pharmacy to collect their medications. Upon registration clients were asked to return within one week for a CD4 count test and then again two weeks later for the test result.

Enrolment and Follow-up

Cohort study. Between January and September 2010, a consecutive sample of all women diagnosed with HIV who reported having been previously unaware of their HIV status and were ≥ 15 years attending Naivasha Hospital pregnancy-related services were invited to join the study cohort. Enrolment into the cohort took place on the same day that women were found to be eligible i.e. either on the day of their HIV diagnosis or during a repeat visit to pregnancy-related services.

Face-to-face questionnaires were administered to women at enrolment covering the woman's pregnancy history, experience of HIV illness, testing and care, knowledge and attitudes about HIV care and treatment, and social support. For participants recruited within ANC, research staff were asked to escort study participants to the HIV clinic immediately following their study enrolment.

A follow-up questionnaire was administered by telephone or in person at least three months following enrolment to elicit information from women on pregnancy-related and HIV services accessed since diagnosis, disclosure and levels of social support, and recent illness.

In addition, researchers searched the registration books for attendance by participants at Naivasha Hospital and five additional HIV clinics where women were most often referred for care.

Attrition at each step along the pathway to HIV care and treatment was assessed using health facility records. Univariable logistic regression analysis was used to assess which factors were associated with registration at an HIV clinic within 90 days of HIV diagnosis. All variables associated with the outcome ($p<0.10$) were included in a multivariable logistic regression model, except for 'personally knowing someone with HIV', which was excluded due to colinearity with 'personally knowing someone who has died from AIDS'.

Quantitative data were double-entered into Epi-Data Version 3.1 and any errors resolved. Analysis used Stata 10.1 (Stata Corp, College Station, Texas).

Qualitative sub-study. Face-to-face semi-structured qualitative interviews were carried out to explore the factors affecting women's access to HIV-related services. Attempts were made to contact 38 cohort participants for an interview, of whom half (n = 19) were interviewed. Initially participants with no/low attendance at the HIV clinic were selected but due to difficulties contacting and arranging face-to-face interviews with women with low attendance, the sampling strategy was broadened to also include women with higher HIV clinic attendance.

Interviews lasted 40–90 minutes. Domains of inquiry included: living situation, experience of HIV diagnosis, social support, experiences of discrimination, and health-seeking behaviours. Reasons given by participants for not attending services were probed in detail.

All interviews were carried out by local interviewers in Swahili and digitally recorded, transcribed and then translated into English for analysis. Transcripts were read repeatedly specifically to identify emerging taxonomies and themes. A coding scheme was derived based initially on findings from a literature review and exploratory focus group discussions, and refined based on themes emerging in the interviews. Following the initial analysis, matrices were created in Excel to allow cross-group comparisons between women displaying different attendance patterns at HIV-related services. Continuous and iterative hypothesis generation and testing throughout the analysis allowed for continual refinement of themes and ensured that the insights provided by the data could be captured.

Qualitative data were managed using NVivo Version 8 (QSR International Pty Ltd. 2008).

Results

Cohort Study Enrolment

Figure 1 shows the flow of participants in the cohort.

During the study timeframe, 110 women in Naivasha Hospital were eligible for study participation of whom 105 (95%) were invited to participate. The other five women received their HIV diagnosis on days when no research staff were at the hospital. All women invited to participate in the study consented to take part. Five women were excluded at the time of follow-up because quantitative analyses on HIV clinic attendance were based on health facility records and they reported having attended an HIV clinic that was too far away for the study team to access their records.

Of the 100 women in the cohort, 66 (66%) completed a structured follow-up questionnaire: 18 in person and 48 by telephone. Median time between enrolment and follow-up was 96.5 days (inter-quartile range (IQR): 93–110 days). No follow-up information was available for 18 (18%) women and a further 16 (16%) could not be reached by telephone or in person even though they had registered at an HIV clinic and their HIV clinic records were accessed. There were no significant differences in the baseline characteristics of women completing the follow-up questionnaire versus those who could not be reached, including HIV-related symptoms, distance from home to the hospital, and prior contact with people living with HIV (see Table S1).

Cohort Participant Characteristics

Among 100 women enrolled in the cohort, the median age at enrolment was 26 years (IQR: 23–30) and the majority of women were married (Table 1). Most women had no more than primary education and just over half were in paid employment. The median gestational age at time of HIV diagnosis was 28 weeks. Women reported a median travel time of 35 minutes (IQR: 30, 60) to reach the hospital from their home, and 58% reported having to pay for transport.

Qualitative Sub-study Participant Characteristics

The 19 women who participated in the qualitative sub-study were more likely than the 81 who did not to have started attending ANC before 28 weeks gestation (75% vs. 26%; p = 0.001), more likely to have registered at the HIV clinic within 90 days of their HIV diagnosis (74% vs. 48%; p = 0.045), and more likely to have returned to the HIV clinic for a second visit (58% vs. 33%; p = 0.047).

Client Attrition between Testing HIV-positive and Attending HIV-related Services

Figure 2, based on health facility records, shows client attrition along the pathway to HIV care and treatment services within 90 days of diagnosis with HIV. If no health facility record could be found, it was assumed that the participant had not enrolled in HIV care and treatment.

Client attrition was substantial at each step of this pathway: 47/100 (47%) women were lost between diagnosis and registration at an HIV clinic; a further 26/53 (49%) of those registering at the HIV clinic did not have a CD4 count result in their file. Only 27 of the original 100 women (27%) had a CD4 count result. Among 11

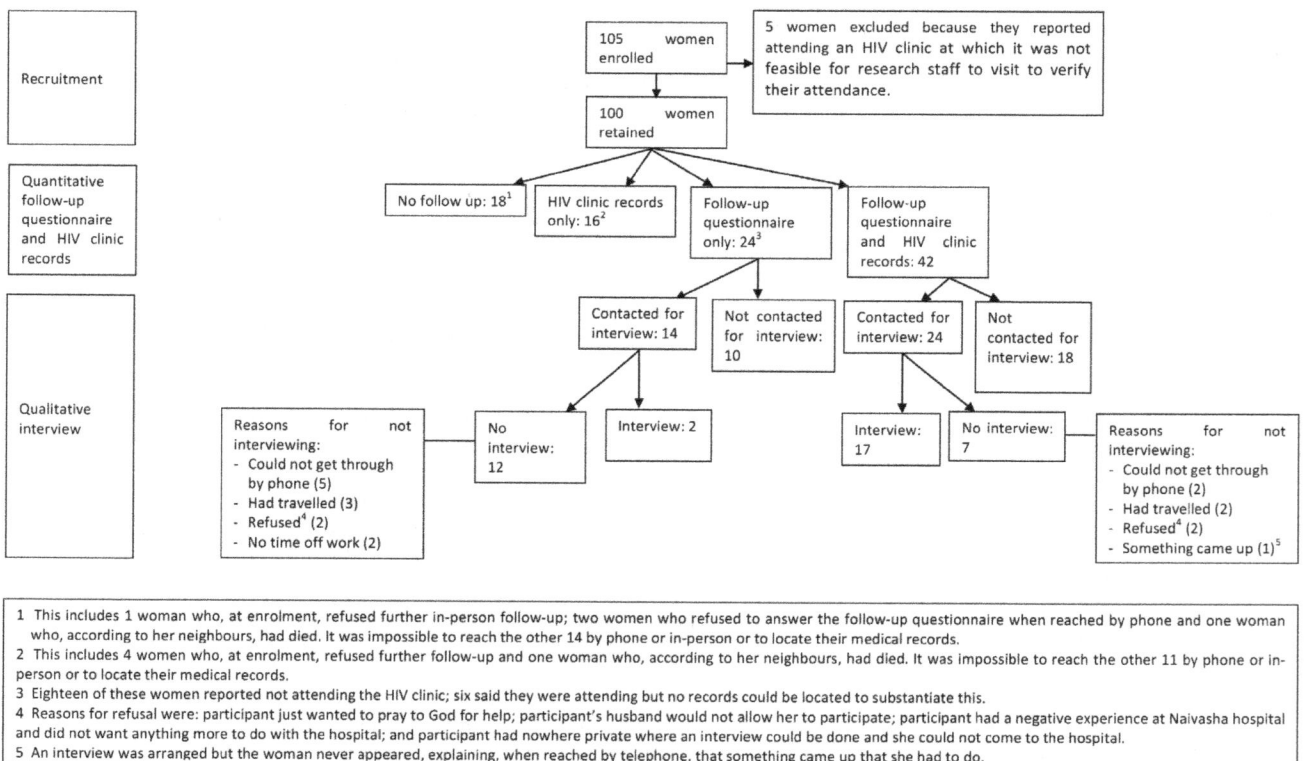

1 This includes 1 woman who, at enrolment, refused further in-person follow-up; two women who refused to answer the follow-up questionnaire when reached by phone and one woman who, according to her neighbours, had died. It was impossible to reach the other 14 by phone or in-person or to locate their medical records.
2 This includes 4 women who, at enrolment, refused further follow-up and one woman who, according to her neighbours, had died. It was impossible to reach the other 11 by phone or in-person or to locate their medical records.
3 Eighteen of these women reported not attending the HIV clinic; six said they were attending but no records could be located to substantiate this.
4 Reasons for refusal were: participant just wanted to pray to God for help; participant's husband would not allow her to participate; participant had a negative experience at Naivasha hospital and did not want anything more to do with the hospital; and participant had nowhere private where an interview could be done and she could not come to the hospital.
5 An interview was arranged but the woman never appeared, explaining, when reached by telephone, that something came up that she had to do.

Figure 1. Cohort recruitment and follow-up.

Table 1. Factors Associated With Attendance At The HIV Clinic Within 90 Days Of HIV Diagnosis Among Women Diagnosed With HIV In Pregnancy-Related Services.

Description	N	Attended HIV clinic (row %)	UnAdjOR*	95%CI	AdjOR*	95%CI
Age			P = 0.980			
15–19	8	4 (50.0)	0.88	0.18, 4.17		
20–24	30	16 (53.3)	1.00			
25–29	35	20 (57.1)	1.17	0.44, 3.11		
30–44	27	15 (55.6)	1.09	0.38, 3.11		
Education			P = 0.521			
None	2	1 (50.0)	0.72	0.04, 12.08		
Some primary	62	36 (58.1)	1.00			
Some secondary	29	16 (55.2)	0.89	0.37, 2.16		
Post-secondary	7	2(28.6)	0.29	0.05, 1.61		
Marital status			P = 0.283			
Not married (single/widowed/separated)	28	13 (46.4)	1.00			
Married	72	42 (58.3)	1.62	0.67, 3.89		
Employment			P = 0.746			
Unemployed	44	25 (56.8)	1.00			
Employed	56	30 (53.6)	0.88	0.40, 1.94		
Gravidity			P = 0.554			
One	29	15 (51.7)	1.00			
Two	22	12 (54.5)	1.12	0.37, 3.40		
Three	31	20 (64.5)	1.70	0.60, 4.78		
Four+	18	8 (44.4)	0.75	0.23, 2.43		
Timing of 1st ANC			P = 0.775			
8–21 weeks	13	7 (53.8)	1.00			
22–27 weeks	8	6 (75.0)	2.57	0.37, 17.83		
28–34 weeks	31	20 (64.5)	1.56	0.42, 5.81		
35–39 weeks	7	4 (57.1)	1.14	0.18, 7.28		
Timing of HIV diagnosis			P = 0.688			
≤28 weeks gestation (ANC)	63	34 (54.0)	1.00			
29+ weeks gestation (ANC)	30	18 (60.0)	1.28	0.53, 3.09		
Delivery	7	3 (42.3)	0.64	0.13, 3.10		
Location of HIV diagnosis			P = 0.788			
ANC	91	50 (54.9)	1.00			
Delivery	8	4 (50.0)	0.82	0.29, 3.48		
Travel time from home to clinic			P = 0.583			
60+ minutes	24	12 (50.0)	1.00			
<60 minutes	76	43 (56.6)	1.25	0.56, 2.78		
Cost of travel to HIV clinic			P = 0.015		P = 0.032	
Not having to pay a transport fare[1]	58	26 (44.8)	1.00		1.00	
Having to pay a fare	42	29 (69.0)	2.75	1.19, 6.32	2.73	1.09, 6.84
HIV symptoms[2]			P = 0.039		P = C.202	
None	60	28 (46.7)	1.00		1.00	
At least one	40	27 (67.5)	2.37	1.03, 5.46	1.83	0.72, 4.62
Ever seen anyone with HIV			P = 0.125			
No	16	6 (37.5)	1.00			
Yes	84	49 (58.3)	2.33	0.78, 7.02		
Personally know anyone with HIV			P = 0.089			
No	31	13 (41.9)	1.00			
Yes	68	41 (60.3)	2.10	0.89, 4.98		
Personally know anyone who died of AIDS			P = 0.037		P = 0.216	

Table 1. Cont.

Description	N	Attended HIV clinic (row %)	UnAdjOR*	95%CI	AdjOR*	95%CI
No	16	5 (31.3)	1.00		1.00	
Yes	84	50 (59.5)	3.24	1.03, 10.15	2.21	0.63, 7.80
Ever cared for anyone with HIV			P = 0.008		P = 0.021	
No	72	34 (47.2)	1.00		1.00	
Yes	26	20 (76.9)	3.73	1.34, 10.36	3.67	1.22, 11.09
Enough information to decide whether or not to test[3]			P = 0.064		P = 0.087	
No	13	4 (30.8)	1.00		1.00	
Yes	86	50 (58.1)	3.13	0.89, 10.94	3.61	0.83, 15.71
Self-perceived ability to refuse to test			P = 0.710			
No	62	35 (56.5)	1.00			
Yes	38	20 (52.6)	0.86	0.38, 1.93		
Receipt of PMTCT prophylaxis			P = 0.245			
Maternal and infant	45	23 (51.1)	1.00			
Maternal only	15	6 (40.0)	0.64	0.19, 2.09		
Infant only	31	19 (61.3)	1.51	0.60, 3.84		
No prophylaxis	9	7 (77.8)	3.35	0.63, 17.90		

*P-values relate to heterogeneity from a likelihood ratio test.
[1]Participants who did not have to pay for transport walked to the hospital.
[2]Participants were asked if they had experienced any of the following symptoms within the previous six months: diarrhoea; big problems with memory or concentration that interfered with normal activities; cough for more than two weeks; high fever; swollen glands; a yeast infection in the mouth or vagina (thrush); numbness, tingling or burning sensations in the arms, legs, hands or feet; substantial weight loss; or a skin rash.
[3]Within a series of questions regarding pre-test counselling, women were asked "Did you feel that you were given enough information to decide whether or not to have an HIV test?".

ART-eligible women, a further 5 (45%) were lost between receiving their CD4 count and actually starting ART. Overall, only six women started ART (15% of the 41 women estimated as likely to have been ART-eligible).

Delays Along the Pathway to HIV Care and Treatment

Among the 53 women who had registered at an HIV clinic during the 90-day follow-up period, 32 (60%) registered on the day of their HIV diagnosis of whom 12 (38%) did not return to the HIV clinic again during the follow-up period. The median time to registration at the HIV clinic among the remaining women who registered at the HIV clinic within 90 days was 21 days (IQR: 11–63).

The median time between registration and having blood taken for a CD4 count was six days (IQR: 0–17). For ART-eligible women, the median time between this blood-draw and initiating ART was 28 days (IQR: 0–37), and the median number of appointments between the visit at which they received their CD4 count result and being started on ART was two (Range: 0–5). Among ART-eligible women who successfully started ART within the 90-day follow-up period, the median time between diagnosis and initiating ART was 48.5 days (IQR: 32–76).

Factors Associated with Uptake of HIV-related Services

Table 1 shows baseline factors associated with HIV clinic registration within 90 days of diagnosis among the 100 women in the cohort. As with Figure 2, this is based on health facility records. In the univariable analysis these factors were: having cared for someone with HIV (OR: 3.73; 95%CI: 1.34, 10.36; p = 0.008), having to pay for transport to the hospital (OR: 2.75; 95%CI: 1.19, 6.32; p = 0.015), personally knowing someone who died of AIDS (OR: 3.24; 95%CI: 1.03, 10.15; p = 0.037), and

having experienced at least one HIV-related symptom in the six months prior to enrolment (OR: 2.37; 95%CI: 1.03, 5.46; p = 0.039). There was also weak evidence of an association with reporting having received enough information to decide to have an HIV test (OR: 3.13; 95%CI: 0.89, 10.94; p = 0.064) and with personally knowing someone with HIV (OR: 2.10; 95%CI: 0.89, 4.98; p = 0.089).

In the multivariable model, factors remaining independently associated with the outcome were: having cared for someone with HIV (aOR:3.67; 95%CI: 1.22, 11.09; p = 0.021) and having to pay for transport to the hospital (aOR:2.73; 95%CI: 1.09, 6.32; p = 0.032). There was also weak evidence of an independent association between the outcome and having received enough information to decide to have an HIV test (aOR:3.61; 95%CI: 0.83, 15.71; p = 0.087).

In the follow-up questionnaire administered to 66 women, 18 (27%) reported not having registered at an HIV clinic. The three most commonly cited reasons for not having registered at an HIV clinic were: women not knowing that they had to register (4/18; 22%), not having had time to register (3/18; 17%), and not feeling ready to do so (2/18; 11%).

Of the 53 women who delivered during the study period and had registered at the HIV clinic, 15 (28%) stopped attending the HIV clinic for at least eight weeks around the time of delivery.

Qualitative Exploration of Reasons Underlying Women's Decisions Regarding Accessing HIV-related Services

The semi-structured interviews corroborated many of the quantitative findings presented above. Three main areas were reported to have affected women's uptake of HIV services for their own care: social support, interactions with health workers and health services-related factors.

Tested + in ANC/delivery	100%	100
Contact with HIV clinic	58%	58
Registered at HIV clinic	53%	53
2nd HIV clinic visit	72%	38
CD4 count result	51%	27
Needed HAART (CD4 <350)	41%	11
Started HAART	55%	6

- If no drop-out, all 100 women would have completed initial screening and received their CD4 count result.
- Of these, assuming that the same proportion would have been HAART-eligible among the 73 women who did not have a CD4 count as among the 27 women who had a CD4 count result, 41 (11/27 = 41%; 100 * 41% = 41) would have been eligible for, and started, HAART.

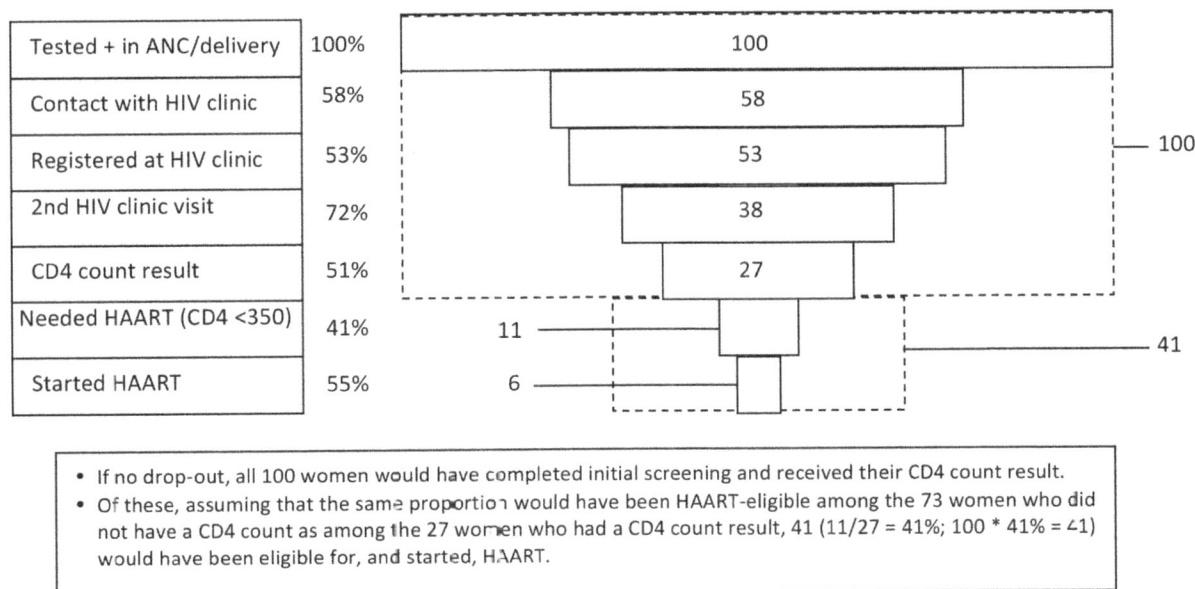

The boxes with solid lines show the actual number of women who completed each step along this pathway. On the left-hand side are the percentages of women completing each step in the cascade; the denominators are the number of women in the previous line of the diagram, with the exception of the percentage of women who registered at the HIV clinic for which the denominator is the total number of women diagnosed with HIV in ANC/delivery, and the percentage of women who had a CD4 count result available for which the denominator is the number of women registered at the HIV clinic. The dotted lines show an ideal patient cascade i.e. with no patient drop-out, which is explained in the box underneath the figure.

Figure 2. Client attrition along the pathway to long-term HIV care and treatment services.

Social support. Supportive partners, family and friends facilitated uptake of care by helping around the house, reminding women to take their drugs and providing emotional support:

"*[My husband] tells me that I shouldn't stress myself.... [He says] 'Stop stressing yourself... there are people who love you'.*" (Participant #126, Age 31).

Conversely, many women reported that following disclosure to their partner they had never again discussed their HIV status with him or any other friend or family member, primarily because they perceived a lack of willingness to talk about their HIV status with them. As one woman explained:

"*I went to test. [After the test]... I made a phone call to my husband. He told me that it is my problem. He said he doesn't have [HIV]... I told him and he ran away, and when he came back he told me not to tell him that information again.*" (Participant #218, Age 21).

Some women reported that their husbands did not want them to disclose their status to anyone else. This lack of communication and low level of disclosure beyond partners left some women feeling isolated as they struggled to come to terms with their HIV diagnosis.

Women's perceptions of HIV-related attitudes suggested that, for most, the potential negative social consequences of disclosure still outweighed perceived benefits, which contributed to low levels of attendance at HIV clinics and support groups.

Interactions with health workers. Health workers might be considered another potentially important source of support for women with HIV. Yet many women described suboptimal communications with health workers. In the context of HIV

counselling, many women reported feeling unprepared for being tested:

"*I felt like she just ambushed me and tested me... people are supposed to be given counselling... so that if [the test result] is positive... you won't have to worry a lot.*" (Participant #228, Age 32).

In addition, many women reported being "*talked to badly*" by reception staff at the HIV clinic, with some feeling "*a little despised*". They found this particularly intimidating during early visits to the HIV clinic and some women reported being afraid to attend the clinic again if they had missed an appointment for fear of being reprimanded.

Other instances where interactions with health workers negatively affected uptake of services were also reported. One woman travelled to her rural home for three months where the HIV clinic refused to register her as she lived in Naivasha so she only began attending services when she returned to Naivasha.

"*They said I couldn't [attend the local HIV clinic]. I must be at a permanent place because of my status... I was not from there so they said they wouldn't do a CD4 for me.*" (Participant 116, Age 33).

Another participant was told not to start ART until she had completed three months of treatment for tuberculosis, which she duly did, even though this delay was contrary to national guidelines for HIV treatment initiation.

In several cases, a sudden change in HIV clinic attendance patterns – from regular attendance at scheduled appointments to non-attendance – came immediately following a negative experience within the hospital. One woman, for example, dropped out of care when she was asked to repeat (and re-pay for) her CD4 count test as her result had been lost. Another woman stopped attending following a miscarriage. In addition to associating her miscarriage with having started ART a week before it occurred, she described staff refusal to attend to her during the stillbirth. At the time of the interview, she had not been to the HIV clinic for five months, meaning that she was not receiving cotrimoxazole as recommended.

Conversely, one woman began attending HIV services months after her HIV diagnosis based on a positive interaction with a health worker: she had attempted to abandon her baby and commit suicide but she was caught, arrested, and taken to the hospital where she reported having received great support and encouragement through counselling from the hospital matron.

Health services-related factors. Reflecting the quantitative findings, costs, including transport costs, were frequently mentioned as a barrier to hospital attendance.

"I lacked money to start on ARVs because I was told that I had to have 250 shillings ($2.87) to begin the clinic. It took me time because everyone had deserted me… my neighbours, husband… I had no friends and no money. So it forced me to sell my baby's blanket so that I could afford to start the clinic." (Participant #215, Age 22).

Many women reported that they had delayed or not had a CD4 count blood-draw due to its cost (usually approximately KShs170 ($1.95)). Conversely, antiretrovirals being free proved a very strong motivational factor for many women to attend HIV services.

Women described difficulties navigating the pathway between HIV testing in pregnancy-related services and long-term HIV care and treatment. Women described having to visit multiple departments in a single day with long waiting times and having to visit the hospital on many different days:

"They make you wait the whole day and make you come here another time for something else, it is not good." (Participant #115, Age 20).

Additional challenges included difficulty in understanding directions, poor understanding of the patient pathway and restricted clinic hours.

Discussion

A lower proportion (53%) of women diagnosed with HIV in pregnancy in this cohort registered at the HIV clinic than in previously published studies (62–85%) from elsewhere in sub-Saharan Africa, [9–12] although this might be partially explained by this study's relatively short follow-up period. The higher proportion of women registering at an HIV clinic in this study compared to the retrospective study we carried out in Naivasha Hospital can be largely attributed to improvements in attendance over time and the ability of the prospective cohort to capture women's attendance at a range of HIV clinics outside Naivasha Hospital.

The uptake of ART among known-eligible women diagnosed with HIV in pregnancy-related services reported in previous studies in sub-Saharan Africa has varied enormously (12–95%). [9,10,12–19] A recent meta-analysis that included both observational and intervention studies estimated that 68% of women diagnosed with HIV in pregnancy had a CD4 cell count done and that 61% of the women who were eligible for ART started treatment. [20] Due to attrition at each step along the pathway to treatment, our study found low uptake of ART in comparison to many other studies. [4] The scale of and reasons underlying attrition from long-term HIV care and treatment services around the time of delivery warrant further study in larger studies.

The qualitative finding that lack of social support impeded uptake of long-term HIV care and treatment services echoes previous studies that have found higher levels of social support to facilitate uptake of PMTCT services and adherence to ART.

[21,22] Although nurse escorts to the HIV clinic at Naivasha Hospital might have increased registration at this clinic immediately following diagnosis with HIV in pregnancy-related services, the high proportion of women who never returned for a subsequent visit to the HIV clinic suggests the need for on-going support for women to ensure uptake of CD4 count testing as well as on-going care and treatment services. The association between having cared for someone living with HIV and successful linkage to the HIV clinic is a new finding. Previous studies have shown close personal contact with someone with HIV to be associated with changes in HIV-related risk behaviours, [23,24] but this has not previously been explored with regard to uptake of HIV care and treatment services.

Although an insufficient measure for informed choice, the weak association between women reporting having received enough information to decide whether or not to take an HIV test and registering at an HIV clinic suggests that current counselling in some settings may be insufficient for preparing pregnant women for a potential HIV diagnosis, with implications for their subsequent uptake of care. A study in Uganda found that some women perceive provider-initiated HIV testing and counselling within antenatal care as compulsory and they do not fully understand its potential consequences, [25] but this remains an underexplored area.

Finally, this study confirms previous studies' findings that complicated patient pathways, [11,26,27] low knowledge among clients of the need to attend the HIV clinic, [27] transportation costs, [28–33] and negative experiences in health facilities may adversely affect future uptake of services. [28,34,35].

Limitations

Limitations of this study include its relatively small sample size. We may have over-estimated client losses if some of the 18 women with no follow-up information accessed HIV care outside the study area. On the other hand, observation showed that the hospital's policy that a nurse from the ANC should accompany any HIV-positive woman to the HIV clinic was not always followed so researchers escorting women to the HIV clinic will have improved their initial linkage into care.

The difficulty arranging qualitative interviews with women who had poorer hospital attendance meant that interview participants under-represented this group. Women's primary reason for refusing to be interviewed was that they had travelled to rural areas and would not return for weeks or months, which would equally have impeded their hospital attendance.

Conclusions and Recommendations

Only 15% of women estimated to be ART-eligible in this cohort started ART within 90 days of their HIV diagnosis. Recommendations for increasing uptake of long-term HIV care and treatment services include: appropriate counselling that allows sufficient time and information for women to make informed decisions about if and when to use services; simplifying the pathway to care by reducing the required number of visits and increasing accessibility of CD4 testing, ideally using point-of-care CD4 testing; ensuring the daily availability of ART services within ANC (this is being promoted by the Kenyan government and the WHO); [8,36] ensuring adequate staffing within ANC, delivery and the HIV clinic; linking women to the HIV clinic post-delivery; and improving the quality of interactions between health workers and clients.

The benefits to an individual of timely access to care, coupled with the increased costs to the health system incurred through delayed access, draw attention to the need to address the factors identified as impediments to prompt linkage into HIV care and treatment services.

Acknowledgments

The authors thank the staff and leadership of Naivasha District Hospital and gratefully acknowledge the study participants whose willingness to

participate in the study made this work possible. The authors are grateful to Peter Godfrey-Faussett, Caroline Jones, Karen Edmond and Justin Parkhurst for their advice on the study design, and to Ernestina Coast and Julia Hussein for comments on an earlier draft of this manuscript.

Author Contributions

Conceived and designed the experiments: LF AG KK DR. Performed the experiments: LF SV JO. Analyzed the data: LF JL AG KK DW-J DR. Wrote the paper: LF AG JL KK DW-J SV JO DR.

References

1. Hensen B, Baggaley R, Wong VJ, Grabbe KL, Shaffer N, et al. (2012) Universal voluntary HIV testing in antenatal care settings: a review of the contribution of provider-initiated testing & counselling. Tropical Medicine & International Health 17: 59–70.
2. Abrams E (2010) Eliminating vertical transmission: Rights here, right now. International AIDS Conference. Vienna, Austria.
3. World Health Organisation (2013) Consolidated guidelines on the use of antiretroviral drugs for treating and preventing HIV infection: recommendations for a public health approach. Geneva, Switzerland: WHO.
4. Ferguson L, Grant AD, Watson-Jones D, Kahawita T, Ong'ech JO, et al. (2012) Linking women who test HIV-positive in pregnancy-related services to long-term HIV care and treatment services: a systematic review. Tropical Medicine & International Health 17: 564–580.
5. Ferguson L, Lewis J, Grant AD, Watson-Jones D, Vusha S, et al. (2012) Patient Attrition Between Diagnosis With HIV in Pregnancy-Related Services and Long-Term HIV Care and Treatment Services in Kenya: A Retrospective Study. JAIDS Journal of Acquired Immune Deficiency Syndromes 60: e90–e97 10.1097/QAI.1090b1013e318253258a.
6. Kenya National Bureau of Statistics, I.C.F Macro (2010) Kenya Demographic and Health Survey, 2008–09. Calverton, Maryland, USA.
7. Ministry of Health, Republic of Kenya (2009) National Guidelines for the Prevention of Mother-to-Child Transmission (PMTCT) of HIV/AIDS in Kenya. Third ed. Nairobi, Kenya.
8. Ministry of Health, Republic of Kenya (2010) National Recommendations for Prevention of Mother to Child Transmission of HIV, Infant and Young Child Feeding and Antiretroviral therapy for children, adults and adolescents. Nairobi, Kenya.
9. Balira R (2010) Implementation of Prevention of Mother-to-Child Transmission of HIV and Maternal Syphilis Screening and Treatment Programmes in Mwanza Region, Tanzania: Uptake and Challenges. London: London School of Hygiene & Tropical Medicine. 233 p.
10. Muchedzi A, Chandisarewa W, Keatinge J, Stranix-Chibanda L, Woelk G, et al. (2010) Factors associated with access to HIV care and treatment in a prevention of mother to child transmission programme in urban Zimbabwe. Journal of the International AIDS Society 13: 38.
11. Otieno PA, Kohler PK, Bosire RK, Brown ER, Macharia SW, et al. (2010) Determinants of failure to access care in mothers referred to HIV treatment programs in Nairobi, Kenya. AIDS Care 22: 729–736.
12. Killam WP, Tambatamba BC, Chintu N, Rouse D, Stringer E, et al. (2010) Antiretroviral therapy in antenatal care to increase treatment initiation in HIV-infected pregnant women: a stepped-wedge evaluation. AIDS 24: 85–91.
13. Chi BH, Chintu N, Lee A, Stringer EM, Sinkala M, et al. (2007) Expanded services for the prevention of mother-to-child HIV transmission: field acceptability of a pilot program in Lusaka, Zambia. JAIDS Journal of Acquired Immune Deficiency Syndromes 45: 125–127
14. Chen JY, Ogwu AC, Svab P, Lockman S, Moffat HJ, et al. (2010) Antiretroviral treatment initiation among HIV-infected pregnant women with low CD4(+) cell counts in Gaborone, Botswana. Journal of Acquired Immune Deficiency Syndromes: JAIDS 54: 102–106.
15. Kranzer K, Zeinecker J, Ginsberg P, Orrell C, Kalawe NN, et al. (2010) Linkage to HIV Care and Antiretroviral Therapy in Cape Town, South Africa. PLoS ONE 5: e13801.
16. Stinson K, Boulle A, Coetzee D, Abrams EJ, Myer L (2010) Initiation of highly active antiretroviral therapy among pregnant women in Cape Town, South Africa. Tropical Medicine & International Health 15: 825–832.
17. Tonwe-Gold B, Ekouevi DK, Bosse CA, Toure S, Kone M, et al. (2009) Implementing family-focused HIV care and treatment: the first 2 years' experience of the mother-to-child transmission-plus program in Abidjan, Cote d'Ivoire. Tropical Medicine and International Health 14: 204–212.
18. Mandala J, Torpey K, Kasonde P, Kabaso M, Dirks R, et al. (2009) Prevention of mother-to-child transmission of HIV in Zambia: implementing efficacious ARV regimens in primary health centers. BMC Public Health 9: 314.
19. Clouse K, Pettifor A, Shearer K, Maskew M, Bassett J, et al. (2013) Loss to follow-up before and after delivery among women testing HIV positive during pregnancy in Johannesburg, South Africa. Tropical Medicine & International Health 18: 451–460.
20. Wettstein C, Mugglin C, Egger M, Blaser N, Salazar L, et al. (2012) Missed Opportunities to Prevent Mother-to-Child-Transmission in sub-Saharan Africa: Systematic Review and Meta-Analysis. AIDS (acquired immune deficiency syndrome).
21. Chinkonde JR, Sundby J, Martinson F (2009) The prevention of mother-to-child HIV transmission programme in Lilongwe, Malawi: why do so many women drop out. Reproductive Health Matters 17: 143–151
22. Ware NC, Idoko J, Kaaya S, Biraro IA, Wyatt MA, et al. (2009) Explaining Adherence Success in Sub-Saharan Africa: An Ethnographic Study. PLoS Med 6: e1000011.
23. Palekar R, Pettifor A, Behets F, MacPhail C (2008) Association Between Knowing Someone Who Died of AIDS and Behavior Change Among South African Youth. AIDS and Behavior 12: 903–912.
24. Macintyre K, Brown L, Sosler S (2001) "It's Not What You Know, But Who You Knew": Examining the Relationship Between Behavior Change and AIDS Mortality in Africa. AIDS Education and Prevention 13: 160–174.
25. Larsson EC, Thorson A, Pariyo G, Conrad P, Arinaitwe M, et al. (2012) Opt-out HIV testing during antenatal care: experiences of pregnant women in rural Uganda. Health Policy and Planning 27: 69–75.
26. Levy JM (2009) Women's expectations of treatment and care after an antenatal HIV diagnosis in Lilongwe, Malawi. Reproductive Health Matters 17: 152–161.
27. Watson-Jones D, Balira R, Ross DA, Weiss HA, Mabey D (2012) Missed opportunities: poor linkage into ongoing care for HIV-positive pregnant women in Mwanza, Tanzania. PLoS One 7: e40091.
28. Duff P, Kipp W, Wild TC, Rubaale T, Okech-Ojony J, et al. (2010) Barriers to accessing highly active antiretroviral therapy by HIV-positive women attending an antenatal clinic in a regional hospital in western Uganda. Journal of the International AIDS Society 13: 37.
29. Kaplan R, Orrell C, Zwane E, Bekker L-G, Wood R (2008) Loss to follow-up and mortality among pregnant women referred to a community clinic for antiretroviral treatment. Aids 22: 1679–1681.
30. Miller CM, Ketlhapile M, Rybasack-Smith H, Rosen S (2010) Why are antiretroviral treatment patients lost to follow-up? A qualitative study from South Africa. (Special Issue: Retention of patients in HIV/AIDS care and treatment programs in Sub-Saharan Africa.) Tropical Medicine and International Health 15: 48–54.
31. Mshana GH, Wamoyi J, Busza J, Zaba B, Changalucha J, et al. (2006) Barriers to accessing antiretroviral therapy in Kisesa Tanzania: a qualitative study of early rural referrals to the national program. AIDS Patient Care & STDs 20: 649–657.
32. Nachega JB, Mills EJ, Schechter M (2010) Antiretroviral therapy adherence and retention in care in middle-income and low-income countries: current status of knowledge and research priorities. Current Opinion in HIV and AIDS 5: 70–77.
33. Tuller DM, Bangsberg DR, Senkungu J, Ware NC, Emenyonu N, et al. (2010) Transportation costs impede sustained adherence and access to HAART in a clinic population in southwestern Uganda: a qualitative study. AIDS & Behavior 14: 778–784.
34. Painter TM, Diaby KL, Matia DM, Lin LS, Sibailly TS, et al. (2004) Women's reasons for not participating in follow up visits before starting short course antiretroviral prophylaxis for prevention of mother to child transmission of HIV: qualitative interview study. BMJ 329: 543.
35. Sprague C, Chersich MF, Black V (2011) Health system weaknesses constrain access to PMTCT and maternal HIV services in South Africa: a qualitative enquiry. AIDS Res Ther 8: 10.
36. WHO (2012) Use of antiretroviral drugs for treating pregnant women and preventing HIV infection in infants: Programmatic update. In: Department HA, editor. Geneva: WHO.

20

Daily Oral Emtricitabine/Tenofovir Preexposure Prophylaxis and Herpes Simplex Virus Type 2 among Men Who Have Sex with Men

Julia L. Marcus[1,2], David V. Glidden[3], Vanessa McMahan[1], Javier R. Lama[4], Kenneth H. Mayer[5,6], Albert Y. Liu[7], Orlando Montoya-Herrera[8], Martin Casapia[9], Brenda Hoagland[10], Robert M. Grant[1,3]*

1 Gladstone Institute of Virology and Immunology, San Francisco, California, United States or America, **2** University of California, Berkeley, California, United States of America, **3** University of California San Francisco, San Francisco, California, United States of America, **4** Asociación Civil Impacta Salud y Educación, Lima, Peru, **5** Fenway Institute, Fenway Health, Boston, Massachusetts, United States of America, **6** Beth Israel Deaconess Medical Center, Boston, Massachusetts, United States of America, **7** Bridge HIV, San Francisco Department of Public Health, San Francisco, California, United States of America, **8** Fundación Ecuatoriana Equidad, Guayaquil, Guayas, Ecuador, **9** Asociación Civil Selva Amazónica, Iquitos, Peru, **10** Instituto de Pesquisa Clínica Evandro Chagas, Fundação Oswaldo Cruz, Rio de Janeiro, Brazil

Abstract

Background: In addition to protecting against HIV acquisition, antiretroviral preexposure prophylaxis (PrEP) using topical 1% tenofovir gel reduced *Herpes simplex* virus type 2 (HSV-2) acquisition by 51% among women in the CAPRISA 004 study. We examined the effect of daily oral emtricitabine/tenofovir (FTC/TDF) PrEP on HSV-2 seroincidence and ulcer occurrence among men who have sex with men (MSM) in the iPrEx trial.

Methods: HSV-2 serum testing was performed at screening and every six months. Among HSV-2-seronegative individuals, we used Cox regression models to estimate hazard ratios (HRs) of HSV-2 seroincidence associated with randomization to FTC/TDF. We used multiple imputation and Cox regression to estimate HRs for HSV-2 seroincidence accounting for drug exposure. We assessed ulcer occurrence among participants with prevalent or incident HSV-2 infection.

Results: Of the 2,499 participants, 1383 (55.3%) tested HSV-2-seronegative at baseline, 892 (35.7%) tested positive, 223 (8.9%) had indeterminate tests, and one test was not done. Of the 1,347 HSV-2-seronegative participants with follow-up, 125 (9.3%) had incident HSV-2 infection (5.9 per 100 person-years). Compared with participants receiving placebo, there was no difference in HSV-2 seroincidence among participants receiving FTC/TDF (HR 1.1, 95% CI: 0.8–1.5; $P = 0.64$) or among participants receiving FTC/TDF with a concentration of tenofovir diphosphate >16 per million viable cells (HR 1.0, 95% CI: 0.3–3.5; $P = 0.95$). Among participants with HSV-2 infection, the proportion with ≥1 moderate or severe ulcer adverse event was twice as high in the placebo vs. active arm (5.9% vs. 2.9%, $P = 0.02$), but there were no differences in the proportions with ≥1 clinical examination during which perianal or groin ulcers were identified.

Conclusions: Tenofovir in daily oral FTC/TDF PrEP may reduce the occurrence of ulcers in individuals with HSV-2 infection but does not protect against HSV-2 incidence among MSM.

Editor: D. William Cameron, University of Ottawa, Canada

Funding: This study was supported by the Division of Acquired Immunodeficiency Syndrome, National Institute of Allergy and Infectious Diseases, National Institutes of Health, as a cooperative agreement (UO1 AI64002, to Dr. Grant), by the Bill and Melinda Gates Foundation, and by the Gladstone Institutes. The funders had no role in study design, data collection and analysis, decision to publish, or preparation of the manuscript.

* E-mail: robert.grant@ucsf.edu

Introduction

Herpes simplex virus 2 (HSV-2) is the primary cause of genital ulcer disease worldwide. In 2003, an estimated 536 million people aged 15–49 years were living with the infection, with seroprevalence varying widely across settings and populations.[1] Most infected individuals are unaware of their infections.[2] In symptomatic infections, the virus causes painful ulcerative lesions that can take two to four weeks to heal in primary outbreaks, and recurrences can be frequent. The prevalence of HSV-2 infection in the general population ranges from 10 to 60 percent, with higher prevalences in female sex workers, men who have sex with men (MSM), and certain regions of the world. [3] Among human immunodeficiency virus (HIV)-infected populations, the estimated seroprevalence of HSV-2 is 60–95 percent, [3] and individuals coinfected with HIV have increased susceptibility to HSV-2 shedding and clinical manifestations of HSV-2 disease. [4] Observational studies have found a two-to-three-fold higher risk of HIV acquisition among individuals with HSV-2 infection, [5,6] although randomized trials of HSV-2 treatment have not reduced HIV acquisition or transmission [7,8].

In addition to protecting against HIV acquisition, antiretroviral preexposure prophylaxis (PrEP) using tenofovir has been shown to have a protective effect on HSV-2 in women. Pericoital 1% vaginal tenofovir gel reduced the risk of HSV-2 acquisition by 51% in women participating in the CAPRISA 004 study. [9] In fact, the protection against HSV-2 in that study was higher than the effect of the gel on HIV acquisition, and a mathematical model suggested that its effect on HSV-2 acquisition may have played a role in its success in protecting against HIV. [10] Oral tenofovir-based PrEP also reduced HSV-2 acquisition by 28% among heterosexual men and women who were HIV-negative and HSV-2-seronegative in the Partners PrEP study. [11] The anti-herpetic effects of tenofovir have since been confirmed in vitro [12].

Protection against HSV-2 could enhance the public health impact of tenofovir when used as an antiretroviral agent for HIV prevention or treatment. Daily oral emtricitabine/tenofovir (FTC/TDF) PrEP was shown to reduce HIV acquisition in MSM in the iPrEx trial, [13] but it is unknown whether tenofovir protects against HSV-2 acquisition or disease expression among MSM. Using data from the randomized iPrEx study, our primary aim was to determine the effect of daily oral FTC/TDF on HSV-2 seroincidence; secondarily, we examined the effect of FTC/TDF on ulcer occurrence. To inform the development of HSV-2 prevention interventions among MSM, we also aimed to identify demographic and behavioral risk factors for HSV-2 seroincidence in the iPrEx cohort.

Materials and Methods

Ethics statement

The iPrEx study (ClinicalTrials.gov: NCT00458393) was approved by the Committee on Human Research at the University of California, San Francisco, as well as local institutional review boards (IRBs) at each study site: Comité Institucional de Bioética, Asociación Civil Impacta Salud y Educación, Lima, Peru; Universidad San Francisco de Quito, IRB #1, Quito, Ecuador; Fenway Community Health Institutional Review Board, Boston, MA; Comissão de Ética para Análise de Projetos de Pesquisa, CAPPesq Hospital das Clínicas da Faculdade de Medicina da USP, São Paulo, Brazil; Comitê de Ética em Pesquisa, Hospital Universitario Clementino Fraga Filho/Universidade Federal de Rio de Janeiro, Rio de Janeiro, Brazil; Comitê de Ética em Pesquisa do Instituto de Pesquisa Clínica Evandro Chagas, Rio de Janeiro, Brazil; National IRB: Comissão Nacional de Ética em Pesquisa – CONEP, Ministério da Saúde, Brasília, Brazil; University of Cape Town Research Ethics Committee, Cape Town, South Africa; Human Experimentation Committee, Research Institute for Health Sciences, Chiang Mai, Thailand; Ethical Review Committee for Research in Human Subjects, Department of Medical Services, Ministry of Public Health, Nonthaburi, Thailand; Research Ethics Committee, Faculty of Medicine, Chiang Mai University, Chiang Mai, Thailand. Written informed consent was obtained from each participant prior to enrollment in the study.

Study population and procedures

Details of the iPrEx trial have been previously published. [13] Briefly, the study enrolled 2,499 MSM and transgender women at risk for HIV infection at 11 sites in Peru, Ecuador, Brazil, South Africa, Thailand, and the United States. Participants were randomized to receive either daily oral FTC/TDF or placebo. Monthly visits included medical history and symptom-directed

physical examination, adverse event (AE) assessment, study drug dispensation, HIV testing, risk-reduction counseling, and adherence assessment. Serologic testing for HSV-2 and physical examinations for signs of sexually transmitted infections (STI) were performed by clinicians at screening (baseline), every six months during follow-up, and when the study drug was suspended, or when prompted by symptoms reported during the monthly medical examination. HIV infection status was determined using two rapid antibody tests and confirmed by Western blot or RNA testing. Sexual practices during the previous three months were assessed by interviewer-administered questionnaires at screening and quarterly visits during follow-up. The primary analysis of iPrEx data included visits through the pre-specified cutoff date of May 1, 2010, while the current analyses include follow-up visits through September 30, 2010, the last visit at which participants would have been expected to have had exposure to study drug.

HSV-2 infection status was determined using ELISA (Herpe-Select, Focus Diagnostics). A negative HSV-2 test was defined as having an index ratio (i.e., the ratio of the optical density of the color generated by the sample to the optical density of a standard calibrator; IR) <0.9, while a positive HSV-2 test was defined as having an IR ≥3.5. [14] Tests with an IR ≥0.9 and <3.5 were classified as indeterminate; participants with an IR <3.5 were retested at the next testing time point. The date of HSV-2 seroconversion was the date of the first positive HSV-2 test. Perianal and groin ulcers were recorded if there was any ulcerative lesion identified during STI examination, which may have included ulcers associated with herpes, syphilis, chancroid, lymphogranuloma venereum, or excoriation. Ulcer AEs were identified by a clinician as an increase in ulcer severity or frequency from baseline, including new onset of ulcers in individuals without preexisting ulcer disease; severity was defined according to the infection criteria in the National Institutes of Health Division of AIDS Table for Grading the Severity of Adult and Pediatric Adverse Events, December 2004. Only clinical AEs that were Grade 2 or above were reported in iPrEx, per protocol; thus, Grade 1 ulcers were not reported as ulcer AEs. Ulcer AEs were identified during STI examination, or were self-reported by participants and not confirmed on clinical examination if symptoms resolved before the examination visit. Additionally, ulcers that were self-reported but confirmed to be a different clinical manifestation during examination were not classified as ulcers or included in this analysis. In a subset of participants assigned to the active arm, levels of FTC and tenofovir were measured in plasma and peripheral blood mononuclear cells (PBMCs). Participants with drug level tests were 1) in the DEXA substudy, which evaluated the impact of FTC/TDF on bone and body composition at seven sites in Peru, Brazil, South Africa, Thailand, and the United States; and/or 2) matched active-arm controls in the case-control substudy of HIV seroconverters (from nine iPrEx sites with active-arm seroconversions). Approximately one-third of the cohort had at least one drug level test.

Statistical analyses

For HSV-2 prevalence analyses, the dependent variable was HSV-2 status at the screening visit, and independent variables were randomization group and other baseline characteristics, including age, level of education, transgender identity, number of alcoholic drinks on days when drinking in the past month, and sexual behaviors in the past three months. Sexual behavior variables were number of anal sex partners, any receptive anal intercourse with a condom (cRAI), any receptive anal intercourse with no condom (ncRAI), any insertive anal intercourse with a condom (cIAI), and any insertive anal intercourse with no condom (ncIAI). We used chi-square tests and log-binomial models to identify factors associated with HSV-2 prevalence at baseline. We also examined the association of age with HSV-2 prevalence and HSV-2 seroincidence using chi-square tests for trend.

For HSV-2 seroincidence analyses, the dependent variable was time to HSV-2 seroconversion during follow-up, and independent variables were randomization group and the demographic and behavioral variables examined in HSV-2 prevalence analyses. We calculated crude rates of HSV-2 seroincidence by randomization group and baseline demographic and behavioral characteristics, including only participants who tested seronegative for HSV-2 at the screening visit. Person-time at risk included time from study enrollment to the first of HSV-2 infection, study drug discontinuation, or loss to follow-up. We estimated the time-to-event distribution by randomization group using Kaplan-Meier methodology. We used Cox regression models to estimate unadjusted and adjusted hazard ratios (HRs) for time to HSV-2 seroincidence. An intent-to-treat analysis included only randomization group; to identify factors associated with time to HSV-2 seroincidence, a multivariable model additionally included demographic and behavioral variables that were statistically significant at the $P<0.05$ level in unadjusted analyses. Sexual behavior variables were time-updated in models at approximately three-month intervals, while other covariates were treated as fixed. All models were stratified by study site.

Among the same participants, we also conducted an as-treated analysis that accounted for study drug use among participants receiving FTC/TDF. Because drug level testing was only conducted in a subset of participants and visits, drug levels were imputed for participants in both arms at any monthly visit missing drug level data using chained equations and predictive means matching. Predictors in the imputations included study week, study site, baseline number of sexual partners, baseline ncRAI, transgender identity, body mass index, weight, report of an STI in the six months before screening, secondary education, circumcision, baseline HSV-2 infection, age, and number of drinks on days when the participant drank in the prior month. Covariates were used to predict the probability of having detectable drug and the probability that the level of tenofovir diphosphate (TFV-DP) in PBMCs was >16 fmol per million viable cells, the concentration associated with an estimated 90% reduction in HIV acquisition. [15] Drug levels were multiply imputed [16] for visits at which drug level testing was not conducted but the participant was still taking study drug, with 200 imputations per observation. [17] We then used site-stratified Cox regression to estimate HRs for HSV-2 seroincidence associated with being randomized to the FTC/TDF arm and having detectable drug with TFV-DP ≤16 or being randomized to the FTC/TDF arm and having detectable drug with TFV-DP >16. Unadjusted models included only a time-dependent covariate for drug detection, while adjusted models also included age, level of education, transgender identity, number of alcoholic drinks on days when drinking in the past month, and sexual behaviors in the past three months (number of anal sex partners, cRAI, ncRAI, cIAI, and ncIAI). Sexual behavior variables were time-updated at approximately three-month intervals.

To examine the effect of FTC/TDF on HSV-2 disease expression, we analyzed the occurrence of ulcers among those who tested seropositive for HSV-2 at baseline or during follow-up. To eliminate the potential effect of HIV infection on ulcer occurrence, participants were excluded if the HSV-2 diagnosis occurred at or after HIV seroconversion, and ulcers were excluded if they occurred at or after HIV seroconversion. We estimated the proportion of participants with ≥1 ulcer AE classified as Grade 2

or above (i.e., moderate, severe, or potentially life-threatening), ≥1 STI examination during which a perianal ulcer was detected, and ≥1 STI examination during which a groin ulcer was detected, using chi-square tests to compare proportions by randomization group. We assessed the proportion of visits at which symptoms were reported that prompted an STI examination, using a chi-square test for comparison by randomization group. We also examined ulcers occurring after HIV seroconversion to determine whether there were differences in ulcer occurrence by randomization group in the absence of study drug.

All analyses were conducted in SAS 9.3 or Stata 12.

Results

Study participants

Characteristics of the 2,499 iPrEx participants have been described previously. [13] Briefly, all participants were born male and 313 (13.0%) identified as transgender or as women. The mean age at enrollment was 25 years (range 18–67), and the majority of participants were enrolled at the three study sites in Peru (1,400, 56.0%). At baseline, over half of participants (59.4%) reported having had ncRAI in the past three months. Among participants with prevalent or incident HSV-2 infection, 11.6% used acyclovir or valacyclovir during study follow-up.

HSV-2 prevalence

Of the 2,499 participants, 1383 (55.3%) tested negative for HSV-2 at baseline, 892 (35.7%) tested positive, 223 (8.9%) had indeterminate tests, and one test was not done. Of the 223 with indeterminate tests at baseline, 114 (51.1%) tested positive for HSV-2 infection at some point during follow-up. Factors associated with testing seropositive for HSV-2 at baseline included older age (P trend <0.001; Figure 1a), transgender identity (prevalence ratio [PR] 2.0, 95% confidence interval [CI]: 1.8–2.2; $P<0.001$), and not having a secondary education (PR 1.4, 95% CI: 1.2–1.5; $P<0.001$). The prevalence of HSV-2 infection was highest among participants living in Peru (46.0%), Brazil (37.8%), and Ecuador (37.3%), with lower prevalence among participants living in Thailand (6.4%), South Africa (17.6%), and the United States (27.1%; $P<0.001$). Randomization group was not associated with HSV-2 prevalence at baseline ($P=0.44$). In multivariable analysis, all factors remained significantly associated with HSV-2 prevalence with the exception of level of education.

FTC/TDF and time to HSV-2 seroincidence

Characteristics of 1,383 participants who tested seronegative for HSV-2 at baseline are presented by randomization group in Table 1. There were no differences in baseline characteristics by randomization group, with the exception of cRAI in the past three months being reported more frequently in the placebo arm ($P=0.01$).

Of the 1,383 participants who tested seronegative for HSV-2 at baseline, 36 (2.6%) did not contribute person-time to incidence analyses because they were retrospectively found to be HIV-infected at baseline, tested seropositive for HSV-2 at the enrollment visit subsequent to screening, or were lost to follow-up after enrollment. Of the remaining 1,347 seronegative participants, 125 (9.3%) were diagnosed with HSV-2 during follow-up, representing an incidence of 5.9 per 100 person-years (Table 2). In unadjusted analysis, HSV-2 incidence decreased with age, with the highest rate among participants aged <25 years (7.1 per 100 person-years) and the lowest rate among participants aged ≥40 years (1.6 per 100 person-years; P trend = 0.001). Country of residence was also associated with HSV-2 incidence, with the

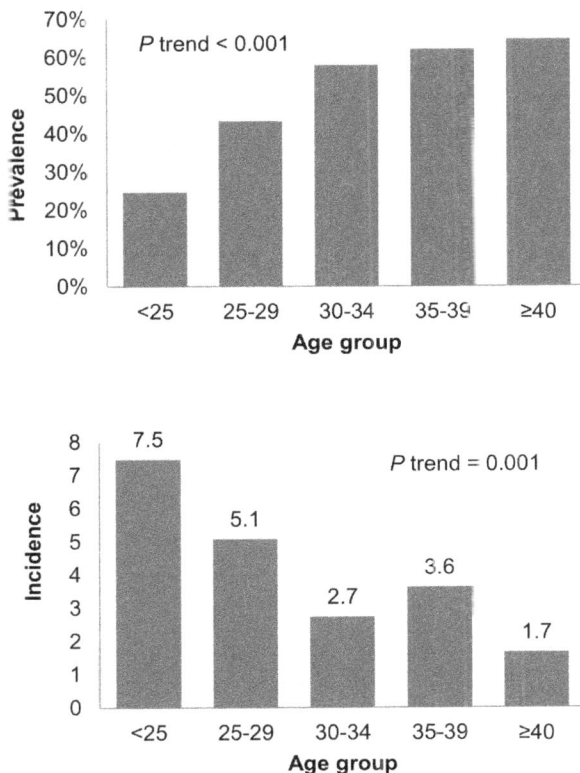

Figure 1. Baseline prevalence of HSV-2 and incidence of HSV-2 during study follow-up by age at enrollment. Figure 1a shows HSV-2 prevalence at baseline by age group at enrollment, while Figure 1b shows HSV-2 incidence during follow-up by age group at enrollment. HSV-2, herpes simplex virus type 2.

highest rate among participants living in Ecuador (9.7 per 100 person-years) and the lowest rate among participants living in Thailand (1.7 per 100 person-years). The only behavioral factor associated with time to HSV-2 incidence was ncRAI in the past three months (HR 2.0, 95% CI: 1.4-3.0; $P<0.001$). In multivariable analysis, younger age and ncRAI remained associated with time to HSV-2 incidence, while level of education, transgender identity, alcohol use, and other sexual behaviors were not associated with time to HSV-2 seroincidence.

Of those who acquired HSV-2 during follow-up, 65 were in the FTC/TDF group (incidence of 6.1 per 100 person-years) and 60 were in the placebo group (incidence of 5.6 per 100 person-years). There was no significant difference in time to HSV-2 incidence among participants assigned to the FTC/TDF arm compared with those assigned to the placebo arm (HR 1.1, 95% CI: 0.8-1.5; $P=0.64$; Figure 2). Compared with participants in the placebo arm, there was also no difference in time to HSV-2 incidence among participants in the FTC/TDF group with a detectable drug level and ≤16 TFV-DP (HR 1.0, 95% CI: 0.4-2.5; $P=0.97$), with similar results among those in the FTC/TDF group with >16 TFV-DP (HR 1.0, 95% CI: 0.3-3.5; $P=0.95$). Results did not change after adjustment for age, education, transgender identity, alcohol use, or sexual behaviors.

FTC/TDF and ulcer occurrence

A total of 1,019 participants tested seropositive for HSV-2 at baseline or during follow-up; of those, 22 (2.2%) tested seropositive for HSV-2 after HIV seroconversion. Among the remaining 997,

there were 72 ulcer AEs classified as Grade 2 or above, with 43 participants (4.3%) having ≥1 ulcer AE. Among the 72 ulcer AEs, 23 (31.9%) were confirmed on STI examination; for the remainder, symptoms resolved before an examination was conducted. Compared with participants in the placebo arm, the proportion of participants with ≥1 ulcer AE was reduced by half among participants in the FTC/TDF arm (2.9% vs. 5.9%, $P=0.02$; Figure 3). There were no differences by randomization group in the proportion of participants with ≥1 STI examination during which a perianal ulcer (FTC/TDF 3.5% vs. placebo 4.7%, $P=0.37$) or groin ulcer (FTC/TDF 2.5% vs. placebo 1.9%, $P=0.51$) was identified; results were similar after excluding participants with a positive syphilis rapid plasma reagin test at the same visit. However, symptoms that prompted STI examination were less common in the FTC/TDF arm compared with the placebo arm (3.7% vs. 7.4%, $P=0.01$).

Among the 89 participants with prevalent or incident HSV-2 infection who also seroconverted to HIV during study follow-up, 6.7% had ≥1 ulcer AE, 6.7% had ≥1 STI examination during which a perianal ulcer was identified, and 5.6% had ≥1 STI examination during which a groin ulcer was identified after HIV seroconversion, and thus after stopping study drug. The proportions with each type of ulcer did not differ between participants in the FTC/TDF arm and participants in the placebo arm.

Finally, the iPrEx protocol did not use the HSV-2 test manufacturer's suggested cutoffs for indeterminate (IR ≥0.9 and ≤1.1) or positive (IR>1.1) tests, but conducting the incidence and ulcer analyses using the cutoffs from the package insert yielded similar results.

Discussion

In this analysis of participants in the iPrEx trial of daily oral FTC/TDF PrEP, we found no association between FTC/TDF and incidence of HSV-2 infection, even after accounting for actual use of FTC/TDF using drug level test results in a subset. The proportion of participants in the FTC/TDF arm with at least one ulcer AE classified as Grade 2 or above was half of that seen in the placebo arm, and this association was no longer present among participants who had stopped study drug after HIV seroconversion; however, this finding was not confirmed by ulcers identified during STI examinations and may have included ulcers of nonherpetic etiologies. In contrast to the 51% reduction in HSV-2 incidence among women randomized to use a 1% tenofovir topical gel in CAPRISA 004, [9] our results suggest that tenofovir in daily oral FTC/TDF may reduce the occurrence of ulcers in individuals with HSV-2 infection but does not protect against HSV-2 incidence among MSM.

The difference between the effects on HSV-2 incidence seen in CAPRISA and iPrEx may be due to differences in the route of transmission, method of drug delivery, or level of drug exposure. We found that the primary risk factor for incident HSV-2 infection in iPrEx was receptive anal intercourse without a condom, a finding that has been reported in several studies of behavioral risk factors for HSV-2 acquisition in MSM. [13,19,20] The rectal mucosa and cervicovaginal mucosa may differ in their susceptibility to HSV-2 infection. Additionally, although oral dosing of tenofovir achieves drug concentrations that are 20-100 times higher in rectal tissue than in vaginal and cervical tissue, [21,22] topical application of tenofovir achieves a more than 100-fold higher concentration of the drug in the genital tract than oral dosing; [23,24] furthermore, the inhibitory concentration for tenofovir is substantially higher for HSV-2 relative to HIV. [12] Drug concentration is also affected by adherence; while iPrEx

Table 1. Characteristics of participants testing HSV-2 seronegative at baseline by randomization group.[a]

	FTC/TDF (n = 692)	Placebo (n = 691)	P-value
Age group			0.11
<25	413 (60)	449 (65)	
25–29	139 (21)	123 (18)	
30–34	61 (9)	52 (8)	
35–39	28 (4)	34 (5)	
≥40	51 (7)	33 (5)	
Completed secondary education			0.38
Yes	557 (82)	571 (84)	
No	126 (18)	114 (17)	
Transgender identity			0.50
Yes	40 (6)	46 (7)	
No	652 (94)	645 (93)	
No. alcoholic drinks on drinking days, past month			0.11
0–4	323 (48)	294 (43)	
≥5	354 (52)	383 (57)	
Number of anal sex partners, past 3 months			0.87
0–1	90 (13)	85 (12)	
2–5	291 (42)	287 (42)	
≥6	311 (45)	319 (46)	
Insertive anal intercourse with condom, past 3 months			0.94
Yes	343 (50)	350 (51)	
No	349 (50)	341 (49)	
Insertive anal intercourse with no condom, past 3 months			0.57
Yes	419 (61)	408 (59)	
No	273 (39)	283 (41)	
Receptive anal intercourse with condom, past 3 months			0.01
Yes	292 (42)	340 (49)	
No	400 (58)	351 (51)	
Receptive anal intercourse with no condom, past 3 months			0.11
Yes	329 (48)	358 (52)	
No	363 (52)	333 (48)	

[a]HSV-2, herpes simplex virus type 2. Ns may not add up to column totals due to missing data.

participants reported taking over 90% of study drug doses, drug was detectable in the blood specimens of only 50% of participants tested in a random subsample.[13] Although we did not observe an effect of FTC/TDF even after accounting for drug levels, it may be that oral FTC/TDF will be shown to have an impact on HSV-2 incidence in settings where drug exposure is higher as a result of more consistent pill taking, such as the Partners PrEP study.[11]

We found that FTC/TDF was associated with a reduction in moderate or severe ulcer AEs among participants with HSV-2 infection, although this was not confirmed by clinical examination findings. Given the inhibition of HSV-2 replication observed after administration of tenofovir, it is biologically plausible that FTC/TDF reduced the frequency or severity of ulcers. Unlike acyclovir, tenofovir does not require the presence of the herpes virus for drug activation, suggesting that it may suppress ulcers before phosphorylation occurs. However, topical dosing may be required to achieve a concentration of drug in tissue sufficient to inhibit HSV-2 shedding, [12] and a study of adults coinfected with HIV and HSV-2 found no impact of oral tenofovir on rates of HSV-2 shedding. [25] More information is needed about the impact of oral and topical tenofovir on the clinical expression of HSV-2 infection.

There are several limitations of our analysis. First, although our intent-to-treat incidence analysis by treatment arm was strengthened by randomization, our findings may have been diluted by low levels of adherence among participants. While drug levels were not available for all participants or visits, we were able to conduct an incidence analysis that accounted for drug exposure but was subject to the limitations of multiple imputation of a substantial amount of missing data, potential unmeasured confounding, and wide confidence intervals. Of participants with prevalent or incident HSV-2, a small proportion were prescribed acyclovir or valacyclovir during study follow-up; if use of these medications biased our analysis toward the null, it is possible that the effect of FTC/TDF on ulcers is stronger than what we observed in our study. Our behavioral risk factor analysis included number of anal sex partners, position during anal sex, and condom use in the last

Table 2. Baseline characteristics by time to HSV-2 seroincidence.[a]

	n (%)	Events/PY	Incidence density	Unadjusted HR[b] (95% CI)	Adjusted HR (95% CI)	P-value
	1347 (100)	125/2134	5.9			
Age group						0.02
<25	809 (60)	94/1322	7.1	1	1	
25–29	271 (20)	21/412	5.1	0.7 (0.4, 1.1)	0.7 (0.4, 1.1)	
30–34	121 (9)	5/188	2.7	0.3 (0.1, 0.8)	0.3 (0.1, 0.8)	
35–39	63 (5)	3/87	3.5	0.4 (0.1, 1.3)	0.4 (0.1, 1.5)	
≥40	83 (6)	2/125	1.6	0.2 (0.0, 0.7)	0.2 (0.0, 0.8)	
Completed secondary education						
Yes	1103 (83)	107/1741	6.1	1.3 (0.8, 2.2)		
No	230 (17)	18/362	5.0	1		
Transgender identity						
Yes	85 (6)	10/126	8.0	1.5 (0.8, 2.9)		
No	1262 (94)	115/2008	5.7	1		
Treatment assignment						
FTC/TDF	671 (50)	65/1062	6.1	1.1 (0.8, 1.5)	1.2 (0.8, 1.7)	0.41
Placebo	676 (50)	60/1071	5.6	1	1	
No. alcoholic drinks on drinking days, past month						
0–4	608 (46)	56/926	6.0	1		
≥5	711 (54)	65/1155	5.6	0.9 (0.6, 1.3)		
Number of anal sex partners, past 3 months[c]						
0–1	169 (13)	18/231	7.8	1		
2–5	563 (42)	42/846	5.0	0.6 (0.4, 1.1)		
≥6	615 (46)	65/1056	6.2	0.7 (0.4, 1.4)		
Insertive anal intercourse with condom, past 3 months						
Yes	681 (51)	52/1060	4.9	0.9 (0.9, 1.0)		
No	666 (49)	73/1074	6.8	1		
Insertive anal intercourse with no condom, past 3 months						
Yes	802 (60)	77/1304	5.9	1.0 (0.7, 1.4)		
No	545 (40)	48/829	5.8	1		
Receptive anal intercourse with condom, past 3 months						
Yes	617 (46)	67/961	7.0	1.0 (1.0, 1.0)		
No	730 (54)	58/1172	4.9	1		
Receptive anal intercourse with no condom, past 3 months						
Yes	671 (50)	86/1091	7.9	2.0 (1.4, 3.0)	2.0 (1.3, 2.9)	<0.001
No	676 (50)	39/1042	3.7	1	1	

[a]HSV-2, herpes simplex virus type 2; PY, person-years; HR, hazard ratio. Among participants testing HSV-2 seronegative at baseline. Ns may not add up to column totals due to missing data.
[b]Unadjusted HRs were derived from univariable models, while adjusted HRs were derived from multivariable models including variables that were statistically significant at the P<0.05 level in unadjusted analyses. Models were stratified by study site.
[c]Sexual behavior variables are shown at baseline for incidence estimates and were time-updated in models.

three months, but we did not include oral sex as a potential risk factor for HSV-2 seroincidence; however, because HSV-2 is infrequently transmitted through oral sex, we expect this had a negligible effect on our analysis. There may have been some misclassification of HSV-2 results, particularly among participants with HSV-1 antibody, [26] but there is no expectation that this would differ by randomization arm. Some ulcer AEs were identified by self-report, which may be subject to inaccuracy or low sensitivity for HSV-2 recurrences, and we were not able to use HSV PCR to confirm that ulcers were herpetic. Finally, AEs only captured ulcers that increased in severity or frequency; thus, the reduction in ulcers associated with FTC/TDF may have been greater than what we observed.

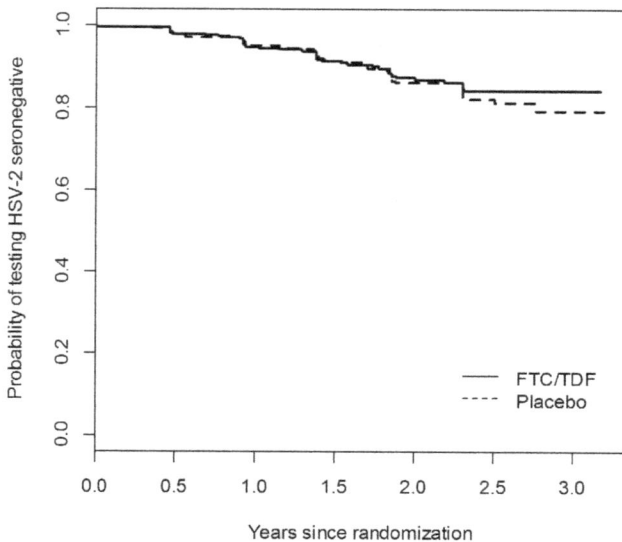

Figure 2. Probability of testing HSV-2 seronegative by randomization group. By Kaplan-Meier analysis. HSV-2, herpes simplex virus type 2.

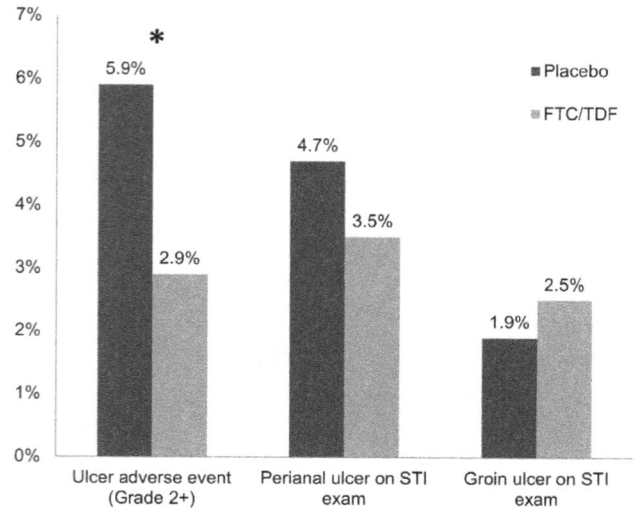

Figure 3. Proportion of prevalent or incident HSV-2 cases with ≥1 ulcer by randomization group. HSV-2, herpes simplex virus type 2; STI, sexually transmitted infection. Asterisk indicates $P<0.05$.

To our knowledge, this is the first analysis of the effect of daily oral FTC/TDF PrEP on HSV-2 incidence and ulcer occurrence among MSM. In our study, oral FTC/TDF did not reduce the acquisition of HSV-2 infection. Although we found that FTC/TDF was associated with a reduction in ulcer AE occurrence, this finding was not confirmed by ulcers identified on clinical examination and should be replicated in settings where ulcer etiology can be confirmed.

Acknowledgments

We thank the participants for their dedication to HIV prevention and the study, as well as the site investigators and their staff for following the cohort and collecting the data. We also thank Maya Petersen, M.D., Ph.D. from the Division of Epidemiology, School of Public Health, University of California, Berkeley, for her helpful comments on the manuscript.

Author Contributions

Conceived and designed the experiments: DVG VM JRL KHM AYL OMH MC BH RMG. Performed the experiments: VM JRL KHM AYL OMH MC BH RMG. Analyzed the data: JLM DVG. Wrote the paper: JLM.

References

1. Looker KJ, Garnett GP, Schmid GP (2008) An estimate of the global prevalence and incidence of herpes simplex virus type 2 infection. Bulletin of the World Health Organization 86: 805–812, A
2. Xu F, Sternberg MR, Gottlieb SL, Berman SM, Markowitz LE, et al. (2010) Seroprevalence of herpes simplex virus type 2 among persons aged 14–49 years — United States, 2005-2008. MMWR 59: 456–459.
3. Gupta R, Warren T, Wald A (2007) Genital herpes. Lancet 370: 2127–2137.
4. Paz-Bailey G, Ramaswamy M, Hawkes SJ, Geretti AM (2007) Herpes simplex virus type 2: epidemiology and management options in developing countries. Sexually transmitted infections 83: 16–22.
5. Wald A, Link K (2002) Risk of human immunodeficiency virus infection in herpes simplex virus type 2-seropositive persons: a meta-analysis. The Journal of infectious diseases 185: 45–52.
6. Freeman EE, Weiss HA, Glynn JR, Cross PL, Whitworth JA, et al. (2006) Herpes simplex virus 2 infection increases HIV acquisition in men and women: systematic review and meta-analysis of longitudinal studies. AIDS 20: 73–83.
7. Celum C, Wald A, Lingappa JR, Magaret AS, Wang RS, et al. (2010) Acyclovir and transmission of HIV-1 from persons infected with HIV-1 and HSV-2. The New England journal of medicine 362: 427–439.
8. Celum C, Wald A, Hughes J, Sanchez J, Reid S, et al. (2008) Effect of aciclovir on HIV-1 acquisition in herpes simplex virus 2 seropositive women and men who have sex with men: a randomised, double-blind, placebo-controlled trial. Lancet 371: 2109–2119.
9. Abdool Karim Q, Abdool Karim SS, Frohlich JA, Grobler AC, Baxter C, et al. (2010) Effectiveness and safety of tenofovir gel, an antiretroviral microbicide, for the prevention of HIV infection in women. Science 329: 1168–1174.
10. Boily MC, Dimitrov D, Masse B (2011) How much of the overall microbicide effectiveness against HIV is due to the protection of TFV gel against HSV-2? The CAPRISA-004 trial. 18th Conference on Retroviruses and Opportunistic Infections. Boston, MA.
11. Celum C, Morrow R, Donnell D, Hong T, Fife K, et al. (2013) Daily oral tenofovir and emtricitabine/tenofovir pre-exposure prophylaxis and prevention

of herpes simplex virus type 2 acquisition among heterosexual men and women. 20th Conference on Retroviruses and Opportunistic Infections. Atlanta, GA.
12. Andrei G, Lisco A, Vanpouille C, Introini A, Balestra E, et al. (2011) Topical tenofovir, a microbicide effective against HIV, inhibits herpes simplex virus-2 replication. Cell host & microbe 10: 379–389.
13. Grant RM, Lama JR, Anderson PL, McMahan V, Liu AY, et al. (2010) Preexposure chemoprophylaxis for HIV prevention in men who have sex with men. N Engl J Med 363: 2587–2599.
14. LeGoff J, Mayaud P, Gresenguet G, Weiss HA, Nzambi K, et al. (2008) Performance of HerpeSelect and Kalon assays in detection of antibodies to herpes simplex virus type 2. Journal of clinical microbiology 46: 1914–1918.
15. Anderson PL, Glidden DV, Liu A, Buchbinder S, Lama JR, et al. (2012) Emtricitabine-tenofovir concentrations and pre-exposure prophylaxis efficacy in men who have sex with men. Sci Transl Med 4: 151ra125.
16. Rubin DB (1987) Multiple Imputation for Nonresponse in Surveys. New York: Wiley and Sons.
17. White IR, Royston P, Wood AM (2011) Multiple imputation using chained equations: Issues and guidance for practice. Statistics in medicine 30: 377–399.
18. van de Laar MJ, Termorshuizen F, Slomka MJ, van Doornum GJ, Ossewaarde JM, et al. (1998) Prevalence and correlates of herpes simplex virus type 2 infection: evaluation of behavioural risk factors. International journal of epidemiology 27: 127–134.
19. Lupi O (2011) Prevalence and risk factors for herpes simplex infection among patients at high risk for HIV infection in Brazil. International journal of dermatology 50: 709–713.
20. Okuku HS, Sanders EJ, Nyiro J, Ngetsa C, Ohuma E, et al. (2011) Factors associated with herpes simplex virus type 2 incidence in a cohort of human immunodeficiency virus type 1-seronegative Kenyan men and women reporting high-risk sexual behavior. Sexually transmitted diseases 38: 837–844.
21. Hendrix CW (2012) The clinical pharmacology of antiretrovirals for HIV prevention. Current opinion in HIV and AIDS 7: 498–504.

22. Patterson KB, Prince HA, Kraft E, Jenkins AJ, Shaheen NJ, et al. (2011) Penetration of tenofovir and emtricitabine in mucosal tissues: implications for prevention of HIV-1 transmission. Science translational medicine 3: 112re114.
23. Tan D (2012) Potential role of tenofovir vaginal gel for reduction of risk of herpes simplex virus in females. International journal of women's health 4: 341–350.
24. Hendrix CW, Chen BA, Guddera V, Hoesley C, Justman J, et al. (2013) MTN-001: randomized pharmacokinetic cross-over study comparing tenofovir vaginal gel and oral tablets in vaginal tissue and other compartments. PLoS One 8: e55013.
25. Tan DH, Kaul R, Raboud JM, Walmsley SL (201_) No impact of oral tenofovir disoproxil fumarate on herpes simplex virus shedding in HIV-infected adults. AIDS 25: 207–210.
26. Golden MR, Ashley-Morrow R, Swenson P, Hogrefe WR, Handsfield HH, et al. (2005) Herpes simplex virus type 2 (HSV-2) Western blot confirmatory testing among men testing positive for HSV-2 using the focus enzyme-linked immunosorbent assay in a sexually transmitted disease clinic. Sexually transmitted diseases 32: 771–777.

21

Increasing HIV and Decreasing Syphilis Prevalence in a Context of Persistently High Unprotected Anal Intercourse, Six Consecutive Annual Surveys among Men Who Have Sex with Men in Guangzhou, China, 2008 to 2013

Fei Zhong[1,2,3], Boheng Liang[2], Huifang Xu[2], Weibin Cheng[2], Lirui Fan[2], Zhigang Han[2], Caiyun Liang[2], Kai Gao[2], Huixia Mai[2], Faju Qin[2], Jinkou Zhao[4], Li Ling[1,3]*

1 School of Public Health, Sun Yat-sen University, Guangzhou, China, 2 Department of HIV/AIDS Control and Prevention, Guangzhou Center for Disease Control and Prevention, Guangzhou, China, 3 Sun Yat-sen Center for Migrant Health Policy, Sun Yat-sen University, Guangzhou, China, 4 The Global Fund to fight AIDS, Tuberculosis and Malaria, Geneva, Switzerland

Abstract

Introduction: Previous studies have reported a possibly increasing HIV prevalence among men who have sex with men (MSM) in China. However there have been limited systematic analyses of existing surveillance data to learn the trend of HIV prevalence and factors driving the trend. The aims of this study were to examine the trend of HIV prevalence among MSM in Guangzhou and to explore the role of unprotected anal intercourse (UAI) in the trend.

Methods: Snow-ball sampling was applied in the subject recruitment for the annual serological and behavioral surveys among MSM from 2008 to 2013. Data collected in the behavioral survey include demographic information, HIV related sexual behavior with men and women, access to HIV prevention services, and symptoms of sexually transmitted infections. Chi-square test was used to analyze the trend of HIV prevalence. Multivariate logistic regression was conducted to test the factors associated with HIV infection.

Results: HIV prevalence increased significantly from 5.0% in 2008 to 11.4% in 2013 while syphilis prevalence decreased from 17.4% to 3.3% in the same period. UAI rates were high and stable in every single year, ranging from 54.5% to 62.0%. Those who were having UAI (OR = 1.80, 95% confidence interval (CI): 1.26–2.58), being migrants, having more than 10 partners, and infected with syphilis had higher risk for HIV infection.

Conclusions: HIV epidemic is expanding in Guangzhou. The persistently high UAI may have played a major role in the increasing trend of HIV prevalence. Targeted prevention program should be conducted among MSM who are migrants, low educational level, syphilis infected, or having multiple partners to encourage HIV test and change UAI behavior. The general high UAI calls for tailored intervention program to promote healthy culture and form a safe sex social norm in the MSM community.

Editor: Marti Vall, Catalan Health Institute, Spain

Funding: This research has been supported by the China Medical Board (12-111), Medical Scientific Research Foundation of Guangdong Province (A2013539), Medical Scientific Program of Guangzhou (20131A011114), and Science and Technology Program of Guangzhou (2012Y2-00021). The funders had no role in study design, data collection and analysis, decision to publish, or preparation of the manuscript.

Competing Interests: The authors have declared that no competing interests exist.

* Email: lingli@mail.sysu.edu.cn

Introduction

During the past decade, the HIV epidemiology has changed in China, from predominantly driven by injection drug use and unsafe plasma collection to by unprotected sex [1]. Among reported HIV/AIDS cases in China, the proportion of men who have sex with men (MSM) increased from 7.3% in 2005, to 11.0% in 2007 and 17.4% in 2011 [2]. Unprotected sex between men has become one of the major HIV transmission modes in China, accounting for 29.4% of estimated annual new HIV infection in China in 2011 [2].

Guangzhou, the capital of Guangdong province and one of the largest cities located in southern China, is remarkable for its rapid economic growth during the past three decades, thanks to the open-door policy since 1978 [3]. The open-door policy brought the opportunities not only for economic development, but for multiple culture environments. Guangzhou gradually became socially tolerant city, which attracts MSM from all over the country and other surrounding Asian cities. During the past decade, lots of gay cruising areas and partner hunting ways emerged, such traditional ones as gay bars, sauna, tea house, parks, public toilets and clubs, and modern ones as gay website, internet chat-room, instant chatting groups, and mobile networking. In addition, highways and high speedy trains make partner hunting very easy for MSM between Guangzhou and its neighboring cities. Easy mobility, together with advanced modern networking tools, incubates spreading of sexually transmitted diseases including HIV when sex is unprotected.

Unprotected anal intercourse (UAI) might have played a key role in the spread of HIV among MSM in Guangzhou. The relationship between UAI and HIV infection and sexually transmitted infections (STIs) is biologically plausible and approved by numerous studies in the United States and Australia [4–6]. Reports in different Chinese cities indicated that UAI has increased or maintained at a high level, despite a high level of knowledge about HIV/AIDS, since early 2000s when most of the studies were conducted [7].

Previous surveys have reported a possibly increasing average HIV prevalence among MSM in China, from 0.9% in 2003, 1.3% in 2004, 3.0% in 2006 and 5.0% in 2008 [8]. Increased HIV prevalence has been reported in big Chinese cities. In Beijing, HIV prevalence of MSM increased from 0.4% in 2004 to 5.8% in 2006, and 8.0% in 2009 [9,10]. In Harbin, the prevalence of HIV increased from 1.0% in 2006 to 7.5% in 2010 [11]. The HIV prevalence was reported to be increasing in some medium-sized cities like Hangzhou (from 1.8% in 2006 to 8.3% in 2009) [12], Jinan (from 0.05% in 2007 to 3.1% in 2008) [13], Suzhou (from 7.1% in 2008 to 8.2% in 2012) [14,15]. This increase is in the context of a regional increase in Asia such as from 17.3% in 2003 to 28.3% in 2005 in Bangkok [16], from 2.5% in 2002 to 8.0% in 2007 in Jakarta [17], from 9.4% in 2006 to 20% in 2010 in Hanoi [18].

There might be an increase in HIV prevalence in Guangzhou. However, there have been limited systematic analyses of existing surveillance data to examine the trend of HIV prevalence and factors driving the trend [11]. Taking advantage of being part of 61 cities' survey among MSM in China organized by Chinese Center for Disease Control and Prevention (China CDC) [19], Guangzhou started the annual biological and behavioral surveys among MSM since 2008 using an identical survey protocol and the same questionnaire, implemented by the same group of interviewers at the same survey site.

In the present study, we examined the trend of HIV prevalence and behaviors using annual biological and behavioral surveys from 2008 to 2013. We also explored the role of UAI in the trend of HIV prevalence.

Materials and Methods

Participants and recruitment

Subjects included in the surveys were men who had anal or oral sex with men in the last 12 months, at least 18 years old and had lived in Guangzhou for at least 6 months prior to the survey year.

Snow-ball sampling was applied in the subject recruitment. An incentive, including a gift (worth about 2 US dollars) and 20 Chinese Yuan cash (approximately 3 US dollars), was given for participation in the questionnaire survey and the provision of 5 ml blood for serological testing. Pre- and post-test counseling services were provided to each of subjects participating in the study. Referral services were provided to HIV or syphilis positive cases.

The sample size was estimated based on the following formula [20]:

$$n = \frac{DEFF \times Np(1-p)}{\dfrac{d^2}{Z_{1-\alpha/2}^2}(N-1) + p(1-p)}$$

The MSM population size (N) in Guangzhou was estimated to be about 35,000 (Personal communication, Huifang Xu, unpublished data based on capture-recapture exercise in 2008). HIV prevalence among MSM (p) was 5.2% in 2008 [21], confidence limit (d) of 5%, a design effect ($DEFF$) of 2, and an alpha (α) of 0.05. Given these conditions, the required smallest sample size would be 152. The sample size was increased to 400 to allow for greater representativeness and possible refusals during the recruitment.

The study protocol was developed by Guangzhou CDC and approved by its Ethics Committee. All subjects provided written informed consents.

Data collection

After written informed consent obtained from each of the eligible subjects, 5 ml intravenous blood was drawn prior to the questionnaire interview. Face to face questionnaire interviews were conducted by the same interviewers using an identical structured questionnaire in a private room at the voluntary counseling and testing (VCT) clinic of Guangzhou CDC.

Data collected in the questionnaire include demographic information, knowledge and attitudes towards HIV or AIDS, access to HIV prevention services, and sexual behavior with men and women in the past 6 months, and symptoms of STIs in the past 12 months. The questionnaire interviews were administered anonymously but such contact information as mobile phone numbers, QQ (Instant messaging software) account or email address were collected to inform the laboratory test results and referral services when necessary.

HIV screening was conducted by using two enzyme-linked immunoassays (ELISAs; Diagnostic Kit for Antibody to Human Immunodeficiency Virus, BioMérieux, Boxtel, The Netherlands, Beijing BGI-GBI Biotech, Beijing, China). If the result of one ELISA was positive, a Western Blot (WB) test was conducted for confirmation (WB;MP Biomedicals Asia Pacific Pte Ltd, Singapore). Syphilis screening was performed by rapid plasma regain (RPR; Shanghai Kehua Bioengineering Co. Ltd, Shanghai, China) to test anticardiolipin. Specimens testing positive by RPR were confirmed by the treponema pallidum particle agglutination test (TPPA; Livzon Group Reagent Factory, Zhuhai, China) to test treponema pallidum antibody. Specimen which is positive in both RPR and TPPA can be diagnosed to be syphilis infection.

Data analysis

Although the sampling method of survey was a non-probability sample, the sample size was considered large enough to be representative of the population. In this study, UAI was defined as failure to consistently use a condom during the past 6 months

Table 1. Demographic characteristics and key behaviors of MSM in Guangzhou, China, 2008–2013.

Characteristics	2008 (N=379) n (%)	2009 (N=385) n (%)	2010 (N=405) n (%)	2011 (N=400) n (%)	2012 (N=401) n (%)	2013 (N=633) n (%)	χ^2 value	p^a
Age (years)							22.80	0.299
<20	14 (3.7)	10 (2.6)	13 (3.2)	15 (3.8)	9 (2.2)	15 (2.4)		
20–29	217 (57.3)	227 (59.0)	245 (60.5)	250 (62.5)	228 (56.9)	385 (60.8)		
30–39	111 (29.3)	113 (29.4)	120 (29.6)	101 (25.3)	128 (31.9)	174 (27.5)		
40–49	35 (9.2)	27 (7.0)	23 (5.7)	25 (6.3)	24 (6.0)	49 (7.7)		
≥50	2 (0.5)	8 (2.1)	4 (1.0)	9 (2.3)	12 (3.0)	10 (1.6)		
Marital status							40.73	<0.001
Married	79 (20.8)	69 (17.9)	74 (18.3)	89 (22.3)	69 (17.2)	76 (12.0)		
Cohabiting with male partner	67 (17.7)	69 (17.9)	62 (15.3)	46 (11.5)	63 (15.7)	104 (16.4)		
Single	214 (54.5)	232 (60.3)	256 (63.2)	260 (65.0)	258 (64.3)	430 (67.9)		
Divorced or widowed	19 (5.0)	15 (3.9)	13 (3.2)	5 (1.3)	11 (2.7)	23 (3.6)		
Hukou (registered permanent residence)							57.46	<0.001
Guangzhou	105 (27.7)	122 (31.7)	122 (30.1)	115 (28.8)	134 (33.4)	235 (37.1)		
Other city in Guangdong province	85 (22.4)	84 (21.8)	90 (22.2)	67 (16.8)	94 (23.4)	186 (29.4)		
Outside Guangdong province	189 (49.9)	179 (46.5)	193 (47.7)	218 (54.5)	173 (43.1)	212 (33.5)		
Han nationality	362 (95.5)	369 (95.8)	382 (94.3)	381 (95.3)	389 (97.0)	614 (97.0)	6.37	0.272
Education level							64.16	<0.001^b
Junior high school or lower	72 (19.0)	47 (12.2)	66 (16.3)	53 (13.3)	49 (12.2)	35 (5.5)		
Senior high school	111 (29.3)	99 (25.7)	115 (28.4)	140 (35.0)	103 (25.7)	110 (17.4)		
College or higher	196 (51.7)	239 (62.1)	224 (55.3)	207 (51.8)	249 (62.1)	488 (77.1)		
Monthly income (CNY)							131.60	<0.001^b
0	49 (12.9)	54 (14.0)	46 (11.4)	39 (9.8)	56 (14.0)	84 (13.3)		
≤2000	125 (33.0)	88 (22.8)	99 (24.5)	65 (16.3)	27 (6.7)	47 (7.4)		
2001–3000	85 (22.4)	95 (24.7)	94 (23.2)	112 (28.0)	78 (19.5)	98 (15.5)		
3001–4000	60 (15.8)	60 (15.6)	69 (17.0)	86 (21.5)	72 (18.0)	112 (17.7)		
>4000	60 (15.8)	88 (22.9)	97 (24.0)	98 (24.5)	168 (41.9)	292 (46.1)		
Self-perceived sexual orientation							26.23	0.003
Homosexual	232 (61.2)	247 (64.2)	264 (65.2)	260 (65.0)	247 (61.6)	451 (71.2)		
Bisexual	106 (28.0)	109 (28.3)	117 (28.9)	120 (30.0)	119 (29.7)	148 (23.4)		
Uncertain	41 (10.8)	29 (7.5)	24 (5.9)	20 (5.0)	35 (8.7)	34 (5.4)		
Venues for meeting partners							170.40	<0.001
Bar, disco, tea house or club	28 (7.4)	31 (8.1)	25 (6.2)	27 (6.8)	22 (5.5)	22 (3.5)		
Bath house, sauna or massage	25 (6.6)	15 (3.9)	14 (3.5)	9 (2.3)	6 (1.5)	8 (1.3)		
Park, public toilet	57 (15.0)	25 (6.5)	24 (5.9)	18 (4.5)	40 (10.0)	5 (0.8)		
Internet	247 (65.2)	273 (70.9)	298 (73.6)	309 (77.3)	282 (70.3)	564 (89.1)		

Table 1. Cont.

Characteristics	2008 (N=379) n (%)	2009 (N=385) n (%)	2010 (N=405) n (%)	2011 (N=400) n (%)	2012 (N=401) n (%)	2013 (N=633) n (%)	χ^2 value	p^a
Other	22 (5.8)	41 (10.6)	44 (10.9)	37 (9.3)	51 (12.7)	34 (5.4)	1.97	0.161[b]
Age of first sex with male (years)								
<19	66 (17.4)	88 (22.9)	63 (15.6)	62 (15.5)	70 (17.5)	118 (18.6)		
19–24	195 (51.5)	178 (46.2)	181 (44.7)	179 (44.8)	192 (48.0)	364 (57.5)		
≥25	118 (31.1)	119 (30.9)	161 (39.8)	159 (39.8)	138 (34.5)	151 (23.9)	7.70	0.006[b]
Years of being MSM								
≤1	24 (6.3)	47 (12.2)	38 (9.4)	24 (6.0)	37 (9.2)	44 (7.0)		
1.1–3.0	82 (21.6)	100 (26.0)	99 (24.4)	99 (24.8)	83 (20.7)	139 (22.0)		
3.1–5.0	86 (22.7)	74 (19.2)	94 (23.2)	112 (28.0)	80 (20.0)	105 (16.6)		
5.1–10.0	124 (32.7)	115 (29.9)	130 (32.1)	111 (27.8)	120 (31.9)	226 (35.7)		
>10	63 (16.6)	49 (12.7)	44 (10.9)	54 (13.5)	73 (18.2)	119 (18.8)		
Have anal sex with male in the past 6 months	336 (88.7)	348 (90.4)	360 (88.9)	369 (92.3)	363 (90.5)	574 (90.7)	3.95	0.556
Number of male partners in the past 6 months							7.45	0.006[b]
1	94 (28.0)	123 (35.3)	121 (33.6)	123 (33.3)	136 (37.5)	184 (32.2)		
2	80 (23.8)	92 (26.4)	96 (26.7)	98 (26.6)	97 (26.7)	159 (27.8)		
3	69 (20.5)	66 (19.0)	63 (17.5)	66 (17.9)	72 (19.8)	112 (19.6)		
4–9	69 (20.5)	38 (10.9)	60 (16.7)	68 (18.4)	40 (11.1)	105 (18.4)		
≥10	24 (7.1)	29 (8.3)	20 (5.6)	14 (3.8)	18 (5.0)	12 (2.1)		
UAI[c]	233 (61.5)	210 (54.5)	240 (59.3)	248 (62.0)	227 (56.6)	361 (57.0)	7.10	0.213
UVI[c]	58 (15.3)	49 (12.7)	64 (15.8)	52 (13.0)	60 (15.0)	53 (8.4)	18.05	0.003
HIV test in the past 12 months	62 (16.4)	274 (71.2)	178 (44.0)	177 (44.7)	198 (49.7)	338 (53.4)	247.15	<0.001
Coverage of HIV intervention	287 (75.7)	338 (87.8)	301 (74.3)	283 (70.8)	334 (83.3)	538 (85.0)	60.94	<0.001
STI symptoms in the past 12 months[c]	85 (22.4)	85 (22.1)	61 (15.1)	64 (16.0)	57 (14.2)	87 (13.7)	23.39	<0.001
Syphilis infection	66 (17.4)	32 (8.3)	28 (6.9)	25 (6.2)	36 (9.0)	21 (3.3)	67.45	<0.001

[a] Pearson chi-square test.
[b] Linear-by-linear association chi-square test.
[c] UAI, unprotected anal intercourse; UVI, unprotected vaginal intercourse; STI, sexually transmitted infection.

Table 2. HIV prevalence by demographic characteristics and sexual behaviors among MSM in Guangzhou, 2008–2013.

Characteristics	2008 % (n)	2009 % (n)	2010 % (n)	2011 % (n)	2012 % (n)	2013 % (n)	χ^2 value	p^a
Overall	5.0 (19)	3.9 (15)	7.7 (31)	9.3 (37)	10.0 (40)	11.4 (72)	25.42	<0.001
Age (years)								
<20	0.0 (0)	0.0 (0)	0.0 (0)	6.7 (1)	0.0 (0)	20.0 (3)	8.98	0.110[b]
20–29	4.1 (9)	3.5 (8)	8.6 (21)	10.0 (25)	9.2 (21)	12.2 (47)	20.31	0.001
30–39	8.1 (9)	5.3 (6)	7.5 (9)	8.9 (9)	10.9 (14)	8.0 (14)	2.69	0.748
40–49	2.9 (1)	3.7 (1)	4.3 (1)	4.0 (1)	20.8 (5)	10.2 (5)	7.75	0.170[b]
≥50	0.0 (0)	0.0 (0)	0.0 (0)	11.1 (1)	0.0 (0)	30.0 (3)	8.50	0.131[b]
Marital status								
Married	5.1 (4)	0.0 (0)	5.4 (4)	7.9 (7)	14.5 (10)	11.8 (9)	13.76	0.017
Cohabiting with male partner	9.0 (6)	7.2 (5)	4.8 (3)	13.0 (6)	17.5 (11)	14.4 (15)	7.68	0.175
Single	3.7 (8)	3.0 (7)	8.2 (21)	9.2 (24)	6.2 (16)	10.5 (45)	18.79	0.002
Divorced or widowed	5.3 (1)	20.0 (3)	23.1 (3)	0.0 (0)	27.3 (3)	13.0 (3)	5.46	0.363[b]
Hukou (registered permanent residence)								
Guangzhou	1.0 (1)	0.8 (1)	4.9 (6)	5.2 (6)	4.5 (6)	8.1 (19)	13.55	0.019
Other city in Guangdong province	5.9 (5)	0.0 (0)	8.9 (8)	10.4 (7)	9.6 (9)	10.2 (19)	10.11	0.072
Outside Guangdong province	6.9 (13)	7.8 (14)	8.8 (17)	11.0 (24)	14.5 (25)	16.0 (34)	13.76	0.017
Han nationality	5.0 (18)	3.3 (12)	7.1 (27)	9.4 (36)	10.0 (39)	11.6 (71)	29.62	<0.001
Education level								
Junior high school or lower	9.7 (7)	12.8 (6)	12.1 (8)	18.9 (10)	22.4 (11)	8.6 (3)	6.16	0.291
Senior high school	5.4 (6)	4.0 (4)	9.6 (11)	12.1 (17)	14.6 (15)	20.0 (22)	19.22	0.002
College or higher	3.1 (6)	2.1 (5)	5.4 (12)	4.8 (10)	5.6 (14)	9.6 (47)	22.03	0.001
Monthly income (CNY)								
0	2.0 (1)	1.9 (1)	2.2 (1)	12.8 (5)	10.7 (6)	8.3 (7)	10.51	0.062[b]
≤2000	8.8 (11)	4.5 (4)	15.2 (15)	10.8 (7)	11.1 (3)	10.6 (5)	6.14	0.293
2001–3000	4.7 (4)	4.2 (4)	5.3 (5)	12.5 (14)	11.5 (9)	17.3 (17)	15.94	0.007
3001–4000	1.7 (1)	5.0 (3)	2.9 (2)	8.1 (7)	12.5 (9)	14.3 (16)	13.95	0.016
>4000	3.3 (2)	3.4 (3)	8.2 (8)	4.1 (4)	7.7 (13)	9.2 (27)	6.80	0.236
Self-perceived sexual orientation								
Homosexual	5.2 (12)	2.8 (7)	8.3 (22)	10 (26)	10.1 (25)	10.9 (49)	18.66	0.002
Bisexual	5.7 (6)	7.3 (8)	7.7 (9)	9.2 (11)	10.1 (12)	11.5 (17)	3.38	0.642
Uncertain	2.5 (1)	0.0 (0)	0.0 (0)	0.0 (0)	9.7 (3)	17.6 (6)	16.02	0.007[b]
Venues for meeting partners								
Bar, disco, tea house or club	3.6 (1)	16.1 (5)	4.0 (1)	11.1 (3)	13.6 (3)	18.2 (4)	5.57	0.350[b]
Bath house, sauna or massage	8.0 (2)	20.0 (3)	14.3 (2)	0.0 (0)	16.7 (1)	37.5 (3)	6.73	0.241[b]

Table 2. Cont.

Characteristics	2008 % (n)	2009 % (n)	2010 % (n)	2011 % (n)	2012 % (n)	2013 % (n)	χ^2 value	p^a
Park, public toilet	3.5 (2)	4.0 (1)	0.0 (0)	16.7 (3)	22.5 (9)	0.0 (0)	16.68	0.005[b]
Internet	5.7 (14)	1.8 (5)	7.7 (23)	9.4 (29)	7.4 (21)	10.5 (59)	22.09	0.001
Other	0.0 (0)	2.4 (1)	11.4 (5)	5.4 (2)	11.8 (6)	17.6 (6)	10.97	0.052[b]
Number of male partners in the past 6 months								
1	4.3 (4)	2.4 (3)	6.6 (8)	7.3 (9)	8.8 (12)	9.2 (17)	7.33	0.197
2	2.5 (2)	3.3 (3)	7.3 (7)	6.1 (6)	9.3 (9)	8.8 (14)	6.35	0.274
3	1.4 (1)	4.5 (3)	7.9 (5)	16.7 (11)	8.3 (6)	11.6 (13)	12.52	0.028
4–9	5.8 (4)	2.6 (1)	10.0 (6)	11.8 (8)	15.0 (6)	18.1 (19)	10.19	0.070
≥10	16.7 (4)	17.2 (5)	20.0 (4)	7.1 (1)	11.1 (2)	25.0 (3)	2.24	0.815[b]
UAI[c]								
Yes	6.4 (15)	3.8 (8)	9.2 (22)	10.1 (25)	11.5 (26)	15.5 (56)	25.12	<0.001
No	2.7 (4)	4.0 (7)	5.5 (9)	7.9 (12)	8.0 (14)	5.9 (16)	6.48	0.262
UVI[c]								
Yes	3.4 (2)	2.0 (1)	7.8 (5)	11.5 (6)	10.0 (6)	11.3 (6)	7.11	0.213[b]
No	5.3 (17)	4.2 (14)	7.6 (26)	8.9 (31)	10.0 (34)	11.4 (66)	20.21	0.001
HIV test in the past 12 months								
Yes	3.2 (2)	2.6 (7)	6.2 (11)	8.5 (15)	7.6 (15)	10.4 (35)	16.54	0.005
No	5.4 (17)	7.2 (8)	8.8 (20)	10.0 (22)	12.7 (25)	12.5 (37)	12.76	0.026
STI symptoms in the past 12 months[c]								
Yes	2.4 (2)	8.2 (7)	14.8 (9)	10.9 (7)	10.5 (6)	18.4 (16)	13.17	0.022
No	5.8 (17)	2.7 (8)	6.4 (22)	8.9 (30)	9.9 (34)	10.3 (56)	21.04	0.001
Syphilis infection								
Yes	13.6 (9)	12.5 (4)	21.4 (6)	16.0 (4)	19.4 (7)	23.8 (5)	2.25	0.813
No	3.2 (10)	3.1 (11)	6.6 (25)	8.8 (33)	9.0 (33)	10.9 (67)	31.30	<0.001

[a]Pearson chi-square test.
[b]Likelihood ratio chi-square test.
[c]UAI, unprotected anal intercourse; UVI, unprotected vaginal intercourse; STI, sexually transmitted infection.

Table 3. Factors associated with HIV infection among MSM in Guangzhou, 2008–2013, by Logistic regression model.

Factor	B	Wald	p	OR (95% CI)
UAI[a]	0.59	10.41	0.001	1.80 (1.26–2.58)
Hukou (registered permanent residence)				
Guangzhou				1.00
Other city in Guangdong province	0.36	2.19	0.139	1.43 (0.89–2.29)
Outside Guangdong province	0.70	10.81	0.001	2.02 (1.33–3.07)
Education level				
Junior High school or lower				1.00
Senior high school	−0.03	0.01	0.905	0.97 (0.63–1.52)
College or higher	−0.61	7.07	0.008	0.54 (0.34–0.85)
Syphilis infection	1.00	19.33	<0.001	2.72 (1.74–4.26)
HIV test in the past 12 months	−0.32	3.84	0.050	0.73 (0.53–1.00)
Number of male partners in the past 6 months				
1				1.00
2	−0.21	0.93	0.336	0.81 (0.52–1.25)
3	0.08	0.11	0.738	1.08 (0.69–1.69)
4–9	0.33	2.12	0.145	1.39 (0.89–2.16)
≥10	0.74	5.67	0.017	2.10 (1.14–3.87)
Year				
2008				1.00
2009	0.41	1.08	0.299	1.50 (0.70–3.25)
2010	1.02	8.94	0.003	2.78 (1.42–5.44)
2011	1.20	12.62	<0.001	3.31 (1.71–6.41)
2012	1.37	16.27	<0.001	3.92 (2.02–7.60)
2013	1.80	31.14	<0.001	6.07 (3.22–11.43)

[a]UAI, unprotected anal intercourse.

when having anal sex. Having no anal sex reported was considered to be safe. UAI was categorized as 'No' if there was no anal intercourse or a condom was used every time, and 'Yes' if a condom was not used all the time. Unprotected vaginal intercourse (UVI) was categorized in the same method. Coverage of prevention services was defined as receiving any service including condom distribution, lubricant distribution, peer education, STI diagnosis or treatment, HIV counseling or testing, or AIDS/STI educational materials in the past 12 months.

Data were double entered and cleaned using EpiData (version 3.1, Denmark). SPSS (version 17.0, LEAD Technologies Inc.) was used to perform Pearson chi-square test, linear-by-linear association chi-square test, likelihood ratio chi-square test, and multivariate logistic regression analysis. The multivariate forward stepwise logistic regression was conducted to test the factors associated with HIV infection. The independent variable input in the regression model of HIV infection included age, marital status, Hukou (registered permanent residence), education level, ethnicity, monthly income, age at first sex with male, years of being MSM, sexual orientation, venues for meeting partners, UAI, UVI, HIV testing history, preventive intervention services received, STI symptoms in the past 12 months, syphilis infection, and with survey year as dummy variable. All statistical significance test results are reported as p-values, where less than 0.05 was used to define significance.

Results

From 2008 to 2013, 379, 385, 405, 400, 401 and 633 subjects were recruited respectively during April to July each year. The demographic characteristics and key behaviors of the participants are shown in Table 1. From 2008 to 2013, along with the development of economy and culture in China, the increasing trends were found in some demographic data, including increased proportions of being single, having higher educational level and income, and being internet surfers for meeting partners. There was an increase in the rates of HIV testing and coverage of HIV intervention during the past 12 months from 2008 to 2013. In the meantime, the proportion of subjects, who reported STI symptoms during the past 12 months, with multiple partners, or having UVI in the past 6 months, decreased statistically. Syphilis prevalence decreased from 17.4% in 2008 to 3.3% in 2013 during the same period of time. However, across the six years, the most commonly reported risk behavior remained stable, the percentage of UAI still range 54.5% to 62.0% (p>0.05) (Table 1).

HIV prevalence increased significantly from 5.0% in 2008 to 11.4% in 2013 (p<0.001). The increasing trend of HIV prevalence was also found among most of subgroups (Table 2). While in some groups, the rates have been stable over six years. HIV prevalence did not increase significantly in those who cohabited with male partners, having educational level of junior high school or lower, having monthly income lower than 2000 Chinese Yuan, meeting sex partners in bar or bath house, having 4 or more male partners, and syphilis infected, and prevalence

Table 4. UAI rates of HIV-positive and HIV-negative MSM in Guangzhou stratified by the factors associated with HIV infection, 2008-2013.

Factor	UAI rate[a] (%)		χ^2 value	p[b]
	HIV positive	HIV negative		
Total	71.0	57.2	15.4	<0.001
Age (years)				
<20	100.0	72.2	2.52	0.112[c]
20–29	74.8	57.6	14.75	<0.001
30–39	63.9	57.3	1.02	0.314
40–49	64.3	49.7	1.10	0.294
≥50	50.0	48.8	0.01	0.963[c]
Hukou (registered permanent residence)				
Guangzhou	66.7	56.2	1.67	0.197
Other city in Guangdong province	81.3	56.5	11.19	0.001
Outside Guangdong province	68.5	58.4	4.76	0.029
Education level				
Junior high school or lower	60.0	63.9	0.25	0.615
Senior high school	73.3	59.7	5.22	0.022
College or higher	74.5	55.0	13.62	<0.001
Syphilis infection				
Yes	88.6	57.8	11.82	0.001
No	67.6	57.2	7.38	0.007
HIV test in the past 12 months				
Yes	68.2	54.4	6.15	0.013
No	72.9	59.8	8.36	0.004
Number of male partners in the past 6 months				
1	69.8	58.5	2.61	0.106
2	78.0	62.3	4.09	0.043
3	74.4	66.7	0.94	0.333
4–9	88.6	69.3	7.12	0.008
≥10	78.9	72.4	0.35	0.557

[a]UAI, unprotected anal intercourse.
[b]Pearson chi-square test.
[c]Likelihood ratio chi-square test.

among them was higher than average rate in each single year. In another aspect, HIV prevalence did not increase in subgroups those who having income higher than 4000, having less than 2 partners, and having no UAI in the past 6 months, and prevalence in these groups was lower than average rate.

Factors associated with HIV infection were reported in Table 3. Those having UAI (OR = 1.80, 95% CI: 1.26–2.58), without Guangdong Province Hukou (OR = 2.02, 95% confidence interval (CI): 1.33–3.07, compared with those with Guangzhou local Hukou), having more than 10 partners (OR = 2.10, 95% CI: 1.14–3.87, compared with those having only 1 partner), and being syphilis positive (OR = 2.72, 95% CI: 1.74–4.26) were associated with higher risk for HIV infection. Having a college or higher education level (OR = 0.54, 95% CI: 0.34–0.85) and having HIV test in the past 12 months (OR = 0.73, 95% CI: 0.53–1.00) were associated with lower risk for HIV infection. After adjusting for demographic characteristics and key behaviors of the participants, the survey year remained an associated factor for HIV infection, indicating an increasing trend in HIV prevalence over years.

UAI rates were high and stable in every single year, ranging from 54.5% to 62.0%. In Table 4, further analysis indicated the UAI among HIV-positive MSM was higher than that among HIV-negative MSM (71.0% versus 57.2%, p<0.001). UAI was generally higher among HIV positive cases in many subgroups especially those having a Hukou in other cities in Guangdong Province, having a college or higher education level, being syphilis positive, and having multiple male partners (Table 4).

Discussion

Results from 6 consecutive annual surveys indicated an increasing HIV prevalence among MSM in Guangzhou. The increase is a continuation of increasing trend since 2006 [21], coincides with the increase in the neighboring cities like Shenzhen [22], in similar Chinese metropolitan cities [9,11,23–25] and in the Asian region [17,18,26,27]. Studies in similar metropolises such as Beijing and Shenyang also reported the high HIV incidence of 8.1 and 5.4 per 100 person-year, respectively [28,29]. The increase of epidemic in China is different from the trend in

San Francisco where HIV epidemic stabilized among MSM during the past decade in a context of decreasing HIV incidence and increased survival of HIV positive individuals due to ART [30].

The increase in HIV prevalence was also found in the most subgroups, by most demographic variables and related behaviors. This is consistent with our previous studies and the results from some studies in China [15,31–32]. Stable prevalence over years was only found in some groups with high risk factors (having educational level of junior high school or lower, having 4 or more male partners, and syphilis infected) or protective factors (having less than 2 partners and no UAI), remaining high or low prevalence, respectively. In our study, after adjusting for years, UAI, migrant, multiple male partners, and syphilis infection were independent related risk factors of HIV infection, while higher educational level and taking an HIV test were protective factors.

Contrary to the trend of HIV prevalence, decreasing syphilis prevalence was found among MSM in Guangzhou from 2008 to 2013. Syphilis is a treatable disease which is passed on through sexual intercourse, therefore syphilis infection can be viewed as a marker for high-risk sexual practices, such as unprotected sex and/or multiple partners, and can also be controlled through screening and treatment. Previous study showed receiving HIV test is a protective factor of syphilis infection among MSM in Guangzhou [21], because when they take an HIV test, they can also receive free syphilis screening and referral services of treatment besides behavior intervention at the same time. Although there is limited data of syphilis screening and treatment among MSM in Guangzhou, our study showed the rate of having HIV test in the past 12 months has increased significantly during six years, arriving 53.4% in 2013, thus the rise of HIV test rate may contribute to control syphilis infection among these MSM. From 2008 to 2013, risk factors found associated with HIV infection decreased while protective factors increased across years. However, UAI, being consistently high and stable from 2008 to 2013, did not change from the level observed in our previous surveys and were not different from those observed in other studies in China [11,15,25,31–33]. The consistently high level of UAI may explain the steady increase in HIV prevalence since UAI is the only biologically plausible but uncontrolled risk factor related to HIV during the past six years. HIV positive cases have higher UAI than those not infected yet. The finding, of 100% UAI among those aged below 20 years, is of a particular concern. This 100% UAI in the younger age group, together with high level of UAI in all subgroups, indicates an unhealthy culture environment and incorrect social norm in the MSM community. Social norms refer to expectations of acceptable behavior or attitudes within a community or peer group prescribed by the respective members

[34]. The social norms of MSM community are to protect himself and his partners anytime having sex. Research among Chinese MSM found that stronger endorsement of positive social norms around condom use strongly predicted lower prevalence of HIV infection [10]. Therefore intervention program which focus on positive social norms and condom using may protect MSM from being infected with HIV.

This study has some limitations. Despite the snow-ball sampling applied, the majority of the sampled MSM were from venues or internet. This may bias the samples towards the relatively active MSM subgroups. Similar to other behavioral surveys, behavioral information was relied on self-reporting, recall bias and social desirability bias may exist. Information bias may also exist given the nature of sensitive sex-related questions. To address these possible biases, the same group of trained interviewers conducted all six surveys at the same site using an identical questionnaire. Consistency was ensured in the methodology and implementation of questionnaire interviews, biases may be towards one direction across years. The risk behaviors, such as UAI, reported by interviewees may be conservative due to social desirability bias. Despite these limitations, the present study is one of the few studies in China to examine the trend of the prevalence of HIV and behaviors among MSM for 6 consecutive years. In further research, cohort study will be conducted to measure incidences of HIV and syphilis among MSM and to modify cause inference.

In conclusion, HIV epidemic is expanding in Guangzhou. The persistently high UAI may have played a major role in the increasing trend of HIV prevalence. Targeted prevention program should be conducted among MSM who are migrants, low educational level, syphilis infected, or having multiple partners to encourage HIV test and change UAI behavior. The general high UAI calls for tailored intervention program to promote healthy culture and form a safe sex social norm in the MSM community.

Acknowledgments

We would like to thank colleagues in Department of AIDS Control and Prevention, Guangzhou Center for Disease Control and Prevention, for the implementation of surveys. We also feel grateful for MSM volunteers of Lingnan Partner Health Center who help the mobilization and organization efforts during the field surveys and participants for their voluntary participation.

Author Contributions

Conceived and designed the experiments: FZ HX WC LF ZH. Performed the experiments: FZ WC LF ZH CL KG HM FQ. Analyzed the data: FZ BL. Contributed to the writing of the manuscript: FZ BL JZ LL.

References

1. Lu F, Wang N, Wu Z, Sun X, Rehnstrom J, et al. (2006) Estimating the number of people at risk for and living with HIV in China in 2005: methods and results. Sex Transm Infect 82: iii 87–91.
2. Ministry of Health of the People's Republic of China (2012) National report for HIV/AIDS estimation in China, 2011 [In chinese]. Beijing: Chinese Center for Disease Control and Prevention.
3. Bui TX YD, Jones WD, Li JZ (2003) China's economic powerhouse: economic reform in Guangdong Province. New York, NY: Palgrave Macmillan. 288p.
4. Chris B, Andrea LW, Damian W, Benjamin J, Frangiscos S, et al. (2011) The Global HIV Epidemics Among Men who Have Sex with Men. Washington DC: The World Bank. 350p.
5. Ackers ML, Greenberg AE, Lin CY, Bartholow BN, Goodman AH, et al. (2012) High and persistent HIV seroincidence in men who have sex with men across 47 U.S. cities. PloS one 7:e34972.
6. Jin F, Prestage GP, Zablotska I, Rawstorne P, Imrie J, et al. (2009) High incidence of syphilis in HIV-positive homosexual men: data from two community-based cohort studies. Sex Health 6:281–284.

7. Liu J, Qu B, Ezeakile MC, Zhang Y (2012) Factors associated with unprotected anal intercourse among men who have sex with men in Liaoning Province, China. PloS one 7:e50493.
8. Wang L, Norris JL, Li DM, Guo W, Ding ZW, et al. (2012) HIV prevalence and influencing factors analysis of sentinel surveillance among men who have sex with men in China, 2003–2011 [In chinese]. Chin Med J (Engl) 125:1857–1861.
9. Ma X, Zhang Q, He X, Sun W, Yue H, et al. (2007) Trends in prevalence of HIV, syphilis, hepatitis C, hepatitis B, and sexual risk behavior among men who have sex with men. Results of 3 consecutive respondent-driven sampling surveys in Beijing, 2004 through 2006. J Acquir Immune Defic Syndr 45:581–587.
10. Fan S, Lu H, Ma X, Sun Y, He X, et al. (2012) Behavioral and serologic survey of men who have sex with men in Beijing, China: implication for HIV intervention. AIDS Patient Care STDS 26:148–155.
11. Wang K, Yan H, Liu Y, Leng Z, Wang B, et al. (2012) Increasing prevalence of HIV and syphilis but decreasing rate of self-reported unprotected anal intercourse among men who had sex with men in Harbin, China: results of five consecutive surveys from 2006 to 2010. Int J Epidemiol 41:423–432.

12. Zhang RS, Shang CX (2011) Investigation on the infection of HIV and Sex Transmitted Diseases in the man who have sex with man from 2006 to 2009 in Hangzhou [In chinese]. Chinese J of Health Laboratory Technology 21:732–733.

13. Ruan S, Yang H, Zhu Y, Wang M, Ma Y, et al. (2009) Rising HIV prevalence among married and unmarried among men who have sex with men: Jinan, China. AIDS Behav 13:671–676.

14. Bai H, Huan X, Tang W, Chen X, Yan H, et al. (2011) A survey of HIV infection and related high-risk factors among men who have sex with men in Suzhou, Jiangsu, China. J Biomed Res 25:17–24.

15. Hao C, Lau JT, Zhao X, Yang H, Huan X, et al. (2014) Associations Between Perceived Characteristics of the Peer Social Network Involving Significant Others and Risk of HIV Transmission Among Men Who Have Sex with Men in China. AIDS Behav 18:99–110.

16. Centers for Disease Control and Prevention (CDC) (2006) HIV prevalence among populations of men who have sex with men—Thailand, 2003 and 2005. Morb Mortal Wkly Rep 55:844–848.

17. Morineau G, Nugrahini N, Riono P, Nurhayati, Girault P, et al. (2011) Sexual risk taking, STI and HIV prevalence among men who have sex with men in six Indonesian cities. AIDS Behav 15:1033–1044.

18. Garcia MC, Meyer SB, Ward P (2012) Elevated HIV prevalence and risk behaviours among men who have sex with men (MSM) in Vietnam: a systematic review. BMJ Open 2:pii: e001511.

19. Lau JT, Lin C, Hao C, Wu X, Gu J (2011) Public health challenges of the emerging HIV epidemic among men who have sex with men in China. Public Health 125:260–265.

20. Scheaffer RL, Mendehall W, Ott RL, Gerow KG (2011) Elementary Survey Sampling, Seventh Edition. Boston, Cengage Learning. 448p.

21. Zhong F, Lin P, Xu H, Wang Y, Wang M, et al. (2011) Possible increase in HIV and syphilis prevalence among men who have sex with men in Guangzhou, China: results from a respondent-driven sampling survey. AIDS Behav 15:1058–1066.

22. Zhao J, Cai WD, Gan YX, Zhang Y, Yang ZR, et al. (2012) A comparison of HIV infection and related risk factors between money boys and noncommercial men who have sex with men in Shenzhen, China. Sex Transm Dis 39:942–948.

23. Zhou C, Raymond HF, Ding X, Lu R, Xu J, et al. (2012) Anal Sex Role, Circumcision Status, and HIV Infection Among Men Who Have Sex with Men in Chongqing, China. Arch Sex Behav 42:1275–1283.

24. Wang Z, Lau JT, Hao C, Yang H, Huan X, et al. (2013) Syphilis-related perceptions not associated with risk behaviors among men who have sex with men having regular male sex partner(s) in Nanjing, China. AIDS Care 25:1010–1017.

25. She M, Zhang HB, Wang J, Xu J, Duan YW, et al. (2012) Investigation of HIV and syphilis infection status and risk sexual behavior among men who have sex with men in four cities of China [In chinese]. Zhonghua Yu Fang Yi Xue Za Zhi 46:324–328.

26. Centers for Disease Control and Prevention (CDC) (2013) HIV and Syphilis Infection Among Men Who Have Sex with Men - Bangkok, Thailand, 2005–2011. Morb Mortal Wkly Rep 62:518–520.

27. Mimiaga MJ, Biello KB, Sivasubramanian M, Mayer KH, Anand VR, et al. (2013) Psychosocial risk factors for HIV sexual risk among Indian men who have sex with men. AIDS Care 25:1109–1113.

28. Li D, Li S, Liu Y, Gao Y, Yu M, et al. (2012) HIV incidence among men who have sex with men in Beijing: a prospective cohort study. BMJ Open 2: e1810–e1829.

29. Xu JJ, Zhang M, Brown K, Reilly K, Wang H, et al. (2010) Syphilis and HIV seroconversion among a 12-month prospective cohort of men who have sex with men in Shenyang, China. Sex Transm Dis 37: 432–439.

30. Raymond HF, Chen YH, Ick T, Scheer S, Bernstein K, et al. (2013) A new trend in the HIV epidemic among men who have sex with men, San Francisco, 2004–2011. J Acquir Immune Defic Syndr 62:584–589.

31. Zhang L, Chow EP, Jing J, Zhuang X, Li X, et al. (2013) HIV prevalence in China: integration of surveillance data and a systematic review. Lancet Infect Dis 13:955–963.

32. Meng X, Zou H, Beck J, Xu Y, Zhang X, et al. (2013) Trends in HIV prevalence among men who have sex with men in China 2003-09: a systematic review and meta-analysis. Sex Health 10:211–219.

33. Guy RJ, Wand H, Wilson DP, Prestage G, Jin F, et al. (2011) Using population attributable risk to choose HIV prevention strategies in men who have sex with men. BMC Public Health 11:247.

34. Peterson JL, Rothenberg R, Kraft JM, Beeker C, Trotter R (2009) Perceived condom norms and HIV risks among social and sexual networks of young African American men who have sex with men. Health Educ Res 24: 119–127.

22

Increased Severity and Mortality in Adults Co-Infected with Malaria and HIV in Maputo, Mozambique

Aase Berg[1,2,3]*, Sam Patel[2], Pål Aukrust[4], Catarina David[2], Miguel Gonca[2], Einar S. Berg[5], Ingvild Dalen[6], Nina Langeland[3]

1 Department of Medicine, Stavanger University Hospital, Stavanger, Norway, 2 Department of Medicine, The Central Hospital of Maputo, Maputo, Mozambique, 3 The Faculty of Medicine, The University of Bergen, Bergen, Norway, 4 Section of Clinical Immunology and Infectious Diseases, Oslo University Hospital Rikshospitalet, Oslo, Norway, 5 Department of Virology, The Norwegian Institute of Public Health, Oslo, Norway, 6 Department of Research, Stavanger University Hospital, Stavanger, Norway

Abstract

Background: Co-infection with falciparum malaria and HIV-1 increases the severity and mortality of both infections in unstable malaria-transmission areas. In contrast, in stable transmission areas, HIV co-infection increases the severity of both infections but has not been found to influence malaria mortality.

Methods: In a prospective cross-sectional study, clinical and laboratory data were consecutively collected for all adults admitted with fever and/or suspected malaria to the medical department of the Central Hospital of Maputo, Mozambique, during two malaria seasons from January 2011. Malaria and HIV PCRs were performed, and risk factors for fatal outcomes were analysed. The impact of HIV on the clinical presentation and mortality of malaria was assessed.

Findings: A total of 212 non-pregnant adults with fever and/or suspected malaria and 56 healthy controls were included in the study. Of the 131 patients with confirmed falciparum malaria, 70 were co-infected with HIV-1. The in-hospital mortality of the co-infected patients was 13.0% (9/69) compared with 1.7% (1/59) in the patients without HIV (p = 0.018). Malaria severity (p = 0.016) and co-infection with HIV (p = 0.064) were independent risk factors for death although the association with HIV did not reach statistical significance. The co-infected patients had significantly more frequent respiratory distress, bleeding disturbances, hypoglycaemia, liver and renal failure and high malaria parasitemia compared with the patients with malaria alone.

Interpretations: HIV co-infection is associated with increased disease severity in and mortality from malaria in an area of stable malaria transmission. This finding was not observed earlier and should motivate doctors working in malaria-endemic areas to consider early HIV testing and a closer follow-up of patients with malaria and HIV co-infection.

Editor: Abdisalan Mohamed Noor, Kenya Medical Research Institute - Wellcome Trust Research Programme, Kenya

Funding: Funding was provided by the Western Norway Regional Health Authority to AB. Economical support was also received from the National Center for Tropical Medicine and Imported Infectious Diseases in Bergen, Norway, and The Norwegian Medical Association for Infectious Diseases. The funders had no role in study design, data collection and analysis, decision to publish, or preparation of the manuscript.

Competing Interests: The authors have declared that no competing interests exist.

* E-mail: beaa@sus.no

Introduction

Despite decreasing prevalence, malaria is one of the most important infectious diseases worldwide. In 2010, approximately 1.24 million people died of malaria globally, the majority of whom were in sub-Saharan Africa, including 52000 people in Mozambique. Of these individuals, 47% were above five years of age, which is more than previously assumed [1]. Malaria is meso-endemic in this country, with stable transmission of more than 95% due to *Plasmodium falciparum (P. falciparum)* [2,3]. Mozambique has an estimated national human immunodeficiency virus type 1 (HIV1) prevalence in adults of 15–49 years of age of 11.5% in general and of 22.5% in Maputo (2009), with one of the highest global incidences of co-infection with malaria and HIV [4,5,6].

Several studies have suggested that people infected with HIV have more frequent and more severe episodes of malaria and *vice versa*, as parameters of HIV disease progression worsen in individuals during acute malaria episodes, with unknown long-term effects [7,8,9,10,11,12]. While there is increased mortality in adults co-infected with malaria and HIV in areas with unstable malaria transmission, this phenomenon has not been established in areas with stable malaria transmission [13,14,15,16].

In the present study, we examined the impact of co-infection with HIV on (i) clinical manifestations and (ii) outcome in hospitalised adult patients in Maputo with *P. falciparum* malaria.

Methods

Study design and participants

The Central Hospital of Maputo is a public quaternary care teaching hospital that serves Maputo's 1.2 million citizens and is a national referral hospital for the 22 million people in Mozambique. From 8th January 2011 to 31st March 2011 and from 7th November 2011 to 14th March 2012, a prospective cross-sectional study was performed on all patients consecutively admitted to the Medical Emergency Department at the Central Hospital in Maputo during workdays. All non-pregnant adults of 18 years or more and with an axillary temperature equal to or more than 38.0°C and/or suspected malaria were included, provided a given consent from the patient or from the next of kin if the patient was mentally confused or unconscious. "Suspected malaria" was defined as a history of fever, chills, headache, mental confusion, vomiting and/or diarrhoea, dyspnoea, myalgia and/or general malaise in the absence of symptoms, findings upon clinical examination or additional diagnostic tests indicating other infections. Additional diagnostic tests and exams were basic laboratory tests (e.g., Hemoglobin (Hb), WBC, differential count, ESR, AST, ALT, ALP, bilirubin, LDH, creatinine); other blood tests (e.g., bacteriological and fungal culture and antigen/antibodies for HIV-1, HIV-2, CMV, EBV, hepatitis B and C); urine analysis (stix, micro, culture); Cerebrospinal fluid (CSF) analysis (erythrocytes, WBC, differential count, protein, glucose, chloride, syphilis and cryptococcal tests, bacteriological and fungal culture); sputum analysis for *M. Tuberculosis* with microscopy (AAFB) and culture; stool analysis (e.g., microscopy for ova and cysts, bacteriological culture); and cytological/histological and different radiological exams, if indicated. In addition, health workers at the hospital and their family and friends were included as controls, provided that these individuals had a subjective feeling of wellbeing and a healthy appearance, as evaluated by the researchers. Female controls were excluded in the case of suspected or confirmed pregnancy.

Procedures

A predefined set of clinical data was recorded from the patient files, which were compiled as a part of the routine clinical examination and follow-up at admission and during the hospital stay. Each file included the duration of symptoms, the presence of clinical criteria for severe malaria and HIV, the treatment given and the status at discharge (alive or dead) [17,18]. If an inexperienced medical doctor had recorded the primary data, the researchers crosschecked these data. Fever was measured by a digital thermometer. (Bastos Medical, Valeo Corporation, Taipei, Taiwan.) Some of the patients who were both admitted and discharged directly from the Emergency Department had limited observations and laboratory findings. Survival data were crosschecked with the nurses' and the ward statistic manager's registries of deaths. For the healthy controls, only age and sex were recorded.

According to the hospital's routine, and consistent with standard procedures in the hospital's laboratory, we performed HIV testing (Determine, Alere Medical Co. Ltd; Chiba, Japan and Unigold, Trinity Biotech plc, Bray, Ireland), an HRP-2 Rapid Diagnostic Test (RDT) for malaria (2010–2011 First Response® Malaria antigen *P. falciparum*, Premium Medical Corporation Ltd., Daman, India; 2011–2012 ICT Malaria P.f.®, ICT Diagnostics Cape Town, South Africa), thick blood smears for malaria (Giemsa 20% for 5 minutes) and other routine laboratory tests. Parasitemia in a thick smear was categorised as +, which correlates to 1–10 parasites/100 fields; ++, or 11–100 parasites/100 fields; +++, or 1–10 parasites/field; ++++, or 11–100 parasites/field; or +++++, or >100 parasites/field [19]. In addition, blood samples were separately collected for HIV and malaria PCR analyses. The total nucleic acids were extracted from blood cell fractions [20]. Using 25% reduced sample volume; HIV-1 RNA was detected using an HIV-1 RG quantitative RT-PCR kit (Professional Biotech Pvt Ltd., New Delhi, India). Inhibitory samples were diluted 10 times and retested. Non-inhibitory, weakly positive samples were retested in a full-scale sample volume. Malaria PCR was performed using malaria plasmodium mitochondria- and species-specific 18S PCR. Divergent results were resolved by DNA sequencing [21] An HCG urine pregnancy test was performed for female patients at fertile age with Quick Vue® (Quidel Corp., San Diego, California, USA).

Malaria positivity was defined as all patients with a positive malaria PCR test. Malaria PCR was not performed for two patients. These patients had positive HRP2 antigen tests and positive slides with parasitemia of 3+ or 5+ and were also defined as malaria positive. HIV positivity was defined as having a positive HIV serological test and/or a positive HIV PCR test. Malaria severity was categorised according to the number of criteria fulfilled for severe malaria, as defined by the WHO, and is given in Table 1 [22]. HIV disease severity was categorised according to the WHO's clinical HIV staging of I–IV [18].

Statistical analysis

Categorical or dichotomous data were presented as counts and percentages, and comparisons between groups of malaria patients were performed using Chi-squared tests. Continuous data were presented as medians and ranges and compared using Mann-Whitney tests. The effects of possible risk factors for fatal outcome are evaluated in terms of odds ratios (ORs) with corresponding 95% confidence intervals (CIs) and p-values from Wald tests and simple and multiple binary logistic regression analyses. For analyses involving variables for which certain subjects/patients had missing observations, these subjects were excluded, and the number of included subjects was indicated in the result tables. When calculating number of fulfilment of the total ten severity criteria for malaria in table 1 and figure 1, patients were included even if missing few criteria done only on suspicion of actual organ involvement as bilirubin. All statistical analysis was performed with SPSS-21.

Ethical consideration

Written consent or fingerprinting was obtained from patients or next of kin. The National Ethical Committee at the Ministry of Health in Mozambique and the Regional Ethical Committee in Eastern Norway approved the study. The institutional review board approved the use of health care workers as healthy controls.

Results

Characteristics of the study population

A total of 212 non-pregnant adults with fever and/or suspected malaria and 56 healthy controls were included in the study. In contrast, 48 eligible patients were excluded for different reasons (e.g., a lack of informed consent, leaving the hospital or not available within the hospital). In the entire patient group, the median age was 37 years (range: 18–84), 47% were women, and 99% were ethnic Mozambicans. Among the healthy controls, the median age was 26 years (range: 18–56), 41% were women, and 96% were ethnic Mozambicans. Most of the patients and most of the healthy controls came from the more peripheral suburbs of Maputo city. (Estimated ≥90%). Of the 212 patients with fever

Table 1. Malaria severity in relation to HIV status.

Malaria severity criteria[1]	Falciparum malaria		
	HIV+	HIV–	p[2]
n	70	61	
Hypotension, systolic BP<70	0 (0/63)	2 (1/52)	0.269
Respiratory distress, RR>30	25 (15/61)	6 (3/52)	0.006
Hyperpyrexia temp ≥40°C	6 (3/54)	12 (6/50)	0.243
GCS[3]<11 and/or convulsions	9 (6/70)	8 (5/61)	0.939
Bleeding disturbances and/or haemolysis	13 (9/70)	2 (1/61)	0.016
Jaundice and/or se-bilirubin >43 µmol/L	17 (13/70)	5 (3/61)	0.017
Hb<5 g/dL	15 (10/67)	5 (3/55)	0.092
Se-Glucose ≤2.2 mmol/L	8 (5/62)	0 (0/47)	0.046
Se-Creatinine >265 µmol/L	24 (15/63)	7 (3/46)	0.016
Malaria parasitemia of 4+ or 5+	52 (33/64)	30 (16/53)	0.020
Malaria severity score (mean and proportion of patients with severe malaria)[4]	1.46 (55/66)	0.44 (24/52)	<0.001

The data are percentage (the proportion of patients with given condition/the patients observed) unless otherwise indicated. Boldface type indicates statistical significance. To convert values for glucose levels to mg/dL, divide by 0.05551; to convert values for creatinine levels to mg/dL, divide by 88.4; and to convert values for bilirubin levels to mg/dL, divide by 17.1.
[1]Malaria severity criteria modified from the malaria severity criteria given by the WHO.
[2]The p-values are from Chi-squared tests (dichotomous data) and Mann-Whitney tests (malaria severity score).
[3]Glascow Coma Scale.
[4]Missing data 13 patients.

and/or suspected malaria, 131 (62%) had malaria and 70 of these patients (53%) were co-infected with HIV (Figure 2 and table 2). There was a significant difference in the HIV rate in malaria patients treated in and discharged from the Emergency Department compared with the admitted patients, with a rate of 29% (4/14) in those patients who were discharged and of 57% (60/106) in the patients who were admitted. (p = 0.048, missing data 10 patients). Of the healthy controls, four people were HIV positive, including one person who also had co-infection with *P. ovale*. All malaria patients were infected with *P. falciparum*. In addition, two patients had a double infection with *P. vivax* or *P. malariae*,

respectively. All HIV-infected patients tested positive for HIV-1, except for one patient who had positive Determine and Unigold tests for HIV-2 but had an HIV PCR positive for HIV-1. Age and gender gave no significant difference between the malaria patients with and without HIV co-infection or between the HIV-positive patients with and without malaria. The median duration of symptoms in malaria patients with HIV was twice that of the malaria patients without HIV (8.6 vs.4.2 days) with a much wider range, although not significant. There was a significant difference in the median duration of symptoms for the HIV patients with and without malaria, from 8.6 days in the malaria- and HIV-infected

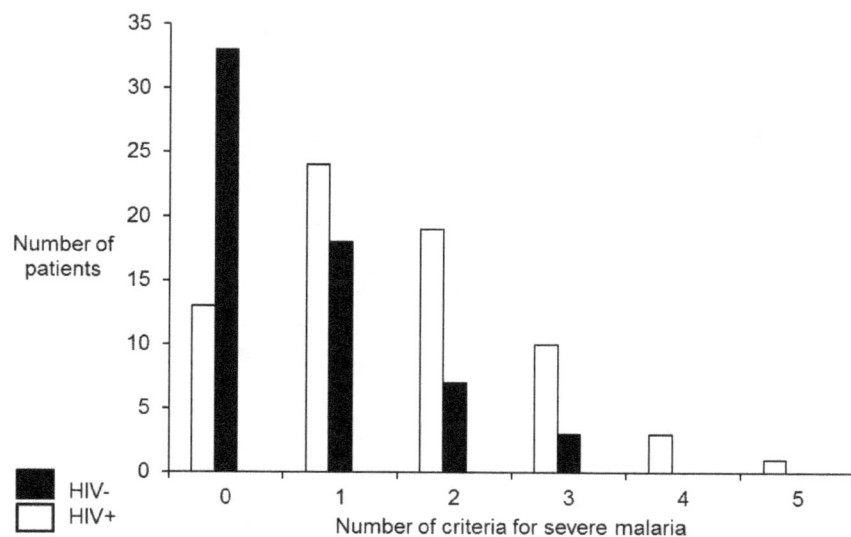

Figure 1. Malaria severity in patients with or without HIV-co-infection. Expressed in number of criteria fulfilled for severe malaria, as outlined in Table 2. (n = 118, missing 13 patients).

Table 2. The characteristics of the study population[1].

Characteristic	Malaria+ HIV+[2]	Malaria+ HIV-	Malaria-HIV+	p[3,4]	p[5]
n	70	61	58		
Case-fatality rate % (proportion)	13.0 (9/69)	1.7 (1/59)	29.1 (16/55)	0.017	0.030
Age in years, median (range)	40 (20–65)	40 (18–79)	38 (20–84)	0.487	0.233
Females, % (proportion)	50 (35/70)	39 (24/61)	50 (29/58)	0.223	1.0
Duration of symptoms in days, median (range)	8.6 (1–180)	4.2 (1–28)	7 (1–365)	0.191	0.001
Severe HIV[6], % (proportion)	59 (41/70)	n.a.	83 (48/58)	n.a.	0.003
HIV viral load in copies/mL (median)	1.8×10^4	n.a.	1.3×10^4	n.a.	0.184
Median CD4 lymphocyte count in cells/µL[7]	206	n.a.	136	n.a.	0.215
Effective ART[8] prior to admission % (proportion)	14 (9/64)	n.a.	19 (10/53)	n.a.	0.485

Boldface type indicates statistical significance.
[1]98.5% of the study population were ethnic Mozambicans.
[2]One patient with a positive malaria PCR test died of other causes than malaria, so his death is categorised as malaria negative.
[3]The p-values are from Mann-Whitney tests (continuous data) or Chi-squared tests (dichotomous data).
[4]Comparison of malaria patients with and without HIV co-infection (columns 1 and 2).
[5]Comparison of HIV patients with and without malaria (columns 1 and 3).
[6]Severe HIV = HIV WHO stage 3 or 4.
[7]Please note the small numbers: n = 11 and n = 8.
[8]ART = antiretroviral therapy = HIV treatment. "Effective" is defined as "Previous known ART and undetectable HIV-RNA in the plasma". In relation to all HIV-patients with and without malaria.

patients to 7 days in the patients with HIV alone (p = 0.001). Of the malaria patients with HIV co-infection, 59% (41/70) had severe HIV infection, with HIV WHO stage 3 or 4, compared with 83% (48/58) of the HIV patients without malaria (p = 0.003). The median HIV viral load for the HIV patients with and without malaria was 1.8×10^4 HIV RNA copies/mL plasma (range: 0 – 8.3×10^6) (n = 61) and 1.3×10^4 HIV RNA copies/mL plasma (range: $0–5.1 \times 10^6$) (n = 58), respectively, without a significant difference (p = 0.184). Unfortunately, data on CD4 T cell counts were lacking in all except 11 and eight HIV patients with and without malaria, respectively, who had a median CD4 T cell count of 206 cells/µL (range: 14–632) and CD4 136 cells/µL (range: 10–196), respectively (p = 0.215). (Table 2)

Clinical manifestations

Despite a history of fever, at admission, 50% (54/108) of the malaria patients presented with no fever, without a significant difference according to HIV status. The patients co-infected with HIV and malaria had significantly more frequent respiratory distress, bleeding disturbances and/or haemolysis, jaundice and/or elevated bilirubin levels, low serum glucose levels, renal failure and high malaria parasitemia compared with the patients with malaria alone. In line with this phenomenon, malaria patients with HIV co-infection had a significantly higher malaria severity score (= number of criteria for severe malaria) (p<0.001) (Table 1 and Figure 1). However, although those patients who were co-infected with HIV had an increased frequency of bleeding disturbance and/or haemolysis, there were no significant differences between the two groups in relation to platelet counts ($<100 \times 10^9$/L) or reduced haemoglobin levels (<5 g/dL). Moreover, there was no significant difference regarding the occurrence of cerebral confusion between the two groups (data not shown).

Case-fatality rates

The in-hospital mortality rate of the patients with malaria and HIV was significantly higher than the mortality rate of the patients with malaria alone (13.0% (9/69) vs. 1.7% (1/59), p = 0.018), with

missing data for two patients. In fact, of the 10 malaria patients who died, nine (90%) were HIV infected, and the tenth was 65 years of age. Patients admitted with fever of other causes than malaria had a HIV rate 72% (59/82) and a case fatality rate of 24% (19/78). Mortality was even higher for the patients with HIV alone (29.1% (16/55), p = 0.030) (Table 2). In total, 67% (77/115) had severe malaria, and 13% (10/77) died (p = 0.020), with missing data for 16 patients. Among the malaria patients, men had an increased risk of dying from malaria, with a crude odds ratio of 3.74 (0.76–18.35), but the difference from women in case-fatality rate was not significant (p = 0.086). The causes of death for the 10 malaria patients were cerebral malaria (three patients), complicated malaria with renal failure (three patients), coagulation disturbances (two patients), liver failure (one patient) and severe anaemia (one patient). Two of these patients had other severe comorbidity consisting of respectively longstanding pronounced alcohol abuse and lymphoma with recent chemotherapy. Although the co-morbidities could have contributed to the fatal outcome in these patients, these patients' histories, clinical findings, laboratory results and malaria parasitemia of 2+ (after quinine i.v. treatment for some days at the referring hospital) or 5+ suggested that malaria was the main cause of death. Moreover, exclusion of those two patients still resulted in significant increased mortality in the HIV-malaria patient group compared to the patients with malaria only (p = 0.042). A third patient had HIV and tuberculous meningoencephalitis according to history, clinical examination and laboratory investigation, but in addition, he had a *P. falciparum*-positive PCR result. This patient's cause of death was classified as meningoencephalitis and not malaria.

Malaria severity was the most important factor associated with increased in-hospital mortality. The patients who met three or more of the criteria for severe malaria had a crude odds ratio of 9.7 for death and a 95% CI of 2.43–38.91 (p<0.001) that persisted in multivariable analyses with an adjusted odds ratio of 6.3 and a 95% CI of 1.40–27.88 (p = 0.016) (Table 3 and Figure 1). The second most important factor associated with death was co-infection with HIV, with a crude odds ratio of 8.7 and a 95% CI of 8.7 (1.07–70.85) (p = 0.018). In multivariable analyses, the

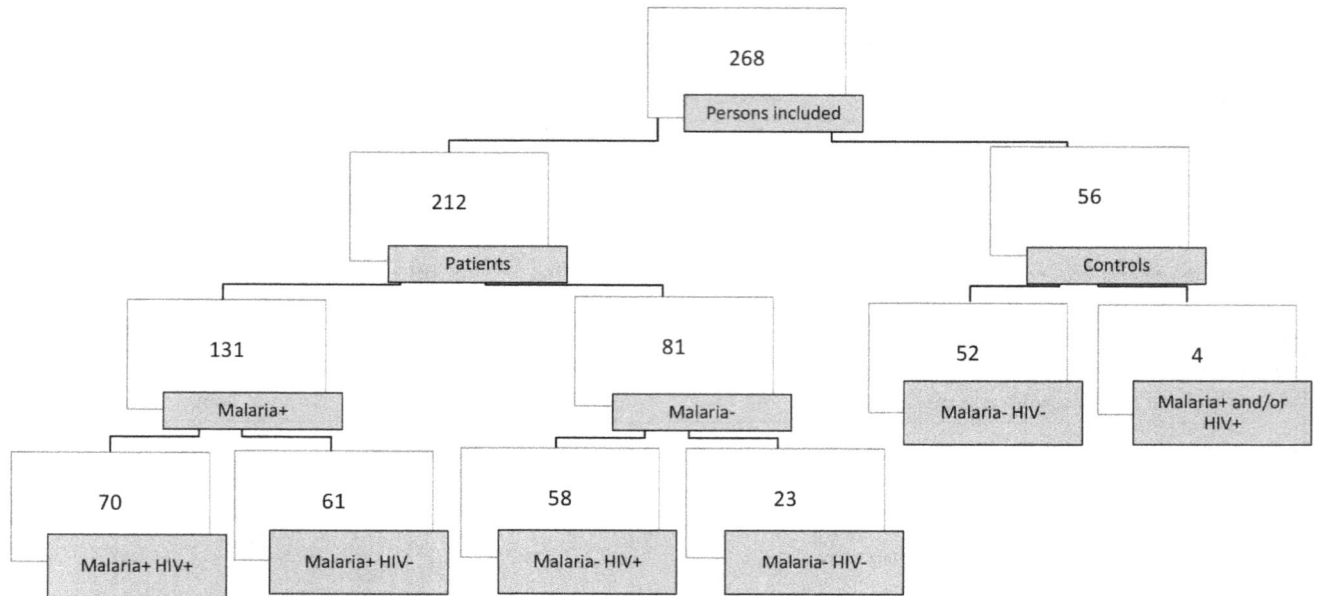

Figure 2. Flow diagram of the study population*. *Number of patients.

difference was not significant (p = 0.064), with an adjusted odds ratio of 8.0 and a 95% CI of 0.89–71.99.

Treatment

Of the malaria patients, 92% received quinine intravenously as a first-line therapy, 4% received artemether intramuscularly, and the rest were treated with oral artemisinin combinations, without any significant differences in mortality. In total, 28% of the patients received antimicrobial therapy (ceftriaxone 27%, ampicillin 18%, penicillin 24% and other 31%). There was no statistically significant difference between the patients with and without HIV in receiving antimicrobials with a potential antimalarial effect, i.e., cotrimoxazole, ciprofloxacin, doxycycline and azithromycin [23,24]. In total, 11% of the patients (14/131) received supplementary corticosteroid treatment, with no influ-

ence on outcome and with no difference between patients with and without HIV co-infection. At admission, 42% (54/128) of the HIV patients had a known HIV diagnosis. Of these patients, 56% (30/54) were on antiretroviral therapy (ART), of whom 63% (19/30) had undetectable HIV-RNA in the plasma (p = 0.001). The ARTs used were stavudine, lamivudine, efavirenz, zidovudine and/or nevirapine. Only eight patients reported receiving cotrimoxazole prophylaxis. There was no significant difference in the number of HIV-infected patients with and without malaria on the use of effective ART (i.e., with undetectable HIV-RNA) prior to admission, with respectively 69% (9/13) and 59% (10/17) (p = 0.558). Surprisingly, there was no significant difference in HIV severity or mortality in the patients with effective ART compared with those patients without ART. (Respectively p = 0.850 and p = 0.141). Of the HIV patients, 60% (44/74) were

Table 3. Risk factors for fatal outcome in malaria patients.

Characteristics		Case-fatality rate[1] %	Crude OR[2] (95% CI)	p[3]	Adjusted OR (95% CI[4])	p[5]
Overall		7.8 (10/128)				
Age	18–49 years	6.3 (6/95)				
	50–79 years	12.1 (4/33)	1.26 (0.31–5.17)	0.752	2.3 (0.46–11.91)	p = 0.308
Sex	Women	3 (2/59)				
	Men	13.0 (9/69)	3.74 (0.76–18.35)	0.086	4.2 (0.76–3.40)	p = 0.100
HIV co-infection	No	1.7 (1/59)				
	Yes	13.0 (9/69)	**8.7 (1.07–70.85)**	**0.018**	8.0 (0.89–71.99)	p = 0.064
Malaria severity score	<3	4.5 (5/112)				
	≥3	31.3 (5/16)	**9.7 (2.43–38.91)**	**<0.001**	**6.3 (1.40–27.88)**	**p = 0.016**

Boldface type indicates statistical significance.
[1]Deaths/number at risk in percentage and proportion.
[2]OR = odds ratio.
[3]The p-values are from Mann-Whitney tests.
[4]CI = confidence interval.
[5]The adjusted OR and p-values are from binary logistic regression.

not receiving ART, despite an indication for ART*, due to a lack of HIV diagnosis before admission (*WHO HIV clinical stage 3 or 4). Of those patients with a known HIV diagnosis prior to admission, 86% (19/22) had an indication for ART but had failed to receive the HIV treatment.

Discussion

In the present study, malaria patients co-infected with HIV had significantly more severe malaria compared with patients with malaria alone (Figure 1), which is consistent with several earlier studies [8,9,10,11,12]. Co-infection with HIV was significantly associated with increased in-hospital mortality. With more advanced immunodeficiency due to HIV, one would have expected increased mortality independent of the transmission area. This because primarily cellular immunity, but also humoral immunity, which are both important in malaria, are progressively affected by deterioration due to HIV disease [9]. However, several studies have failed to find increased mortality in endemic areas, which is in contrast to the findings of the present study [9,13,14,15,16]. These apparent discrepancies may have several explanations. First, in most of the previous studies, the sample size was relatively low (n<70) [9,13,14,15,16]. Second, the degree of HIV severity and the use of ART varied between the different studies [13,15]. Third, in several of the previous studies, the ability to exclude relevant differential diagnoses was poor [9,13]. Fourth, treatment for severe malaria varied between the different studies, with quinine used in most studies (including here) and artesunate used in other reports. This difference clearly could have influenced the outcome because artesunate is more effective than quinine [9,13,14,15].

There was even higher mortality in the patients admitted with HIV without malaria, with 29.1% (16/55) compared with 13.2% (9/68) of the patients co-infected with HIV and malaria, which is most probably due to their advanced HIV-infection. (Table 2). The median duration of symptoms before admittance was 8.6, 4.2 and 7 days respectively in patients with malaria and HIV, malaria only and HIV only. HIV and malaria co-infected patients had a median duration of symptoms twice as long as HIV negative patients with malaria, although this was not statistically significant. Even if the median duration of symptoms between HIV-infected patients with and without malaria was rather modest, it reached statistical significance (Table 2). This again reflects the severity of disease in those two patient groups. The median viral load was about the same in the HIV-malaria group compared with the HIV group, despite less severe HIV disease. It is known that co-infection with malaria temporarily may boost HIV viremia [25]. There were also no significant differences in the median CD4 lymphocyte count or fraction on effective ART before admission, but the number of patients with known CD4 count was low (n = 8 and n = 11).

In comparison with the present investigation, a 2006 study on 51 patients with presumptive malaria, recruited at the same hospital as in the present study (Central Hospital of Maputo), had more severely ill patients, fewer patients on ART, a lower standard of care in the ward and a higher prevalence of both HIV and malaria. While there was no HIV-related increased malaria mortality, the diagnostic accuracy was poorer, the study group was smaller, and the treatment for severe malaria was artesunate rather than quinine [14]. Other studies also failed to find increased mortality, except for one retrospective study from Senegal on cerebral malaria [9,15,26]. However, the present study is, to the best of our knowledge, the first prospective study to show increased mortality in malaria patients co-infected with HIV in an area with stable malaria transmission. Importantly, the present study included patients with a wide spectrum of HIV-related immunodeficiency and had high diagnostic accuracy for both HIV and malaria.

Another possible reason for increased mortality in relation to co-infection with HIV in the present as opposed to the previous studies is that malaria transmission has decreased in Maputo, causing a gradual loss of malaria immunity [7]. This phenomenon would be expected to first be observed in immune-compromised patients, since it seems reasonable that an eventual reduction in the "average immunity" in the population will first be observed in patients with reduced immunity. However, most of the malaria patients in the current study came from the more peripheral parts of Maputo, rather than the city centre, where there is regular malaria exposure, and thus a lower risk of reduced immunity due to urban life. Whereas most literature has reported diminishing malaria prevalence in Mozambique, a recent WHO publication reported a steady increase in the number of confirmed malaria cases since 2009, but a reduction in hospital admissions and malaria-related deaths [27].

Another important point is whether positive malaria PCR may have been an incidental finding in several of the patients suffering from a different condition who happened to receive a malaria diagnosis after being subclinical carriers. In Manhiça in southern Mozambique, nearly half of the population was found to be carriers of P. falciparum, and most individuals were asymptomatic, with decreasing parasitemia with increasing age [28]. In contrast, in the Maputo area, there was a low prevalence of subclinical carriage, with 1.8% falciparum PCR positivity compared with 13.7% in the Mocuba District in Zambezia province [4]. Several studies have had similar findings, although asymptomatic falciparum carriage is particularly described in children, less in adolescents and usually even less in adults, but more in HIV positive persons [2,4,28,29]. Asymptomatic carriage has likely not been a substantial problem in this case, since alternative diagnoses were not identified with a relatively effective diagnostic armamentarium. Second, only one of 56 healthy controls was a subclinical carrier (and then with P. ovale and not P. falciparum) in addition to being HIV positive. Third, the diagnosis at discharge agreed very well with the malaria PCR positivity (Cohen s kappa = 0.88, data not shown).

Despite a history of fever, only 50% of the malaria PCR-positive malaria patients presented with a temperature of 38°C or more at admission, measured with the same reliable thermometer by the researchers. Could this be an indication, despite what was discussed above, that there is substantial subclinical carriage in this area, in certain subgroups differing from the healthy controls in this study. If so, we would have expected positive blood culture results in another parallel study of patients with fever. There is missing data for the use of paracetamol or other antipyretics, which may have influenced our findings. Alternatively, because the patients were admitted with a history of fever, these individuals may be in the stage of shifting from the cold to the warm phase or the opposite in the malaria cycle. If this was the case, similar studies may have lost patients if these studies used fever upon admittance as an inclusion criterion.

The only HIV-negative patient who died was 65 years of age, which is consistent with the known increased risk of malaria death with higher age in non-endemic areas [30]. In endemic areas, increased risk with age is not known, although there seems to be more frequent malaria in the age group above 50 years [31].

An important question in low-resource settings is whether there is a clinical entity of symptoms, signs and simple laboratory observations indicating that a patient is co-infected with HIV. In the current study, the co-infected patients had significantly more respiratory distress, bleeding disturbances, hypoglycaemia, liver and renal failure and high malaria parasitemia compared with patients with malaria alone. In several studies, the co-infected patients had more respiratory distress, renal failure, abdominal pain, diarrhoea or anaemia, whereas in other studies, there was no difference in clinical presentation [8,13,32]. The common denominator of these studies may well be that there is no specific clinical entity typical of co-infection with HIV and malaria; rather, there may be different indicators of disease severity, as also suggested by others [26].

The strength of the present study is its prospective nature, with the consecutive inclusion of a relatively large number of patients compared with similar studies and a high diagnostic accuracy for HIV and malaria. The main limitation is a possible selection bias of not including the poorest and the wealthiest patients because the wealthiest prefer private health care, and the poorest cannot pay the admission fee of approximately 5 USD if they do not have a referral letter. Because poverty is associated with an increased risk of malaria but a lower risk of HIV, this bias may have resulted in a potential loss of HIV-negative malaria patients, which could have influenced the observed mortality both ways [33]. The PCR method may have yielded false-positive malaria patients after treatment or false-negative HIV patients if these individuals were on ART without admitting its use during the hospital stay. The first mentioned issue could have given a too-low mortality rate, and the second issue could have yielded a too-high mortality rate. However, we assume that the second did not have a very important impact on the mortality data because there was supplementary HIV serology for most of the patients and a close follow-up in the ward. Two of the patients with severe malaria were not ethnic Mozambicans, but because both survived, this finding represents no bias. Lastly, even if most patients were severely ill, relatively few died, and the sample size may have been too low to detect other factors related to death.

Conclusions

HIV co-infection is associated with increased mortality from malaria in an area of stable malaria transmission, in which both malaria severity and HIV are risk factors for death. The patients with HIV and malaria co-infection had significantly more frequent respiratory distress, bleeding disturbances, hypoglycaemia, liver and renal failure and high malaria parasitemia compared with the patients with malaria alone. Hence, early HIV testing should always be considered in patients with suspected malaria, and particularly with severe malaria, independent of the type of malaria transmission area. We hypothesise that this alertness of the physician may contribute to the increased survival of patients co-infected with HIV and malaria, due to awareness of potential complications at an early stage. As part of the search for improved therapy, future research is recommended to first confirm the present findings and to then elucidate the underlying immune mechanisms resulting in the observed HIV-associated increased malaria mortality.

Acknowledgments

The authors are indebted to all of the patients and their next of kin who participated in this study; to the healthy controls; to the medical doctors; to the nurses and nurses' aids in the medical wards; to the Intensive Care Unit; and to the laboratory coordinators and personnel in both the General Laboratory and the Microbiological Laboratory of the Central Hospital of Maputo, Mozambique. The authors offer a particular thanks to Christel Haanshuus at the National Centre for Tropical Medicine and Imported Diseases, Bergen, Norway, for performing the malaria PCR and sequencing.

Author Contributions

Conceived and designed the experiments: AB SP CD MG PA ESB NL. Performed the experiments: AB SP CD MG. Analyzed the data: AB PA ESB ID NL. Contributed reagents/materials/analysis tools: AB ESB. Wrote the paper: AB SP PA CD MG ESB ID NL.

References

1. Murray CJ, Rosenfeld LC, Lim SS, Andrews KG, Foreman KJ, et al. (2012) Global malaria mortality between 1980 and 2010: a systematic analysis. Lancet 379: 413–431.
2. Mabunda S, Casimiro S, Quinto L, Alonso P (2008) A country-wide malaria survey in Mozambique. I. Plasmodium falciparum infection in children in different epidemiological settings. Malar J 7: 216.
3. Funk-Bauman M (2001) Geographic Distribution of Malaria at Traveller Destinations; P S, editor. Ontario, Canada: BC Decker. p 76 p.
4. Noormahomed EV, Orlov M, do Rosario V, Petersen BW, Guthrie C, et al. (2012) A cross-sectional study of sub-clinical Plasmodium falciparum infection in HIV-1 infected and uninfected populations in Mozambique, South-Eastern Africa. Malar J 11: 252.
5. UNAIDS (2010-2011) Global AIDS Response Report 2012. Available: http://www.unaids.org/en/media/unaids/contentassets/documents/epidemiology/2012/gr2012/20121120_unaids_global_report_2012_with_annexes_en.pdf Accessed 2014 Jan 12.
6. Brentlinger PE, Behrens CB, Kublin JG (2007) Challenges in the prevention, diagnosis, and treatment of malaria in human immunodeficiency virus infected adults in sub-Saharan Africa. Archives of Internal Medicine 167: 1827–1836.
7. Flateau C, Le Loup G, Pialoux G (2011) Consequences of HIV infection on malaria and therapeutic implications: a systematic review. Lancet Infect Dis 11: 541–556.
8. Cohen C, Karstaedt A, Frean J, Thomas J, Govender N, et al. (2005) Increased prevalence of severe malaria in HIV-infected adults in South Africa. Clinical Infectious Diseases 41: 1631–1637.
9. Diallo AH, Ki-Zerbo G, Sawadogo AB, Guiguemde TR (2004) [Severe malaria and HIV in adult patients in Bobo-Dioulasso, Burkina Faso]. Medecine Tropicale 64: 345–350.
10. Chalwe V, Van geertruyden JP, Mukwamataba D, Menten J, Kamalamba J, et al. (2009) Increased risk for severe malaria in HIV-1-infected adults, Zambia. Emerg Infect Dis 15: 749; quiz 858.
11. Francesconi P, Fabiani M, Dente MG, Lukwiya M, Okwey R, et al. (2001) HIV, malaria parasites, and acute febrile episodes in Ugandan adults: a case-control study. AIDS 15: 2445–2450.
12. French N, Nakiyingi J, Lugada E, Watera C, Whitworth JA, et al. (2001) Increasing rates of malarial fever with deteriorating immune status in HIV-1-infected Ugandan adults. AIDS 15: 899–906.
13. Hendriksen IC, Ferro J, Montoya P, Chhaganlal KD, Seni A, et al. (2012) Diagnosis, Clinical Presentation, and In-Hospital Mortality of Severe Malaria in HIV-Coinfected Children and Adults in Mozambique. Clinical Infectious Diseases 55: 1144–1153.
14. Berg A, Patel S, Langeland N, Blomberg B (2008) Falciparum malaria and HIV-1 in hospitalized adults in Maputo, Mozambique: does HIV-infection obscure the malaria diagnosis? Malar J 7: 252.
15. Leaver RJ, Haile Z, Watters DA (1990) HIV and cerebral malaria. Transactions of the Royal Society of Tropical Medicine and Hygiene 84: 201.
16. Niyongabo T, Deloron P, Aubry P, Ndarugirire F, Manirakiza F, et al. (1994) Prognostic indicators in adult cerebral malaria: a study in Burundi, an area of high prevalence of HIV infection. Acta Tropica 56: 299–305.
17. Trampuz A, Jereb M, Muzlovic I, Prabhu RM (2003) Clinical review: Severe malaria. Crit Care 7: 315–323.
18. WHO (2007) HIV/AIDS Programme. Available: http://www.who.int/hiv/pub/guidelines/HIVstaging150307.pdf Accessed 2014 Jan 12.
19. Tiago AD, Calú N, Caupers P, Mabunda S (2011) Normas de Tratamento da Malaria em Moçambique; Ministerio da Saúde DNdSP, Programa Nacional de Controlo de Malária, editor. p 16.
20. Stevens W, Erasmus L, Moloi M, Taleng T, Sarang S (2008) Performance of a novel human immunodeficiency virus (HIV) type 1 total nucleic acid-based real-time PCR assay using whole blood and dried blood spots for diagnosis of HIV in infants. Journal of Clinical Microbiology 46: 3941–3945.
21. Haanshuus CG, Mohn SC, Morch K, Langeland N, Blomberg B, et al. (2013) A novel, single-amplification PCR targeting mitochondrial genome highly sensitive and specific in diagnosing malaria among returned travellers in Bergen, Norway. Malar J 12: 26.
22. WHO (2011) Guidelines for the treatment of malaria, second edition. Available: http://whqlibdoc.who.int/publications/2010/9789241547925_eng.pdf Accessed 2014 Jan 12.

23. Dahl EL, Rosenthal PJ (2007) Multiple antibiotics exert delayed effects against the Plasmodium falciparum apicoplast. Antimicrobial Agents and Chemotherapy 51: 3485–3490.

24. Puri SK, Dutta GP (1982) Antibiotics in the chemotherapy of malaria. Progress in Drug Research 26: 167–205.

25. Kublin JG, Patnaik P, Jere CS, Miller WC, Hoffman IF, et al. (2005) Effect of Plasmodium falciparum malaria on concentration of HIV-1-RNA in the blood of adults in rural Malawi: a prospective cohort study. Lancet 365: 233–240.

26. Soumare M, Seydi M, Diop SA, Diop BM, Sow PS (2008) [Cerebral malaria in adults at the Infectious Diseases Clinic in the Fann Hospital in Dakar, Senegal]. Bulletin de la Societe de Pathologie Exotique 101: 20–21.

27. WHO (2013) World Health Statistics 2013. Available: http://www.who.int/gho/publications/world_health_statistics/EN_WHS2013_Full.pdf. Accessed 2014 Jan 12.

28. Mayor A, Aponte JJ, Fogg C, Saute F, Greenwood B, et al. (2007) The epidemiology of malaria in adults in a rural area of southern Mozambique. Malar J 6: 3.

29. Gudo ES, Prista A, Jani IV (2013) Impact of asymptomatic Plasmodium falciparum parasitemia on the imunohematological indices among school children and adolescents in a rural area highly endemic for Malaria in southern Mozambique. BMC Infect Dis 13: 244.

30. Muhlberger N, Jelinek T, Behrens RH, Gjorup I, Coulaud JP, et al. (2003) Age as a risk factor for severe manifestations and fatal outcome of falciparum malaria in European patients: observations from TropNetEurop and SIMPID Surveillance Data. Clinical Infectious Diseases 36: 990–995.

31. Erhabor O, Azuonwu O, Frank-Peterside N (2012) Malaria parasitaemia among long distance truck drivers in the Niger delta of Nigeria. Afr Health Sci 12: 98–103.

32. Saracino A, Nacarapa EA, da Costa Massinga EA, Martinelli D, Scacchetti M, et al. (2012) Prevalence and clinical features of HIV and malaria co-infection in hospitalized adults in Beira, Mozambique. Malar J 11: 241.

33. Thang ND, Erhart A, Speybroeck N, Hung le X, Thuan le K, et al. (2008) Malaria in central Vietnam: analysis of risk factors by multivariate analysis and classification tree models. Malar J 7: 28.

23

Consequences of Missed Opportunities for HIV Testing during Pregnancy and Delayed Diagnosis for Mexican Women, Children and Male Partners

Tamil Kendall*

Women and Health Initiative and Takemi Program in International Health, Department of Global Health and Population, Harvard School of Public Health, Boston, Massachusetts, United States of America

Abstract

Introduction: HIV testing during pregnancy permits prevention of vertical (mother-to-child) transmission and provides an opportunity for women living with HIV to access treatment for their own health. In 2001, Mexico's National HIV Action Plan committed to universal offer of HIV testing to pregnant women, but in 2011, only 45.6% of women who attended antenatal care (ANC) were tested for HIV. The study objective was to document the consequences of missed opportunities for HIV testing and counseling during pregnancy and late HIV diagnosis for Mexican women living with HIV and their families.

Methods: Semi-structured-interviews with 55 women living with HIV who had had a pregnancy since 2001 were completed between 2009 and 2011. Interviews were analyzed thematically using *a priori* and inductive codes.

Results: Consistent with national statistics, less than half of the women living with HIV (42%) were offered HIV testing and counseling during ANC. When not diagnosed during ANC, women had multiple contacts with the health-care system due to their own and other family members' AIDS-related complications before being diagnosed. Missed opportunities for HIV testing and counseling during antenatal care and health-care providers failure to recognize AIDS-related complications resulted in pediatric HIV infections, AIDS-related deaths of children and male partners, and HIV disease progression among women and other family members. In contrast, HIV diagnosis permitted timely access to interventions to prevent vertical HIV transmission and long-term care and treatment for women living with HIV.

Conclusions: Omissions of the offer of HIV testing and counseling in ANC and health-care providers' failure to recognize AIDS-related complications had negative health, economic and emotional consequences. Scaling-up provider-initiated HIV testing and counseling within and beyond antenatal care and pre-service and in-service trainings on HIV and AIDS for health-care providers can hasten timely HIV diagnosis and contribute to improved individual and public health in Mexico.

Editor: Claire Thorne, UCL Institute of Child Health, University College London, United Kingdom

Funding: This research was supported by a Canadian Institutes of Health Research Postdoctoral Fellowship (http://www.cihr-irsc.gc.ca/e/193.html), a Pierre Elliott Trudeau Foundation Doctoral and Post-Doctoral Scholarship (http://www.trudeaufoundation.ca/en), a Social Sciences and Humanities Research Council Canada Vanier Canada Graduate Scholarship (http://www.vanier.gc.ca/eng/home-accueil.aspx), and a grant from UNIFEM (now UNWOMEN) sub-regional office for Mexico, Central America, Cuba and the Dominican Republic (http://www.unwomen.org/). The funders had no role in study design, data collection and analysis, decision to publish, or preparation of the manuscript.

Competing Interests: The author declares that no competing interests exist.

* Email: tkendall@hsph.harvard.edu

Introduction

Prevention of vertical (mother-to-child) transmission of HIV is recognized as an important action to achieve the Millennium Development Goals, particularly the health-related goals of reducing child and maternal mortality and turning the tide of the HIV epidemic [1,2]. Antenatal HIV testing is necessary to prevent vertical HIV transmission and also offers an opportunity for women and other family members to learn their HIV status and access treatment for their own health [3]. In 2012 only 38% of pregnant women in low and middle-income countries were tested for HIV; in the Americas the proportion was 62% [4]. This is despite the fact that in 2001, member countries of the United Nations committed to providing antiretroviral prophylaxis to

prevent vertical HIV transmission to 80% of women who needed it by 2011 [5].

After endorsing the United Nations Political Declaration on HIV and AIDS in 2001, Mexico, like many other countries around the world, strengthened domestic policies to prevent vertical HIV transmission. The 2001 Mexican National Action Plan on HIV and AIDS established the universal offer of HIV testing to pregnant women; the 2007–2012 National Action Plan on HIV and AIDS reaffirmed this objective [6,7]. The most important operational intervention to promote HIV testing during antenatal care (ANC) after 2001 was the national distribution of 800,000 rapid HIV tests to primary care clinics that serve the population without employer-provided health insurance at the end of 2006 and beginning of 2007 with the instruction to offer HIV testing to all pregnant women [8]. However, Mexican HIV legislation was not modified to include the obligation of health-care services to offer HIV testing to all pregnant women until 2010 [9] and, as of June 2014, the national ANC legislation still stated that antenatal HIV testing should only be offered to "high risk women–those who have received blood transfusions, drug addicts, and prostitutes" [10]. This disjuncture between the commitment to offer of HIV testing to all pregnant women in the HIV National Action Plan and the legislative frameworks for HIV and reproductive health care, combined with the vertical organization of HIV and reproductive health services, assignation of the responsibility for prevention of vertical HIV transmission to the HIV program, and competing priorities in both HIV and reproductive health have been identified as policy and political barriers to the scale-up of HIV testing among pregnant women in Mexico, as well as other Latin American countries [11,12]. Additional operational barriers to antenatal HIV testing identified in Mexico between 2001 and 2011 included a limited number of health workers trained in HIV testing and counseling in reproductive health services and insufficient availability of commodities [12].

Mexico's national prenatal care legislation has recommended a minimum of five ANC visits since 1993 and the national HIV action plan introduced universal offer of HIV testing in 2001 [6,10]. Since 2006, 81.5% of women have begun ANC during the first trimester and beginning in 2009 national guidelines for antiretroviral management recommended HIV testing during the first trimester of pregnancy or as soon as possible thereafter [13,14]. However, when the current study began in 2009, despite 95.8% of Mexican women attending at least one ANC visit and 86.3% of women attending four or more ANC visits [15], only 42.1% of Mexican women who attended ANC were tested for HIV [16]. In 2011 when the study concluded, only 45.6% of women who attended ANC were tested for HIV [16]. The objective of this analysis is to describe missed opportunities for HIV diagnosis during pregnancy and document the consequences for the health and well-being of women living with HIV and their families.

Methods

Ethics statement

The design and conduct of this study was reviewed and approved annually by the University of British Columbia-Okanagan Behavioural Research Ethics Board and the Mexican National AIDS Program (CENSIDA) Ethics Board. To ensure confidentiality, pseudonyms were assigned to all women living with HIV who participated in the research, and physicians and decision-makers are identified only by their professional role.

Data collection and analysis

The analysis draws on semi-structured interviews with 55 Mexican women of reproductive age living with HIV conducted between July 2009 and January 2011. The criteria for women's inclusion in the study were: living with HIV, speaking Spanish, being at least 18 and of reproductive age (18–49 years of age), and having had a pregnancy since 2001 when universal offer of HIV testing during ANC was first included in the Mexican National Action Plan on HIV and AIDS. Women living with HIV were recruited from eight ambulatory HIV clinics in Central Mexico (Mexico State, Morelos, and Mexico City) that serve the population without employer-provided health insurance. The population attending these health services is generally economically disadvantaged. Reported monthly family incomes of the

women living with HIV ranged from 200 pesos (USD 16) to 10,000 pesos (USD 777) per month, with a median family income of 3000 pesos per month (USD 233) and a mean income of 3500 pesos per month (USD 272). All of the women living with HIV reported monthly household incomes below the Mexican national mean of USD 950 a month [17]. The exchange rate of 12.86 Mexican pesos for a US Dollar was calculated using the Federal Reserve Rate on the first day of each month between July 2009 and December 2010 (http://www.federalreserve.gov). Based on the cost of the basic monthly food basket in urban areas in 2008, which Mexico uses to estimate poverty, two-thirds of the women faced food insufficiency at the household level even before taking into account the cost of rent and other living expenses [18].

Women of reproductive age living with HIV were given a written invitation to participate by clinic staff. If they met the selection criteria and wished to participate clinic staff made an appointment to conduct an interview. Interviews were conducted in Spanish by the author, who has been doing qualitative research with Mexican women living with HIV for more than a decade, or a female Mexican anthropologist experienced in reproductive health research who was trained by the author about HIV and in the use of the interview guide. A site which afforded sufficient privacy was chosen by the woman living with HIV; most interviews were conducted in a private office at the HIV clinic. Research participants were given 100 pesos (approximately eight dollars) to pay for their travel and childcare. All research participants signed written informed consent prior to the interview. As one of the study objectives was to analyze implementation of the Mexican program to prevent vertical HIV transmission, and consequences of successful or failed implementation for women and their families, this was a purposive sample of women living with HIV diagnosed during ANC as well as women who were diagnosed in other settings. Sample size was determined by the principle of saturation, which refers to the point at which additional interviews do not provide novel information about the primary areas of interest [19]. Interviews were continued until saturation was reached with respect to women's narratives about the offer of HIV testing during antenatal care, the circumstances of their HIV diagnosis, and referral to services to prevent vertical HIV transmission. Numerical balance between women living with HIV diagnosed during ANC and those diagnosed in other settings was not sought.

Interviews with women living with HIV ranged from one to two hours in length and included questions about the circumstances of the HIV diagnosis, pregnancy history, sexual and reproductive practices and desires before and after the HIV diagnosis, experience of and management of HIV disease, prevention of vertical HIV transmission, interactions with the health-care system and health-care providers, and social and economic situation. This analysis focuses on the experiences of women living with HIV however data from 60 additional interviews with health-care providers, policymakers and other experts about prevention of vertical HIV transmission in Mexico between 2001 and 2011 are drawn upon to contextualize women's experiences.

All interviews were audiotaped and transcribed verbatim. The author conducted analysis during fieldwork and modified the interview guide to explore emerging issues. Interviews were coded thematically by the author, using a combination of predefined codes related to areas of interest and codes which were generated inductively from the interviews. Examples of a priori codes were HIV diagnosis during ANC and circumstances of the HIV diagnosis; examples of inductive codes include diagnosis because of AIDS-related morbidity or mortality of a child or a male partner, diagnosis when women developed AIDS-related complications, or through provider-initiative testing and counseling outside of ANC. Data were managed using the qualitative analysis package Atlas-ti 6.0.

Results

In total, 48 of the 55 women living with HIV attended ANC without knowledge of their diagnosis between 2001 and 2009. Figure 1 describes two routes to HIV diagnosis for these 48 women who attended ANC after 2001 and were diagnosed subsequently with HIV: 1) provider initiated testing and counseling (PITC) as part of ANC or intrapartum care, or 2) missed opportunities for HIV diagnosis during ANC/intrapartum care and subsequent HIV testing in another setting, usually when the woman, her child(ren), or the male partner developed AIDS-related complications.

As shown in Figure 1, all 14 pregnant women who were offered PITC and tested positive during ANC or intrapartum care received interventions to prevent vertical HIV transmission, as did another seven women who were diagnosed with HIV during pregnancy outside of ANC (21/48). Of the 34 women who were not diagnosed in ANC/intrapartum care, 27 were diagnosed after delivery and did not receive any interventions to prevent vertical HIV transmission (27/48). Four women who were offered and accepted PITC during ANC or intrapartum care had an initial negative test result. These four women, two women who refused HIV testing during ANC, and twenty-four women not offered PITC in ANC were subsequently diagnosed when the woman, her child(ren), or the male partner became ill with AIDS-related complications (30/48).

Seven women living with HIV were excluded from Figure 1 because they were already aware of their HIV diagnosis before becoming pregnant and accessing ANC post-2001. Their routes to HIV diagnosis were similar to other women who were not diagnosed during ANC: the woman becoming ill with AIDS-related complications, the male partner becoming ill or dying of AIDS-related complications, or PITC of asymptomatic women in other settings e.g. at work or prior to surgery.

HIV diagnosis during pregnancy

On average, women went to 6.5 ANC visits in the pregnancy prior to HIV-diagnosis or the pregnancy during which they were diagnosed [range 1–10], providing ample opportunities for health workers to offer HIV testing. Nevertheless, of the 48 women who attended ANC after 2001 but before being diagnosed with HIV, only 20 (42%) were offered HIV testing during ANC or labor and delivery (Figure 1). Many of the women who reported antenatal HIV testing were pregnant during 2007 and 2008 (after the national distribution of rapid tests to public primary care clinics), however other women who attended ANC in those years were not offered testing. The haphazard offer of HIV testing and counseling during ANC is exemplified by Nancy's experience. In 2008, she attended ANC at the public primary health care center "in my neighborhood, where my mother lives" and was not offered HIV testing and counseling. Nancy only learned she was living with HIV during pregnancy because, by chance, she went to an ANC visit at a different public primary health care center in the same city and was offered an HIV test.

Of the 20 women who received PITC during ANC, two refused testing, for an acceptance rate similar to the 85–90% identified in other Mexican studies [20,21]. Women who refused testing said they had not received specific information about preventing vertical HIV transmission as part of counseling. The perception among a few women that HIV testing was compulsory during pregnancy also suggests that the quality of counseling was sub-optimal. For instance, Jacinta wanted to be tested but understood HIV testing to be "a requirement of the health center to receive prenatal care".

Four of the women tested during ANC received negative test results (Figure 1). While one woman reported that she acquired HIV from a partner who she met after the index pregnancy, the other three women had the same male partner at the time of diagnosis as during the index pregnancy and were diagnosed shortly after delivery. This finding indicates that repeat HIV testing in the third trimester of pregnancy could provide additional benefit for identifying women living with HIV, preventing vertical HIV transmission, and enabling women's timely referral to long-term care.

Another group of women (n = 7) were not offered HIV testing as a routine part of ANC but were diagnosed during pregnancy. Among these women, four were diagnosed because their male partner became ill with AIDS-related complications during the pregnancy, one male partner disclosed his HIV status after his female partner became pregnant, one woman's husband received PITC as part of his application for work, and one woman happened to test at a street testing fair held in her neighbourhood.

Provision of interventions to prevent vertical HIV transmission and linkage to long-term HIV care and treatment

Once women had an HIV-positive test result, health-care providers and administrators reported that they expedited confirmation of pregnant women's HIV test results and access to interventions to prevent vertical HIV transmission, including antiretroviral prophylaxis. The head of a state HIV Program, explained "we consider a pregnant woman an emergency so we don't wait to have the viral load and CD4, we start the [prophylactic antiretroviral] regimen immediately." These efforts were reflected in women's reported experiences. Of the 21 women who learned their HIV status during pregnancy, all took steps to prevent vertical HIV transmission: 17/21 received antiretroviral prophylaxis; one woman diagnosed at 38 weeks gestation delivered by cesarean section and her child was given antiretroviral prophylaxis; none of the three women diagnosed during labor received antiretroviral prophylaxis for themselves or their children but two delivered by caesarean section; and none of the women breastfed. Of the 21 women who learned their diagnosis during ANC or intrapartum, 16 had children with an HIV-negative diagnosis, three children were too young to have a confirmed diagnosis, and two women were pregnant at the time of the interview.

With respect to linkage to and uptake of long-term HIV care, whether they were diagnosed during prenatal care or in another context, most women reported a relatively smooth and speedy transition from initial diagnosis to being referred to a public HIV clinic, confirmatory testing of HIV status and receiving the first CD4 and viral load count. At the time of the interview, all of the participants were enrolled in long-term HIV care and treatment for their own health. Sara's experience was typical of that reported by most participants, in that during the month after her child was born she "started to go to the [HIV] clinic with the doctor, my medical visits, my medications, and did everything to take care of myself." However, 7 of 55 women (12.7%) reported delaying seeking care and treatment after their diagnosis (from a few months up to several years), suspending HIV care for a period before they were treatment eligible, and temporarily stopping treatment during the postpartum period; only one of these women was diagnosed during pregnancy. Reasons given by women for

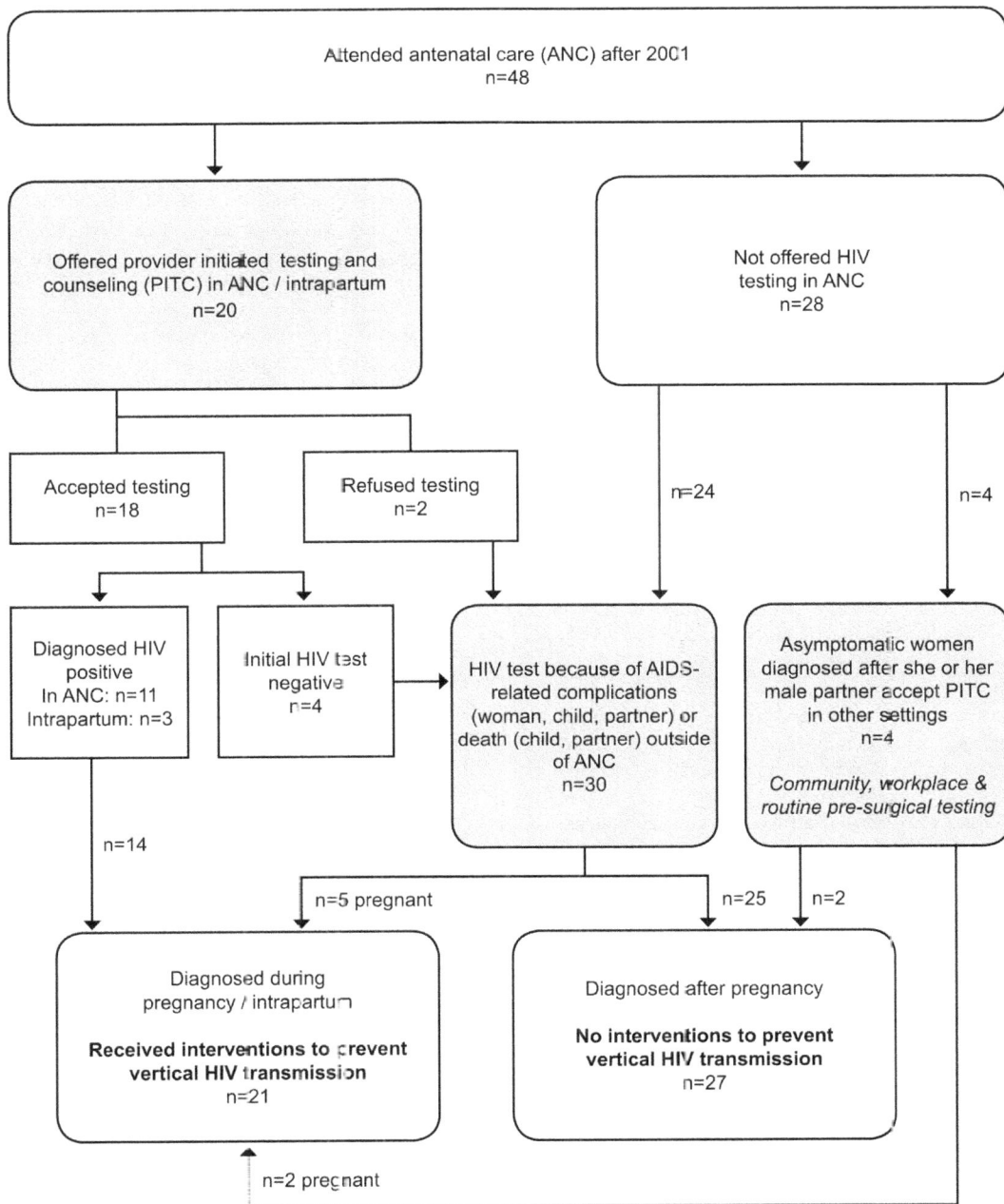

Figure 1. Routes to HIV diagnosis for Mexican women who attended antenatal care (ANC) after 2001.

delaying or suspending HIV care and treatment included lack of knowledge about HIV disease and treatment, perceived lack of empathy from health-care providers, antiretroviral side effects, prioritizing a child's treatment over their own health, and the cost of transportation. For example, Amparo said that before she was eligible for treatment she "stopped coming for about a year. I thought 'I'm fine, the doctor doesn't even give me a check-up, so why I am paying for transport and leaving my little kid."

Health, economic and emotional consequences of missed opportunities for HIV testing and delayed diagnosis

When the opportunity to offer HIV testing during ANC was missed, the most common route to the HIV diagnosis was when women or their family members experienced AIDS-related complications (Figure 1). As discussed in more detail below, the health, economic and emotional consequences of missing the opportunity to diagnose HIV during pregnancy were frequently exacerbated by health-care providers' failure to recognize HIV and AIDS-related complications among children, male partners, and women.

AIDS-related morbidity and mortality among children

In this sample, only women who were not diagnosed with HIV during pregnancy had children who were known to be living with HIV, or who had died from complications that were known or suspected to be AIDS-related. Four of the women interviewed experienced the death of a child who tested positive for HIV, three lost a child who had symptoms that could be due to AIDS without a diagnosis, and ten were mothers of children living with HIV. Children's AIDS-related illness or death was a common way for women to learn their HIV diagnosis. The tragedy of the preventable child death due to vertical HIV transmission is compounded by the fact that the parents invariably sought medical care for their children without receiving a timely HIV diagnosis. Itzel and her husband were typical in this respect. Despite their limited income (she is a maid and he is a day labourer), they sought specialized medical care in the public and private sectors for their son, and became deeply indebted. Itzel said:

> Test after test, they pricked him wherever they wanted and they never did this one [HIV], until the very last days when he had a convulsion and then, according to them, they wanted to do a more advanced test. By then we had gone through everything. Paediatricians and paediatricians, private ones, and the best–we spent so much money. [...] And we got deeply into debt. And for what? Nothing. Doctors and doctors and nothing. Why did it not occur to them to think just for a minute about [HIV]? And we did not either because, well, we never could have imagined it.

By the time of her son's death from AIDS-related complications at two years of age in 2008, Itzel had also progressed to AIDS. Mother and child had the same clinical symptoms: extreme weight loss (wasting), vomiting, and diarrhoea. Itzel explained that it "seemed strange to me that I had the same symptoms as him, you understand? I had totally lost weight, a lot of diarrhoea, and everything that we ate, I threw up, and that was how he was." If Itzel's husband had not taken the initiative to track down the physician who had ordered the HIV test for their son because he wanted to know what his son had died of, even their son's death would not have resulted in them learning their HIV diagnosis.

Similar to Itzel, Karen sought health-care for her son but did not learn he was living with HIV until shortly before he died. Karen's son died of AIDS-related complications at three years of age, and her younger daughter is HIV-positive. The history of Karen's pregnancies and the AIDS-defining illnesses experienced by the family illustrate that health-care providers had multiple opportunities and indications for recommending HIV testing. During her first pregnancy in 2004, Karen and her husband were both public sector employees with health insurance. Yet despite attending eight ANC visits and doing "eight ultrasounds with my son, every month I did one," Karen was not offered HIV testing and counseling. Her son was born vaginally and she breastfed exclusively for three months after which time she fed him with formula and breast milk. He was a sickly child and was being hospitalized regularly for infections and respiratory problems when she became pregnant with her daughter. During her second pregnancy in 2006 Karen attended six ANC visits but was not offered HIV testing. Her son's repeated illnesses, her husband's AIDS-defining illness (oesophageal candidiasis) and both of them being hospitalized did not result in health-care providers recommending HIV testing. Karen said she feels "impotent about my son because we knew that my husband got sick a lot from this.

He was hospitalized several times and they never, ever diagnosed anything". Just as her husband's symptoms did not provoke suspicion of HIV, her son was also misdiagnosed. Karen was told her son "had adenoiditis, and that was why he was always getting sick in his throat. So we finally got together enough money, and my father also lent us [money], so that he could have an operation." After the operation, Karen's son became acutely ill and remained hospitalized. At the same time, his younger sister became ill and was hospitalized. Karen related that "when they saw the two little siblings hospitalized, they asked why. It seemed strange to them, and they started to do tests". The simultaneous hospitalization of Karen's two children led to Karen, her husband and their two children learning that they were living with HIV.

Three other women living with HIV had lost children due to symptoms that could be AIDS-related but who died without a diagnosis. For example, Lilia miscarried and then, "in 2005, I had another baby who died at twenty-seven days old. He got pneumonia in one of his little lungs." Antonina's daughter died, but "even now, three years later, I don't know what killed her. She was sick to her throat. We took her to the doctor, but never found out what was wrong with her."

AIDS-related morbidity and mortality among male partners

Another route to the HIV diagnosis for women was when a male partner became ill with AIDS-related complications. In Carmen's case, health-care services missed the opportunity to diagnose her in 2003 while she was pregnant, but when her husband became ill with AIDS-related complications in 2009, they were both diagnosed. Similarly, Luisa was not offered HIV testing and counseling though she attended ANC during three pregnancies between 2002 and 2006. She learned she was HIV-positive in 2008 when her husband "started to get sick with fever, his whole body hurt, his bones, and when we came to the hospital for a vaccine, because he felt sick, the doctor told me that he did not have anemia, that probably he had AIDS." She and her husband both tested positive for HIV, and he died shortly afterwards. Very late diagnosis and deaths from AIDS-related complications were a hallmark of the family medical histories of women who participated in the research.

Women's HIV disease progression

The other common route to diagnosis was when a woman presented symptoms of HIV disease or AIDS-related complications. However, these diagnoses were frequently delayed. Over and over again, women reported that they had sought health care for a variety of HIV-related ailments without physicians ever suggesting an HIV test. Paola's story exemplifies the difficulty that women have receiving an HIV diagnosis despite being symptomatic. She said that

> for almost a year I was doing tests. I was going to urologists and other specialists because it seemed that I had a urinary tract infection. I had pain that wouldn't go away. I went to several different physicians but none sent me to do the [HIV] test. It was only when I felt really sick, I had a lot of diarrhoea and fever, I went to a doctor who knows my father, a family doctor. And because I trusted him, and based on the symptoms, the medicines [I had taken], and that I hadn't gotten better, he sent me to do an ELISA [Enzyme-linked immunosorbent assay].

Research has shown a close relationship between gynaecological disorders and HIV among women, yet despite her symptomology and determined health seeking, Paola progressed to the third clinical stage of HIV disease before she received her diagnosis [22]. Noemi had different symptoms than Paola, but she also experienced a long period of health-care seeking and became very ill before she was diagnosed.

They told me that it was pneumonia. They controlled it, I was okay, and then I got sick again. After that, they did tests but they never did one of these [HIV] tests. Because they did not think that it could be this [HIV]. They said that no, well it was just pneumonia, it was pneumonia, and they prescribed medicine, and I got better, and then again.

Noemi presented with recurrent pneumonia, an AIDS-defining illness, for years without an HIV test being suggested. When Noemi was finally tested for HIV, she was extremely ill:

They put me in intensive care because I had third grade dehydration; they said I arrived weighing thirty kilos (66 lbs.). By then I had pneumonia, dehydration, I was in the third stage of HIV. And as well, I had genital herpes, and also in the mouth. I was at the end. In fact, they [the physicians] told my family to come and say goodbye because they couldn't do anything for me.

Women living with HIV repeatedly narrated becoming very ill—losing weight, having fevers and diarrhoea, a chronic chest infection or pneumonia, or on-going gynaecological complications, and consulting a variety of physicians without receiving the recommendation of an HIV test.

Economic consequences

Futile health-care seeking that included consultations with specialists who ordered numerous laboratory tests but never recommended HIV testing, prescribed medicines and performed surgical interventions to treat AIDS-related symptoms and disease progression that limited women and men's ability to work had negative economic consequences for families. In many cases, the families of these women living with HIV simply could not afford their odyssey through the health system, and became indebted in order to pay their medical bills. Itzel explains that when seeking a diagnosis for her now deceased son, "sometimes my husband said, or I said: 'Well, now there is no money.' And then he'd say: 'well, we'll get it from wherever we can, what's important is that he's healthy and well.'" When men and women experienced AIDS-related complications, they became unable to work, digging their families into an ever deeper economic hole. For instance, Pamela was not diagnosed with HIV during her first pregnancy. While she was pregnant with their second child, her husband became ill with AIDS-related complications. The family was forced to migrate from another state to live with her male partner's family, increasing the economic precariousness of two households. Pamela said her greatest fear was her husband getting

sick again, right now he is in bed, and he cannot do almost anything .... He will not be able to work until I don't know when. We rely on my father-in-law. And it's not the same as before. Before, my husband gave me my money, and I could buy what I wanted–things for my daughter. And now it is

very different. We are dependent on my father-in-law, and with him it's only food, and hospital bills.

Death or abandonment by the male partner also left women and children in difficult economic situations. For example, at the time of the interview in March 2010, Anel was the only economic support for her family. She described being the sole breadwinner and the primacy of her job as a burden and a barrier to her HIV treatment: "I arrive too early for my appointments, and I apologize a million times, because at work they don't give me time off. And if I lose [my job] how do I eat? It is the only thing I have to support my kids."

Emotional consequences

The emotional costs of the failure to prevent vertical HIV transmission were also high, both for those women who had children living with HIV and those whose children had died of AIDS-related complications. A psychologist working in an ambulatory HIV clinic called the transmission of HIV to a child a "double grief" for their mothers.

I am speaking about part of the Mexican culture in which the value of maternity is channelled into moral questions, questions of values, of virtues, right? A good woman is a good mother, a good mother gives everything for her child, and a good mother who gives everything for her child would not forgive herself for an irresponsible act or let herself be, let herself be-I don't know how I can express this–to not provide protection to avoid that the child be born infected. Based on my work experience, this is how I could sum it up: when children are born infected because they did not realize in time, the mothers experience a double grief and they have to work doubly hard to accept [the diagnosis]. First, to accept that they are the ones who are alive. And afterwards to work out the guilt that they were the ones who infected their children.

Women's guilt because they had, unknowingly, transmitted HIV to their children was a recurrent theme of the interviews. Gisela said that having a child who is living with HIV "isn't nice, because they are going to suffer. Right now my daughter is little and everything, but when she is bigger, she is going to say that it is my fault." Karen, who was inconsolable about the AIDS-related death of her son and wept for most of the two hour long interview, said that "it hurts me because he was a child and he wasn't guilty of anything. I feel that I am [guilty] because I did not take care of myself, and I never realized that he was sick [with AIDS-related complications]." Karen never suspected she could be living with HIV, assiduously sought health-care services during pregnancy and to promote her son's health, and still blames herself for his death. The cultural construction of motherhood that condemns women for their children's ill health, irrespective of women's circumstances and efforts to promote their children's well-being, is made clear by Lourdes' experiences with health-care providers when seeking care for her son before either of them were diagnosed with HIV. Lourdes went to the regional hospital with

a bag of [his] medicines and prescriptions and I don't know what all. And even then the doctors who were there hit me with everything they had. They said, 'What an irresponsible mother. How is it possible that she is just letting this child die? Can you believe it?' 'No Miss, [Lourdes responded], I am not letting him die. Here are all of his prescriptions, all of his medicines, everything that I am giving him, and he just doesn't get better.' 'Why?' I also wanted to know what was wrong with my child.

Vertical HIV transmission, disability and death among children is mainly attributable to health-care providers' failure to offer HIV testing and counseling during pregnancy and failure to recognize AIDS-related complications among children, yet women living with HIV experienced guilt and were blamed by health-care providers for their children's ill-health.

Discussion

One of the central findings of this study is that these women were in regular contact with the health-care system for ANC and on multiple other occasions while seeking a diagnosis for AIDS-related complications for themselves or other family members and that often HIV counseling and testing was not offered. For more than half of the women living with HIV, the first failure to offer HIV testing and counselling occurred when they attended ANC during pregnancy. This omission of the offer of HIV testing and counselling was then frequently repeated when women and their families subsequently sought health-care for HIV and AIDS-related complications. Consequences of the omission of the offer of HIV testing and counseling during ANC and then during repeated contacts with the health care system included: new pediatric HIV infections, including younger siblings becoming infected with HIV because the woman wasn't diagnosed during the earlier pregnancy, disease progression of women, children and male partners, and deaths due to AIDS-related causes among children and male partners. The women living with HIV who participated in the research had survived these omissions. Beyond negative health consequences, futile health-care seeking and delayed diagnoses had negative economic and emotional consequences for women living with HIV and their families.

The serious health, economic and emotional consequences of the failure to offer HIV testing and counseling during ANC and delayed HIV diagnoses for women and their families could be averted by: 1) routine PITC in ANC and 2) improved recognition of AIDS-related complications by health-care providers.

To address low levels of HIV testing during ANC internationally, both the Centers for Disease Control and Prevention in the United States and the World Health Organization have advocated routine PITC [23,24]. Studies in both high- and low-income countries have demonstrated that antenatal PITC results in significantly higher HIV screening rates and increased implementation of programs to prevent vertical HIV transmission without a corresponding drop in clinic attendance because of fears of HIV testing [25–28]. The high uptake of PITC described in this study reiterates other Mexican studies that have found that PITC in ANC is acceptable to a large proportion of pregnant women with HIV (85–90%) and emphasizes the importance of counseling that informs pregnant women that vertical HIV transmission exists, that it can be prevented, and that there is effective and free treatment for HIV disease available for women's own health [20,21]. The need to improve and monitor the quality of counseling is also highlighted by the finding that a few women understood testing during pregnancy to be compulsory, substantiating concerns that PITC can contravene principles of informed consent; it is crucial to monitor PITC to ensure informed consent and confidentiality [24,29,30].

This research also suggests that the failure to offer HIV testing and counseling in Mexico is not simply an issue of financial constraints-either for the health-care system or for individual families. Frequently ANC included many tests and procedures which are more expensive than an HIV test. In fact, some of the care provided could be considered superfluous. The most dramatic example of this was reported by Karen who underwent eight ultrasounds during ANC but was not offered an HIV test–this omission resulted in the death of her son from AIDS, the subsequent transmission of HIV to her younger daughter, and delayed her and her husband's HIV diagnosis until he was experiencing AIDS-related complications. In response to AIDS-related complications, these low-income families actively sought health-care in both the for-profit and not-for-profit sectors, and paid for physician visits, laboratory tests, medications, and surgery.

Late HIV diagnosis is a serious individual and public health problem in Mexico and around the globe. For individuals living with HIV, late diagnosis (lower CD4 count, higher viral load, or an AIDS-defining illness) has been associated with a greater probability of progression to AIDS and death [31]. In Mexico, half of those people newly diagnosed with HIV in 2011 were categorized as having AIDS [32]. Similarly, a study from a tertiary level Mexico City hospital categorized 61% of people as late-testers because within six months of diagnosis, they had CD4 counts below 200 and/or they had experienced an AIDS-defining illness [27]. Free lifelong antiretroviral treatment for people living with HIV has been available to beneficiaries of the Social Security Institutes for private and public sector workers since the late 1990 s and those without employer-provided health insurance since 2003 [33]. However, many of the women living with HIV who participated in this study and their family members weren't able to take advantage of freely available antiretroviral treatment in a timely fashion because of delayed HIV diagnosis. This study makes a novel contribution to the literature by documenting how missed opportunities to offer HIV testing and counseling to women when they attend ANC during pregnancy and to recognize the symptoms of HIV and AIDS when women and other family members seek health-care resulted in late diagnosis.

After the HIV diagnosis, women's experiences of linkage to and uptake of health-care services suggest both the existence of a relatively strong referral system within the public health-care system and women's strong motivation to prevent vertical HIV transmission and access long-term HIV care and treatment for themselves and other family members. At the time of the interview, all of the women living with HIV were participating in long-term HIV care and treatment. A small proportion of women (7 of 55, 12.7%) reported that they had delayed or interrupted HIV care and treatment for their own health. Reasons given, such as lack of knowledge about HIV disease and treatment, not having symptoms, negative interactions with health-care providers, and transportation costs have also been identified in other settings and should be addressed [34,35]. Research from sub-Saharan Africa has raised concerns about the large proportion of women (ranging from 38% to 88% depending on the study) who do not enroll in care and treatment for their own health after being diagnosed with HIV during pregnancy [35,36].

Study limitations

The experiences of women attending public HIV clinics located in three Central Mexican States may not be relevant for women of different socioeconomic status, or those who live in other areas of the country. Despite increasing coverage of HIV testing during the period under study, omission of HIV testing in ANC remains a significant problem in Mexico. The most recently published national statistics indicate that in 2012 only 59.8% of pregnant women who attended ANC were tested for HIV [16]. In addition, as women were reporting on events that could have occurred up to a decade prior to the interview, recall bias may have influenced their responses. Finally, as this study recruited women living with HIV from care and treatment clinics, it cannot provide insight into the linkage to and uptake of long-term HIV care and treatment by all women testing for HIV during ANC. Studies to explore this issue should be considered a priority for HIV research in Mexico and other Latin American countries.

Conclusions

A decade after universal HIV testing for pregnant women was included in Mexico's National Action Plan on HIV and AIDS, less than half of Mexican women attending ANC were tested for HIV [6,16]. The seriousness of the negative health, economic and emotional consequences of this omission for women and their families and the high acceptance rate of HIV testing by pregnant Mexican women are compelling arguments firstly to create a favorable policy environment by harmonizing ANC legislation with existing HIV legislation and secondly to make the necessary investments in health-care provider training, commodities, supervision and monitoring to rapidly accelerate scale-up of routine provider-initiated HIV testing and counseling during ANC. This research also documents the need to undertake national education campaigns for health-care workers about the HIV epidemic and the symptoms of AIDS in collaboration with medical and nursing

schools, health-care institutions, and professional associations. There is an urgent need for both pre-service and in-service training to increase health-care providers' awareness of HIV as well as their abilities to provide HIV testing and counseling, identify HIV and AIDS-related complications, and appropriately refer people to HIV care and treatment. PITC within and beyond ANC and more pre-service and in-service medical education about HIV will not only prevent vertical HIV transmission but will reduce extremely late HIV diagnosis and facilitate timely access to free, lifesaving antiretroviral treatment for women and other family members.

Acknowledgments

This research was only possible thanks to the generosity of all of those who gave of their time and knowledge to participate, particularly the women living with HIV who shared their stories. The author received institutional support during the research and preparation of the manuscript from the Mexican non-governmental organization Balance, as well as from the Takemi Program in International Health and the Women and Health Initiative at the Harvard School of Public Health. Thanks are also due to Lauren Ng and Rebecca Hope for their helpful comments.

Author Contributions

Conceived and designed the experiments: TK. Analyzed the data: TK. Contributed reagents/materials/analysis tools: TK. Wrote the paper: TK.

References

1. UNAIDS (2011) Countdown to Zero: Global Plan Towards the Elimination of New HIV Infections Among Children by 2015 and Keeping Their Mothers Alive, 2011–2015. Geneva.
2. WHO (2010) Towards Universal Access: Scaling up priority HIV/AIDS intervention in the health sector. Progress Report 2010. Geneva.
3. UNAIDS (2012) UNAIDS World AIDS Day Report 2012. Geneva.
4. WHO UNICEF, UNAIDS (2013) Global update on HIV treatment 2013: results, impact and opportunities, June 2013 Brief summary. Geneva. WHO/HIV/2013.9 WHO/HIV/2013.9.
5. UN (2001) Declaration of Commitment on HIV/AIDS: United Nations General Assembly Special Session on HIV/AIDS, 25–27 June 2001, UNAIDS/02.31E. Geneva: UNAIDS. 92-9173-190-0 92-9173-190-0.
6. Secretaría de Salud (2002) Programa de Acción: VIH/SIDA e Infecciones de Transmisión Sexual (ITS) (2001–2006). Mexico City.
7. Secretaría de Salud (2008) Programa de Acción Específico 2007–2012 en respuesta al VIH/SIDA e ITS. Mexico City: Secretaría de Salud.
8. Godinez Leal L (2007) Tiene Censida pruebas rápidas de VIH para embarazadas. CIMAC Noticias. Mexico City, Mexico: CIMAC.
9. Secretaría de Salud (2010) Norma Oficial Mexicana NOM-010-SSA2-2010, Para la prevención y control de la infección por de Inmunodeficiencia Humana. Mexico City: Secretaría de Salud.
10. Secretaría de Salud (1993) Norma Oficial Mexicana NOM-007-SSA2-1993, Atención de la mujer durante el embarazo, parto y puerperio y del recién nacido. Criterios y procedimientos para la prestación del servicio. Mexico City: Secretaría de Salud: Secretaría de Salud.
11. Kendall T, López-Uribe E (2010) Improving the HIV Response for Women in Latin America: Barriers to Integrated Advocacy for Sexual and Reproductive Health and Rights. Global Health Governance 4.
12. Kendall TR (2012) Prevention of Vertical HIV Transmission and the HIV Response for Women in Latin America [PhD]. Kelowna, British Columbia: University of British Columbia. 242 p.
13. Guttierez J, Rivera-Donmarco J, Shamah-Levy T, Villalbando-Hernandez S, Franco A, et al. (2013) Encuesta Nacional de Salud y Nutrición Resultados Nacionales 2012; Oropeza-Abundez C, editor. Cuernavaca: Instituto Nacional de Salud Pública.
14. CENSIDA (2009) Guía de manejo de antirretroviral de las personas con VIH, cuarta edición Mexico City: Secretaría de Salud.
15. United Nations Statisctics Division (2011) Millenium Development Goals Indicators: The official United Nations site for the MDG Indicators. In: United Nations Statisctics Division, editor.
16. CONASIDA (2013) Boletin del Grupo de Informacion Sectorial en VIH/SIDA No. 10. Mexico City: Secretaría de Salud.
17. INEGI (2009) El INEGI da a conocer los resultados de la Encuesta Nacional de Ingresos y Gastos de los Hogares (ENIGH) 2008. Comunicado numero 191/09.
18. CONEVAL (2011) Measurement: Frequently Asked Questions. Mexico City: CONEVAL.
19. Charmaz K (2005) Grounded Theory in the 21st Century: Applications for Advancing Social Justice Studies. In: Denizen NK, Lincoln YS, editors. The Sage Handbook of Qualitative Research. 3 ed. Thousand Oaks, CA: Sage Publications. 507–535.
20. Romero-Gutierrez G, Delgado-Macias AA, Mora-Escobar Y, Ponce-Ponce de Leon AL, Amador N (2007) Mexican women s reasons for accepting or declining HIV antibody testing in pregnancy. Midwifery 23: 23–27.
21. Vera Gamboa L, Gongora Biachi RA, Pavia Ruz N, Gaber Osorno J, Lara Perera D, et al. (2005) Aceptabilidad para la detección de anticuerpos contra el VIH en un grupo de mujeres embarazadas de Yucatán, México. Ginecol Obstet Mex 73: 355–359.
22. Squires KE (2007) Gender differences in the diagnosis and treatment of HIV. Gend Med 4: 294–307.
23. Branson BM, Handsfield HH, Lampe MA, Janssen RS, Taylor AW, et al. (2006) Revised Recommendations for HIV Testing of Adults, Adolescents, and Pregnant Women in Health-Care Settings. Atlanta: Centers for Disease Control and Prevention 1–17 p.
24. WHO UNAIDS (2007) Guidance on Provider-Initiated HIV Testing and Counselling in Health Facilities. Geneva.
25. Creek TL, Ntumy R, Seipone K, Smith M, Mogodi M, et al. (2007) Successful introduction of routine opt-out HIV testing in antenatal care in Botswana. J Acquir Immune Defic Syndr 45: 102–107.
26. Manzi M, Zachariah R, Teck R, Buhendwa L, Kazima J, et al. (2005) High acceptability of voluntary counselling and HIV-testing but unacceptable loss to follow up in a prevention of mother-to-child HIV transmission programme in rural Malawi: scaling-up requires a different way of acting. Trop Med Int Health 10: 1242–1250.
27. Moses A, Zimba C, Kamanga E, Nkhoma J, Maida A, et al. (2008) Prevention of mother-to-child transmission: program changes and the effect on uptake of the HIVNET 012 regimen in Malawi. Aids 22: 83–87.
28. Walmsley S (2003) Opt in or opt out: what is optimal for prenatal screening for HIV infection? CMAJ 168: 707–708.
29. Rennie S, Behets F (2006) Desperately seeking targets: the ethics of routine HIV testing in low-income countries. Bull World Health Organ 84: 52–57.
30. Maman S, King E (2008) Changes in HIV testing policies and the implications for women. J Midwifery Womens Health 53: 195–201.
31. Egger M, May M, Chene G, Phillips AN, Ledergerber B, et al. (2002) Prognosis of HIV-1-infected patients starting highly active antiretroviral therapy: a collaborative analysis of prospective studies. Lancet 360: 119–129.
32. CENSIDA (2012) El VIH/SIDA en México 2012. Mexico City, Mexico: Secretaria de Salud.
33. Saavedra-Lopez J, Bravo-Garcia E (2006) Panorama del VIH/SIDA en el 2006. In: Rodríguez CM, Bárcenas HB, Kenefick SB, editors. SIDA: Aspectos de Salud Pública. Cuernavaca: Instituto Nacional de Salud Pública. 3–14.
34. Ferguson L, Grant AD, Lewis J, Kielman K, Watson-Jones D, et al. (2014) Linking women who test HIV-positive in pregnancy-related services to HIV care

and treatment services in Kenya: A mixed methods prospective cohort study. PLoS One 9: e89764.

35. Ferguson L, Grant AD, Watson-Jones D, Kahawita T, Ong'ech JO, et al. (2012) Linking women who test HIV-positive in pregnancy-related services to long-term HIV care and treatment services: a systematic review. Tropical Medicine & International Health 17: 564–580.

36. Watson-Jones D, Balira R, Ross DA, Weiss HA, Mabey D (2012) Missed opportunities: poor linkage to ongoing care for HIV-positive pregnant women in Mwanza, Tanzania. PLoS One 7: e40091.

24

Indices to Measure Risk of HIV Acquisition in Rakai, Uganda

Joseph Kagaayi[1,2]*, Ronald H. Gray[3], Christopher Whalen[5], Pingfu Fu[2], Duncan Neuhauser[2],
Janet W. McGrath[4], Nelson K. Sewankambo[6], David Serwadda[6], Godfrey Kigozi[2], Fred Nalugoda[2],
Steven J. Reynolds[7,8], Maria J. Wawer[3], Mendel E. Singer[2]

1 Rakai Health Sciences Program, Entebbe, Uganda, 2 Department of Epidemiology and Biostatistics, Case Western Reserve University, Cleveland, Ohio, United States of America, 3 Department of Epidemiology, Johns Hopkins Bloomberg School of Public Health, Baltimore, Maryland, United States of America, 4 Department of Anthropology, Case Western Reserve University, Cleveland, Ohio, United States of America, 5 Department of Epidemiology and Biostatistics, University of Georgia, Athens, Georgia, United States of America, 6 Makerere University College of Health Sciences, Kampala, Uganda, 7 Division of Intramural Research, National Institute of Allergy and Infectious Diseases, National Institutes of Health, Bethesda, Maryland, United States of America, 8 Johns Hopkins School of Medicine, Baltimore, Maryland, United States of America

Abstract

Introduction: Targeting most-at-risk individuals with HIV preventive interventions is cost-effective. We developed gender-specific indices to measure risk of HIV among sexually active individuals in Rakai, Uganda.

Methods: We used multivariable Cox proportional hazards models to estimate time-to-HIV infection associated with candidate predictors. Reduced models were determined using backward selection procedures with Akaike's information criterion (AIC) as the stopping rule. Model discrimination was determined using Harrell's concordance index (c index). Model calibration was determined graphically. Nomograms were used to present the final prediction models.

Results: We used samples of 7,497 women and 5,783 men. 342 new infections occurred among females (incidence 1.11/100 person years,) and 225 among the males (incidence 1.00/100 person years). The final model for men included age, education, circumcision status, number of sexual partners, genital ulcer disease symptoms, alcohol use before sex, partner in high risk employment, community type, being unaware of a partner's HIV status and community HIV prevalence. The Model's optimism-corrected c index was 69.1 percent (95% CI = 0.66, 0.73). The final women's model included age, marital status, education, number of sex partners, new sex partner, alcohol consumption by self or partner before sex, concurrent sexual partners, being employed in a high-risk occupation, having genital ulcer disease symptoms, community HIV prevalence, and perceiving oneself or partner to be exposed to HIV. The models optimism-corrected c index was 0.67 (95% CI = 0.64, 0.70). Both models were well calibrated.

Conclusion: These indices were discriminative and well calibrated. This provides proof-of-concept that population-based HIV risk indices can be developed. Further research to validate these indices for other populations is needed.

Editor: Matthew Law, University of New South Wales, Australia

Funding: The study was supported by National Institute of Child Health and Human Development of the National Institutes of Health; grant number RO1HD050180; and National Institutes of Health; grant number U01AI075115; and in part (SJR) by the Division of Intramural Research, National Institute of Allergy and Infectious Diseases, National Institutes of Health. The funders had no role in study design, data collection and analysis, decision to publish, or preparation of the manuscript.

Competing Interests: The authors have declared that no competing interests exist.

* E-mail: jxk597@case.edu

Introduction

Identifying individuals most-at-risk for HIV and targeting them with specific preventive interventions has been shown to be cost-effective [1–7]. These groups could be targeted with behavioral interventions combined with voluntary HIV testing and counseling (VCT), voluntary medical male circumcision (VMMC), and pre-exposure prophylaxis (PrEP) with antiretroviral drugs.

Moreover, the effectiveness of some preventive programs was shown to be higher among people most-at-risk of HIV. For example, male circumcision (MC) was more effective in studies of men deemed to be at high risk of HIV such as men recruited from

clinics treating sexually transmitted infections and among truck drivers [8], or HIV uninfected men in discordant relationships with HIV-positive women [9]. Higher efficacy of MC was also suggested for men with many partners or genital ulcers in the Rakai circumcision trial [10].

With respect to PrEP, mathematical models suggest higher cost-effectiveness of oral PrEP among most-at-risk groups [11,12].

Unlike countries where the HIV epidemic is limited to specific groups (concentrated epidemics) and high-risk groups are readily identified, in sub-Saharan Africa (SSA) with a generalized epidemic, identifying high-risk groups to target is especially challenging.

Table 1. Description of potential predictors, Rakai, 2003–2011.

Demographics	Type	Description
Age	Continuous	
Marital status	Categorical	Monogamous, polygamous, divorced/separated, never married
Education	Categorical	Primary/no education, at or above secondary level
Behaviors		
Number of sexual partners in last 12 months	Ordinal Categorical	1,2,3+ for males and 1,2+ for females
Frequency of condom use in last 12 months	Categorical	Always, sometimes and never
Alcohol before sex	categorical	Taking alcohol before sex, (Yes/No)
Casual sex	Categorical	sex with a non-regular, non-cohabiting partner (yes/no)
Transactional sex	categorical	Engagement in sex where money or gifts were exchanged as a condition for having sexual relations (Yes/No)
Biomedical factors		
Genital ulcers		Yes/No
Circumcision		Yes/No
Hormonal contraception		Taking hormonal pills, injectable, implanted hormonal contraceptives (Yes/No)
VCT		
HIV Testing in last 12 months	Categorical	Yes/No
Sexual Partner variables		
Used alcohol before sex	Categorical	As reported by partner (Yes/No)
Perceived partner's exposure to HIV	Categorical	As a response to the question: "How likely is it that your partner has been exposed to HIV, the virus that causes HIV/AIDS infection" Yes (very likely or likely), No (very unlikely or unlikely)
High risk employment	Categorical	Yes, if working in a bar, brewing alcohol, working in a restaurant, working in a hotel or guest house, fishing, truck or taxi driver, motor-cycle taxi rider (locally called boda-boda cyclist), market vending, housekeeper, trading which required one to work away from their community, and being in the army, police, or security work, No Otherwise
Unaware of partner's HIV status	Categorical	Yes/No
Domestic violence situation	Categorical	Involves violence received or perpetuated. (including verbal and physical insults)
Contextual variables		
Residence	Categorical	Village/Trading center
Recent immigration	Categorical	Yes/No (Moved to community within last 2 years)
Community HIV prevalence	Continuous	Prevalence of HIV in one's community

Prediction indices have been used successfully to predict the risk for chronic diseases such as coronary heart disease and cancer [13,14] but have had limited application to HIV infection. To-date research into indices to predict HIV risk in SSA has been limited to discordant couple relationships [15,16]. Development of indices for the general population is especially critical for SSA where identifiable discordant couple relationships contribute only modestly to HIV incidence [17,18].

We developed gender-specific indices to predict the risk of HIV acquisition based on the general population of sexually active individuals who participated in the Rakai Community Cohort Study (RCCS) in Rakai district, Uganda.

Methods

Ethics statement

The Rakai Community cohort study (RCCS) was approved by the Science and Ethics Committee of Uganda Virus Research Institute, the Uganda National Council of Science and Technology and US-based Western IRB. Written consent was obtained from all research participants. Participants less than 18 years had their parents, caretakers, or guardians provide written consent for them in addition to their own written assent. Consent procedures were approved by the Science and Ethics Committee of Uganda Virus Research Institute, the Uganda National Council of Science and Technology and US-based Western IRB.

Population

Derivation of the indices was based on data from the Rakai Community Cohort Study (RCCS), in Rakai district, South-Western Uganda. The cohort has been described previously [19,20]. Briefly, the RCCS is an open population-based prospective cohort of approximately 15,000 consenting participants aged 15–49 years who were interviewed in surveys conducted every 12–20 months since 1994. Participants provided information in structured interviews and provided blood samples for HIV serology. The data collected included demographics, sexual behaviors, health and contextual characteristics. We used longitudinal data collected from 2003 to 2011. The maximum follow-up time was 7.7 years. The indices were limited to sexually active individuals who reported sexual intercourse in the previous 12 months.

Table 2. Characteristics of Sexually active Participants, Rakai Cohort, 2003–2011.

	Men		Women	
	Number/Mean	Percent/SD	Number/Mean	Percent/Sd
All	5,783	100	7,497	100
Age (years, SD)	28.3	8.0	27.0	7.8
Marital status				
Monogamous	3,179	55.0	4,342	57.9
Polygamous	549	9.5	1,228	16.4
Separated/Divorced	242	4.2	778	10.4
Never married	1,813	31.3	1,149	15.4
Education				
Primary/No education	3,899	67.4	5,100	68.0
Post-primary education	1,884	32.6	2,397	32.0
Recent migrant to community	1,102	19.1	2,430	32.4
Community type				
Village	4,881	84.4	6,119	81.2
Trading center	902	15.6	1,378	18.4
Number of sexual partners				
1	3,308	57.2	7027	94.0
2	1,667	28.8	-	-
2+	-	-	446	6.0
3+	808	14.0	-	-
New sex partner	3,013	52.1	1,970	26.3
Transactional sex	145	2.5	43	0.5
Casual sex	662	11.5	111	1.5
Concurrent sexual partners	2,137	37.0	267	3.6
Frequency of condom use				
Always	862	14.9	593	7.9
Sometimes	2,215	38.3	1,692	22.6
Never	2,706	46.8	5,212	69.5
Alcohol use before sex	2,166	37.5	2,971	39.6
Genital ulcers	618	10.7	904	12.1
Perception of risk of exposure	1,691	29.2	3,011	40.2
Domestic violence	1,606	27.8	2,106	28.1
Circumcised	1,332	23.0	1332	23.1
Uncircumcised sexual partner	-	-	5212	69.7
Hormonal contraception	-	-	1522	20.3
VCT in last 12 months	1,852	32.0	2,935	39.2
Any partner of unknown HIV status	4,523	78.8	5,868	78.3
Partner in a high risk employment	636	11.0	3,083	41.1
Has high risk employment	1,986	34.3	973	13.0
Community HIV prevalence	11.7	3.6	11.9	3.8

Potential predictor variables

The variables considered included participant demographics (age, marital status, education); sexual behaviors in the previous twelve months including number of sexual partners, frequency of condom use, use of alcohol before sex by either partner, casual sex, transactional sex, concurrent sexual partners and self-perception of exposure to HIV or perception of exposure by partner (for unmeasured risk factors); biomedical factors including genital ulcer symptoms, men's circumcision status, and use of hormonal contraception by women; HIV testing and counseling in the previous twelve months; contextual factors including community type (trading center versus village), whether one migrated to the community within the previous 2 years, Community HIV prevalence, whether or not the participant's employment type was associated with high risk of acquiring HIV); and partner characteristics including use of alcohol before sex, perception of partner's exposure to HIV, whether partner had a high risk employment type and whether the partner's HIV status was

Table 3. Association between variables and HIV acquisition by Gender, Rakai, Uganda 2003–2011: Unadjusted analyses.

Characteristic	Men			Women		
	Relative Hazard	95% CI	p-value	RelativeHazard	95% CI	P-value
Age (linear, years)	1.27	1.05–1.44	0.002	0.98	0.96–0.99	0.001
Age (squared)	99.51	99.24–99.79	0.001	-	-	-
Marriage						
Monogamous	1	-	-	1	-	
Polygamous	1.38	0.90–2.12	0..140	1.01	0.79–1.52	0.569
Separated	2.42	1.47–3.98	0.001	2.73	2.05–3.63	<0.001
Never married	1.38	1.03–1.86	0.034	2.23	1.68–2.96	<0.001
Education						
Primary/None	1	-	-	1	-	
Post-primary	0.55	0.40–0.77	<0.001	0.88	0.69–1.11	0.284
Recent migration to community	1.12	0.79–1.59	0.522	1.50	1.20–1.88	<0.001
Community type						
Village	1			1		
Trading center	1.81	1.33–2.45	<0.001	1.24	0.96–1.62	0.102
Number of sexual partners						
1	1	-	-	1	-	-
2	1.36	1.00–1.86	0.053			
2+	-	-	-	3.96	2.99–5.25	<0.001
3+	2.71	1.97–3.72	<0.001	-	-	-
New sex partner	1.53	1.17–2.00	0.002	2.56	2.06–3.19	<0.001
Transactional sex	2.21	1.21–4.05	0.010	2.82	1.05–7.55	0.040
Casual sex	1.44	0.99–2.08	0.055	2.61	1.39–4.91	0.003
Frequency of condom use						
Always	1	-	-	1	-	-
Sometimes	1.20	0.81–1.78	0.363	1.25	0.83–1.88	0.276
Never	0.75	0.50–1.12	0.157	0.60	0.41–0.89	0.011
Concurrency	1.61	1.24–2.09	<0.001	4.26	3.07–5.93	<0.001
Alcohol use before sex	1.46	1.12–1.89	0.005	1.38	1.12–1.71	0.003
Perception of exposure to HIV	1.70	1.30–2.23	<0.001	1.75	1.42–2.16	<0.001
Genital ulcers	2.31	1.68–3.19	<0.001	1.96	1.49–2.56	<0.001
VCT in last 12 months	0.83	0.62–1.09	0.179	0.74	0.59–0.92	0.007
Circumcision	.56	0.39–0.82	0.003	-	-	-
Use of hormonal contraception	-	-	-	1.06	0.88–1.29	0.518
Partner of unknown HIV status	2.18	1.48–3.21	<0.001	1.44	1.09–1.90	0.011
High risk employment	1.17	0.89–1.52	0.262	1.65	1.26–2.16	<0.001
Partner in high risk employment	2.53	1.83–3.50	<0.001	1.09	0.88–1.35	0.425
Community HIV prevalence	1.05	1.01–1.08	0.003	1.04	1.01–1.07	0.002

unknown. These factors have been associated with HIV risk in published literature [10,21–31]. A full description of the variables and their coding is shown in table 1.

Statistical methods

We performed frequency tabulations of potential categorical variables and summaries of continuous variables. We used a correlational matrix to determine pairwise correlations between potential variables. Highly correlated variables were combined if they measured similar domains of HIV risk. For this reason, use of alcohol before sex by oneself and one's sexual partner were

combined into one variable. The same was done for self-perception of exposure to HIV and perception of exposure to HIV by sexual partners. Two percent of males and about three percent of females had at least one of the candidate variables missing. To avoid possible selection bias we imputed missing values using the aregImpute (Hmisc) R function. This function conducts multiple imputation by using the bootstrap samples for each of the multiple imputations and fits a flexible additive model on a sample with replacement from the original data and this model is used to predict all of the original missing and non-missing values for the variables being imputed [32].

Table 4. Multivariable Associations between variables and HIV acquisition by Gender, Rakai, Uganda 2003–2011.

	Men				Women			
	Hazard Ratio	95% CI	Coefficients	χ^2	HazardRatio	95% CI	Coefficients	χ^2
Age (linear)	1.23	1.04–1.44	0.2084	16.7	0.97	0.95–0.99	−0.0300	11.0
†Age (square)	99.57	99.30–99.86	−0.0042	8.8	-			
Marital status								
Monogamous	-	-	-	-	1	1	0	
Polygamous	-	-	-	-	1.10	0.79–1.54	0.0988	23.7
Separated	-	-	-	-	2.08	1.44–2.80	0.6987	
Never married	-	-	-	-	1.72	1.26–2.33	0.5404	
Education								
Primary/Never	1	-	0	11.7	1	-	0	
Post-primary	0.56	0.41–0.78	−0.5732		0.83	0.65–1.06	−0.1873	2.2
No of sexual partners								
1	1	-	0		1	-	0	
2	1.21	0.88–1.66	0.1879	14.2	-			
2+	-	-	-		1.59	0.97–2.63	0.4665	3.3
3+	1.90	1.36–2.67	0.6434		-			
New sex partner					1.45	1.09–1.92	0.3703	6.7
Either partner drunk alcohol before sex	1.28	0.96–1.71	0.2469	2.9	1.44	1.15–1.80	0.3617	9.9
Concurrent relationships					1.50	0.87–2.60	0.4058	2.2
Perception of HIV risk	-				1.49	1.20–1.86	0.4001	12.7
Gud	1.78	1.28–2.48	0.5939	12.5	1.75	1.33–2.31	0.5627	16.3
Circumcision	0.61	0.41–0.90	−0.4973	6.3	-	-	-	-
Community type								
Village	1	-	0	9.9	-			
Trading center	1.67	1.21–2.31	0.5148		-	-	-	-
Partner with unknown HIV	1.82	1.22–2.70	0.5790	8.2	-	-	-	
Community HIV prevalence	1.03	0.99–1.07	0.0319	3.3	1.03	1.01–1.06	0.0369	7.7
Having a high risk occupation	-				1.32	0.99–1.75	0.2788	3.7
Partner in high risk occupation	1.89	1.34–2.67	0.6135	12.4	-	-	-	-

We used Cox proportional hazards regression to model time-to-HIV infection as a function of candidate predictor variables. Since HIV infection was only detected at the time of the survey visits, the exact time of HIV infection was not known so the time of infection was assumed to be the middle of the interval between the last negative and first positive HIV test.

Analyses were stratified by gender because some of the important variables, such as circumcision status and use of hormonal contraception were gender-specific.

We assessed unadjusted associations between variables and HIV acquisition. To determine the optimal form for continuous variables (age and community HIV prevalence), we compared deviances of nested models of polynomials including linear, square, and cubic terms; as well as restricted cubic splines with 3–5 knots. As a result, age was modeled using a square term for men and a linear term for women. Community HIV prevalence was modeled using a linear term.

The global and variable-specific proportional hazards assumption was checked using the cox.zph R function [33] which examines the correlation coefficient between transformed survival time and scaled Schoenfeld residuals as well as the slope of the time-dependent coefficient.

In view of the evidence of higher effectiveness of male circumcision among high risk men [8,10], we included an interaction term between number of sex partners and circumcision status in the full multivariable men's model. We used a main effects model for women. A reduced model was obtained using backward selection procedures with AIC as stopping rule. For statistical inference, the AIC criteria requires that the increase in model χ^2 for a given variable be greater than two times the degrees of freedom for the variable and a χ^2 p-value not greater than 0.157 for one degree of freedom [34,35].

Model performance

Model discrimination was assessed by using Harrell's concordance index (c index) for survival data and its 95 percent confidence interval [36]. We also examined discrimination graphically using a plot of cumulative HIV incidence by quartiles of predicted HIV risk score.

Model calibration was assessed graphically using a plot of 4-year observed versus predicted survival for groups of participants with different survival probabilities.

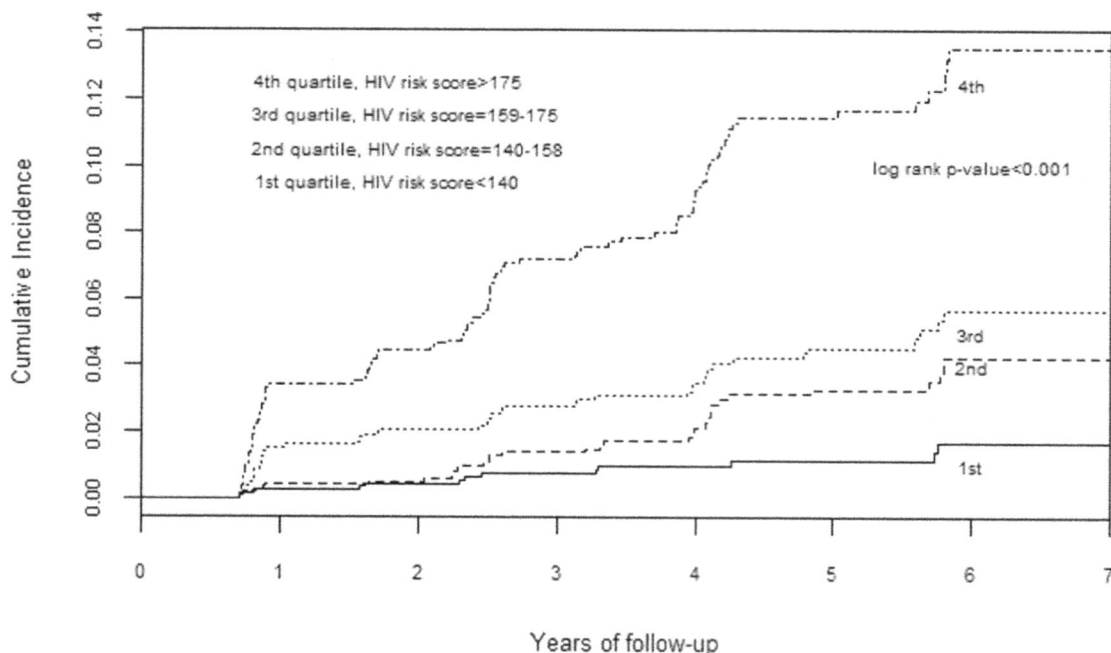

Figure 1. Cumulative HIV incidence by predicted quartile of HIV risk score for sexually active men.

Internal Validation

A bias-corrected (corrected for possible over-fitting) c index was obtained using bootstrap resampling validation procedures [36] with 200 bootstrap samples from the original sample. The bias-corrected c index gives the best estimate of discrimination if the coefficients from this model were applied to another sample to predict HIV acquisition.

Proportion of new infections due to most-at-risk status

We determined the proportion of cumulative new infections contributed by the most-at-risk group. We used various thresholds of HIV risk scores to define most-at-risk status, including the upper quintile, upper two quintiles, upper quartile, upper third and upper half of the risk scores as possible thresholds.

The model was presented as a nomogram using Harrell's nomogram R function [37]. The nomogram provides scores

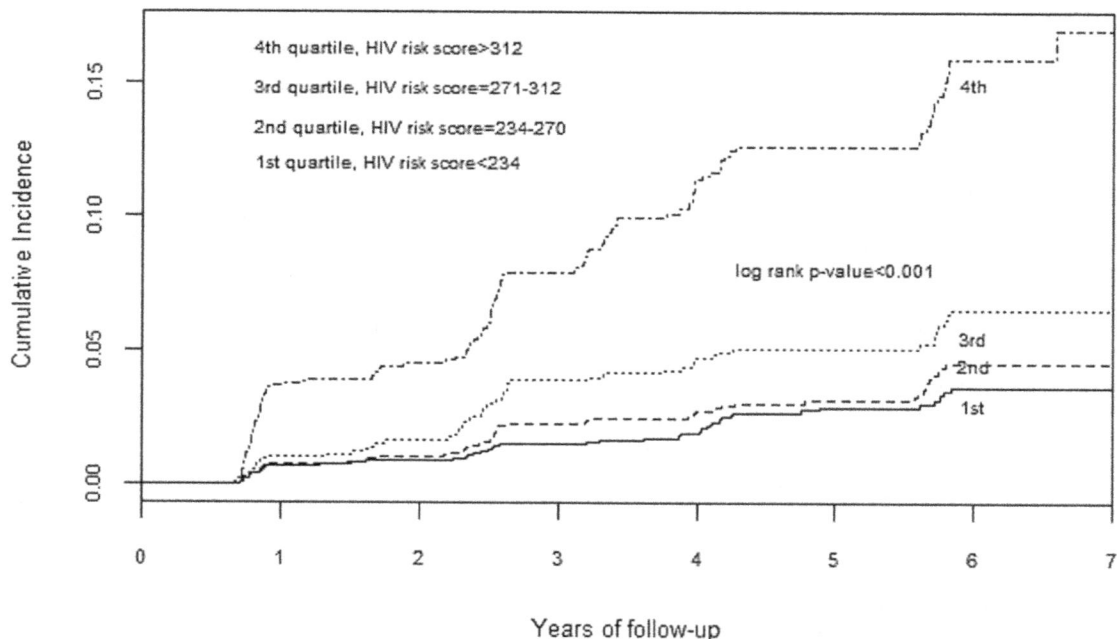

Figure 2. Cumulative HIV incidence by predicted quartile of HIV risk score for sexually active women.

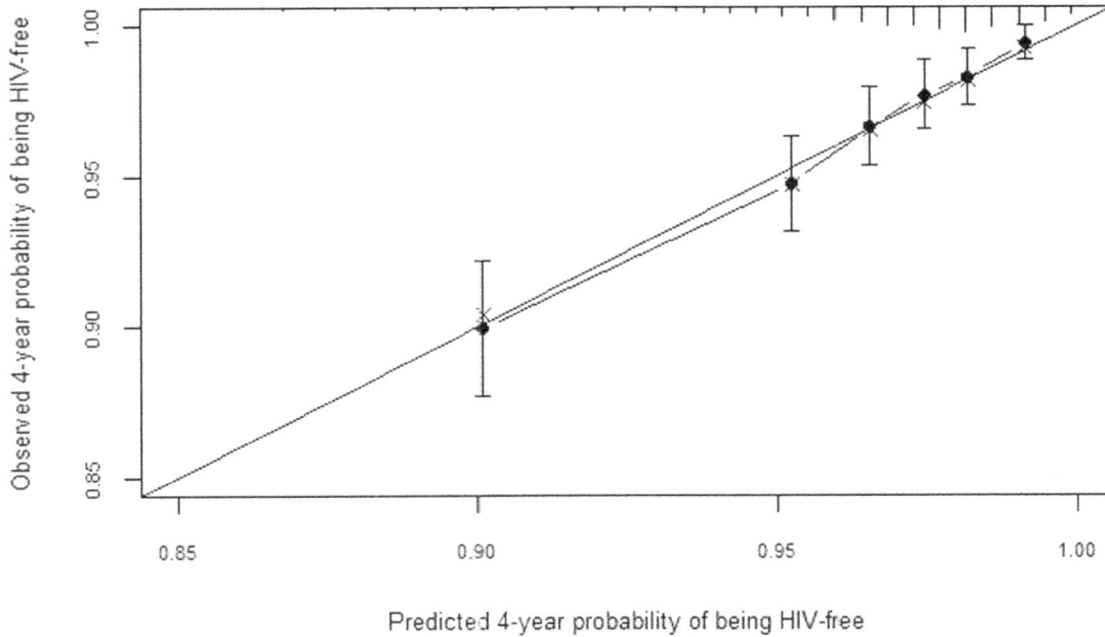

Figure 3. Observed vs predicted probabilities of being HIV-free at 4 years of follow-up. The figure provides bias-corrected calibration of the men's prediction model.

associated with levels of predictors in the final model. Total points for a given subject are obtained by summing across scores from all variables.

Analyses used STATA 10.0 (StataCorp, College Station, TX) and R version 2.15.2 (The R Project for Statistical Computing).

Results

Sample

There were a total of 30771 participants in the RCCS surveys from 2003 to 2011. Of these, 4,181 were newly enrolled into the cohort at the last survey and so did not provide follow-up for outcome analyses. Of the remaining 26,590, other participants

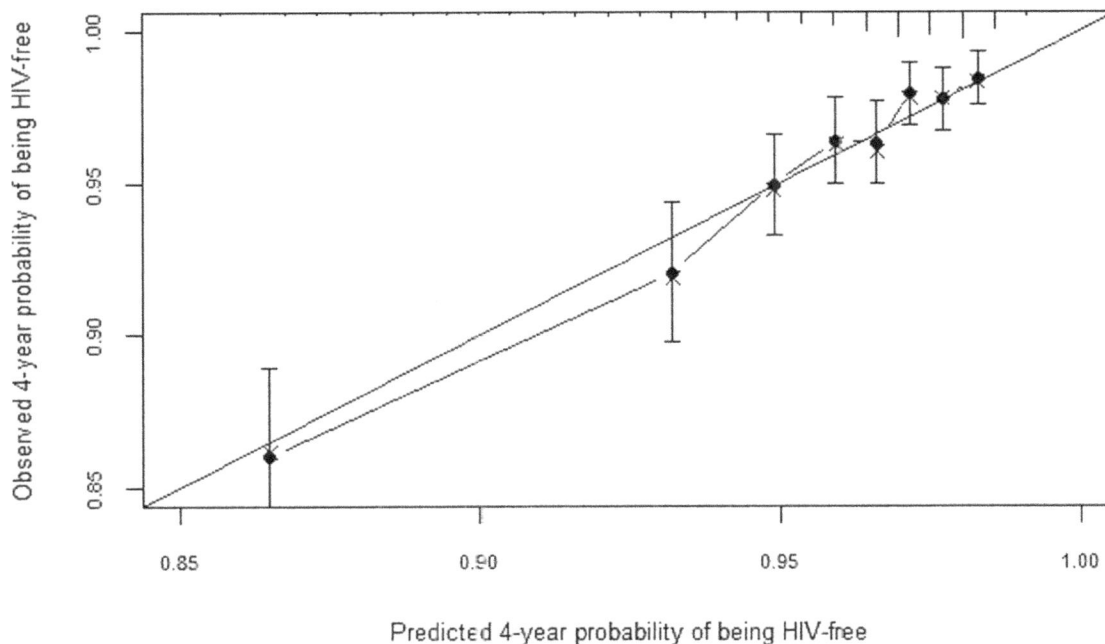

Figure 4. Observed vs predicted probabilities of being HIV-free at 4 years of follow-up. The figure provides bias-corrected calibration of the women's prediction model.

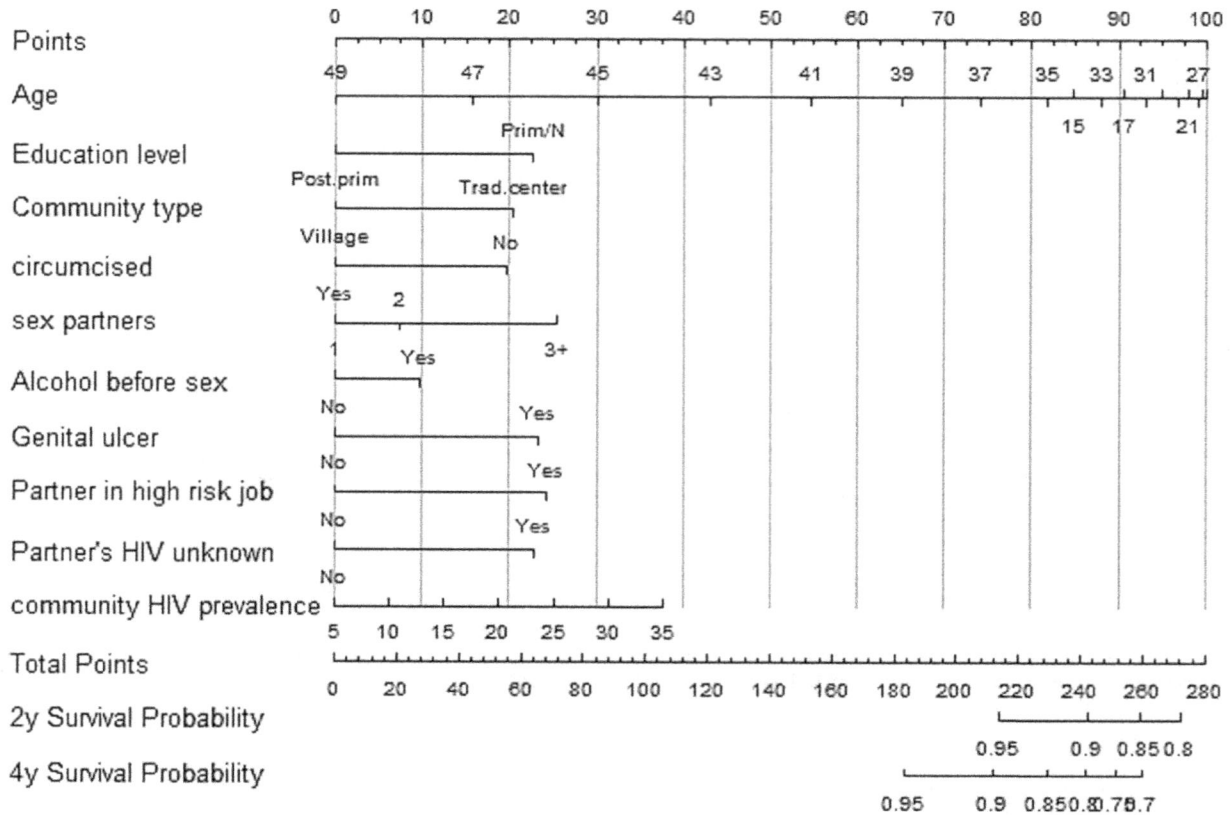

Figure 5. Nomogram of HIV risk for sexually active men developed using the Rakai cohort, Uganda 2003–2011.

were excluded for the following reasons: 7,555 (28.4 percent) were seen only at one survey and so did not contribute to the incident outcome analyses; 2,620 (10.0 percent) were not sexually active during the study period; 2,013 (7.6 percent) were prevalent cases of HIV; and 1,122 (4.2 percent) had no HIV tests or had only one HIV test and therefore could not contribute to the outcome analysis. Therefore we used 13,280 initially HIV uninfected participants with follow up visits to develop the indices. Of these, 7,497 (56.4 percent) were women and 5,783 (43.6 percent) were men. The mean follow-up time was 4.0 years (SD = 1.98) with a maximum of 7.7 years.

A total of 567 incident cases of HIV occurred in this sample (incidence rate = 1.06 per 100 person years, 95% CI = 0.97–1.15); 342 among females (incidence = 1.11 per 100 person years, 95% CI = 1.00–1.24) and 225 among the males (incidence rate = 0.98 per 100 person years, 95% CI = 0.86–1.12)

Table 2 shows the distribution of baseline characteristics of the population, stratified by gender.

Time trends in HIV risk

We tested for time trends in HIV risk by comparing HIV incidence rates in two time periods 2003–2006 and 2007–2011, stratified by gender. 2003–2006 represented a period just before the roll-out of antiretroviral therapy and subsequent early roll-out (the peri-HAART period), and a period prior to the availability of male circumcision services. The period 2007–2011 was characterized by rapid scale-up of HAART and early roll-out of a male circumcision services in the Rakai communities. The difference in HIV incidence rate between the two time periods was not statistically significant. HIV incidence among men in the 2003–

2006 period was 0.84 per 100 person years (95% CI = 0.68–1.04) and 0.86 per 100 person years (95% CI = 0.71–1.03) in the second time period. The difference in incidence rate was −0.02 per 100 person years (95 percent CI = −0.20, 0.25). Among the females, HIV incidence in the 2003–2006 period was 0.99 per 100 person years (95% CI = 0.83–1.16) and 1.07 per 100 person years (95% CI = 0.92–1.23) in the second time period. The difference in incidence rate was −0.08 per 100 person years (95 percent CI = is −0.30, 0.14)

Unadjusted analyses

For men, all of the variables we tested were significantly associated with HIV acquisition in the unadjusted analyses at $p \leq 0.157$ (table 3) except high risk employment and recent migration to the community. For the women, non-significant variables included education, having a partner in high risk occupation, and hormonal contraception.

Multivariable analyses and final model discrimination

In the multivariable analysis 10 factors were selected in the men's model. These factors included age, education, circumcision status, number of sexual partners, alcohol consumption by self or partner, genital ulcers, being unaware of a partner's HIV status, community type, having a partner with a high-risk employment type and community HIV prevalence (table 4). Because age was modeled using a quadratic term, to obtain the effect of age, we differentiated the regression equation with respect to age and obtained the following equation: $\frac{d(\ln \lambda_1/\lambda_0)}{d(age)} = 0.2084292 -$ $2 * 0.0042433 * age$. This equation shows that the effect of age on

Points
Age
Marital Status
Education
Sexual partners
New sexual partner
Concurrency
Genita ulcer
Alcohol before sex
Perception of HIV risk
In a high risk job
Community HIV prevalence
Total Points
2y Survival Probability
4y Survival Probability

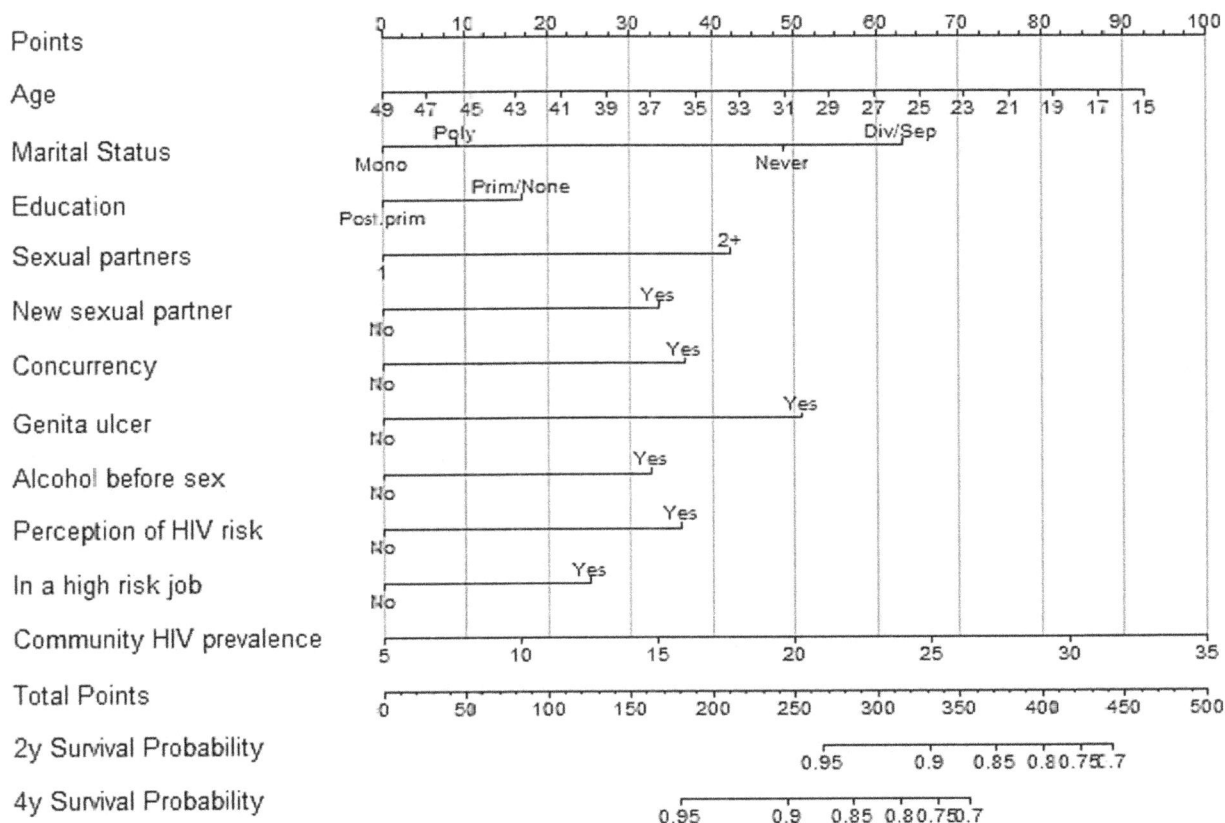

Figure 6. Nomogram of HIV risk for sexually active women developed using the Rakai cohort, Uganda 2003–2011.

the hazards of HIV acquisition is a function of age. The hazard increases more rapidly at age 15 and less rapidly thereafter and tends to reduce after 25 years of age. Men with post-primary education had 43 percent lower hazards of HIV infection compared to men with primary education or no education. Being circumcised was associated with 39 percent lower hazards compared to being non-circumcised. Compared to having one sexual partner in the previous 12 months, having two partners was associated with 21 percent higher hazards and 90 percent higher hazards for having three or more partners. Alcohol consumption before sex by self or partner was associated with 28 percent higher hazards. Having genital ulcers was associated with 81 percent higher hazards. Being unaware of a partner's HIV status was associated with 78 percent higher hazards. Living in in a trading

center was associated with 67 percent higher hazards compared to living in the village. Having a partner with a high risk employment type was associated with 85 percent higher hazards. Every unit increase in community HIV prevalence was associated with three percent higher hazards.

A similar reduced model for the women included the following 11 factors: age, marital status, education, number of sex partners, having a new sex partner, alcohol consumption by self or partner before sex, having concurrent relationships, being employed in a high-risk occupation, having genital ulcers, community HIV prevalence, and perceiving oneself or partner to have been exposed to HIV infection (table 4). Each year increase in age was associated with a three percent reduction in hazard of HIV acquisition. Post-primary education was associated with 17

Table 5. Proportion of Cumulative Incidence Contributed by Different Definitions of Most-at-risk status.

	Men			Women		
Threshold	Nomogram Score range	Proportion Cumulatve incidence(%)	95% confidence interval	Nomogram Score ange	Proportion Cumulatve incidence(%)	95% confidence interval
Upper quintile	>179	46.7	40.1–53.2	>325	40.1	35.3–45.8
Upper two quintiles	>164	70.2	64.2–76.1	>286	63.2	58.0–68.2
Upper quartile	>175	55.1	48.6–61.6	>314	48.0	42.7–53.2
Upper third	>169	63.1	56.7–69.4	>298	55.6	50.3–60.8
Upper half	>158	73.7	73.3–84.0	>271	68.7	63.8–73.6

percent lower hazards compared with primary education. Compared to monogamous marriage, being in a polygamous relationship was associated with 10 percent higher hazards of HIV acquisition, being separated or divorced was associated with two times the hazard, and women who were never married had 72 percent higher hazards. Compared to having one sexual partner in the previous 12 months, having two or more partners was associated with twice the hazards of infection. Having a new sexual partner in the previous 12 months was associated with 59 percent higher hazards. Concurrent relationships were associated with 50 percent higher hazards. Having genital ulcers was associated with 76 percent higher hazards. High risk employment type was associated with 32 percent higher hazards. Every unit increase in community HIV prevalence was associated with 3.8 percent higher hazards

Discrimination

The final model for the men had a c index equal to 0.73 (95% CI = 0.69–0.75). After internal validation using bootstrap resampling the optimism-corrected c index was 69.1 percent (0.66, 0.73). The final model for the women had a c index equal to 0.69 (95% CI = 0.66–0.72) and the optimism-corrected c index after internal validation was equal to 0.67 (95% CI = 0.64, 0.70).

Discrimination was also demonstrated graphically by plotting the cumulative HIV incidence by quartiles of risk score (a linear combination of products of model coefficients and levels of variables). The plot for men (figure 1) showed good separation of quartiles of risk especially the highest quartile. A similar trend is observed in the women's plot; however the separation is less for the lowest two quartiles (figure 2).

Model calibration

A plot of observed versus predicted probabilities of being HIV-free after four years of follow-up showed excellent agreement between observed and predicted probabilities (figures 3 and 4). Similar results were observed at two years of follow-up (results not shown).

Nomograms

Gender-specific nomograms are shown in figures 5 and 6. A score for each variable is obtained by drawing a vertical line to the top scale and reading off the variable's score for each individual. The total score for an individual is obtained by summing up all the individual variable scores. A scale for the total score and the corresponding 2-year and 4-year probabilities of being HIV-free are given at the bottom of the nomograms.

Proportion of cumulative incidence due to most-at-risk status

In table 5 we provided proportions of cumulative incidence due to most-at-risk status at various thresholds. The upper quartile of nomogram scores contributed 55 percent of incident HIV among men and 48 percent among women; while the upper two quintiles contributed 70 percent among men and 63 percent among women. Proportions at other thresholds are shown in table 5.

Discussion

Gender-specific indices to predict risk of HIV acquisition based on the Rakai cohort in Uganda were discriminative and well calibrated. Through graphical methods we showed that the indices showed better discrimination between the highest quartile of risk

scores and lower quartiles. Also, most-at-risk groups defined by upper thresholds of risk scores contributed substantially to cumulative incidence (table 5). We believe that this property of the indices makes them suitable for identifying individuals most-at-risk of HIV infection.

To the best of our knowledge, this is the first effort to develop indices to predict individual risk of HIV infection in the general population of SSA. Our study has several strengths. We used a population-based longitudinal cohort which provided high quality data on known predictors of HIV acquisition. We tested various transformations of age to obtain the optimal transformation for age and community HIV prevalence. We also used self-perceived exposure or perceived exposure of partner to HIV as a predictor variable to capture unmeasured predictors of HIV infection. In this population self-perceived risk of exposure to HIV was associated with a higher risk of HIV infection [38].

Our study has limitations. All the variables apart from HIV prevalence were self-reported and therefore subject to recall error and social-desirability bias. However, these self-reported variables were found to be predictive of HIV risk. We believe that the ease of obtaining self-reports makes it feasible to use these indices in clinic settings or HIV counseling offices. We also did not validate these indices in other settings; however we noted that the indices performed well during internal validation; which provides a good indication that they are likely to perform well in other similar settings. However, despite the performance with internal validation, we recommend that these indices be externally validated before use in other populations similar to Rakai. To facilitate external validation, we have provided model coefficients in table 4. In settings where these indices may not be sufficiently predictive, techniques are available to re-calibrate them and update them for these news settings [39].

Given successful validation in other populations, these tools could be used in the context of voluntary counseling and testing to identify people most-at-risk of HIV for targeting them with preventive programs. An example of such interventions is oral pre-exposure prophylaxis (PrEP) with Tenofovir and Emtricitabine. In the FEM-PrEP [40] and VOICE (MTN 003) [41] trials, oral PrEP was not efficacious for HIV prevention due to low adherence to medications which was ascribed to low self-perceived risk of HIV [40]. Indices such as ours could help inform individuals of their true risk and thus offset false self-perceptions of risk. Therefore, these prediction indices, in addition to generating demand for HIV preventive services, could help maintain high levels of adherence to these services. Also, the routine use of these indices in HIV counseling may increase the efficiency of counseling by focusing on an individual's risk.

The implementation of these indices would require an HIV counselor to score clients HIV risk during a post-test counseling session using gender-specific nomograms provided in figures 5 and 6. The counselor would then determine the individual's level of HIV risk and provide appropriate risk-reduction counseling. We have provided a simple step-by-step guide in the online supplement to guide the implementation (supplement S1).

Conclusion

We developed and internally validated gender-specific indices to predict risk of HIV infection. Our study provides proof-of-concept that indices to predict individual's risk of HIV infection can be developed to increase the efficiency of HIV prevention programs. Further research to validate these indices for other populations is needed.

Acknowledgments

We wish to thank Betty Nantume, Grace Kigozi, Robert Ssekubugu and the RCCS team for their efforts in data collection. We thank Anthony Ndyanabo, Jessica Nakukumba, Maria Nakafeero and Joseph Sekasanvu for helping with data management. We also thank Richard Musoke for his work on some graphics

Author Contributions

Conceived and designed the experiments: JK RHG CW. Analyzed the data: JK. Contributed reagents/materials/analysis tools: JK PF. Wrote the paper: JK RHG CW PF DN JWM NKS DS GK FN SJR MJW MES.

References

1. Bautista-Arredondo S, Gadsden P, Harris JE, Bertozzi SM (2008) Optimizing resource allocation for HIV/AIDS prevention programmes: an analytical framework. AIDS 22 Suppl 1: S67–74.

2. Herida M, Larsen C, Lot F, Laporte A, Desenclos JC, et al. (2006) Cost-effectiveness of HIV post-exposure prophylaxis in France. AIDS 20: 1753–1761.

3. Hughes D, Morris S (1996) The cost-effectiveness of condoms in the prevention of HIV infection in England and Wales: should condoms be available on prescription? J Health Serv Res Policy 1: 205–211.

4. Juusola JL, Brandeau ML, Owens DK, Bendavid E (2012) The cost-effectiveness of preexposure prophylaxis for HIV prevention in the United States in men who have sex with men. Ann Intern Med 156: 541–550.

5. Kahn JG (1996) The cost-effectiveness of HIV prevention targeting: how much more bang for the buck? Am J Public Health 86: 1709–1712.

6. Long EF, Brandeau ML, Owens DK (2010) The cost-effectiveness and population outcomes of expanded HIV screening and antiretroviral treatment in the United States. Ann Intern Med 153: 778–789.

7. Youngkong S, Teerawattananon Y, Tantivess S, Baltussen R (2012) Multi-criteria decision analysis for setting priorities on HIV/AIDS interventions in Thailand. Health Res Policy Syst 10: 6.

8. Weiss HA, Quigley MA, Hayes RJ (2000) Male circumcision and risk of HIV infection in sub-Saharan Africa: a systematic review and meta-analysis. AIDS 14: 2361–2370.

9. Gray RH, Kiwanuka N, Quinn TC, Sewankambo NK, Serwadda D, et al. (2000) Male circumcision and HIV acquisition and transmission: cohort studies in Rakai, Uganda. Rakai Project Team. AIDS 14: 2371–2381.

10. Gray RH, Kigozi G, Serwadda D, Makumbi F, Watya S, et al. (2007) Male circumcision for HIV prevention in men in Rakai, Uganda: a randomised trial. Lancet 369: 657–666.

11. Abbas UL, Anderson RM, Mellors JW (2007) Potential impact of antiretroviral chemoprophylaxis on HIV-1 transmission in resource-limited settings. PLoS One 2: e875.

12. Cremin I, Alsallaq R, Dybul M, Piot P, Garnett G, et al. (2013) The new role of antiretrovirals in combination HIV prevention: a mathematical modelling analysis. AIDS 27: 447–458.

13. D'Agostino RB Sr, Grundy S, Sullivan LM, Wilson P, Group CHDRP (2001) Validation of the Framingham coronary heart disease prediction scores: results of a multiple ethnic groups investigation. JAMA 286: 180–187.

14. Steyerberg EW, Roobol MJ, Kattan MW, van der Kwast TH, de Koning HJ, et al. (2007) Prediction of indolent prostate cancer: validation and updating of a prognostic nomogram. J Urol 177: 107–112; discussion 112.

15. Kahle EM, Hughes JP, Lingappa JR, John-Stewart G, Celum C, et al. (2012) An empiric risk scoring tool for identifying high-risk heterosexual HIV-1 serodiscordant couples for targeted HIV-1 prevention. J Acquir Immune Defic Syndr.

16. Fox J, White PJ, Weber J, Garnett GP, Ward H, et al. (2011) Quantifying sexual exposure to HIV within an HIV-serodiscordant relationship: development of an algorithm. AIDS 25: 1065–1082.

17. Gray R, Ssempiija V, Shelton J, Serwadda D, Nalugoda F, et al. (2011) The contribution of HIV-discordant relationships to new HIV infections in Rakai, Uganda. AIDS 25: 863–865.

18. Chemaitelly H, Shelton JD, Hallett TB, Abu-Raddad LJ (2013) Only a fraction of new HIV infections occur within identifiable stable discordant couples in sub-Saharan Africa. AIDS 27: 251–260.

19. Wawer MJ, Gray RH, Sewankambo NK, Serwadda D, Paxton L, et al. (1998) A randomized, community trial of intensive sexually transmitted disease control for AIDS prevention, Rakai, Uganda. AIDS 12: 1211–1225.

20. Wawer MJ, Sewankambo NK, Serwadda D, Quinn TC, Paxton LA, et al. (1999) Control of sexually transmitted diseases for AIDS prevention in Uganda: a randomised community trial. Rakai Project Study Group. Lancet 353: 525–535.

21. Arora P, Nagelkerke NJ, Jha P (2012) A systematic review and meta-analysis of risk factors for sexual transmission of HIV in India. PLoS One 7: e44094.

22. Kelly RJ, Gray RH, Sewankambo NK, Serwadda D, Wabwire-Mangen F, et al. (2003) Age differences in sexual partners and risk of HIV-1 infection in rural Uganda. J Acquir Immune Defic Syndr 32: 446–451.

23. Wojcicki JM (2005) Socioeconomic status as a risk factor for HIV infection in women in East, Central and Southern Africa: a systematic review. J Biosoc Sci 37: 1–36.

24. Koenig MA, Lutalo T, Zhao F, Nalugoda F, Kiwanuka N, et al. (2004) Coercive sex in rural Uganda: prevalence and associated risk factors. Soc Sci Med 58: 787–798.

25. Zablotska IB, Gray RH, Koenig MA, Serwadda D, Nalugoda F, et al. (2009) Alcohol use, intimate partner violence, sexual coercion and HIV among women aged 15–24 in Rakai, Uganda. AIDS Behav 13: 225–233.

26. Zablotska IB, Gray RH, Serwadda D, Nalugoda F, Kigozi G, et al. (2006) Alcohol use before sex and HIV acquisition: a longitudinal study in Rakai, Uganda. AIDS 20: 1191–1196.

27. Auvert B, Taljaard D, Lagarde E, Sobngwi-Tambekou J, Sitta R, et al. (2005) Randomized, controlled intervention trial of male circumcision for reduction of HIV infection risk: the ANRS 1265 Trial. PLoS Med 2: e298.

28. Bailey RC, Moses S, Parker CB, Agot K, Maclean I, et al. (2007) Male circumcision for HIV prevention in young men in Kisumu, Kenya: a randomised controlled trial. Lancet 369: 643–656.

29. Denison JA, O'Reilly KR, Schmid GP, Kennedy CE, Sweat MD (2008) HIV voluntary counseling and testing and behavioral risk reduction in developing countries: a meta-analysis, 1990–2005. AIDS Behav 12: 363–373.

30. Matovu JK, Gray RH, Makumbi F, Wawer MJ, Serwadda D, et al. (2005) Voluntary HIV counseling and testing acceptance, sexual risk behavior and HIV incidence in Rakai, Uganda. AIDS 19: 503–511.

31. Commission UNA (2009) Uganda HIV Modes of Transmission and Prevention Response Analysis.

32. Harrell F aregImpute. Available: http://cran.r-project.org/web/packages/Hmisc. Accessed 2013 Mar 25.

33. Therneau PGT (1994) Proportional hazards tests and diagnostics based on weighted residuals. Biometrika 81: 515–526

34. Atkinson AC (1980) A note on the generalized information criterion for choice of a model. Biometrika 67: 413–418.

35. Van Houwelingen JC, Le Cessie S (1990) Predictive value of statistical models. Stat Med 9: 1303–1325.

36. Harrell FE Jr, Lee KL, Mark DB (1996) Multivariable prognostic models: issues in developing models, evaluating assumptions and adequacy, and measuring and reducing errors. Stat Med 15: 361–387.

37. Harrell F Regression modelling strategies. Available:http://cran.r-project.org/web/packages/rms/rms.pdf. Accessed 2013 Mar 25.

38. Santelli JS, Edelstein ZR, Mathur S, Wei Y, Zhang W, et al. (2013) Behavioral, Biological, and Demographic Risk and Protective Factors for New HIV Infections Among Youth in Rakai, Uganda. J Acquir Immune Defic Syndr 63: 393–400.

39. Steyerberg EW (2010) Clinical Prediction Models: A Practical Approach to Development, Validation, and Updating. 233 Spring Street, New York,NY 10013, USA: Springer Science+Business Media.

40. Van Damme L, Corneli A, Ahmed K, Agot K, Lombaard J, et al. (2012) Preexposure prophylaxis for HIV infection among African women. N Engl J Med 367: 411–422.

41. Marrazzo J RG, Nair G (2013) Pre-exposure prophylaxis for HIV in women: daily oral tenofovir, oral tenofovir/emtricitabine, or vaginal tenofovir gel in the VOICE (MTN 003). 20th Conference on Retroviruses and Opportunistic Infections. Atlanta,GA.

25

Host Genetic Factors Associated with Symptomatic Primary HIV Infection and Disease Progression among Argentinean Seroconverters

Romina Soledad Coloccini[1], Dario Dilernia[1], Yanina Ghiglione[1], Gabriela Turk[1], Natalia Laufer[1,2], Andrea Rubio[1], María Eugenia Socías[2,3], María Inés Figueroa[2,3], Omar Sued[2,3], Pedro Cahn[2,3], Horacio Salomón[1], Andrea Mangano[4], María Ángeles Pando[1]*

1 Instituto de Investigaciones Biomédicas en Retrovirus y SIDA (INBIRS), Universidad de Buenos Aires-CONICET, Buenos Aires, Argentina, 2 Hospital Juan A. Fernandez, Buenos Aires, Argentina, 3 Fundación Huésped, Buenos Aires, Argentina, 4 Laboratorio de Biología Celular y Retrovirus, CONICET, Hospital de Pediatría "Prof. Dr. Juan P. Garrahan", Buenos Aires, Argentina

Abstract

Background: Variants in HIV-coreceptor C-C chemokine receptor type 5 (CCR5) and Human leukocyte antigen (HLA) genes are the most important host genetic factors associated with HIV infection and disease progression. Our aim was to analyze the association of these genetic factors in the presence of clinical symptoms during Primary HIV Infection (PHI) and disease progression within the first year.

Methods: Seventy subjects diagnosed during PHI were studied (55 symptomatic and 15 asymptomatic). Viral load (VL) and CD4 T-cell count were evaluated. HIV progression was defined by presence of B or C events and/or CD4 T-cell counts < 350 cell/mm³. CCR5 haplotypes were characterized by polymerase chain reaction and SDM-PCR-RFLP. HLA-I characterization was performed by Sequencing.

Results: Symptoms during PHI were significantly associated with lower frequency of CCR5-CF1 (1.8% vs. 26.7%, p = 0.006). Rapid progression was significantly associated with higher frequency of CCR5-CF2 (16.7% vs. 0%, p = 0.024) and HLA-A*11 (16.7% vs. 1.2%, p = 0.003) and lower frequency of HLA-C*3 (2.8% vs. 17.5%, p = 0.035). Higher baseline VL was significantly associated with presence of HLA-A*11, HLA-A*24, and absence of HLA-A*31 and HLA-B*57. Higher 6-month VL was significantly associated with presence of CCR5-HHE, HLA-A*24, HLA-B*53, and absence of HLA-A*31 and CCR5-CF1. Lower baseline CD4 T-cell count was significantly associated with presence of HLA-A*24/*33, HLA-B*53, CCR5-CF2 and absence of HLA-A*01/*23 and CCR5-HHA. Lower 6-month CD4 T-cell count was associated with presence of HLA-A*24 and HLA-B*53, and absence of HLA-A*01 and HLA-B*07/*39. Moreover, lower 12-month CD4 T-cell count was significantly associated with presence of HLA-A*33, HLA-B*14, HLA-C*08, CCR5-CF2, and absence of HLA-B*07 and HLA-C*07.

Conclusion: Several host factors were significantly associated with disease progression in PHI subjects. Most results agree with previous studies performed in other groups. However, some genetic factor associations are being described for the first time, highlighting the importance of genetic studies at a local level.

Editor: Srinivas Mummidi, South Texas Veterans Health Care System and University of Texas Health Science Center at San Antonio, United States of America

Funding: This research was funded by grants from: Agencia Nacional de Promoción Científica y Tecnológica (grant number 2008-0559), "Fundación Florencio Fiorini" (period: 2009–2010), UBACYT (period: 2010–2012) and CONICET (PIP 2011–2013). The funders had no role in study design, data collection and analysis, decision to publish, or preparation of the manuscript.

* Email: mpando@fmed.uba.ar

Introduction

Research studies on primary HIV infection (PHI) are increasing worldwide to better understand the natural history of HIV infection and to identify the most important disease prognostic markers. As most of these studies were performed in other countries and due to genetic differences in the circulating virus and in the host, local studies are needed to better understand the particular characteristics of HIV infection dynamics [1].

In Argentina, an estimated 110,000 persons live with HIV (approximately 5,000 new cases per year) [2]. The first multicenter follow-up study of PHI (*Grupo Argentino de Seroconversión*) started in 2008. Retrospective and prospective data analyses allowed identifying factors associated with disease progression among untreated subjects. Symptomatic PHI, high VL (≥100,000

RNA copies/ml) or low CD4 T-cell count (≤ 350 cell/mm^3) at baseline were identified as relevant factors for faster progression during the first year follow-up [3]. Data comparisons with other PHI cohorts revealed that VL at baseline in the Argentinean cohort was higher than those found in developed countries [4–5], closer to African and Asian levels [6–7]. Globally, 50–90% of subjects diagnosed during PHI are symptomatic [8–10], reaching 74% in the mentioned Argentinean cohort [3].

Previous studies demonstrated extensive variability in host susceptibility to HIV infection and disease progression [11–13]. Several host genetic factors affecting HIV infection and pathogenesis were identified, like chemokine receptors and HLA alleles [14–17]. Multiple variations were described in the CCR5 gene, in particular the 32 base-pair deletion (CCR5-Δ32). This deletion provides protection against HIV-1 infection with CCR5 tropic viruses in homozygotes and delays progression in heterozygous subjects [16,18–19]. Seven Single Nucleotide Polymorphisms (SNPs) were defined in the cis-regulatory region between -2761 and -1835 of the CCR5 gene: -2733, -2554, -2459, -2135, -2132, -2086 and -1835 (GenBank accession number AF031236 and AF031237) [20]. Based on these variations and on the CCR2-V64I polymorphism, nine polymorphisms, called CCR5 Human Haplotypes (HH)-A, -B, -C, -D, -E, -F (F*1 and F*2), and –G (G*1 and G*2) were defined [15,20–21]. One of the largest studies in the subject demonstrated that the frequency and effect of CCR5-HH differ among different ethnic groups. CCR5-HHA was associated with disease retardation among African-Americans, whereas CCR5-HHC did so among European-Americans. In the same study, specific sequences of CCR5-HHE were associated with higher transcriptional activity, surface expression and HIV/AIDS susceptibility [21]. Another factor associated with disease progression is the dose of the gene encoding CCL3L1 (MIP-1α), a natural ligand of CCR5. A previous study found an association between lower gene dose and disease progression, and this susceptibility is even greater in individuals with CCR5 genotypes associated with disease progression [22].

The HLA system has an impact on several aspects of HIV infection such as transmission, progression and therapeutic response [23–24]. HLA class I molecules are involved in peptide presentation to CD8 cytotoxic T lymphocytes (CTLs), which play a key role in reducing viral replication. HIV specific CD8 T-cell response emerges along with the control of viremia and resolution of clinical symptoms, which varies from person to person and constitutes a strong predictor of disease progression [25–26]. Heterozygosis at HLA class I region is considered to be a selective advantage because those individuals are able to present a greater range of antigenic peptides to CTLs than homozygotes, deferring the emergence of escape mutants and prolonging the period before the development of AIDS [18]. Even when several HLA alleles were associated with disease progression, HLA-B*27 and HLA-B*57 alleles showed a particularly strong association with delayed progression [27] and HLA-B*35 and HLA-B*53 with acceleration to AIDS [28].

Based on the effects of host genetic variations described on HIV disease progression, our aim was to analyze the association of CCR5/CCL3L1 system and HLA in the presence of clinical symptoms during PHI and disease progression within the first year post-infection.

Materials and Methods

Study population

A group of 70 individuals recruited through 2008–2012 was studied. Inclusion criteria for enrolment in the cohort were: >16 years old at first evaluation, PHI confirmed diagnosis, and first medical and laboratory evaluation (i.e., CD4 T-cell count and plasma HIV RNA) within six months of the probable date of infection. Primary HIV infection is defined as: (1) detection of HIV RNA or p24 antigen with a simultaneous negative or indeterminate Western blot assay [12]; or (2) positive Western blot with a negative test within the previous six months. Hence, it includes both acute and recently infected patients [3].

In this study, PHI was defined as symptomatic if one or more of the following symptoms, associated with acute retroviral syndrome, were present: fever, rash, lymphadenopathy, headache, oral ulcers, dysphagia or pharyngitis. Disease progression was defined by clinical B or C events (according to the Centers for Disease Control and Prevention 1993 classification [29]) and/or CD4 T-cell count <350 cells/mm^3 within the first year of infection [3].

Ethics Statement

International and national ethical guidelines for biomedical research involving human subjects were followed. This research study was reviewed and approved by a local Institutional Review Board (IRB), "Fundación Huésped" and was conducted in compliance with all federal regulations governing the protection of human subjects. All potential participants signed an informed consent prior to entering the study.

Study Procedure

Once subjects were identified as PHI, they were included in the cohort. Subjects were evaluated at the time of diagnosis (baseline), at 6 months and at one year. On each visit, HIV plasma VL (branched-DNA, Versant HIV-1 RNA 3.0 assay, Siemmens Healthcare, USA), CD4 T-cell count (flow cytometry double platform, BD FACSCanto, BD Biosciences, USA), and clinical information were updated.

Study samples

Peripheral blood samples were obtained on each visit. Whole blood samples or peripheral blood mononuclear cells (PBMC) were used for DNA extraction using QIAmp DNA Blood Mini Kit (QIAGEN GmbH, Hilden, Germany). Plasma samples from the first visit after HIV diagnosis were used for lipopolysaccharide (LPS) quantification (Limulus Amebocyte Lysate test, LAL assay, QCL-1000, Lonza, DK). HIV tropism was determined by sequencing a region of V3 loop from env gene (HXB2) [30]. Viral DNA was amplified in duplicate by nested PCR and amplicons were sequenced by Big Dye Terminator Kit (Amersham, Sweden). Viral tropism was inferred from Geno2Pheno algorithm (http://coreceptor.bioinf.mpi-inf.mpg.de/index.php) using a false positive rate of 10%.

CCR5 and CCL3L1 characterization

CCR5-Δ32 deletion was identified by differences in PCR products size. CCR2 genotypes and Single Nucleotide Polymorphisms (SNPs) of the CCR5 gene corresponding to positions 29, 208, 627, 630, 676 and 927 (Genbank accession number: AF031236 and AF031237) [31] were determined with Site Directed Mutagenesis-PCR-Restriction Fragment Length Polymorphism (SDM-PCR-RFLP) assay. Primers used in each determination, PCR cycling condition and RFLP assay were reported previously [15,21,32–33]. Haplotype classification (HHA, HHB, HHC, HHD, HHE, HHF*1, HHF*2, HHG*1 and HHG*2) was determined as reported previously [15,20–21]. CCL3L1 Copy Number (CN) was determined by Taqman real-time PCR [22].

HLA characterization

HLA class I characterization was performed by sequencing-based typing (SBT). HLA-A exons 2 and 3 were amplified together. HLA-B and HLA-C exons 2 and 3 were amplified separately as reported in Table S1 and Figure S1 [34–36]. Amplicons were sequenced using the Big Dye Terminator sequencing kit (Amersham, Sweden) [36]. Sequence interpretation was performed using the NCBI SBT Interpretation software (http://www.ncbi.nlm.nih.gov/gv/mhc/sbt.cgi?cmd=main).

Genetic score

Additive genetic score was used to compile host genetic information [37]. In our model, alleles with a previous reported protective effect were added, and risk alleles were subtracted. For CCR5 polymorphisms, Δ32 and CCR2-64I alleles were considered as protective (1) [21]. Regarding CCR5 genotypes, HHC/HHF*2 and HHC/HHG*2 were considered as protective (1), HHC/HHE, HHE/HHE and HHE/HHG*2 as deleterious (−1), and the others as neutral (0) [21,32]. Two CCL3L1 cpg (mean in the Argentinean population) were considered as neutral (0). Lower CCL3L1 CN than the mean was considered as deleterious (−1) and higher CN as protective (1) [22]. HLA-A*02, HLA-A*32, HLA-A*68, HLA-B*15, HLA-B*13, HLA-B*27, HLA-B*32, HLA-B*39, HLA-B*44, HLA-B*51 and HLA-B*57 were considered as protective (1). HLA-A*11, HLA-A*23, HLA-A*24, HLA-B*08, HLA-B*35, HLA-B*53, HLA-C*04 and HLA-C*07 were considered as deleterious (−1). Other HLA alleles were considered as neutral (0) [11–13,23–24,27–28,37–39]. Heterozygosis for HLA was considered as protective (1) and homozygosis as deleterious (−1) [18].

Statistical analysis

Baseline characteristics were described using mean or medians and standard deviation or interquartile ranges [IQRs] for continuous variables respectively, and counts and percentages for categorical data. Chi-square test or Fisher's exact test were used to compare proportions. Differences among continuous variables were analyzed using Student's t-test or Wilcoxon test. Spearman correlation was calculated for genetic score and HIV viral load and CD4 T-cell count (baseline and follow up). All p values were two-sided; p values<0.05 were considered to be statistically significant. Lack of complete data values in table is expressed in numbers. Data analysis was performed using SPSS 15.0, 2007 (Chicago, Illinois).

Results

Characteristics of the study population

We studied 70 HIV-infected adults diagnosed during primary HIV infection (PHI) (49 men and 21 women), 55 were symptomatic and 15 asymptomatic. Sixty of them were also classified according to disease progression within the first year post diagnosis, 18 progressed and 42 did not. Most PHI subjects were recruited during Fiebig stages V and VI [40]. Sexual transmission was reported as the main route: all the women reported heterosexual transmission whereas 82.2% of men reported sexual relationship with other men as the probably route of acquisition of the virus. All subjects were from Buenos Aires City and

surrounding areas. The population of this area is mostly descendent from South Europe [41]. Median HIV VL at diagnosis was 61862 RNA copies/ml, whit significantly higher VL in those who presented symptoms and those who progressed (Table 1). The same trend was observed for VL at 6 months. Baseline CD4 T-cell count was 514 cells/mm^3 without statistical differences between symptomatic and asymptomatic subjects. Significantly higher CD4 T-cell counts (baseline, 6 and 12 months) were observed among subjects who did not progress to disease during the first year (Table 1).

Frequency of CCR5 haplotypes/genotypes and CCL3L1

Similar to the results found in Argentinean children exposed perinatally to HIV (including both HIV infected and not infected) [42] and blood donors [43], the most frequent CCR5 haplotypes in the PHI group were HHE (36.4%) and HHC (30.7%). Frequencies of all the other haplotypes were lower than 10% (Figure 1; Table S2). Regarding CCR5 genotypes, HHC/HHE (21.4%) and HHE/HHE (12.9%) were the most commonly found. Other genotypes were present with frequencies lower than 10% (Table 2 and Table S3). The CCL3L1 gene copy number, one of the main ligands of CCR5, was evaluated in 50 PHI subjects with a median of two copies (IQR25-75, 1–4), as reported in persons of European origin [22].

Frequency of HLA variants

Given the essential role of CTL responses during PHI as well as the description of a strong association among certain HLA-I alleles with virus control, HLA-I frequencies were studied in this cohort finding 17 HLA-A, 27 HLA-B and 14 HLA-C different alleles. The HLA-A alleles most frequently found were HLA-A*02 (27.2%) and HLA-A*24 (12.5%). In HLA-B locus, HLA-B*35 (15.6%) and HLA-B*44 (12.9%) were the most frequent. In HLA-C, HLA-C*07 (27.9%), HLA-C*04 (16.2%) and HLA-C*03 (11.8%) were the most frequent. Other HLA-A, B and C alleles showed frequencies lower than 10% (Table S4). HLA class I alleles were found in homozygosis in the following frequencies: 32.4% for HLA-A, 3.0% for HLA-B and 17.6% for HLA-C (Table S5). The most common combinations for HLA-A were A*02-A*02 (11.8%) and A*02-A*68 (8.8%), for HLA-B were B*15-B*35 (4.5%) and B*35-B*44 (4.5%), and for HLA-C, C*04-C*07 (8.8%), C*07-C*07 (8.8%) and C*03-C*07 (7.4%) (data not shown).

Influence of CCR5 haplotypes/genotypes, CCL3L1 copy number, and HLA variants on symptoms present during acute HIV infection

In order to identify individual host genetic determinants of early HIV disease progression, the PHI cohort was stratified according to the presence/absence of symptoms during the seroconversion period. Regarding the CCR5 coreceptor, HHC was overrepresented (40% vs. 28.2%) and HHE (23.3% vs. 40%) was less frequent in asymptomatic as compared to symptomatic subjects, however without statistical significance (Figure 1). Concerning CCR5 genotypes, HHC/HHF*1 was detected in a significantly higher percentage among asymptomatic subjects (26.7% vs. 1.8%, p = 0.006). Even when it was not statistically significant, genotype HHE/HHF*1 was only found among symptomatic subjects (10.9%) (Table 2 and Table S3). No significant differences were found in the CCL3L1 copy number, even when a higher copy number was detected among asymptomatic (median (IQR25-75); 3 (2–3) and 2 (1–4), respectively). No influence of HLA-A, -B and -C alleles was detected in the presence of symptoms during PHI (Table S4). Likewise, no influence of HLA homozygosis was

Host Genetic Factors Associated with Symptomatic Primary HIV Infection and Disease Progression...

205

Table 1. HIV viral load and CD4 T-cell count of the study population diagnosed during primary HIV infection [PHI] (N = 70).

		Symptomatic PHI			Progressor at one year			All (N = 70)
		Yes (N = 55)	No (N = 15)	p	Yes (N = 18)	No (N = 42)	p	
HIV RNA median copies/ml (IQR)	Baseline	77,080	7,024	**0.003**	193,601	41,402	**0.003**	61,862
		(30,449–386,715)	(2,699–76,466)		(80,545–500,000)	(10,409–154,476)		(17,050–257,524)
	6 month	66,002	9,018	**0.004**	166,812	33,508	**0.001**	40,231
		(17,959–178,030)	(3,820–34,624)		(47,167–321,018)	(8,578–73,231)		(117,17–165,238)
CD4 T-cell count median cells/mm^3 (IQR)	Baseline	502	587	0.322	306	602	**<0.001**	514
		(356–649)	(416–876)		(237–346)	(500–741)		(387–671)
	6 month	499	555	0.694	323	602	**<0.001**	503
		(356–665)	(424–665)		(172–386)	(488–690)		(404–65)
	12 month	491	534	0.296	330	534	**0.001**	501
		(389–615)	(436–672)		(289–504)	(435–643)		(400–619)

PHI: primary HIV infection. IQR: interquartile range. Statistically significant p values are in bold.

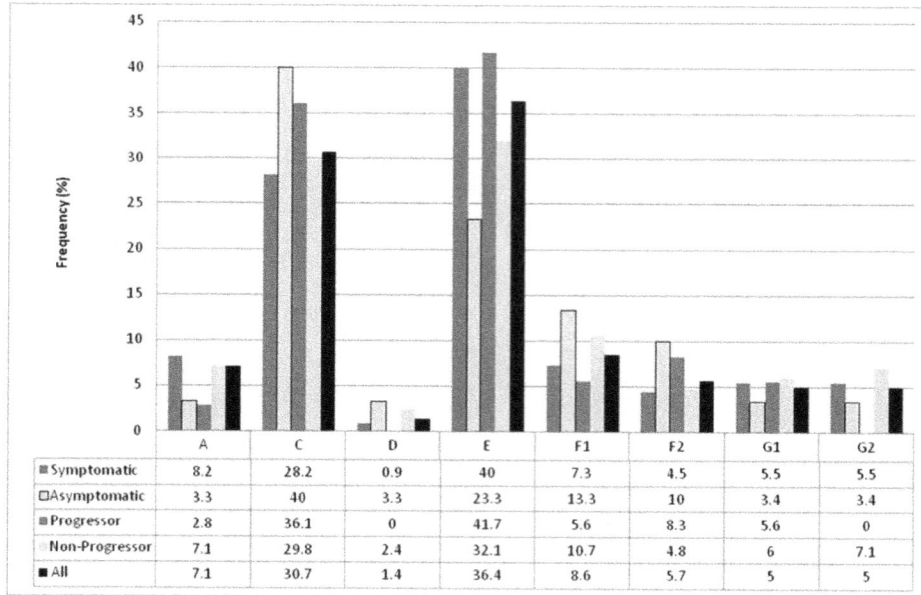

Figure 1. Frequency of CCR5 haplotypes of the study population diagnosed during primary HIV infection [PHI] (N = 70). Full information is available on supplementary material (Table S1).

observed in the presence of symptoms during seroconversion (Table S5). When HLA pairs were compared, HLA-B*35-B*44 was found in a significantly higher frequency among asymptomatic subjects (21.4% vs. 0%, p = 0.007) (data not shown).

Only CCR5 genotypes with a frequency higher than 10% in some of the study groups were included in the table. No significant differences were observed among CCR5 genotypes with frequencies lower than 10%. Full information is on supplementary material (Table S2).

Influence of CCR5 haplotypes/genotypes, CCL3L1 and HLA variants on disease progression within the first year

Additionally, the PHI group was analyzed in order to identify possible genetic factors that might influence the rate of progression within the first year. Several CCR5 haplotypes were most frequently detected in individuals who did not progress (e.g. HHA, HHF*1 and HHG*2) and HHF*2 was most represented in subjects who progressed to disease (Table S2), without statistical differences. Regarding CCR5 genotypes, HHC/HHF*2 was significantly associated with progression (p = 0.024) and a higher, but not significant proportion of subject who progress had HHE/HHE also as compared with those who do not progress (22.2% vs. 7.1%) (Table S3). Regarding HLA alleles, a strong association was found between disease progression and higher frequency of HLA-A*11 (16.7% vs. 1.2%, p = 0.003) and lower frequency of HLA-C*03 (17.5% vs. 2.8%, p = 0.035) (Table S4). No influence of HLA homozygosis was observed in disease progression (Table S5).

Influence of CCR5 haplotypes/genotypes, CCL3L1 and HLA variants on plasma HIV viral load and CD4 T-cell count

As the CD4 T-cell count and HIV plasma VL are good predictors of disease progression [3], the association of these parameters with host genetic factors was also analyzed. Subjects with CCR5 HHE haplotype had higher VL after 6 months

(66,001 copies/ml vs. 31,718 copies/ml, p = 0.039) and also higher baseline VL (98,684 copies/ml vs. 41,402 copies/ml, p = 0.082). On the other hand, HHA was found to be associated with higher baseline CD4 T-cell levels (656 cells/mm^3 vs. 499 cells/mm^3, p = 0.044). Regarding CCR5 genotypes, HHC/HHF*1 was associated with lower VL (6,243 copies/ml vs. 53,997 copies/ml, p = 0.027) and HHC/HHF*2 with lower CD4 T-cell levels at baseline (379 cells/mm^3 vs. 545 cells/mm^3, p = 0.046), at 6 months (355 cells/mm^3 vs. 531 cells/mm^3, p = 0.024) and at 12 months (290 cells/mm^3 vs. 510 cells/mm^3, p = 0.034).

Concerning the HLA influence on CD4 T-cell count and HIV plasma VL, the presence of several alleles was found to be beneficial for HIV subjects, with an association with higher CD4 T-cell count (HLA-A*01, HLA-A*23, HLA-B*07, HLA-B*39 and HLA-C*07) or lower HIV plasma VL (HLA-A*31 and HLA-B*57). Conversely, some alleles were found to be detrimental for subjects, with an association with higher HIV plasma VL (HLA-A*11, HLA-A*24 and HLA-B*53) or lower CD4 T-cell count (HLA-A*24, HLA-A*33, HLA-B*14, HLA-B*53 and HLA-C*08) (Table 3).

Additive genetic score

Additive genetic score was calculated for each subject and average values were calculated considering symptoms during PHI (2.6 for asymptomatic and 1.4 for symptomatic subjects) and disease progression within the first year (1.8 for those who did not progress and 0.6 for those who progressed). Subjects were grouped according to both characteristics: Group 1: Asymptomatic/Non-progressors, Group 2: Asymptomatic/Progressors and Symptomatic/Non-progressors, and Group 3: Symptomatic/Progressors. Mean genetic score was: 2.8, 1.6 and 0.5 for groups 1, 2 and 3, respectively. Correlation analyses revealed a significant negative correlation between genetic score and HIV viral load at baseline (p = 0.008) (Figure 2). No significant association was observed between genetic score and CD4 T-cells count.

Table 2. Frequency of CCR5 human genotypes of the study population diagnosed during primary HIV infection [PHI] (N = 70).

Genotype	Symptomatic PHI			Progressor at one year			All (N = 70)
	Yes (N = 55)*	No (N = 15)*	p	Yes (N = 18)*	No (N = 42)*	p	
HHC/HHC	2 (3.6)	1 (6.7)	0.521	2 (11.1)	1 (2.4)	0.212	3 (4.3)
HHC/HHE	12 (21.8)	3 (20)	1.000	4 (22.2)	9 (21.4)	1.000	15 (21.4)
HHC/HHF*1	1 (1.8)	4 (26.7)	0.006	1 (5.6)	4 (9.5)	1.000	5 (7.1)
HHC/HHF*2	3 (5.5)	1 (6.7)	1.000	3 (16.7)	0	0.024	4 (5.7)
HHC/HHG*1	5 (9.1)	1 (6.7)	1.000	1 (5.6)	5 (11.9)	0.658	6 (8.6)
HHE/HHE	8 (14.5)	1 (6.7)	0.672	4 (22.2)	3 (7.1)	0.220	9 (12.9)
HHE/HHF*1	6 (10.9)	0	0.329	1 (5.6)	4 (9.5)	1.000	6 (8.6)

*Data are no. (%) of CCR5 haplotypes.

Complementary studies

HIV infection has been associated with disruption of mucosal barrier and CD4 T-cell depletion in the gastrointestinal tract. This damage is caused, at least in part, by increased translocation of microbial products, mainly lipopolysaccharides (LPS), a major component of gram-negative bacterial cell walls [44–46]. Since immune activation is a good predictor of disease progression, plasma LPS levels were determined in the baseline sample of 65 individuals finding a median of 39.0 pg/ml (IQR25-75, 26.7–56.8) with significantly higher levels in the symptomatic than the asymptomatic group (43.5 pg/ml vs. 29.0 pg/ml, p = 0.040). No association was found among LPS levels, disease progression, CD4 T-cell count, HIV VL or host genetic factors. HIV tropism was determined given that the presence of X4 tropic viruses was associated with a more rapid disease progression (data not shown). Fourteen out of 59 (23.7%) PHI subjects presented X4 tropic HIV variants. Even when no statistically significant differences were observed, X4 tropic HIV variants were overrepresented among symptomatic subjects (26.1% vs. 15.4%, p = 0.713). No differences were observed among HIV tropism, disease progression, CD4 T-cell count or HIV VL.

Discussion

Other countries reported associations between human genes and HIV susceptibility. However, local studies are needed considering differences in genetic background [14,17,19]. In line with this, for the first time in Argentina, this study reports several human genes associated with early HIV disease progression among adults.

Buenos Aires population is mainly descendant of Southern Europe. The frequency of CCR5 haplotypes reported here correlates with reports in Hispanic and other Argentinean groups [21,43], with HHE and HHC being the most common haplotypes. Regarding CCR5 genotypes, the most common were HHC/HHE and HHE/HHE, with other genotypes having frequencies lower than 10%. In comparison with blood donors, PHI individuals were found to have a higher but not significant frequency of HHE/HHE genotype (5.9% vs. 12.9% respectively). This result is consistent with previous reports evidencing an association between presence of HHE/HHE genotype and enhancement of HIV infection [21,42]. Even when the HHE haplotype and the HHE/HHE genotype were overrepresented among symptomatic subjects and those who progressed, no significant associations were observed, maybe due to sample size. Data on HIV VL also supports the same trend with significantly higher VL at 6 months among subjects carrying HHE. This trend is in line with previous studies that associated disease progression with HHE [21,42]. However, this disease-modified effect was not observed among other ethnic groups (i.e., Africans) where the frequency of HHE haplotype was much lower (≈18%) [21]. As HHE is the most frequent CCR5 haplotype in our cohort, the potential adverse effect of this haplotype deserves special attention.

HHC/HHF*1 genotype was associated with asymptomatic PHI and HHC/HHF*2 with disease progression. In line with these results, we found that the HHC/HHF*1 genotype was associated with lower levels of VL and HHC/HHF*2, with lower CD4 T-cell levels at baseline and during one-year follow-up. Only few studies support these findings, maybe due to the fact that these genotypes were found in low frequency in most cohorts [21,42]. One of the most important studies in the subject found a disease accelerating effect for HHC/HHF*1 among African Americans [21]. However, this study also reports that the effect of HHC haplotypes on HIV disease differed among ethnic groups. While the HHC

Table 3. HIV viral load and CD4 T-cell count of the study population diagnosed during primary HIV infection [PHI] according to HLA alleles (N = 70).

Alleles		CD4 T-cell count median cells/mm³			HIV RNA median copies/ml	
		Baseline	6 months	12 months	Baseline	6 months
HLA-A*01	Yes	902	810	716	5160	4298
	No	500	499	491	64045	40083
	p	**0.022**	**0.019**	0.112	0.241	0.317
HLA-A*11	Yes	347	344	475	477708	166930
	No	525	517	492	52352	38270
	p	0.070	0.071	0.447	**0.020**	0.059
HLA-A*23	Yes	736	637	534	36101	24322
	No	499	497	475	61862	40232
	p	**0.038**	0.072	0.195	0.374	0.290
HLA-A*24	Yes	393	403	483	500000	89517
	No	576	545	500	41402	30591
	p	**0.049**	**0.048**	0.371	**0.001**	**0.004**
HLA-A*31	Yes	602	563	612	24654	19603
	No	502	502	491	67397	56594
	p	0.494	0.616	0.883	**0.032**	**0.038**
HLA-A*33	Yes	387	387	347	67660	67660
	No	535	528	515	55276	39484
	p	**0.046**	0.100	**0.021**	0.818	1.00
HLA-B*07	Yes	535	818	679	378025	133268
	No	525	499	474	52352	38720
	p	0.972	**0.015**	**0.005**	0.177	0.280
HLA-B*14	Yes	466	485	410	213099	117061
	No	575	542	534	52352	37506
	p	0.167	0.135	**0.002**	0.229	0.260
HLA-B*39	Yes	644	780	573	4383	18062
	No	509	497	483	62679	42753
	p	0.098	**0.027**	0.175	0.073	0.085
HLA-B*53	Yes	288	248	286	500000	349244
	No	545	531	509	54286	39033
	p	**0.046**	**0.036**	0.117	0.058	**0.028**
HLA-B*57	Yes	525	495	654	16926	12971
	No	529	528	492	66821	47077
	p	0.819	0.865	0.272	**0.046**	0.058
HLA-C*07	Yes	525	527	534	66821	60546
	No	497	491	449	62679	40083
	p	0.738	0.527	**0.038**	0.584	0.563
HLA-C*08	Yes	437	499	409	184000	163664
	No	519	499	533	61045	40083
	p	0.290	0.200	**0.001**	0.443	0.286

haplotype in African Americans was associated with disease acceleration, in Caucasians and Hispanics it was associated with disease retardation. Regarding the HHF*2 haplotype, a previous report found similar results in individuals carrying the allele with lower CD4 T-cell counts during follow-up [47]. However, these results disagree with previous studies that observed a protective effect against disease progression among subjects carrying the CCR2-64I allele [33]. HHC/HHF*2 genotype was also associated with disease retardation among Argentinean children [42]. Even when no statistically significant association was established, the

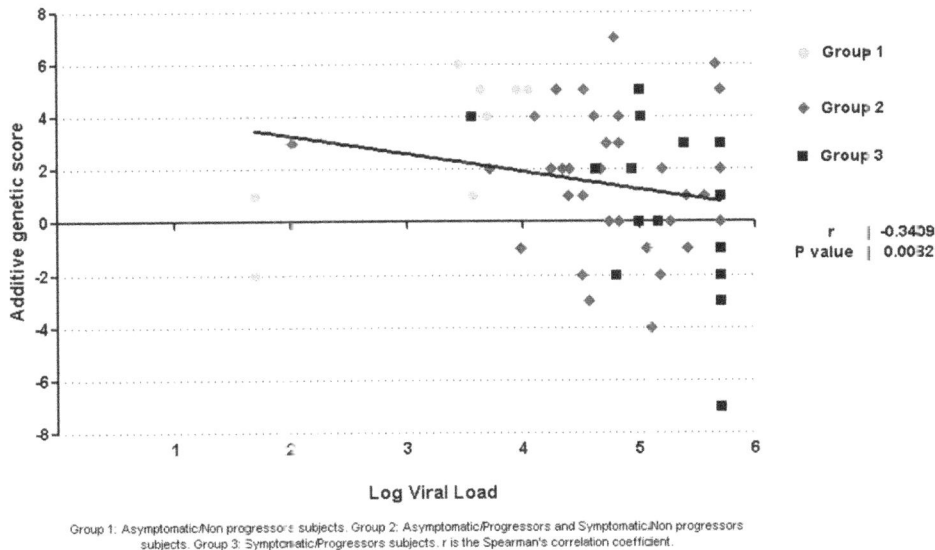

Figure 2. Correlation between baseline HIV viral load and additive genetic score on the study population diagnosed during primary HIV infection [PHI] (N = 70).

CCR5 genotype HHE/HHF*1 was only detected among symptomatic subjects in more than 10% of the group. CCL3L1 copy number distribution in PHI population was similar to that observed in the European population [22] with a median of two copies. Even when no significant differences were observed, asymptomatic individuals had a higher copy number, maybe suggesting that CCL3L1 would have an impact since the HIV infection onset.

Identifying HLA alleles associations with HIV disease progression is complex due to the extreme variability of the loci. In fact, this study identifies 17, 27 and 14 HLA-A, B and C alleles, respectively. Coincident with previous reports, including our blood donors group, the alleles most frequently reported here were HLA-A*02 and HLA-*24, HLA-B*35 and HLA-B*44, and HLA-C*07, HLA-C*04 and HLA-C*03 [41]. Even when it was proposed that heterozygosis on HLA confers advantages on disease progression revealing a greater variety of the immune response [18,48–49], no significant differences in disease progression were detected between heterozygotes and homozygotes at any individual HLA locus or homozygosis at one, two, or all three class I loci.

Several HLA alleles identified in our study were associated with disease progression. Our results adds more evidence to the protective effect of HLA-B*57 allele on disease progression [23], with significantly lower VL at baseline and also lower, but not significant, VL at 6 months. Moreover, the allele was only found among those who did not progress. Even when HLA-B*57 was previously associated with the absence of symptoms during seroconversion, our study failed to confirm these findings [50]. Regarding HLA-B*27, reported as a protective allele [50], we did not observe this trend or evidence, likely due to the low frequency found (1.5% among HIV positive and 2.0% among blood donors). Another HLA allele, several times associated with disease progression is HLA-B*35 [18,23]. However, our study did not find any statistical association or trend even when the frequency of the allele was around 15% in the overall group.

HLA-A*11 was associated with disease progression during the first year and with higher VL at baseline. We also found a trend in the presence of the allele and higher HIV VL at 6 months and

lower CD4 T-cell counts at baseline and during follow-up. These results agree with a previous study that found a higher frequency of HLA-A*1101 among subjects with AIDS compared with other HIV subjects who did not progress [51]. Even when this study performed high resolution HLA-typing, in contrast to our low resolution data it is important to mention that typing studies reported that most of the typed HLA-A*11 are HLA-A*1101 [41,52].

HLA-B*53 was associated with lower CD4 T-cell counts and higher HIV VL levels, even when only two subjects carried that allele. Elevated VL levels among subjects with HLA-B*53 were previously observed among African seroconverters [53]. Although only few subjects carried the HLA-B*53, the potential impact of this allele on disease progression may deserve more investigation. Another interesting allele is HLA-A*24, associated with lower CD4 T-cell counts and higher VL levels at baseline and during follow-up. This allele frequency was also higher (but not significant) among subjects who presented symptoms during seroconversion as compared with those without them. Previous studies also found a deleterious effect of this allele, enhancing HIV infection [54], showing rapid decline in CD4 T-cells [27] and favouring disease progression [55]. HLA-B*39 confers a beneficial effect on disease evolution yielding high CD4 T-cell counts and low VL levels [16,55]. We also observed a trend in higher frequency of HLA-B*39 among asymptomatic vs. symptomatic (10.7% vs. 2.9%) subjects. Controversial results were found in other alleles. While our study suggests that subjects with HLA-B*14 (with significantly lower CD4 T-cell counts at 12 months and a trend of lower levels of CD4 T-cells at baseline and at 6 months and higher VL) progressed faster to disease, others found significant associations between allele and low disease progression [56] and that the allele had enhanced HIV infection [57].

Previous studies showed that plasma LPS levels among subjects with acute HIV infection were similar to non-infected subjects [58]. In fact, our study found similar levels in the PHI group (39.0 pg/ml) and a group of HIV-negative subjects (37.4 pg/ml, data not shown). However, we found that higher plasma LPS levels are significantly associated with presence of symptoms during PHI.

These results suggest higher immune activation in symptomatic subjects since the establishment of infection.

An important limitation of the current research was the low frequency of asymptomatic subjects included due to the difficulty in identifying them during the seroconversion period. The lack of progression data in a group of patients also influenced the possibility of finding significant associations. It is also important to note the difficulty in finding associations when genetic variants are in low frequency. Given these limitations, a score was constructed in order to combine some of the most important human genetic factors previously associated with HIV/AIDS and to look for associations with presence of symptoms, disease progression and other progression markers like HIV viral load and CD4 T-cell count. Results reveal a higher score in asymptomatic and those who did not progress, revealing the presence of more protective genetic factors in these groups. Even more, when data were analysed considering both variables (symptoms and progression) a higher score was observed for those who did not present symptoms during PHI and did not progress at one year. As described by other authors, the genetic score was a useful tool to evaluate the additive influence of human genetic factors with high variability on small groups [37].

Conclusions

This study reveals that some host genetic variants identified previously as disease-modifying factors influence disease progression from the very beginning of the HIV infection. However, here we also described some associations for the first time. Variability of host genetic factors as well as their association with HIV infection and/or disease progression relies strongly on the ethnic population background. Therefore, the population ethnicities are growing it is becoming increasingly difficult to extrapolate results from one study to other populations. In this context, it is important to highlight the need to perform studies at a in this setting not only these genetic differences in the population but also the environmental variance and the circulating virus.

Supporting Information

Figure S1 PCR Cycle conditions for HLA class I characterization.

References

1. Pilcher CD, Eron JJ Jr, Galvin S, Gay C, Cohen MS (2004) Acute HIV revisited: new opportunities for treatment and prevention. J Clin Invest 113: 937–945.
2. Boletín N°30 sobre VIH-sida e ITS en la Argentina (2013) Ministerio de Salud. Presidencia de la Nación. Available: http://www.msal.gov.ar/sida. Accessed 2014 July 3.
3. Socías ME, Sued O, Laufer N, Lázaro ME, Mingrone H, et al. (2011) Acute retroviral syndrome and high baseline VL are predictors of rapid HIV progression among untreated Argentinean seroconverters. J Int AIDS Soc: 14–40.
4. Hubert JB, Burgard M, Dussaix E, Tamalet C, Deveau C, et al. (2000) Natural history of serum HIV-1 RNA levels in 330 patients with a known date of infection. The SEROCO Study Group. AIDS 14: 123–131.
5. Lyles RH, Muñoz A, Yamashita TE, Bazmi H, Detels R, et al. (2000) Natural history of human immunodeficiency virus type 1 viremia after seroconversion and proximal to AIDS in a large cohort of homosexual men. Multicenter AIDS Cohort Study. J Infect Dis 181: 872–880.
6. Salamon R, Marimoutou C, Ekra D, Minga A, Nerrienet E, et al. (2002) Clinical and biological evolution of HIV-1 seroconverters in Abidjan, Côte d'Ivoire, 1997–2000. J Acquir Immune Defic Syndr 29: 149–157.
7. Buchacz K, Hu DJ, Vanichseni S, Mock PA, Chaowanachan T, et al. (2004) Early markers of HIV-1 disease progression in a prospective cohort of seroconverters in Bangkok, Thailand: implications for vaccine trials. J Acquir Immune Defic Syndr 36: 853–860.

Table S1 Sequences of primers used for HLA class I characterization.

Table S2 Frequency of CCR5 haplotypes of the study population diagnosed during primary HIV infection [PHI] (N = 70).

Table S3 Frequency of CCR5 human genotypes among the study population diagnosed during primary HIV infection [PHI] (N = 70).

Table S4 Frequency of HLA class I alleles among the study population diagnosed during primary HIV infection [PHI].

Table S5 Frequency of HLA class I alleles homozygosis among the study population diagnosed during primary HIV infection [PHI].

Acknowledgments

We thank all the physicians of the "Grupo Argentino de Seroconversión" Study Group: Lorena Abusamra, Marcela Acosta, Carolina Acuipil, Viviana Alonso, Liliana Amante, Graciela Ben, M. Belén Bouzas, Ariel Braverman, Mercedes Cabrini, Pedro Cahn, Osvaldo Cando, Cecilia Cánepa, Daniel Cangelosi, Juan Castelli, Mariana Ceriotto, Carina Cesar, María Collins, Fabio Crudo, Darío Dilernia, Andrea Duarte, Gustavo Echenique, María I. Figueroa, Valeria Fink, Claudia Galloso, Palmira Garda, Manuel Gómez Carrillo, Ana Gun, Alejandro Krolewiecki, Natalia Laufer, María E. Lázaro, Alberto Leoni, Eliana Loiza, Patricia Maldonado, Horacio Mingrone, Marcela Ortiz, Patricia Patterson, Héctor Pérez, Norma Porteiro, Daniel Pryluka, Carlos Remondegui, Raúl Román, Horacio Salomón, M. Eugenia Socías, Omar Sued, J. Gonzalo Tomás, Gabriela Turk, Javier Yave, Carlos Zala, Inés Zapiola. Authors also thank Sergio Mazzini for assistance during manuscript preparation.

Author Contributions

Conceived and designed the experiments: RSC AM HS MAP. Performed the experiments: RSC DD YG GT AR. Analyzed the data: MAP RSC. Contributed to the writing of the manuscript: MAP AM RSC. Participants' recruitment: NL MES MIF OS PC.

8. Lavreys L, Thompson ML, Martin HL Jr, Mandaliya K, Ndinya-Achola JO, et al. (2000) Primary human immunodeficiency virus type 1 infection: clinical manifestations among women in Mombasa, Kenya. Clin Infect Dis 30: 486–490.
9. Hightow-Weidman LB, Golin CE, Green K, Shaw EN, MacDonald PD, et al. (2009) Identifying people with acute HIV infection: demographic features, risk factors, and use of health care among individuals with AHI in North Carolina. AIDS Behav 13: 1075–1083.
10. Richey LE, Halperin J (2013) Acute human immunodeficiency virus infection. Am J Med Sci 345: 136–142.
11. O'Brien SJ, Nelson GW (2004) Human genes that limit AIDS. Nat Genet 36: 565–574.
12. Smith MZ, Kent SJ (2005) Genetic influences on HIV infection: implications for vaccine development. Sex Health 2: 53–62.
13. Telenti A, Goldstein DB (2006) Genomics meets HIV-1. Nat Rev Microbiol 4: 865–873.
14. Marmor M, Hertzmark K, Thomas SM, Halkitis PN, Vogler M (2006) Resistance to HIV Infection. J Urban Health 83: 5–17.
15. Mummidi S, Ahuja SS, Gonzalez E, Anderson SA, Santiago EN, et al. (1998) Genealogy of the CCR5 locus and chemokine system gene variants associated with altered rates of HIV-1 disease progression. Nat Med 4: 786–793.
16. Tang J, Shelton B, Makhatadze NJ, Zhang Y, Schaen M, et al. (2002) Distribution of Chemokine Receptor CCR2 and CCR5 Genotypes and Their Relative Contribution to Human Immunodeficiency Virus Type 1 (HIV-1) Seroconversion, Early HIV-1 RNA Concentration in Plasma, and Later Disease Progression. J Virol 76: 662–672.

17. Telenti A, Bleiber G (2006) Host genetics of HIV-1 susceptibility. Future Virology 1: 55–70.

18. Carrington M, Dean M, Martin MP, O'Brien SJ (1999) Genetics of HIV-1 infection: chemokine receptor CCR5 polymorphism and its consequences. Human Molecular Genetics 8: 1939–1945.

19. Smith MZ, Kent SJ (2005) Genetic influence on HIV infection: implications for vaccine development. Sexual Health 2: 53–62.

20. Mummidi S, Bamshad M, Ahuja SS, Gonzalez E, Feuillet PM, et al. (2000) Evolution of human and nonhuman primate CC chemokine receptor 5 gene and mRNA. Potential roles for haplotype and mRNA diversity, differential haplotype-specific transcriptional activity and altered transcription factor binding to polymorphic nucleotides in the pathogenesis of HIV-1 and SIV. J Biol Chem 275: 18946–18961.

21. Gonzalez E, Bamshad M, Sato N, Mummidi S, Dhanda R, et al. (1999) Race-specific HIV-1 disease-modifying effects associated with CCR5 haplotypes. Proc Natl Acad Sci U S A 96: 12004–12009.

22. Gonzalez E, Kulkarni H, Bolivar H, Mangano A, Sanchez R, et al. (2005) The influence of CCL3L1 gene-containing segmental duplications on HIV-1/AIDS susceptibility. Science 307: 1434–1440.

23. Carrington M, O'Brien SJ (2003) The influence of HLA genotype on AIDS. Annu Rev Med 54: 535–551.

24. Goulder PJ, Walker BD (2012) HIV and HLA class I: an evolving relationship. Immunity 37: 426–440.

25. Borrow P, Lewicki H, Hahn BH, Shaw GM, Oldstone MB (1994) Virus-specific CD8+ cytotoxic T-lymphocyte activity associated with control of viremia in primary human immunodeficiency virus type 1 infection. J Virol 68: 6103–6110.

26. Koup RA, Safrit JT, Cao Y, Andrews CA, McLeod G, et al. (1994) Temporal association of cellular immune responses with the initial control of viremia in primary human immunodeficiency virus type 1 syndrome. J Virol 68: 4650–4655.

27. Kaslow RA, Carrington M, Apple R, Park L, Muñoz A, et al. (1996) Influence of combinations of human major histocompatibility complex genes on the course of HIV-1 infection. Nat Med 2: 405–411.

28. Gao X, Nelson GW, Karacki P, Martin MP, Phair J, et al. (2001) Effect of a single amino acid change in MHC class I molecules on the rate of progression to AIDS. N Engl J Med 344: 1668–1675.

29. 1993 revised classification system for HIV infection and expanded surveillance case definition for AIDS among adolescents and adults (1992) MMWR Recomm Rep 14: 1–19.

30. McGovern RA, Harrigan PR, Swenson LC (2010) Genotypic inference of HIV-1 tropism using population-based sequencing of V3. J Vis Exp 46: 2531.

31. Mummidi S, Ahuja SS, McDaniel BL, Ahuja SK (1997) The human CC chemokine receptor 5 (CCR5) gene. Multiple transcripts with 5'-end heterogeneity, dual promoter usage, and evidence for polymorphisms within the regulatory regions and noncoding exons. J Biol Chem 272: 30662–30671.

32. Mangano A, Kopka J, Batalla M, Bologna R, Sen L (2000) Protective Effect of CCR2-64I and Not of CCR5-Δ32 and SDF-1-3' in Pediatric HIV-1 infection. JAIDS 23: 52–57.

33. Smith MW, Dean M, Carrington M, Winkler C, Huttley GA, et al. (1997) Contrasting Genetic Influence of CCR2 and CCR5 Variants on HIV-1 Infection and Disease Progression. Science 277: 959–965.

34. Cereb N, Maye P, Lee S, Kong Y, Yang SY (1995) Locus-specific amplification of HLA class I genes from genomic DNA: locus-specific sequences in the first and third introns of HLA-A, -B, and -C alleles. Tissue Antigens 45: 1–11.

35. Hurley CK, Fernandez-Vina M, Hildebrand WH, Noreen HJ, Trachtenberg E, et al. (2007) A high degree of HLA disparity arises from limited allelic diversity: analysis of 1775 unrelated bone marrow transplant donor-recipient pairs. Hum Immunol 68: 30–40.

36. Dun PPJ, Day S (2001) Sequencing-Based Typing for HLA-A, B and C. International Histocompatibility Working Group (IHWG). Chapter 30 A, 1–5.

37. Casado C, Colombo S, Rauch A, Martínez R, Günthard HF, et al. (2010) Host and viral genetic correlates of clinical definitions of HIV-1 disease progression. PLoS One 5: e11079.

38. Fellay J, Shianna KV, Ge D, Colombo S, Ledergerber B, et al. (2007) A whole-genome association study of major determinants for host control of HIV-1. Science 317: 944–947.

39. Fellay J, Ge D, Shianna KV, Colombo S, Ledergerber B, et al. (2009) Common genetic variation and the control of HIV-1 in humans. PLoS Genet 5: e1000791.

40. Fiebig EW, Wright DJ, Rawal BD, Garrett PE, Schumacher RT, et al. (2003) Dynamics of HIV viremia and antibody seroconversion in plasma donors: implications for diagnosis and staging of primary HIV infection. AIDS 17: 1871–1879.

41. Gonzalez-Galarza FF, Christmas S, Middleton D, Jones AR (2011) Allele frequency net: a database and online repository for immune gene frequencies in worldwide populations. Nucleic Acid Research 39: D913–D919.

42. Mangano A, Gonzalez E, Dhanda R, Catano G, Bamshad M, et al. (2001) Concordance between the CC chemokine Receptor 5 Genetic Determinants That Alter Risks of Transmission and Disease Progression in Children Exposed Perinatally to Human Immunodeficiency Virus. J Infect Dis 183: 1574–1585.

43. Rocco CA, Mangano A, del Pozo A, Sen L (2003) Distribution of CCR5-CCR2 haplotypes in an Argentinean population. AIDS Res Hum Retroviruses 19: 943–945.

44. Brenchley JM, Price DA, Schacker TW, Asher TE, Silvestri G, et al. (2006) Microbial translocation is a cause of systemic immune activation in chronic HIV infection. Nat Med 12: 1365–1371.

45. Hunt PW, Brenchley J, Sinclair E, McCune JM, Roland M, et al. (2008) Relationship between T cell activation and CD4+ T cell count in HIV-seropositive individuals with undetectable plasma HIV RNA levels in the absence of therapy. J Infect Dis 197: 126–133.

46. Tincati C, Bellistri GM, Ancona G, Merlini E, d Arminio Monforte A, et al. (2012) Role of in vitro stimulation with lipopolysaccharide on T-cell activation in HIV-infected antiretroviral-treated patients. Clin Dev Immunol 2012: 935425.

47. Nguyen L, Chaowanachan T, Vanichseni S, McNicholl JM, Mock PA, et al. (2004) Frequent human leukocyte antigen class I alleles are associated with higher viral load among HIV type 1 seroconverters in Thailand. J Acquir Immune Defic Syndr 37: 1318–1323.

48. Tang J, Rivers C, Karita E, Costello C, Allen S, et al. (1999) Allelic variants of human beta-chemokine receptor 5 (CCR5) promoter: evolutionary relationships and predictable associations with HIV-1 disease progression. Genes Immun 1: 20–27.

49. Naruto T, Gatanaga H, Nelson G, Sakai K, Carrington M, et al. (2012) HLA class I-mediated control of HIV-1 in the Japanese population, in which the protective HLA-B*57 and HLA-B*27 alleles are absent. J Virol 86: 10870–10872.

50. Altfeld M, Addo MM, Rosenberg ES, Hecht FM, Lee PK, et al. (2003) Influence of HLA-B57 on clinical presentation and viral control during acute HIV-1 infection. AIDS 17: 2581–2591.

51. Huang X, Ling H, Mao W, Ding X, Zhou Q, et al. (2009) Association of HLA-A, B, DRB1 alleles and haplotypes with HIV-1 infection in Chongqing, China. BMC Infect Dis 9: 201.

52. Li L, Chen W, Bouvier M (2005) A biochemical and structural analysis of genetic diversity within the HLA-A*11 subtype. Immunogenetics 57: 315–325.

53. Prentice HA, Price MA, Porter TR, Cormier E, Mugavero MJ, et al. (2014) Dynamics of viremia in primary HIV-1 infection in Africans: insights from analyses of host and viral correlates. Virology 449: 254–262.

54. de Sorrentino AH, Marinic K, Motta P, Sorrentino A, López R, et al. (2000) HLA class I alleles associated with susceptibility or resistance to human immunodeficiency virus type 1 infection among a population in Chaco Province, Argentina. J Infect Dis 182: 1523–1526.

55. Leslie A, Matthews PC, Listgarten J, Carlson JM, Kadie C, et al. (2010) Additive contribution of HLA class I alleles in the immune control of HIV-1 infection. J Virol 84: 9879–9888.

56. Magierowska M, Theodorou I, Debré P, Sanson F, Autran B, et al. (1999) Combined genotypes of CCR5, CCR2, SDF1, and HLA genes can predict the long-term nonprogressor status in human immunodeficiency virus-1-infected individuals. Blood 93: 936–941.

57. Li S, Jiao H, Yu X, Strong AJ, Shao Y, et al. (2007) Human leukocyte antigen class I and class II allele frequencies and HIV-1 infection associations in a Chinese cohort. J Acquir Immune Defic Syndr 44: 121–131.

58. Douek D (2007) HIV disease progression: immune activation, microbes, and a leaky gut. Top HIV Med 15: 114–117.

Permissions

List of Contributors

Bulbulgul Aumakhan, Chris Beyrer, Lorie Benning and Stephen J. Gange
Johns Hopkins Bloomberg School of Public Health, Baltimore, Maryland, United States of America

Charlotte A. Gaydos
Johns Hopkins University School of Medicine, Baltimore, Maryland, United States of America

Thomas C. Quinn
Johns Hopkins University School of Medicine, Baltimore, Maryland, United States of America Laboratory of Immunoregulation. Division of Intramural Research, National Institute of Allergy and Infectious Diseases, National Institutes of Health, Bethesda, Maryland, United States of America

Howard Minkoff
Maimonides Medical Center and SUNY Downstate, Brooklyn, New York, United States of America

Daniel J. Merenstein
Georgetown University Medical Center, Washington, D. C., United States of America

Mardge Cohen
Cook County Medical Center, Chicago, Illinois, United States of America

Ruth Greenblatt
Schools of Pharmacy and Medicine, University of California San Francisco, San Francisco, California, United States of America

Marek Nowicki
University of Southern California, Los Angeles, California, United States of America

Kathryn Anastos
Albert Einstein College of Medicine, Bronx, New York, United States of America

Victoria Simms
London School of Hygiene and Tropical Medicine, London, United Kingdom Cicely Saunders Institute, King's College London, London, United Kingdom

Nancy Gikaara, Grace Munene, Mackuline Atieno, Jeniffer Kataike, Clare Nsubuga, Geoffrey Banga, Eve Namisango and Richard A. Powell
African Palliative Care Association, Kampala, Uganda

Suzanne Penfold
London School of Hygiene and Tropical Medicine, London, United Kingdom

Peter Fayers
Department of Population Health, University of Aberdeen, Aberdeen, United Kingdom

Irene J. Higginson and Richard Harding
Cicely Saunders Institute, King's College London, London, United Kingdom

Annaléne Nel
International Partnership for Microbicides, Silver Spring, Maryland, United States of America

Cheryl Louw, Martie de Villiers and Jannie Hugo
Madibeng Centre for Research, Brits, South Africa

Elizabeth Hellstrom, Ina Treadwell, Melanie Marais, Inge Paschke and Chrisna Andersen
Be Part Yoluntu Centre, Mbekweni and Paarl, South Africa

Sarah L. Braunstein
New York City Department of Health and Mental Hygiene, New York City, New York, United States of America

Janneke van de Wijgert
Academic Medical Center of the University of Amsterdam and Amsterdam Institute for Global Health and Development, Amsterdam, The Netherlands

Bradley N. Gaynes
Department of Psychiatry, University of North Carolina School of Medicine, Chapel Hill, North Carolina, United States of America

Brian W. Pence
Department of Community and Family Medicine, Duke Global Health Institute, and Center for Health Policy and Inequalities Research, Duke University, Durham, North Carolina, United States of America

Julius Atashili
Department of Public Health and Hygiene, University of Buea, Buea, Cameroon

Julie O'Donnell and Dmitry Kats
Department of Epidemiology, Gillings School of Global Public Health, University of North Carolina, Chapel Hill, North Carolina, United States of America

Peter M. Ndumbe
Department of Biomedical Sciences, University of Buea, and Department of Microbiology and Immunology, University of Yaounde I, Buea, Cameroon

Lauren E. Cipriano and Margaret L. Brandeau
Department of Management Science and Engineering, Stanford University, Stanford, California, United States of America

Gregory S. Zaric
Richard Ivey School of Business, University of Western Ontario, London, Ontario, Canada

Mark Holodniy
Veterans Affairs Palo Alto Health Care System, Palo Alto, California, United States of America
Department of Medicine, Stanford University, Stanford, California, United States of America
Division of Infectious Diseases & Geographic Medicine, Stanford University, Stanford, California, United States of America

Eran Bendavid
Department of Medicine, Stanford University, Stanford, California, United States of America
Division of Infectious Diseases & Geographic Medicine, Stanford University, Stanford, California, United States of America
Division of General Medicine Disciplines, Stanford University, Stanford, California, United States of America
Center for Health Policy and Center for Primary Care and Outcomes Research, Department of Medicine, Stanford University, Stanford, California, United States of America

Douglas K. Owens
Veterans Affairs Palo Alto Health Care System, Palo Alto, California, United States of America
Department of Medicine, Stanford University, Stanford, California, United States of America
Center for Health Policy and Center for Primary Care and Outcomes Research, Department of Medicine, Stanford University, Stanford, California, United States of America

Tudor J. C. Phillips and Andrew S. C. Rice
Department of Anaesthetics, Pain Medicine and Intensive Care, Imperial College London, Chelsea and Westminster Hospital Campus, London, United Kingdom

Catherine L. Cherry
Centre for Virology, Burnet Institute, Melbourne, Australia
Infectious Diseases Unit, Alfred Hospital, Melbourne, Australia
Department of Medicine, Monash University, Melbourne, Australia

Sarah Cox
Chelsea and Westminster NHS Foundation Trust, London, United Kingdom

Sarah J. Marshall
East Kent Hospitals University Foundation Trust and Pilgrims Hospices, Kent, United Kingdom

Jim Todd, Helen A. Weiss, David Mabey and Richard Hayes
Department of Population Health, London School of Hygiene & Tropical Medicine, London, United Kingdom

Gabriele Riedner
Department of Population Health, London School of Hygiene & Tropical Medicine, London, United Kingdom
National Institute for Medical Research - Mbeya Medical Research Programme, Mbeya, Tanzania

Leonard Maboko and Mary Rusizoka
National Institute for Medical Research - Mbeya Medical Research Programme, Mbeya, Tanzania

Michael Hoelscher
Department of Infectious Diseases and Tropical Medicine, Klinikum, Ludwig-Maximilians-University, Munich, Germany

Eligius Lyamuya
Muhimbili University College of Health Sciences, Dar es Salaam, Tanzania

Laurent Belec
Laboratoire de Microbiologie, hôpital Européen Georges Pompidou, Paris, France
Facultéde Médecine Paris Descartes. Université Paris Descartes (Paris V), Paris, France

Mark Berry, Andrea L. Wirtz, Stefan Baral and Chris Beyrer
Johns Hopkins Bloomberg School of Public Health, Department of Epidemiology, Baltimore, Maryland, United States of America

Assel Janayeva and Valentina Ragoza
Amulet Public Organization, Almaty, Kazakhstan

Assel Terlikbayeva and Bauyrzhan Amirov
Global Health Research Center of Central Asia, Almaty, Kazakhstan

Sylvia Adebajo, Otibho Obianwu, George Eluwa, Ayo Oginni and Babatunde Ahonsi
Population Council, Abuja, Nigeria

Lung Vu
Population Services International (PSI), Washington, DC, United States of America

Waimar Tun
Population Council, Washington, DC, United States of America

Meredith Sheehy
Population Council, New York, New York, United States of America

Adebobola Bashorun
Federal Ministry of Health, Abuja, Nigeria

Omokhudu Idogho
Society for Family Health, Abuja, Nigeria

Andrew Karlyn
United States Agency for International Development (USAID), Washington, DC, United States of America

Mohammed Ahmed Yassin
Liverpool School of Tropical Medicine, Liverpool, United Kingdom
Faculty of Medicine, University of Hawassa, Awassa, Ethiopia

Roberta Petrucci, Gregory Harper, Amin Ahmed Bawazir, Nabil Mohamed Abuamer, Luis Eduardo Cuevas
Liverpool School of Tropical Medicine, Liverpool, United Kingdom

Kefyalew Taye Garie and Zelalem Kebede
Faculty of Medicine, University of Hawassa, Awassa, Ethiopia

Isabel Arbide
Bushullo Major Health Centre, Awassa, Ethiopia

Melkamsew Aschalew and Yared Merid
Southern Region Health Bureau, Awassa, Ethiopia

Munyaradzi Dimairo, Tsitsi Bandason, Abbas Zezai, Shungu S. Munyati and Peter R Mason
Biomedical Research and Training Institute, Harare, Zimbabwe

Peter MacPherson and Elizabeth L. Corbett
Wellcome Trust Tropical Centre, University of Liverpool, Liverpool, United Kingdom

Anthony E. Butterworth
Clinical Research Unit, London School of Hygiene and Tropical Medicine, London, United Kingdom

Stanley Mungofa
Harare City Health, Harare, Zimbabwe

Simba Rusikaniko
University of Zimbabwe College of Health Sciences, Harare, Zimbabwe

Katherine Fielding
Infectious Disease Epidemiology Unit, London School of Hygiene and Tropical Medicine, London, United Kingdom

Gabriel Chamie, Tamara D. Clark, Vivek Jain, Elvin Geng and Diane V. Havlir
HIV/AIDS Division, Department of Medicine, San Francisco General Hospital, University of California San Francisco, San Francisco, United States of America
Makerere University-University of California San Francisco (MU-UCSF) Research Collaboration, Uganda
The Sustainable East Africa Research in Community Health (SEARCH) Consortium

Jane Kabami
Makerere University-University of California San Francisco (MU-UCSF) Research Collaboration, Uganda
The Sustainable East Africa Research in Community Health (SEARCH) Consortium

Dalsone Kwarisiima
Makerere University-University of California San Francisco (MU-UCSF) Research Collaboration, Uganda
The Sustainable East Africa Research in Community Health (SEARCH) Consortium
Mulago-Mbarara Joint AIDS Program, Kampala and Mbarara, Uganda

Laura B. Balzer and Maya L. Petersen
The Sustainable East Africa Research in Community Health (SEARCH) Consortium
School of Public Health, University of California, Berkeley, United States of America

Harsha Thirumurthy
The Sustainable East Africa Research in Community Health (SEARCH) Consortium
Gillings School of Global Public Health, University of North Carolina at Chapel Hill, United States of America

Edwin D. Charlebois
Makerere University-University of California San Francisco (MU-UCSF) Research Collaboration, Uganda
The Sustainable East Africa Research in Community Health (SEARCH) Consortium
Center for AIDS Prevention Studies, Department of Medicine, University of California San Francisco, San Francisco, United States of America

Moses R. Kamya
Makerere University-University of California San Francisco (MU-UCSF) Research Collaboration, Uganda
The Sustainable East Africa Research in Community Health (SEARCH) Consortium
Department of Medicine, School of Medicine, Makerere University College of Health Sciences, Kampala, Uganda

Annaléne Nel
International Partnership for Microbicides, Silver Spring, Maryland United States of America

Zonke Mabude and Jenni Smit
MatCH, Department of Obstetrics and Gynecology, University of the Witwatersrand Durban, KwaZulu-Natal, South Africa
International Partnership for Microbicides, Paarl, Western Cape, South Africa

Philip Kotze
Qhakaza Mbokodo Research Clinic, Ladysmith, KwaZulu-Natal, South Africa

Derek Arbuckle
PHIVA Project, Pinetown, KwaZulu- Natal, South Africa

Jian Wu
JW Consulting, Hurstville Grove, New South Wales, Australia

Neliëtte van Niekerk
International Partnership for Microbicides, Paarl, Western Cape, South Africa

Janneke van de Wijgert
Academic Medical Center of the University of Amsterdam and Amsterdam Institute for Global Health and Development, Amsterdam, The Netherlands

Sundhiya Mandalia and Brian Gazzard
NPMS-HHC Coordinating and Analytic Centre, London, United Kingdom
Imperial College, London, United Kingdom
Chelsea and Westminster Hospital, London, United Kingdom

Roshni Mandalia
NPMS-HHC Coordinating and Analytic Centre, London, United Kingdom

Gary Lo
NPMS-HHC Coordinating and Analytic Centre, London, United Kingdom
Chelsea and Westminster Hospital, London, United Kingdom

Tim Chadborn
Health Protection Agency, London, United Kingdom

Peter Sharott
London Specialised Commissioning Group, London Procurement Programme, London, United Kingdom

Mike Youle
NPMS-HHC Coordinating and Analytic Centre, London, United Kingdom
Royal Free Hospital, London, United Kingdom

Jane Anderson
Homerton University Hospital NHS Foundation Trust, London, United Kingdom

Guy Baily
London and Barts Hospitals, London, United Kingdom

Ray Brettle
Edinburgh General Hospital, Edinburgh, United Kingdom

Martin Fisher
Royal County Sussex Hospital, Brighton, United Kingdom

Mark Gompels
Southmead Hospital, Bristol, United Kingdom

George Kinghorn
Royal Hallamshire Hospital, Sheffield, United Kingdom

Margaret Johnson
Royal Free Hospital, London, United Kingdom

Brendan McCarron
James Cook University Hospital, Middlesborough, United Kingdom

Anton Pozniak
Chelsea and Westminster Hospital, London, United Kingdom

Alan Tang
Royal Berkshire Hospital, Berkshire, United Kingdom

John Walsh
St. Mary's Hospital, London, United Kingdom

David White
Birmingham Heartlands Hospital, Birmingham, United Kingdom

Ian Williams
Mortimer Market Centre, London, United Kingdom

Eduard J. Beck
NPMS-HHC Coordinating and Analytic Centre, London, United Kingdom
Chelsea and Westminster Hospital, London, United Kingdom
London School of Hygiene & Tropical Medicine, London, United Kingdom

Damani A. Piggott, Abimereki D. Muzaale, Todd T. Brown and Gregory D. Kirk
Johns Hopkins University School of Medicine, Baltimore, Maryland, United States of America
Johns Hopkins Bloomberg School of Public Health, Baltimore, Maryland, United States of America

Shruti H. Mehta
Johns Hopkins Bloomberg School of Public Health, Baltimore, Maryland, United States of America

Kushang V. Patel
University of Washington School of Medicine, Seattle, Washington, United States of America

Sean X. Leng
Johns Hopkins University School of Medicine, Baltimore, Maryland, United States of America

Amare Deribew
Department of Epidemiology, Jimma University, Jimma, Ethiopia

Nebiyu Negussu
Somali Regional Health Bureau, Jijiga, Ethiopia

Zenebe Melaku
International Center for AIDS Care and Treatment Program (ICAP), Addis Ababa, Ethiopia

Kebede Deribe
Department of General Public Health, Jimma University, Jimma, Ethiopia

Rachel C. Vreeman, Michael L. Scanlon, Matthew Turissini
Children's Health Services Research, Department of Pediatrics, Indiana University School of Medicine, Indianapolis, Indiana, United States of America
USAID-Academic Model Providing Access to Healthcare (AMPATH), Eldoret, Kenya

Ann Mwangi
USAID-Academic Model Providing Access to Healthcare (AMPATH), Eldoret, Kenya

Samuel O. Ayaya, Constance Tenge and Winstone M. Nyandiko
Department of Behavioral Science, School of Medicine, College of Health Sciences, Moi University, Eldoret, Kenya
Department of Child Health and Paediatrics, School of Medicine, College of Health Sciences, Moi University, Eldoret, Kenya

Annelies Van Rie, Kate Clouse and Colleen Hanrahan
Department of Epidemiology, University of North Carolina at Chapel Hill, Chapel Hill, North Carolina, United States of America

Katerina Selibas and Ian Sanne
Clinical HIV Research Unit, University of the Witwatersrand, Johannesburg, South Africa

Sharon Williams and Peter Kim
National Institute of Allergy and Infectious Diseases, National Institutes of Health, Bethesda, Maryland, United States of America

Jean Bassett
Witkoppen Health and Welfare Center, Johannesburg, South Africa

Laura Ferguson
Institute for Global Health, University of Southern California, Los Angeles, California, United States of America
MRC Tropical Epidemiology Group, Department of Infectious Disease Epidemiology, London School of Hygiene and Tropical Medicine, London, United Kingdom
University of Nairobi Institute for Tropical and Infectious Diseases, Nairobi, Kenya

Alison D. Grant
Clinical Research Department, London School of Hygiene & Tropical Medicine, London, United Kingdom

James Lewis and David A. Ross
MRC Tropical Epidemiology Group, Department of Infectious Disease Epidemiology, London School of Hygiene and Tropical Medicine, London, United Kingdom

Karina Kielmann
Institute for International Health & Development, Queen Margaret University, Edinburgh, United Kingdom

Deborah Watson-Jones
Clinical Research Department, London School of Hygiene & Tropical Medicine, London, United Kingdom
Mwanza Intervention Trials Unit, National Institute for Medical Research, Mwanza, Tanzania

Sophie Vusha
University of Nairobi Institute for Tropical and Infectious Diseases, Nairobi, Kenya

John O. Ong'ech
University of Nairobi Institute for Tropical and Infectious Diseases, Nairobi, Kenya
Department of Obstetrics and Gynaecology, University of Nairobi, Nairobi, Kenya

Julia L. Marcus
Gladstone Institute of Virology and Immunology, San Francisco, California, United States or America
University of California, Berkeley, California, United States of America

David V. Glidden
University of California San Francisco, San Francisco, California, United States of America

Vanessa McMahan
Gladstone Institute of Virology and Immunology, San Francisco, California, United States or America

Javier R. Lama
Asociación Civil Impacta Salud y Educación, Lima, Peru

Kenneth H. Mayer
Fenway Institute, Fenway Health, Boston, Massachusetts, United States of America
Beth Israel Deaconess Medical Center, Boston, Massachusetts, United States of America

Albert Y. Liu
Bridge HIV, San Francisco Department of Public Health, San Francisco, California, United States of America

Orlando Montoya-Herrera
Fundación Ecuatoriana Equidad, Guayaquil, Guayas, Ecuador

Martin Casapia
Asociación Civil Selva Amazónica, Iquitos, Peru

Brenda Hoagland
Instituto de Pesquisa Clínica Evandro Chagas, Fundac̨ão Oswaldo Cruz, Rio de Janeiro, Brazil

Robert M. Grant
Gladstone Institute of Virology and Immunology, San Francisco, California, United States or America University of California San Francisco, San Francisco, California, United States of America

Fei Zhong
School of Public Health, Sun Yat-sen University, Guangzhou, China
Department of HIV/AIDS Control and Prevention, Guangzhou Center for Disease Control and Prevention, Guangzhou, China
Sun Yat-sen Center for Migrant Health Policy, Sun Yat-sen University, Guangzhou, China

Boheng Liang, Huifang Xu, Weibin Cheng, Lirui Fan, Zhigang Han, Caiyun Liang, Kai Gao, Huixia Mai and Faju Qin
Department of HIV/AIDS Control and Prevention, Guangzhou Center for Disease Control and Prevention, Guangzhou, China

Jinkou Zhao
The Global Fund to fight AIDS, Tuberculosis and Malaria, Geneva, Switzerland

Li Ling
School of Public Health, Sun Yat-sen University, Guangzhou, China
Sun Yat-sen Center for Migrant Health Policy, Sun Yat-sen University, Guangzhou, China

Aase Berg
Department of Medicine, Stavanger University Hospital, Stavanger, Norway
Department of Medicine, The Central Hospital of Maputo, Maputo, Mozambique
The Faculty of Medicine, The University of Bergen, Bergen, Norway

Sam Patel
Department of Medicine, The Central Hospital of Maputo, Maputo, Mozambique

Pål Aukrust
Section of Clinical Immunology and Infectious Diseases, Oslo University Hospital Rikshospitalet, Oslo, Norway

Catarina David and Miguel Gonca
Department of Medicine, The Central Hospital of Maputo, Maputo, Mozambique

Einar S. Berg
Department of Virology, The Norwegian Institute of Public Health, Oslo, Norway

Ingvild Dalen
Department of Research, Stavanger University Hospital, Stavanger, Norway

Nina Langeland
The Faculty of Medicine, The University of Bergen, Bergen, Norway

Tamil Kendall
Women and Health Initiative and Takemi Program in International Health, Department of Global Health and Population, Harvard School of Public Health, Boston, Massachusetts, United States of America

Joseph Kagaayi
Rakai Health Sciences Program, Entebbe, Uganda
Deparment of Epidemiology and Biostatistics, Case Western Reserve University, Cleveland, Ohio, United States of America

Ronald H. Gray and Maria J. Wawer
Department of Epidemiology, Johns Hopkins Bloomberg School of Public Health, Baltimore, Maryland, United States of America

Christopher Whalen
Department of Epidemiology and Biostatistics, University of Georgia, Athens, Georgia, United States of America

Pingfu Fu, Duncan Neuhauser, Godfrey Kigozi, Fred Nalugoda and Mendel E. Singer
Deparment of Epidemiology and Biostatistics, Case Western Reserve University, Cleveland, Ohio, United States of America

Janet W. McGrath
Department of Anthropology, Case Western Reserve University, Cleveland, Ohio, United States of America

Nelson K. Sewankambo and David Serwadda
Makerere University College of Health Sciences, Kampala, Uganda

Steven J. Reynolds
Division of Intramural Research, National Institute of Allergy and Infectious Diseases, National Institutes of Health, Bethesda, Maryland, United States of America
Johns Hopkins School of Medicine, Baltimore, Maryland, United States of America

Romina Soledad Coloccini, Dario Dilernia, Yanina Ghiglione, Gabriela Turk, Andrea Rubio, Horacio Salomón, María Ángeles Pando
Instituto de Investigaciones Biomédicas en Retrovirus y SIDA (INBIRS), Universidad de Buenos Aires-CONICET, Buenos Aires, Argentina

Natalia Laufer
Instituto de Investigaciones Biomédicas en Retrovirus y SIDA (INBIRS), Universidad de Buenos Aires-CONICET, Buenos Aires, Argentina
Hospital Juan A. Fernandez, Buenos Aires, Argentina

María Eugenia Socías, María Inés Figueroa, Omar Sued and Pedro Cahn
Hospital Juan A. Fernandez, Buenos Aires, Argentina
Fundación Huésped, Buenos Aires, Argentina

Andrea Mangano
Laboratorio de Biología Celular y Retrovirus, CONICET, Hospital de Pediatría "Prof. Dr. Juan P. Garrahan", Buenos Aires, Argentina

Index

www.ingramcontent.com/pod-product-compliance
Lightning Source LLC
Chambersburg PA
CBHW082050190326
41458CB00010B/3497